Pharmaceutical Blending and Mixing

Pharmaceutical Blending and Mixing

Edited by

P.J. CULLEN

School of Chemical Engineering,
University of New South Wales,
Australia

RODOLFO J. ROMAÑACH

Department of Chemistry,
University of Puerto Rico – Mayagüez,
Puerto Rico

NICOLAS ABATZOGLOU

Chemical Engineering and Biotechnological Engineering,
Université de Sherbrooke, Canada

CHRIS D. RIELLY

Department of Chemical Engineering,
Loughborough University, UK

WILEY

This edition first published 2015

Registered Office
John Wiley & Sons, Ltd, The Atrium, Southern Gate, Chichester, West Sussex, PO19 8SQ, United Kingdom

For details of our global editorial offices, for customer services and for information about how to apply for permission to reuse the copyright material in this book please see our website at www.wiley.com.

Library of Congress Cataloging-in-Publication data applied for.

ISBN: 9780470710555

A catalogue record for this book is available from the British Library.

Cover credit: Photograph kindly provided by Gebruder Lodige

Set in 10/12pt Times by SPi Global, Pondicherry, India

1 2015

Contents

Contributor List

Nicolas Abatzoglou Chemical Engineering and Biotechnological Engineering, Université de Sherbrooke, Canada

Mostafa Barigou School of Chemical Engineering, University of Birmingham, UK

Charles L. Cooney Department of Chemical Engineering, Massachusetts Institute of Technology, USA

P.J. Cullen School of Chemical Engineering, University of New South Wales, Australia

David S. Dickey MixTech, Inc., USA

Reuben D. Domike Center for Biomedical Innovation, Massachusetts Institute of Technology, USA; School of Business at the University of Prince Edward Island, Canada

Mojtaba Ghadiri Institute of Particle Science and Engineering, School of Chemical and Process Engineering, University of Leeds, UK

Karen P. Hapgood Monash Advanced Particle Engineering Laboratory, Department of Chemical Engineering, Monash University, Australia

Ali Hassanpour Institute of Particle Science and Engineering, School of Chemical and Process Engineering, University of Leeds, UK

Ian Jones Innopharmalabs, Ireland

Suzanne M. Kresta Department of Chemical and Materials Engineering, University of Alberta, Canada

N.N. Misra School of Food Science & Environmental Health, Dublin Institute of Technology, Ireland

Frans L. Muller AstraZeneca, Hursfield Industrial Estate, UK

Fernando J. Muzzio Department of Chemical and Biochemical Engineering, Rutgers, The State University of New Jersey, USA

Juan G. Osorio Department of Chemical and Biochemical Engineering, Rutgers, The State University of New Jersey, USA

Gül N. Özcan-Taşkın BHR Group (trading name for VirtualPiE Ltd), UK

Andrzej W. Pacek School of Chemical Engineering, University of Birmingham, UK

Chris D. Rielly Department of Chemical Engineering, Loughborough University, UK

Rodolfo J. Romañach Department of Chemistry, University of Puerto Rico, Puerto Rico

Chris Smalley Merck Sharp and Dohme, USA

Rachel M. Smith Chemical and Biological Engineering, Sheffield University, UK

Aditya U. Vanarase Bristol-Myers Squibb Co., USA

Mi Wang Institute of Particle Science and Engineering, School of Chemical and Process Engineering, University of Leeds, UK

Preface

Pharmaceutical Blending and Mixing: Role, Challenges and Trends

Pharmaceutical Blending and Mixing provides a dedicated reference for one of the most critical and ubiquitous unit operations within the pharmaceutical industry. The text aims to cover the unique role and challenges of mixing associated with pharmaceutical manufacture. This book has been prepared as a source of scientific knowledge in support of international Quality by Design (QbD) initiatives which acknowledge that increased process understanding leads to a more reliable and risk free product for patients.

This book covers the underlying principles and mechanisms of mixing necessary for designing and optimising processing thereby assuring final product quality. Equipment design, control strategies and numerical techniques available to advance the scientific understanding of pharmaceutical mixing are detailed. Detailed discussions of the fundamentals of the field are completed by a discussion of several applications from powder blending to emulsions.

Opportunities for Process Analytical Technology (PAT) and imaging strategies to monitor and control the current state of the system are discussed in Chapters 15 and 16. However, this important topic is also discussed in Chapter 4 because (1) the advantages of continuous manufacturing include the opportunity for meaningful PAT and modelling techniques to be implemented for automated process control leading to finished products with improved quality and (2) PAT will be ineffective if process monitoring is biased or affects the process stream. Since PAT is the main tool of QbD, it is more than worth mentioning that there is a high activity in terms of both fundamental and applied research/endeavours and, consequently, there is a continuous flow of mixing/blending knowledge production. A large part of this knowledge becomes public through scientific papers, manuscripts and reports, but the production and actual existence of in-house knowledge must not be ignored. Much of the latter is kept proprietary for at least some years while the rest, although not necessarily publicly available through peer-reviewed material, could be uncovered in conferences specialized on PAT (i.e. IFPAC, ISPE, pan-European PAT and QbD). This book's ambition in this area is to present the development so far as well as the most commonly used and promising PAT tools in Pharmaceutical Blending/Mixing.

Pharmaceutical Blending and Mixing provides 17 chapters describing the current state of the field. We hope that this huge effort will be useful to QbD initiatives, and help to catalyse the incorporation of scientific and technological knowledge in the design, control and validation of pharmaceutical blending processes.

It is envisaged that the reference will complement general references on mixing such as the *Handbook of Industrial Mixing: Science and Practice* (Wiley, 2004).

P.J. Cullen, Rodolfo J. Romañach, Nicolas Abatzoglou and Chris Rielly
March 2015

Part I

Fundamentals of Mixing

1
Mixing Theory

Chris D. Rielly
Department of Chemical Engineering, Loughborough University, UK

1.1 Introduction

Mixing of ingredients, or dispersion of one phase in another, is an essential step in many pharmaceuticals processes. For example, the vast majority of manufacturing routes to form an active pharmaceutical ingredient (API) make use of crystallization, which involves a number of mixing steps in a liquid phase, such as: dispersion and dissolution of solid reagents into a solvent, blending of liquid reagents with the solvent phase, creation of super-saturation through mixing, for example with an anti-solvent addition, chemical reaction, or heat removal and suspension of the API crystals during subsequent growth (Kirwan & Orella, 2002; Paul *et al.*, 2004). Each of these operations involves a mixing step, which is aimed at removing gradients of concentration, temperature or solids mass fraction within the crystallizer vessel, to give a more uniform environment for chemical reaction and/or crystal growth.

A second example may be taken from later in a pharmaceutical manufacturing process: during the formulation of solid dosage forms, dry-powder mixing of an API with excipients (themselves mixtures of binders, diluents, flow modifiers and granulating agents) is required to produce suitable physical, flow and mechanical properties for tableting (for example Lee, 2002). Here, the objective is to remove concentration differences within the dry powder mix, so that each tablet contains a mixture with exactly the same properties and with a tightly-controlled amount of the API. Other forms of oral dosage may involve the

Pharmaceutical Blending and Mixing, First Edition. Edited by P.J. Cullen, Rodolfo J. Romañach, Nicolas Abatzoglou and Chris D. Rielly.

blending of suspensions, emulsions and syrups to give a formulated liquid product; again the objective of mixing is to ensure that each dosage contains almost exactly the same amount of the active ingredient.

These examples demonstrate that in a mixing process the objective is to reduce inhomogeneities in composition to an acceptable level, to provide a more uniform processing environment and/or a more uniform product. The examples also illustrate that there are differences between fluid mixtures of miscible phases and particle mixtures, which can, in principle, unmix; for example, by segregation effects (Sommier *et al.*, 2001). Segregation often occurs in free-flowing powders and is driven by differences in particle size and density. The phenomenon occurs when particulate mixtures are shaken (Rosato *et al.*, 1987), or during flow within or between vessels (e.g. discharge from a vessel). During shaking or shear flow, there is relative motion between particles and small particles can fall into gaps beneath larger particles. Thus, the larger particles tend to rise to the surface, whereas small particles percolate downwards. Therefore, segregation can cause a previously well-mixed material to undergo unmixing into a non-uniform solid form; a way to counteract the tendency to segregate is to introduce a binder or adjust the moisture content to produce cohesion within the particulate mixture. In many processes a granulation operation follows the blending stage to prevent segregation in subsequent processing steps (Fung & Ng, 2003).

A distinction may also be drawn between batch and continuous flow mixing processes, although similar measures of mixing quality may be defined for both. Almost all current pharmaceutical processes operate by transferring batches of material between stages of the manufacturing process, rather than by continuous inflow and outflow to process equipment. Therefore this chapter will focus mainly on batch mixing processes, where the purpose is to use fluid mechanics, molecular diffusion and dispersion effects to produce spatially homogeneous mixtures; up to a point, an increase in the batch time will lead to an improvement in the mixture quality, that is a reduction in the level of spatial inhomogeneities, but thereafter, the degree of mixedness will not improve. The chapter will address the question of what is an 'acceptable' measure of mixedness; the idea of a *scale of scrutiny* of the mixture will be introduced in Section 1.3 and various measures of the quality of a mixture will be discussed. The examples given here consider two rather different situations of mixing (1) between components in a liquid and (2) between different types of solid particles. In this context it is useful to differentiate between fine and coarse-grained mixtures and this is discussed in Section 1.4. Selection of different definitions of the end-point for a mixing process will be considered in Section 1.5, to consider their sensitivity at various stages of mixing and their sensitivity to sampling methods.

Recently the pharmaceuticals industries have paid increasing attention to continuous manufacturing operations, as potentially they could significantly reduce production costs and provide more reliable manufacturing routes; see, for example, Schaber *et al.* (2011). Therefore, the final section (Section 1.6) of this chapter will consider continuous mixing of ingredients. In such operations the mixing objective is to obtain a product with a homogeneous distribution of ingredients in the correct proportions, which requires careful metering of the feed flow rates, as well as achieving a high degree of homogeneity. In continuous flow devices, the output product composition should not vary in time and the processing history of each element of the mixture should be the same. Variations in the feed composition to a continuous flow mixer can be compensated to an extent by allowing 'mixing in time', that is not all elements of fluid spend the same amount in the mixer, allowing materials that have arrived early, to mix with materials that have arrived late. Thus the concept of a residence time distribution will be introduced in Section 1.6 to describe the process of back-mixing, or mixing in time. Furthermore it will be shown that back-mixing can effectively filter out higher frequency variations in feed composition and still give a uniform product. Thus, there are processing advantages and disadvantages in having some width to the residence time distribution.

Throughout this chapter, the term *concentration* will be used quite generally to described the composition of a material within a mixture; for a single liquid phase the term can be interpreted as mass (or mole) fraction, or mass (or moles) per unit volume of a specific component; for particulate mixtures it could represent mass fraction, number fraction or volume fraction of one type of solid; for a multi-phase mixture it could be the volume or mass fraction of a specific phase. In general, the mixedness will be judged from a statistical measure of the distribution of concentrations of key components within samples drawn from a mixture.

1.2 Describing Mixtures

In practice, the whole of the composition of a mixture cannot be determined at a single time, so sampling is often used to assess the state of mixedness; sampling at an appropriate scale of scrutiny will be discussed in Section 1.3, but first the degree of uniformity between samples will be considered. The average concentration of a species in the whole mixture is determined by the amounts of all components added and can be calculated straightforwardly from a mass balance. The average species concentrations obtained from samples drawn from this mixture ought to have values distributed about the average for the whole mixture; it is the width of this distribution that provides information about the quality of the mixture, not the average value from the various samples.

Figure 1.1 shows an example of an idealized mixture comprising 50% white particles and 50% black particles. The whole mixture is divided into 36 samples, each containing 16 particles. Figure 1.1(a) is a homogeneous, but non-random mixture; each sample contains exactly eight white particles (or 50% white particles), which is exactly the same as the mean concentration of the mixture. Figure 1.1(b) shows the number of particles in each sample and indicates that there are no spatial differences in concentration; hence the mixture can be regarded as perfectly mixed. This mixture is 'perfect' in the sense that each sample contains *exactly* the same concentration as the whole mixture average; in other words there is no vari ance between the samples. The probability of forming such a mixture by a stochastic process is rather small, so this situation is very unlikely to occur in a conventional mixing process.

In contrast, Figure 1.1(c) shows a mixture that has been generated entirely randomly by giving each particle an equal probability of being black or white; the overall composition of the whole mixture is still 50% white particles, but each sample now shows deviations from the whole mixture mean, as shown in Figure 1.1(d). Some samples contain as few as four particles, whereas others have 12 or 13, compared to the expected eight, which might lead to the conclusion that the material is not well mixed. However, further mixing, or randomization, of the particles will not lead to any significant improvement in the distribution of white particles between the samples. Figure 1.1(c) represents a more realistic picture of a perfectly mixed material, yet it is highly likely that a given sample concentration will show a large difference from the mean value, particularly when the number of particles in the sample is small.

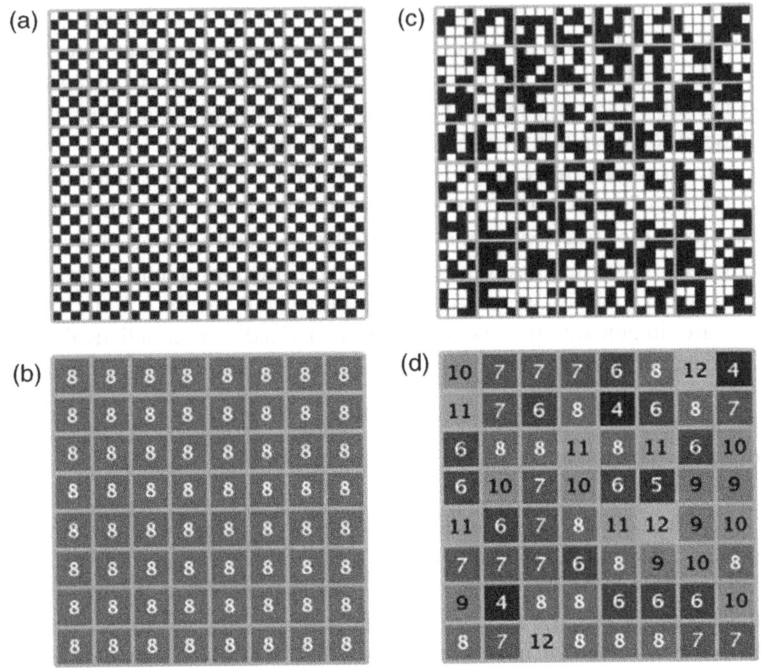

Figure 1.1 *Idealized mixtures of 50% white and 50% black particles (a) non-random perfect mixture, (b) number of white particles in each 4 × 4 sample of the non-random mixture (c) random mixture and (d) number of white particles in each 4 × 4 sample of the random mixture*

A simple definition of 'complete mixing' could be defined as the state where there are equal concentrations of components in each sample, which is the same as in the mixture overall. However, this example shows that statistical variations between samples in a fully random mixture leads to the conclusion that such a simple definition is of no practical use. Therefore, the principle applied later in this chapter to define the 'well-mixed' state will make use of a comparison back to the best state that can be achieved by random distribution processes, for example a mixture of the sort shown in Figure 1.1(c). Essentially, this will be what is regarded as 'well-mixed' since any further mixing would yield no statistical improvement in the mixture quality. Thus any description of the quality of a mixture must be able to distinguish between the sample-to-sample variations that can occur for a fully randomized mixture and those that result from incomplete mixing.

1.3 Scale of Scrutiny

The previous section described how sampling is required to assess the variability of the concentrations in a mixture, which begs the question, 'What is an appropriate size for each sample?' The end use for a mixed product determines the quality of mixing that will be required and this can only be established by viewing samples of the mixture at an appropriate *scale of scrutiny*. Danckwerts (1953a) defined this scale of scrutiny to be the 'minimum size of regions of segregation which would cause the mixture to be regarded as unmixed', Scrutinizing a mixture on the scale of a whole batch of formulated product is essentially useless: if the correct proportions of ingredients have been charged in the first place, then the whole mixture must have the required average composition. At the other extreme, scrutiny at the scale of a single particle will show a completely segregated mixture. What is required is to scrutinize a sample of the mixture at an appropriate scale, determined by the end use of the product. For example, a pharmaceutical product is designed to deliver a fixed amount of a key component, usually the API, in each unit dose taken by the patient. Thus, the scale of scrutiny could be the mass contained in one tablet of the product, which could lie between 10 mg and 5 g in typical human patient dosages (Berthiaux *et al.*, 2008). *In-situ s*ampling of particulate mixtures from within a blender at this scale of scrutiny is not straightforward to achieve and involves removal of a representative mass from within a flowing bed, for example using a thief probe. Muzzio *et al.* (2003) provide a detailed discussion of the requirements of various designs of thief probe and highlighted the difficulties in obtaining accurate composition data for their use in determining mixture quality. Thief probes cause a disruption to the powder mixture and there can be uneven flow of the different powder species into the probe; segregation of different components can occur as the mixture is sampled. These problems are compounded in continuous systems and with cohesive materials that do not flow easily in the sample cavity. Thus the issues with sampling are to obtain (1) an appropriate mass of the mixture, corresponding to the scale of scrutiny and (2) a representative sample, with the same composition as within the mixer.

Figure 1.2 illustrates the effect of changing the scale of scrutiny on the mixture quality in an idealized mixture. The left-hand sample appears to be homogeneous and on this scale of scrutiny the mixture is completely mixed; there are no visual signs of concentration differences. Increasing the magnification at which the first sample is viewed shows up differences in concentration, until at the highest magnification, the mixture appears to be completely segregated, since individual particles can be clearly identified. In all cases the sample contains the same proportions of the key component, since it is the same mixture. It appears that this mixture quality would be acceptable at the left-hand scale of scrutiny, but completely unacceptable at the right-hand scale of scrutiny.

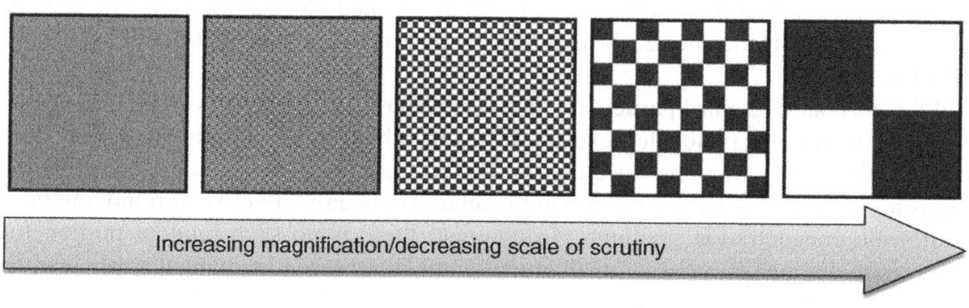

Figure 1.2 *The effect of decreasing the scale of scrutiny on the perceived quality of the mixture*

As described previously, once the scale of scrutiny has been determined, then samples at this scale can be obtained from the mixture and assessed for their homogeneity using the statistical measures described later in Section 1.5. Thus, the scale of scrutiny determines the sample mass required for any off-line analysis of product quality. For example, the FDA (2003) make recommendations about the analysis of samples drawn from blenders or from intermediate bulk containers; the guidelines state that sample sizes between 1 and 10 times the dosage unit should be investigated. Thus, the scale of scrutiny (that is the sample mass) is often taken as three times the dose mass.

In-line assessment of the homogeneity of a blend using a Process Analytical Technology (PAT) instrument would require an assessment of the effective sampling mass to justify that the FDA requirements are satisfied. Pernenkil and Cooney (2006) provided an example of such as assessment for a NIR PAT assessment of two-component powder blending, by estimating the sample size from the probe diameter and the measurement penetration depth. The mass of powder scanned per sample was estimated and compared to the mass in a single dose; hence the number of samples to be scanned and averaged to equate to a scale of scrutiny of 3 times the dose size could be calculated.

1.4 Quantifying Mixedness for Coarse and Fine-Grained Mixtures

1.4.1 Coarse and Fine-Grained Mixtures

The mixtures discussed in the previous section and shown schematically in the right-hand images of Figure 1.2 are examples of *coarse-grained* mixtures. When examined at these scales of scrutiny, a sample contains a relatively small (countable) number of discrete particles, which can be individually identified. Figure 1.3(a) shows a coarse-grained mixture comprising light and dark particles; the material appears highly segregated and the composition changes abruptly from point to point, when moving from a light particle to a dark particle. In contrast Figure 1.3(b) shows a *fine-grained* mixture. At the same scale of scrutiny, a sample contains such a large number of particles that the material can be treated as a continuum. In this case the concentration varies smoothly from point to point and finite concentration gradients exist within the mixture. Fluids behave as fine-grained mixtures, since each sample will contain a very large number of molecules and for practically useful scales of scrutiny the material can be regarded as a continuum. Mixtures of very finely-divided powders may also be considered to be fine-grained, since each sample will contain a very large number of individual particles.

Fluid and coarse-grained particulate mixtures differ in other respects. With the former, random motion of the molecules leads to diffusion, which causes a flux of material down concentration gradients to produce a more uniform mixture. However, molecular diffusion is a slow process and so this mixing mechanism is only effective at removing very small scale concentration gradients. In contrast, there is no such random motion for coarse particles and moreover, in practice small differences in diameter can lead to unmixing or segregation effects (see Section 1.1); small particles tend to percolate through the interstices created between larger particles, creating an unmixing effect based on size.

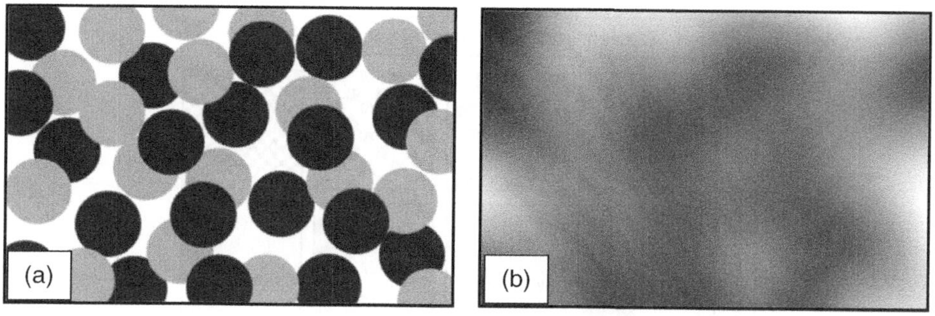

Figure 1.3 (a) a coarse-grained mixture and (b) a fine-grained mixture

1.4.2 Scale and Intensity of Segregation

Danckwerts (1953a) proposed that two measures are required to quantify the mixedness, namely a *length scale of segregation* and an *intensity of segregation*. The former indicates the physical size of the unmixed regions in an imperfect mixture, whereas the latter represents the degree to which there are variations in concentration between samples. Both measures are affected by the selection of the sample size or scale of scrutiny (see Section 1.3), as will be illustrated with some examples. The top left image in Figure 1.4 shows a highly segregated mixture (coarse-grained), in which individual regions of distinctly different concentration are visible: in qualitative terms, the length scale of segregation is large, because the regions of unmixed material have a significant size compared to the scale of scrutiny. Moving to the right in Figure 1.4, the size of the unmixed regions becomes smaller (the length scale of segregation decreases), although the mixture remains highly segregated between black and white areas. Moving downwards in Figure 1.4, the regions of unmixed material remain of the same size, but the concentration gradients are increasingly smeared out, that is the intensity of segregation decreases. The effect is created here by blurring the interface regions between black and white regions, in a process analogous to diffusion. The combination of decreases in intensity and length scale of segregation results in the mixture becoming increasingly more fine-grained as it approaches the perfectly mixed (uniform concentration) state, as shown in the bottom right image of Figure 1.4. Here, individual particles are not visible and neither are concentration gradients. In other words, the mixture is well-mixed.

Danckwerts (1952) provided quantitative definitions for the intensity and length scale of segregation based on measurements of the concentration fields. Consider an imperfect binary mixture of components A (white) and B (black), containing mass fractions a and b, respectively, at any point in the mixture. A mass fraction $a = 1$ would represent pure component A at that point in the mixture, whereas $a = 0$ would represent pure component B and for a binary components $a + b = 1$. The average mass fraction of A in the mixture would be given by

$$\bar{a} = \frac{1}{n}\sum_{i=1}^{n} a_i \tag{1.1}$$

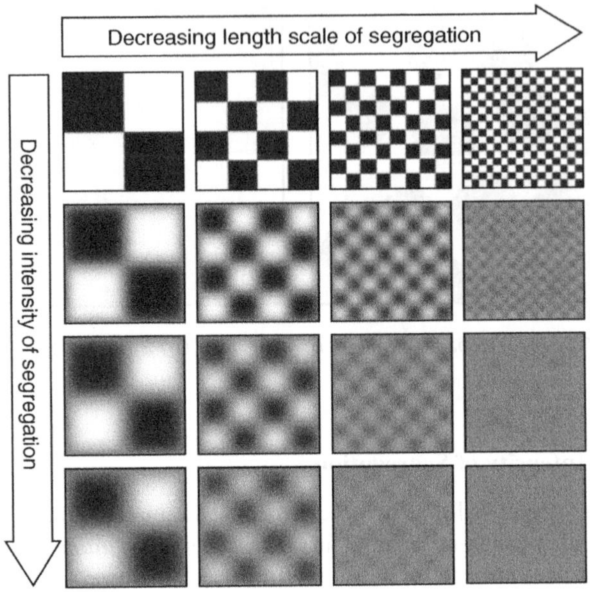

Figure 1.4 The effects of changing scale and intensity of segregation on the quality of the mixture

where a_i is the concentration of A in sample i drawn from the mixture and n is the number of samples. The sample size should be less than or equal to the required scale of scrutiny, as discussed in Section 1.3. The mean composition $\bar{a}$ provides almost no useful information about the quality of the mixture, only that it contains the correct proportions of A and B. In contrast, the variance of the sample concentrations, a_i, provides a useful statistic to characterize differences from the mean, $\bar{a}$, and is defined by

$$\sigma^2 = \frac{1}{n-1}\sum_{i=1}^{n}(a_i - \bar{a})^2 \quad (1.2)$$

A perfect mixture might be thought to have a variance of zero, but as Figure 1.1 illustrates, this is unlikely to happen in practice. Lacey (1943) showed that for a fully randomized binary mixture of the same-sized particles, the variance is given by

$$\sigma_r^2 = \frac{\bar{a}(1-\bar{a})}{n_p} \quad (1.3)$$

where n_p is the number of particles in each sample (determined by the required scale of scrutiny). Returning to the random mixture shown in Figure 1.1(c), the samples shown each contain 16 particles and the variance calculated from equation (1.2) is $\sigma^2 = 0.018$, which compares well with the value of $\sigma_r^2 = 0.017$ from equation (1.3). Thus further randomization of the mixture in Figure 1.1(c) would not result in an improvement in its uniformity and hence σ_r^2 represents the lowest variance that can practically be achieved.

The maximum variance for a binary mixture occurs for a completely segregated mixture in which each sample contains only one particle and so this represents the worst case.

$$\sigma_0^2 = \bar{a}(1-\bar{a}) \tag{1.4}$$

Hence, Danckwerts (1952) defined his intensity of segregation as one measure of mixedness, according to

$$I = \frac{\sigma^2}{\sigma_0^2} = \frac{\sigma^2}{\bar{a}(1-\bar{a})} \tag{1.5}$$

so that for a completely segregated mixture $I=1$ and for a perfectly uniform mixture $I=0$. Note that Danckwert's definition does not include the variance, σ_r^2 of a fully random mixture containing n_p particles, given by equation (1.3) and hence the minimum value of the intensity of segregation is in practice given by σ_r^2/σ_0^2. Therefore one way to characterize the quality of a mixture would be to take repeated samples of a given size and then calculate the variance from equation (1.2) and the intensity of segregation from equation (1.5). Specifications may then be prescribed for the satisfactory uniformity of the mixture in terms of a suitable range of the intensity of segregation.

The length scale of segregation provides information about the size of unmixed regions and is calculated from an autocorrelation coefficient, defined as

$$R(r) = \frac{\overline{(a(\mathbf{x})-\bar{a})(a(\mathbf{x}+\mathbf{r})-\bar{a})}}{\overline{(a(\mathbf{x})-\bar{a})^2}} \tag{1.6}$$

where $a(\mathbf{x})$ is the concentration at position $\mathbf{x}$ (taken over at a suitable scale of scrutiny), whereas $a(\mathbf{x}+\mathbf{r})$ is the concentration at distance r away (at the same scale of scrutiny), as shown in Figure 1.5. The overbars in equation (1.6) represent an average over the whole mixture, for various positions $\mathbf{x}$ and distances r. In Figure 1.5, the average concentration is $a = 0.5$.

Consider a position $\mathbf{x}$ centred in circle C_1, which is a region of approximately uniform, below-average concentration, $(a(\mathbf{x})-\bar{a})<0$. Here it is assumed that the scale of scrutiny is small, such the position $\mathbf{x}$ represents a point. Moving small distances away from $\mathbf{x}$ within the circle gives $(a(\mathbf{x}+\mathbf{r})-\bar{a})<0$, so that the product in the numerator of equation (1.6) on average remains positive in this region. If the radius r extends outside the circle C_1, then $(a(\mathbf{x}+\mathbf{r})-\bar{a})$ could be either negative or positive so that, when averaged over many positions, the numerator becomes close to zero. This is also true for other regions of approximately constant concentration, for example areas C_2 and C_3. Within these regions the concentrations are fairly well correlated with each other, but when the pairs of points lie too far apart there is almost no correlation. The denominator in equation (1.6) simply normalizes the autocorrelation so that it falls in the range $-1 < R(r) < 1$. So, the correlation function decreases from 1 to around zero at large distances r, as shown in Figure 1.6.

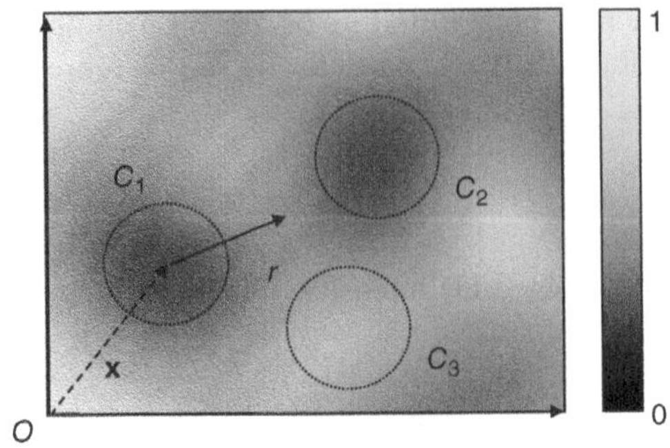

Figure 1.5 An illustration of the calculation of the autocorrelation function for a mixture

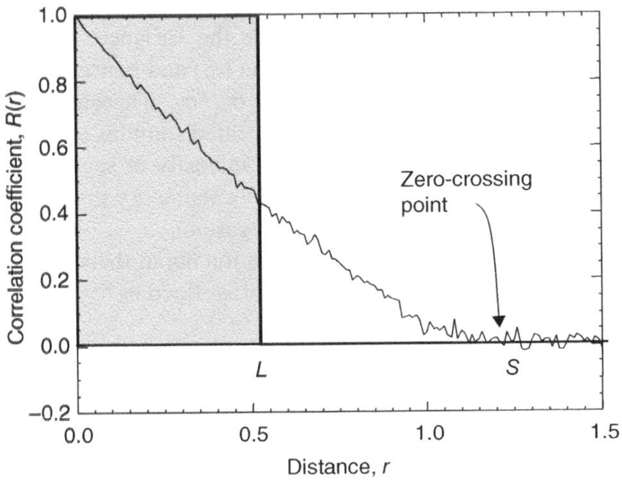

Figure 1.6 The autocorrelation function for a mixture showing the definition of the length scale of segregation

Using these ideas of spatial correlation of concentration fields, the length scale of segregation was defined by Danckwerts (1957) as

$$S = \int_0^{\infty} R(r)\ dr \approx \int_0^{\xi} R(r)\ dr \tag{1.7}$$

In practice, the correlation function does not remain exactly at zero for large distances r and hence the upper limit is usually replaced by the first zero-crossing point $r = \xi$, as shown in Figure 1.6. The figure also provides an interpretation of the length scale L: the real correlation function is replaced by a region of perfect correlation over a distance S, signifying the size of the unmixed regions of almost uniform concentration.

A volume of segregation may also be defined as

$$V = 2\pi\int_0^{\infty} r^2 R(r)\ dr \approx 2\pi\int_0^{\xi} r^2 R(r)\ dr \tag{1.8}$$

and for a linear correlation function

$$V = \frac{4\pi}{3} S^3 \tag{1.9}$$

which indicates that S will represent the radius of the unmixed regions.

The length scale of segregation is a useful concept for coarse-grained mixtures in which individual particles may be distinguished; however, it conveys little information about variations in concentration between different samples from the mixture, which is why the intensity of segregation is also required.

Figure 1.7 shows an analysis of a 50:50 binary mixture that is fully randomized; in the left hand picture, the mixture is viewed at the scale of scrutiny of a single particle; moving towards the right, the sample sizes increase, showing the effects of choosing different scales of scrutiny. Here the correlation coefficient has been obtained using a Monte-Carlo technique; the mixture is sample at 5000 pairs of points a distance r apart ($r = 1$ corresponds to the length of the side of one of the black or white particles that form the mixture). For a sample containing a single particle, $n_p = 1$, the mixture is completely segregated, and hence the intensity of segregation is $I = 1$. For larger scales of scrutiny, the intensity of segregation is always close to the theoretical value given by equation (1.3) and hence it decreases as the number of particles in the sample increases. For a well-mixed system,

$$I \approx \frac{\sigma_r^2}{\sigma_0^2} = \frac{1}{n_p} \tag{1.10}$$

The values show in Figure 1.7 correspond almost exactly to equation (1.10), with any minor differences caused by the numerical calculation method. Visually, the mixture

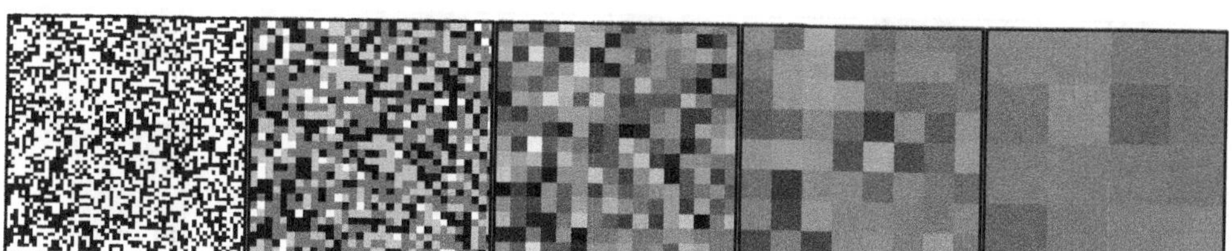

Sample	1x1	2x2	4x4	8x8	16x16
Intensity	1.00	0.25	0.06	0.01	0.00
Scale	0.5	0.9	1.8	3.1	6.1

Figure 1.7 *The effect of the scale of scrutiny on the intensity and length scale of segregation for a fully random mixture (lengths scales are multiples of the particle size)*

becomes less segregated as the sample size (scale of scrutiny) increases. The length scale of segregation for the left-hand image ($n_p = 1$) is about half the particle size and remains at approximately half the length scale of each sample. From this point of view the mixture is well-mixed; the size of the unmixed regions is comparable with the radius of the sample size.

Figure 1.8 shows a incompletely mixed situation, with intensities of segregation that are considerably higher than for the equivalent sample size in Figure 1.7; even as the scale of scrutiny increases, there are noticeable differences in concentration between samples drawn from the same mixture. Furthermore, the length scale of scrutiny for $n_p = 1$ (left hand image) is considerably larger than half the particle size, indicating that there are regions of unmixed concentrations. Increasing the scale of scrutiny (moving to the right) decreases the intensity of segregation, but the values are considerably larger than for the equivalent sample size in Figure 1.7. In Figure 1.8 the length scale also increases with the sample size; it is only for the $n_p = 16 \times 16$ sample, that the length scale of segregation approaches half the sample size; that is, the sample size is now close to the size of the unmixed regions, which are clearly visible in the left hand image.

So the last two examples, illustrate how when viewed at an appropriate scale of scrutiny (that is the required sample size which will depend on the end use for the mixture), then the concepts of length scale and intensity of segregation can be used to obtain quantitative information about the quality of the mixture, in terms of both the size of the unmixed regions and their uniformity. The mixture of Figure 1.7 is coarse grained and so when the sample size is small, it appears as being segregated, even though it is in fact fully randomized. The intensity of segregation is high for $n_p = 1$ and $n_p = 4$, because Danckwerts's definition of the intensity does not account for the variance of a random mixture with sample size n_p. Other workers have included this effect in their definition of mixedness quantities, as described in the next section.

In practice, in batch mixing operations, the length scale of segregation is difficult to obtain, as the spatial autocorrelation function is required by equations (1.6) and (1.7), that is it requires pairs of concentrations to be measured, at known distances apart (Rielly *et al.*, 1994). Consequently the majority of workers have tended to focus on the intensity of segregation, or similar measures of mixedness (see Section 1.5); the intensity of segregation is more easily obtained from an assessment of the variance between samples withdrawn from

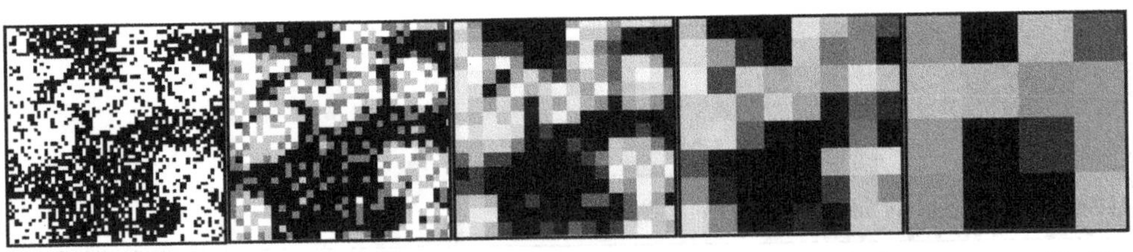

Sample	1x1	2x2	4x4	8x8	16x16
Intensity	1.00	0.48	0.31	0.21	0.11
Scale	1.9	3.7	5.1	6.4	8.3

Figure 1.8 *The effect of the scale of scrutiny on the intensity and length scale of segregation for a poorly mixed mixture (lengths scales are multiples of the particle size)*

the batch, without knowledge of their spatial positions. In contrast, for continuous blenders, the definition of the correlation function can be applied in the time domain to samples that are continuously monitored at the exit from the mixer. Weinekötte and Reh (1995) redefined the scale of segregation in terms of a temporal autocorrelation function when written in the form

$$R(\tau) = \frac{\overline{\left(a(t)-\bar{a}\right)\left(a(t+\tau)-\bar{a}\right)}}{\overline{\left(a(t)-\bar{a}\right)^2}} \tag{1.11}$$

where τ is the time delay and $a(t)$ is the concentration at time t. The scale of segregation can then be calculated by adapting equation (1.7)

$$S = \dot{m} \int_0^\infty R(\tau)\ d\tau \tag{1.12}$$

where $\dot{m}$ is the mass flow rate leaving the mixer. In this case, the scale of segregation represents the mass of the unmixed regions. The definition of the intensity of segregation for a continuous blender remains the same as in equation (1.5), but with the variance calculated from the temporal variation of the outlet concentration, $a(t)$. Weinekötte and Reh (1995) also showed how both the scale and intensity of segregation can be conveniently obtained from the power spectral density of the outlet concentration from a continuous mixer.

1.5 *Determining the End-Point of Mixing:* Comparison of Mixing Indices

The previous section describes two methods to characterize the end-point of a mixture, which could be applied to samples withdrawn from a batch blender or from measurements at the exit from a continuous mixer. In this section, a number of these statistical measures of mixedness will be compared and critically reviewed to determine their effectiveness in establishing an end point of mixing.

The definition of mixing indices dates back to Lacey (1943) who proposed various statistical measures to represent the closeness of approach to the randomly mixed state. In general, mixing indices are defined as

$$M = \frac{\text{amount of mixing that has occurred}}{\text{amount of mixing that could occur}} \tag{1.13}$$

The most extreme conditions are given by an initially fully segregated mixture with variance σ_0^2 given by equation (1.4) and a fully randomized sample with a variance of σ_r^2 given by equation (1.3). Hence, Lacey (1943) proposed

$$M = \frac{\sigma_0^2 - \sigma^2}{\sigma_0^2 - \sigma_r^2} \tag{1.14}$$

which varies between 0 (completely segregated) and 1 (fully randomized). This definition has been criticized in the past (Harnby, 1985), because even in a poor quality mixture the variance is closer to σ_r^2 than σ_0^2 and hence the useful range is restricted to $0.75 < M < 1$. A feature of this definition of a mixing index is that it shows some sensitivity to the number of particles in a sample, through the variance of a fully randomized sample, with σ_r^2 given by equation (1.3). Therefore a small improvement in the degree of homogeneity could be obtained by grinding or crushing the particles, whilst still containing the same scale of scrutiny in terms of the mass of the sample. In practice, however, grinding to particle sizes below about 1 μm becomes ineffective, because cohesive interactions cause multi-particle agglomerates to form. As a consequence zero variance mixtures are still difficult to achieve (Staniforth, 1982).

Many other mixing indices have been proposed in the literature, but they all take a similar form to that originally defined by Lacey (1943). Rielly *et al.* (1994) and Fan *et al.* (1990) have reviewed the range of mixing indices available, as summarized in Table 1.1. In the majority of cases a mixing index of 0 represents a fully segregated mixture, whereas a mixing index of unity corresponds to a fully mixed situation.

Table 1.1 *Definitions of mixing indices from the literature for use with particulate systems*

Source	Mixing index	Fully segregated	Full mixed
Rose and Robinson (1965)	$M_1 = 1 - \frac{\sigma}{\sigma_0}$	0	$1 - \frac{\sigma_r}{\sigma_0}$
Miles (1962)	$M_2 = 1 - \frac{\sigma^2}{\sigma_0^2}$	0	$1 - \frac{\sigma_r^2}{\sigma_0^2}$
Lacey (1954)	$M_3 = \frac{\sigma_0^2 - \sigma^2}{\sigma_0^2 - \sigma_r^2}$	0	1
Weidenbaum and Bonilla (1955)	$M_4 = \frac{\sigma_r}{\sigma}$	σ_r / σ_0	1
Beaudry (1948)	$M_5 = \frac{(\sigma_0 / \sigma) - 1}{(\sigma_0 / \sigma_r) - 1}$	0	1
Yano *et al.* (1956)	$M_6 = \frac{\sigma}{\sigma_0}$	1	σ_r / σ_0
Ashton and Valentin (1966)	$M_7 = \sqrt{\frac{\ln\sigma_0^2 - \ln\sigma^2}{\ln\sigma_0^2 - \ln\sigma_r^2}}$	0	1
Lacey (1943)	$M_8 = \frac{\sigma_0 - \sigma}{\sigma_0 - \sigma_r}$	0	1
Westmacott and Lineham (1960)	$M_9 = \frac{\sigma^2}{\sigma_0^2}$	1	σ_r^2 / σ_0^2

Although these definitions relate to coarse particulate mixtures, they could also be applied to fine-grained or fluid systems, in which case the variance σ_r^2 would be taken to equal zero. These analyses of the end point of a particulate blending operation are often conducted for a binary mixture of particles with equal sizes and hence there is no difference between a mass- or number-based definition of the concentration. In practice, however, mixtures will often contain a range of particle sizes and will be characterized by mass concentrations of particular species. In this case Poole *et al.* (1964) has shown that the random variance, σ_r^2, is given by

$$\sigma_r^2 = \frac{\bar{a}(1-\bar{a})}{W}\left[(1-\bar{a})\sum_i (f_i W_i)_A + \bar{a}\sum_i (f_i W_i)_B\right] \tag{1.15}$$

where $\bar{a}$ is the mass fraction of A in a mixture with total sample mass of W, f_i is the mass fraction of particles of A in size range i with mean particle mass of W_i (and similarly for species B. Mixtures containing particles with different sizes are often subject to segregation and hence mixing indices do not always increase monotonically with increasing time. For example, Harnby (1985) present mixing index data for a Rotocube, in which Lacey's definition of M_3 (see Table 1.1) initially increases with time, passes through a maximum and then decreases to an asymptotic value of around 0.85 as a result of particle segregation. The tumbling action of batch mixers such as the Rotocube will initially provide some blending of dry powders, but at later stages will result in a degree of segregation, such that the fully random state is never achieved with non-uniformly sized particles.

Rielly *et al.* (1994) compared the mixing indices of Table 1.1 by examining a simplified model that described the evolution of the concentration variance of a binary mixture of uniformly sized particles. In general blending between binary components occurs by a combination of mechanisms:

1. Convection and shear mixing, in which groups of particles are displaced or slip relative to each other over large distances. Convection without shear or relative displacement of particles is not effective for mixing.
2. Diffusion, in which particles move relative to each other over small scales, as a result of random collisions; in general, there will be a flux of particles down the concentration gradient, because of random collisions.

In a batch mixer, a diffusion type model may be used to describe the rate at which binary particles mix. For example, in a rotating cylinder mixer, of length L, the following axial diffusion equation may be written:

$$\frac{\partial a}{\partial t} = D\frac{\partial^2 a}{\partial z^2} \tag{1.16}$$

where a is the concentration of particles of A at axial distance z from the end of the mixer and at time t; D is an axial diffusion coefficient. In equation (1.16) is assumed that radial diffusion is very fast (due to cylinder rotation), whereas axial diffusion is much slower. Initially the mixer is fully segregated containing equal concentrations of A and B particles in the left and right hand ends of the mixer. Therefore, the initial and boundary conditions for equation (1.16) are

$$\text{at } t = 0, \qquad a = a_0 \ \text{ for } 0 < z < L/2 \qquad a = 0 \ \text{ for } L/2 < z < L \tag{1.17}$$

$$\text{at } t > 0, \qquad \frac{\partial a}{\partial z} = 0 \ \text{ at } z = 0 \text{ and } z = L \tag{1.18}$$

There is an analytical solution to equation (1.16) for $a(z,t)$, subject to these boundary conditions, from which the variance of the concentration distribution of A particles may be calculated from

$$\sigma^2 = \frac{2}{\pi^2} \sum_{j=1}^{\infty} \left(\frac{\sin(j\bar{a}\pi)}{j} \right)^2 \exp\left(-\frac{2j^2\pi^2 Dt}{L^2} \right) \tag{1.19}$$

where $\bar{a}$ is the mean concentration of species A in the mixer. The variance from equation (1.19) is plotted in Figure 1.9(a) for the case of binary mixture with mean concentration, $\bar{a} = 0.5$, giving an initial fully segregated variance of $\sigma_0^2 = 0.25$. The calculated variance fall rapidly at first (note the logarithmic axis) and then becomes asymptotic to zero at long times, which is realistic only for fine-grained mixtures in which the scale of scrutiny contains a very large number of particles. In other words, the mixture can attain $\sigma_r^2 \approx 0$. Figure 1.9(b) shows the various mixing indices plotted against dimensionless time for a sample containing a large number of particles. Mixing indices M_6 and M_9 decrease with increasing time, starting from an initial value of unity and falling towards a final value of zero; they show poor sensitivity at long times. Mixing indices M_2 and M_3 become equal for the special case of $\sigma_r^2 \approx 0$ and follow the more usual convention of starting at 0 (fully segregated) and finishing at 1 (fully mixed). However, neither of these indices show much sensitivity during the final stages of mixing. Similarly indices M_1 and M_8 become equal for

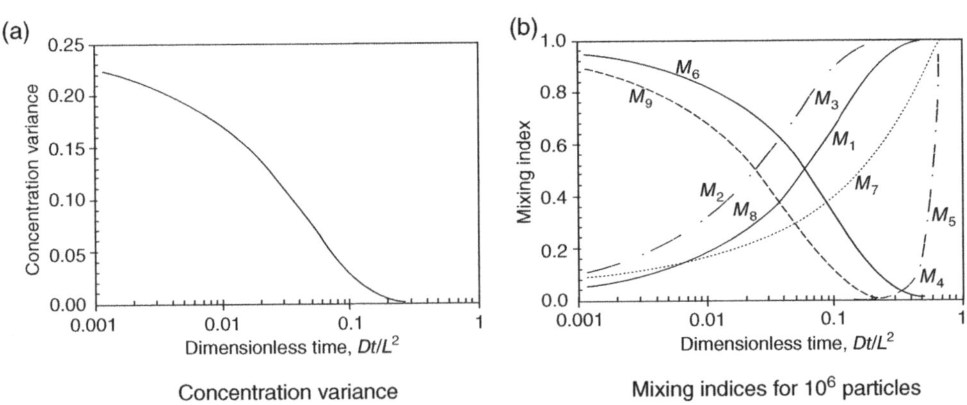

Figure 1.9 *Comparison of the variance from equation (1.19) for the diffusion model and some commonly used mixing indices for a sample size of 10^6 particles*

samples containing large numbers of particles, but also show poor sensitivity in the final stages of mixing. M_4 and M_5 show no sensitivity at early times, and extreme sensitivity in the final stages of mixing. They also highlight one of the problems with the diffusion model, which is that it predicts variances that are below σ_r^2 and hence can yield values of M_4 and M_5 greater than 1; as will be shown later, both M_4 and M_5 show significant dependence on the number of particles in the sample, that is they depend on the scale of scrutiny. Ashton and Valentin (1966) proposed the use of logarithms in their definition of M_7 to overcome such problems; Figure 1.9(b) shows that indeed M_7 shows good sensitivity to changes in the degree of mixedness in both the early and late stages of mixing and therefore is one of the better mixing indices that can be selected.

An alternative model for the kinetics of the mixing process may be formulated. Oyama and Ayaki (1955) proposed a first-order dependence for the decrease of the concentration variance towards the randomized variance, σ_r^2, as indicated in

$$\frac{d\sigma^2}{dt} = -k\left(\sigma^2 - \sigma_r^2\right) \tag{1.20}$$

where k^{-1} may be regarded as a time-constant. Integrating equation (1.20) gives

$$\frac{\sigma^2 - \sigma_r^2}{\sigma_0^2 - \sigma_r^2} = \exp(-kt) \tag{1.20}$$

which is illustrated in Figure 1.10 for the case of a sample containing 10 particles. In contrast to the diffusion model (Figure 1.9), the first-order model shows that the variance becomes asymptotic to a non-zero value at long times. The variance also depends on the number of particles within the sample, since this affects the fully randomized variance, σ_r^2, through equation (1.3). Figure 1.10(b)–(d) show that both M_4 and M_5 show sensitivity at large times, but also exhibit significant dependence on the number of particles in the sample, that is they depend on the scale of scrutiny.

This is a disadvantage, as these mixing indices are affected by the chosen scale of scrutinty; the only become independent of sample size, when the number of particles becomes very large. The indices M_2 and M_3 are almost indistinguishable for samples containing 100 or mode particles, as are the mixing indices represented by M_1 and M_8. All of these indices are relatively insensitive in the final stages of mixing. However, as noted in connection with the diffusion model (Figure 1.9), the use of logarithms in the definition of M_7 gives good discrimination over the full range of mixing times and hence is recommended.

1.6 Continuous Flow Mixers

1.6.1 Idealized Mixing Patterns

The majority of this chapter has focussed on mixing in batch process systems, where the spatial distribution of components approaches a well-mixed condition with increasing batch time. Batch processes are inherently unsteady and are often best suited to small scale production, or for multi-product manufacturing processes; hence the vast majority of

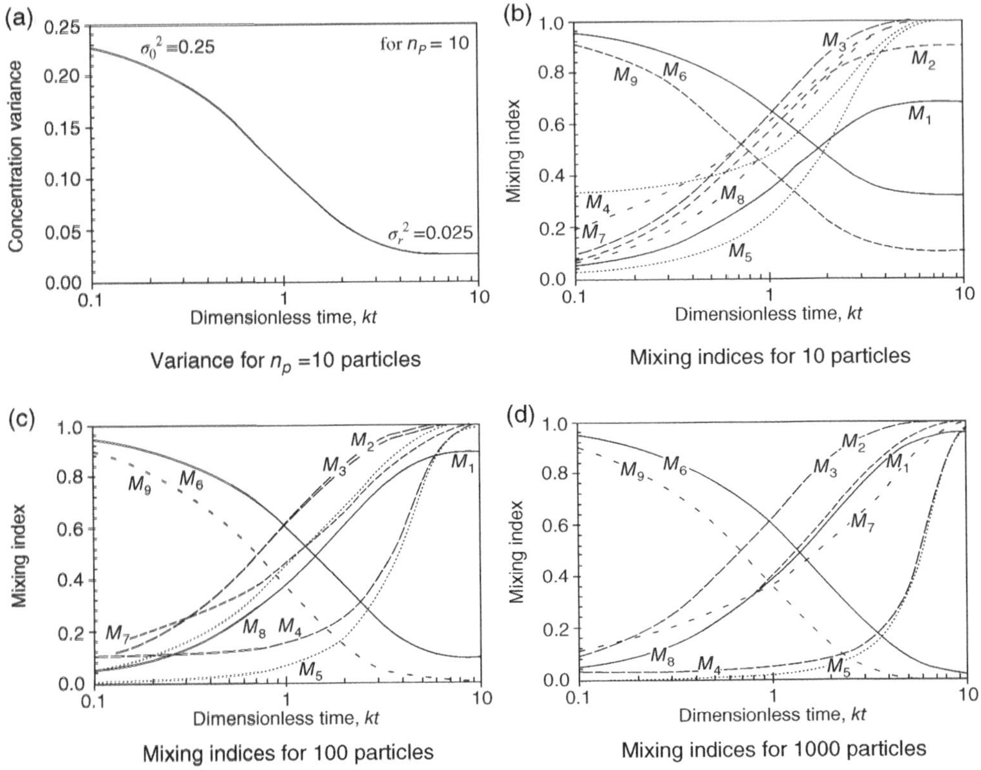

Figure 1.10 *Comparison of the variance and some commonly used mixing indices for diferent sample sizes. The concentration variance is assumed to decrease by a first-order process with time constant* k^{-1}

pharmaceutical operations are conducted as batch processes. Recently, however, pharmaceutical companies have become more interested in continuous flow processes that can be intensified and applied even for small scale production runs.

Continuous processes are designed to operate under steady conditions and the well-mixed state is usually approached with increasing *residence time* within a mixer. The residence time may be defined as the time that a fluid (or solid) element remains within the mixer, or the age of an element in the device. The plug flow reactor (PFR) has an idealized mixing pattern, in which all ingredients in the mixture experience exactly the same residence time and hence receive equal amounts of processing within the mixer. Figure 1.11 shows that a PFR exhibits perfect mixing in the radial direction, but no mixing in the axial direction. Consider an experiment in which an input pulse of tracer material is injected into the plug flow; it mixes immediately in the radial direction and will be advected axially at a velocity, u. With no mixing in the axial direction, the concentration distribution is independent of position z in the mixer, (or the age of the fluid element, $\tau = z / u$) and the pulse of tracer propagates along the mixer without change of shape.

For many operations, for example reaction, crystallization, heat treatment and sterilization, this is the ideal flow pattern to ensure a consistent product, so long as there are

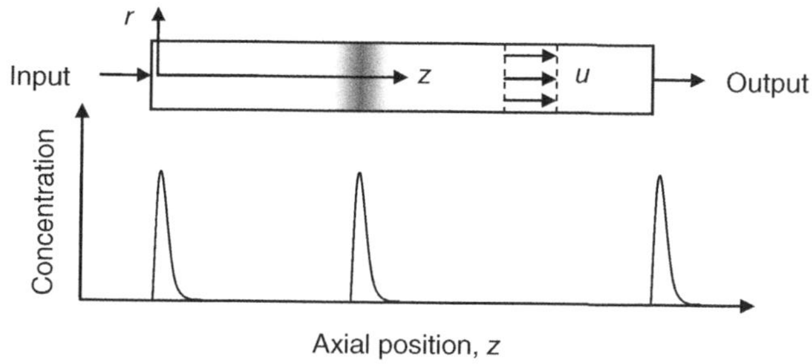

Figure 1.11 An idealized plug flow device

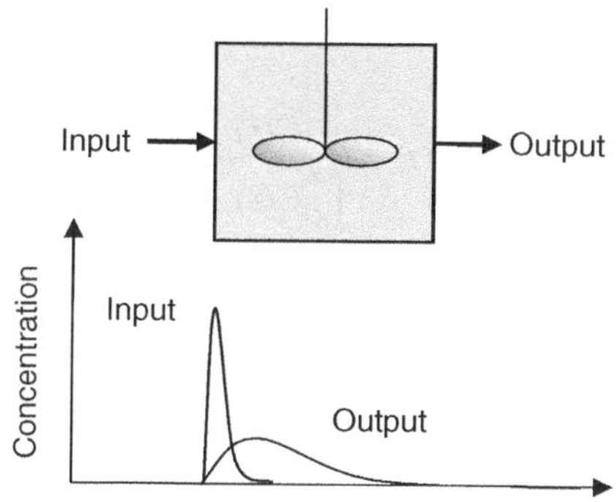

Figure 1.12 An idealized continuous stirred tank reactor

negligible variations in the feed composition, since each fluid element receives experiences exactly the same history within the device.

In contrast, the continuous flow stirred tank reactor (CSTR) is the other extreme of idealized mixer. As soon as feed enters the device it becomes instantly mixed with fluid already inside the CSTR. At any instant in time, the contents of the CSTR are spatially homogeneous and the outlet stream contains the same composition as is in the vessel. Figure 1.12 shows that as soon as a pulse of tracer enters the CSTR, the output concentration starts to rise; mixing with lower concentrations already present within the tank, causes dilution and a reduction in concentration, in comparison with the input. The CSTR is characterized by a broad range of residence times; all ages of fluid inside the vessel have an equal probability of leaving through the outlet. Therefore, some fluid elements leave very shortly after they have arrived inside the CSTR and others remain for a very long time. In this way variations in the feed composition are smoothed out by the process of mixing in time, which will be described in the next section. Such a process is also described as back-mixed, because fluid elements of different age mix with each other.

1.6.2 Residence Time Distributions

The idealized mixing patterns of the PFR and CSTR have different distributions of the residence time. Danckwerts (1953b) defined the residence time distribution (RTD) in the same way as a probability density function: $E(t)\ dt$ is the probability that a fluid element will have an residence time between t and $t+dt$. The cumulative probability that the fluid has a residence time less than T is

$$\Pr(t<T)=\int_0^T E(t)\ dt \tag{1.21}$$

and hence

$$\Pr(t<\infty)=\int_0^\infty E(t)\ dt=1 \tag{1.22}$$

The RTD can be easily measured for process equipment by introducing a pulse of tracer (mathematically this is a Dirac delta function, $\delta(t)$) at the inlet to the device and measuring the outlet concentration as a function of time. The RTD may then be obtained from

$$E(t)=\frac{C(t)}{\int_0^\infty C(t)\ dt} \tag{1.23}$$

Normalization using the integral in the denominator of equation (1.23) simply ensures that equation (1.22) is satisfied.

Figure 1.13 shows a typical residence time distribution, of a device that exhibits a considerable degree of back-mixing, or mixing in time, as well as a time delay or plug flow component – the latter is evident because there is an initial delay in the $E(t)$. The cumulative probability (see equation (1.23)) for $T=10\text{s}$ is given by the area under the curve and in this case is 85%. The mean residence for the device may be obtained from the first moment of the RTD

$$\tau=\int_0^\infty tE(t)\ dt=\frac{V}{q} \tag{1.24}$$

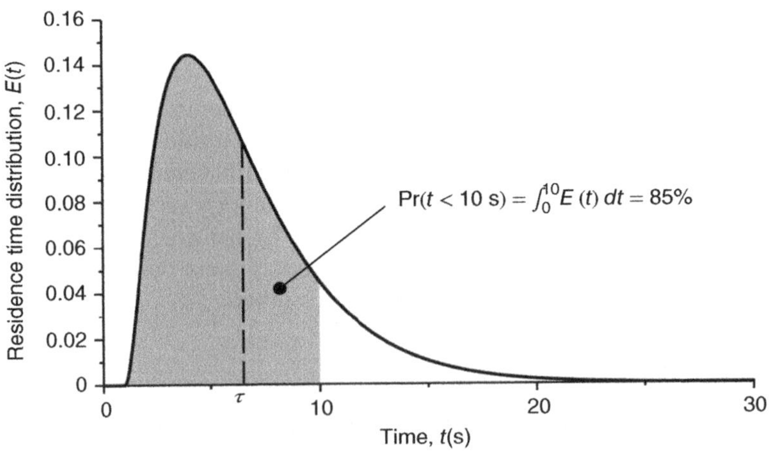

Figure 1.13 *The residence time distribution function*

where V is the volume of the vessel and q is the volumetric flow rate passing through the vessel.

1.6.3 Back-Mixing and Filtering of Disturbances Using a CSTR

Knowledge of the RTD, $E(t)$, allows calculation of the output response, $C_1(t)$ of the system to any variation in the input or feed concentration, $C_1(t)$, using the principle of convolution given by

$$C_1(t) = \int_0^t E(t')\, C_0(t-t')dt' \tag{1.25}$$

Back-mixing allows continuous flow mixers to produce more consistent product compositions, even when the feed composition is varying; effectively these mixers filter disturbances that have a much shorter time scale than the mean residence time. As an example, consider a pulse disturbance in the feed concentration to a PFR and a CSTR, each with a mean residence time of $\tau = 5$s. The RTDs for these idealized mixers are

$$\text{PFR} \qquad E(t) = \delta(t-\tau) \tag{1.26}$$

$$\text{CSTR} \qquad E(t) = \frac{e^{-t/\tau}}{\tau} \tag{1.27}$$

Applying the convolution integral of equation (1.25) and (1.26) for a square pulse of 1 s width, using the RTDs given by equations (1.26) and (1.27), gives the results shown in Figure 1.14. The pulse is unchanged by passing through the PFR, whereas it effect is attenuated and filtered by passing through the CSTR. This will be the case for pulse widths that are small compared to the mean residence time of the CSTR. This simple example illustrates why CSTRs are used as buffer tanks to smooth out disturbances in continuous flow processes.

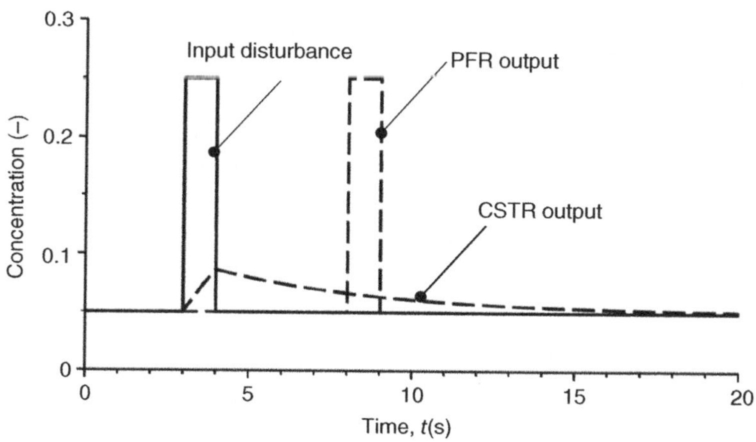

Figure 1.14 *The response of a PFR and CSTR to a disturbance*

References

Ashton. M.D. and Valentin, F.H.H. (1966) 'The mixing of powders and particles in industrial mixers,' *Trans.I.Chem.E.*, **44**, pp.166–188.

Beaudry, J.P. (1948) 'Blender efficiency,' *Chemical Engineering*, **55**, pp.112–113.

Berthiaux, H., Marikh, K. and Gatumel, C. (2008) 'Continuous mixing of powder mixtures with pharmaceutical process constraints,' *Chemical Engineering and Processing*, **47**, pp.2315–2322.

Danckwerts, P.V. (1952), 'The definition and measurement of some characteristics of mixtures,' *Applied Science Research*, **3A**, p.279.

Danckwerts, P.V. (1953a) 'Theory of mixtures and mixing,' *Research (London)*, **6**, pp.355–361.

Danckwerts, P.V. (1953b). 'Continuous flow systems. Distribution of residence times.,' *Chem. Eng. Sci.* **2**, pp.1–13.

Fan, L.T., Chen, Y.-M. and Lai, F.S. (1990), 'Recent developments in solids mixing,' *Powder Technology*, **61**, pp.255–287.

FDA (2003) *Guidance for Industry. Powder Blends and Finished Dosage Units – Stratified In-Process Dosage Unit Sampling and Assessment.*

Fung, K.Y. and Ng, K.M. (2003), 'Product-centered processing: pharmaceutical tablets and capsules,' *A.I.Ch.E.J.*, **49**(5), pp.1193–1215.

Harnby, N. (1985), 'Characterisation of powder mixtures' in '*Mixing in the Process Industries*', Harnby, N., Edwards, M.F. and Nienow, A.W. (eds), London, Butterworths, pp.23–38.

Kirwan, D.J. and Orella, C.J. (2002) 'Crystallization in the pharmaceutical and bioprocessing industries,' Chapter 11 in *Handbook of Industrial Crystallization*, Myerson, A.S. (ed.), Butterworth-Heineman, Woburn, MA, USA, pp.253–256.

Lacey, P.M.C. (1954) 'Developments on the theory of particle mixing,' *J. App. Chem.*, **4**, pp.257–268.

Lacey, P.M.C. (1943) 'The mixing of solid particles,' *Trans.I.Chem.E.*, **21**, pp.53–59.

Lee, B.J. (2002) 'Pharmaceutical preformulation: physicochemical properties of excipients and Powders And Tablet Characterisation,' Chapter 6.1, Vol. 10 Of *Pharmaceutical Manufacturing Handbook: Production and Processes*, Gad, S.C. (ed.), John Wiley & Sons, Inc., Hoboken, New Jersey, pp.881–931.

Miles, S.R. (1962) 'Heterogeneity of seed lots,' *Proc. Int. Seed Testing Assoc.*, **27**(2), pp.407–413

Muzzio, F.J., Goodridge, C.L., Alexander, A., Arratia, P., Yang, H., Sudah, O. and Mergen, G. (2003) 'Sampling and characterization of pharmaceutical powders and granular blends,' *Int. J. Pharmaceutics*, **250**, pp.51–64.

Oyama, Y. and Ayaki, K, (1956), 'Studies on the mixing of particulate solids,' *Kagaku Kogaku*, **20**, p.148.

Paul, E.L., Midler, M. and Sun, Y., (2004), 'Mixing in the fine chemicals and pharmaceuticals industries,' Chapter 9 in *Handbook of industrial Mixing, Science and Practice*, Paul, E. L., Atiemo-Obeng, V.A., Kresta, S. M. (eds), John Wiley & Sons, Inc., Hoboken, New Jersey, pp.1028–1029.

Pernenkil, L. and Cooney, C.L. (2006) 'A review of continuous blending of powders,' *Chem. Eng. Sci.*, **61**, pp. 720–742.

Poole, K.R., Taylor, R.F. and Wall, G.P. (1964) 'Mixing powders to fine scale homogeneity: studies of batch mixing,' *Trans. I. Chem. E.*, **42**, p.305.

Rielly, C.D., Smith, D.L.O., Lindley, J.A., Niranjan, K. and Phillips, V.R. (1994) 'Mixing Processes for Agricultural and Food Materials: Part 4, *Assessment and Monitoring of Mixing Systems*, **59**, pp.1–18.

Rosato, A., Strandberg, K.J., Priz, F. and Swendesn, R.H. (1987) 'Why the Brazil nuts are on top: Size segregation of particulate matter by shaking,' *Physical Review Letters*, **58**(10). pp.1038–1040.

Rose, H.E. and Robinson, D.J. (1965) 'The application of the digitial computr to the study of some problems in the mixing of powders,' *A.I.Ch.E.J.*, **10**, p.61.

Schaber, S.D., Gerogiorgis, D.I., Ramachandran, R., Evans, J.M.B., Barton, P.I. and Trout, B.L. (2011), 'Economic analysis of integrated continuous and batch pharmaceutical manufacturing: a case study,' *Ind. Eng. Chem. Res.*, **50**(17), pp.10083–10092.

Sommier, N., Porion, P., Evesque, P., Leclerc, B., Tchoreloff, P. and Couarraze, G. (2001), 'Magnetic resonance imaging investigation of the mixing-segregation process in a pharmaceutical blender,' *International Journal of Pharmaceutics*, **222**(2), pp.243–258.

Staniforth, J.N. (1982) 'Investigation of methods for identifying formation of ordered powder,' *Proc. 4th Eur. Conf. on Mixing*, Leewenhorst, Netherlands, BHRA, Cranfield, UK, pp.181–194.

Weidenbaum, S.S. and Bonilla, C.F.A. (1955) 'A fundamental study of the mixing of particulate solids,' *Chem. Eng. Prog.*, **51**, p.27.

Weinekötter, R. and Reh, L. (1995) 'Continuous mixing of fine particles,' *Particle and Particle Systems Characterization* **12**(1), pp.46–53.

Westmacott, M.H. and Lineham, P.A. (1960) 'Measurement of uniformity in seed bulks,' *Proc. Int. Seed Testing Assoc.*, **25**, p.151.

Yano, T., Kanise, I. and Tanaka, K. (1956) 'Mixing of powders by the V-type mixer,' *Kagaku Kogaku*, **20**, p.20.

2

Turbulent Mixing Fundamentals

Suzanne M. Kresta
Department of Chemical and Materials Engineering, University of Alberta, Canada

2.1 Introduction

Mixing is perhaps one of the most intuitive and appealing of all of the steps in a chemical process. We first meet mixing as young children – playing in the mud or watching the patterns cream makes when it is poured into coffee. Who has not watched the plume of water vapor condense and disperse from a power plant on a cold winter's day – or discovered that you can gently shake a bowl of mixed nuts to make the Brazil nuts move to the surface? All of these mixing examples, and many more, have analogs in pharmaceutical processing.

In order to make sense of turbulent mixing, it is useful to have a good technical definition of what we mean by "well mixed." Any mixing requirement actually has three parts (Kukukova et al., 2009):

- Achieve uniform concentration, or reduce the *intensity of segregation.*
- Reduce the length scale of either striations (particularly in laminar mixing) or of bubbles, drops, or particles of a segregated second phase (dispersion of oil in water for pharmaceutical creams, or disperse a gaseous reagent into a liquid). This mixing specification addresses reduction in the *scale of segregation.*
- Achieve a *specified mixing rate*. This specification may require the mixing time *at a specific scale* of turbulence. The simplest example is the blending of completely soluble liquids in a basic formulation. In this case, the macro-scale blend time defines the process result. In a second example, a reagent is fed to a process where it is critical to avoid

Pharmaceutical Blending and Mixing, First Edition. Edited by P.J. Cullen, Rodolfo J. Romañach, Nicolas Abatzoglou and Chris D. Rielly.

the formation of by-product in a competing side reaction. In this case, the dispersion of a plume of reagent must be faster than the rate of the side reaction. The rate of reaction is set by the *local concentration of reagent,* not the average concentration. If the reagent is fed at the surface of the vessel, the plume dispersion time, or meso-mixing rate, will dominate. If the feed is moved to the impeller, the mixing will be much faster, and the micro-mixing time will dominate. In both of these cases, the *local mixing time* is more important than the blend time for the tank.

From this point, we could consider at least three branches of mixing fundamentals: powder mixing, where particle-particle adhesion and solids demixing must be considered; laminar mixing, where chaos theory and the evolution of stretching and folding patterns determine the mixing rate; and turbulent mixing, where mixing occurs against a backdrop of turbulent eddies. Turbulent mixing, the subject of this chapter, is mainly done in stirred tanks and pipes.

2.2 The Velocity Field and Turbulence

The turbulent eddy is familiar to anyone who has trailed a stick through the water to watch the patterns made in its wake (Figure 2.1), or who has watched a mountain stream burble and churn its way over the rocks in a creek bed. More formally, an eddy is a packet of fluid that is at least reasonably coherent over a region of eddy size L, for a period of time τ. We usually sketch eddies as if they were spherical and rotating, but in fact eddies can take on any arbitrary shape, and large eddies can also contain smaller eddies. One of the most remarkable images of eddies in their full range of behavior was compiled recently by NASA in their animation of ocean currents over several years, *Perpetual Ocean* (www.nasa.gov/topics/earth/features/perpetual-ocean.html). If you watch this video, notice that

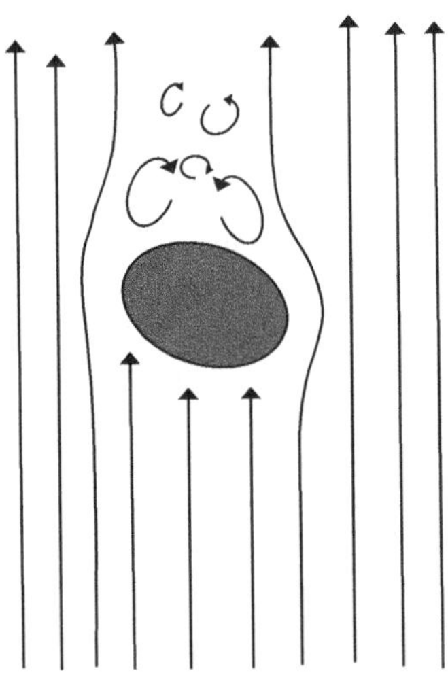

Figure 2.1 Eddies in the wake of an obstacle (Reproduced with permission from Paul et al. 2004).

the scale of the largest eddies matches the scale of nearby land features, with the flows around Cuba and Florida giving particularly good examples. Similar large eddies form around obstacles in a stirred tank, such as baffles, dip pipes, and heat exchanger tubes.

These large eddies typically fall close to what is known as the *integral scale of turbulence.* Because the eddies can have an arbitrary shape, the integral scale of turbulence, L_{t}, is actually an average length scale, taken over all of the dimensions of all of the largest eddies based on an autocorrelation spectrum of the fluctuating velocity signal over time (Rao and Brodkey, 1972). This scale usually lies somewhere close to the size of the equipment (the pipe diameter, or impeller blade width). The smallest eddies in the flow, or the Kolmogorov eddies, $\eta = \left(\nu^3 / \varepsilon\right)^{1/4}$ fall at the point where the average lifetime of the small eddy is exactly the same as the time it takes to dissipate the energy in the eddy by viscous friction, $\tau_K = (\nu/\varepsilon)^{1/2}$.

The *rate of dissipation of turbulent kinetic energy per unit mass, or the dissipation,* ε, is one of the most important variables for mixing characterization. This is the amount of energy available to do the work of turbulent mixing: for example drop break-up, dispersion of additives by eddy dispersion, or solids suspension off the bottom of the tank. Historically, the average dissipation over the volume of the tank, $(P/\rho V_{TANK})$ has been used to characterize the dissipation. The power, in this case, is calculated from the power number for the impeller, the impeller diameter, and the rotational speed of the impeller ($P = N_P \rho N^3 D^5$). Note that because impeller diameter is raised to the power of 5, a 10% error in the impeller diameter will result in a 50% error in the calculation of power. For small changes of scale and perfect geometric similarity, the average dissipation is often sufficient, but for large changes of scale or for difficult problems with many competing rates, the maximum local dissipation, ε_{MAX}, *and its location in the tank,* are needed (Machado et al., 2012; Zhou and Kresta, 1996).

Given the mixing specifications for the process, the integral scale of the largest eddies in the turbulent spectrum, the Kolmogorov scale of the smallest eddies, and the average and maximum dissipation, what is needed to use turbulence characteristics to predict mixing performance? First, the tank must be well mixed on the macro-scale, meaning there is active circulation throughout the region where mixing is needed, with no dead zones. This constraint is related to the bulk circulation or mean flow patterns in the tank. Second, the flow throughout the tank must be fully turbulent if the results are to scale-up correctly and provide robust operation (Machado et al., 2013). Third, the process requirements must be fully satisfied by the available levels of dissipation, particularly at the point of injection of any additives to the flow. Fourth and last, the scales of turbulence must provide a good match to the scales of segregation required by the process. Fortunately, several of these requirements can be combined using some fairly straightforward constraints on the process.

2.3 Circulation and Macro-Mixing

Stirred tanks are classically designed with one impeller, ($0.25 < D/T < 0.6$) situated between ($0.25 < C/T < 0.5$) with four vertical, flat, rectangular baffles of width ($W = T/10$ or $W = T/12$). While conical bottoms are common in the pharmaceuticals industry, the deep part of the cone is often poorly mixed. Flat bottom, or preferably curved bottom (ASME torispherical heads) are preferred. For historical reasons related to the limitations of glass coating technology, glass lined vessels often use a retreat blade impeller, shaped like a pump impeller and placed close to the bottom of the tank with one or more rounded baffles suspended from the roof of the vessel. This is not an efficient mixing configuration, providing mostly rotational flow with very little top to bottom circulation. Current glass coating technology allows a fully baffled tank with modern impellers. Where possible, the latter configuration should be used for new processes.

The Rushton turbine (RT), shown in Figure 2.2, is an energy intensive radially pumping impeller that provides high ε_{MAX} and strong circulation throughout the tank. It is typically placed at a clearance of (C = T/2). It is not recommended for solids suspension off the tank bottom (Ayranci et al., 2011), but is the classical impeller for gas dispersion. More modern impellers (Figure 2.3b and c) provide more stable gas dispersion operation. Rushton turbines can fill a tank of liquid height (H = T) with strong circulation and flow.

A whole family of impellers has been designed to pump liquid toward the bottom of the tank, producing good top to bottom circulation and axial flow (PBT shown in Figure 2.2a, and hydrofoils, for example A310 and A315 shown in Figure 2.3a and b). These impellers provide low to moderate local turbulence, good solids suspension, and in some specialized

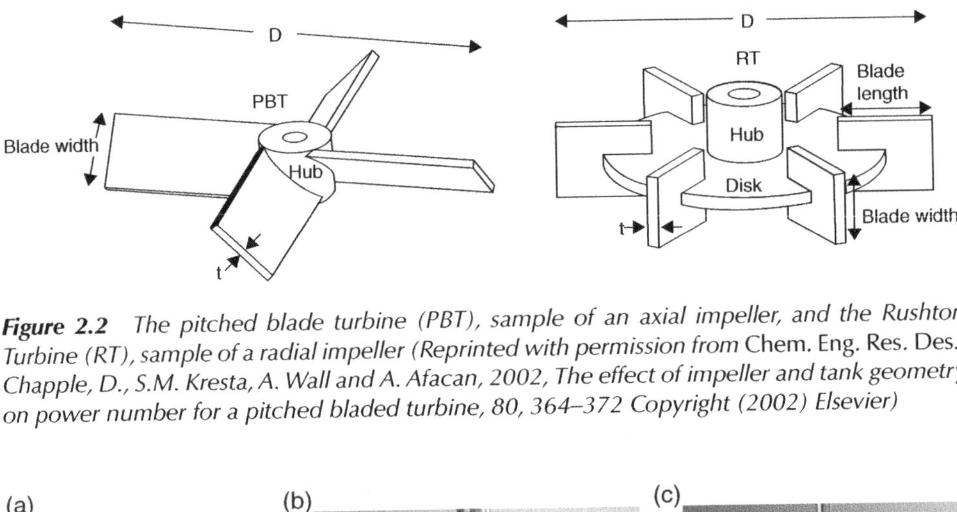

Figure 2.2 *The pitched blade turbine (PBT), sample of an axial impeller, and the Rushton Turbine (RT), sample of a radial impeller (Reprinted with permission from* Chem. Eng. Res. Des., *Chapple, D., S.M. Kresta, A. Wall and A. Afacan, 2002, The effect of impeller and tank geometry on power number for a pitched bladed turbine, 80, 364–372 Copyright (2002) Elsevier)*

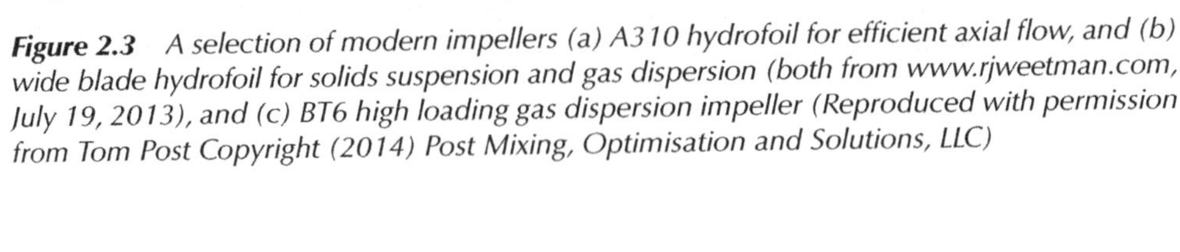

Figure 2.3 *A selection of modern impellers (a) A310 hydrofoil for efficient axial flow, and (b) wide blade hydrofoil for solids suspension and gas dispersion (both from www.rjweetman.com, July 19, 2013), and (c) BT6 high loading gas dispersion impeller (Reproduced with permission from Tom Post Copyright (2014) Post Mixing, Optimisation and Solutions, LLC)*

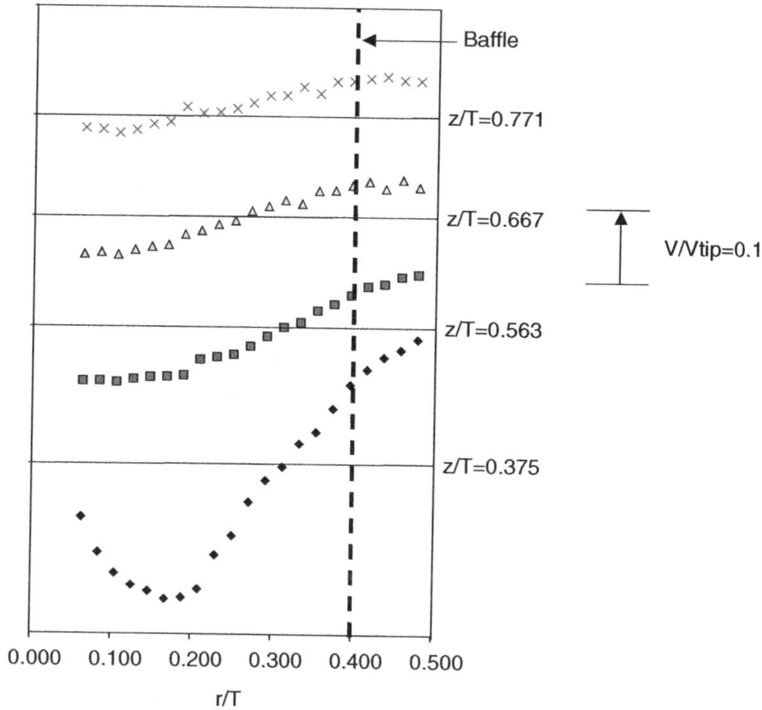

Figure 2.4 *Axial velocity profiles in a stirred tank with an A310 impeller. The impeller diameter is (D = 0.58T) and the off-bottom clearance is (C = 0.68D = 0.4T). By a height of 0.667T, the upwards flow has essentially stopped (Reprinted with permission from* Chem. Eng. Sci., *Active volume of mean circulation for stirred tanks agitated with axial impellers, Bittorf, K.J. and Suzanne M. Kresta, 55, 1325–1336. Copyright (2000) Elsevier)*

cases with wide impeller blades (Figure 2.3b), good gas dispersion. Axial impellers produce active circulation in one loop that extends from the tank bottom to a liquid height of (z = 0.67T), as shown in Figure 2.4. Because of very large scale instabilities, particularly for the PBT, these impellers can often be successfully used for liquid heights up to (H = 1.2T), but if there are strong mixing requirements in the top third of the tank, addition of a second, up-pumping impeller close to the surface ($0.2T < S < 0.4T$) is recommended (e.g. Motamedvaziri and Armenante (2012, for an RT $S_{crit}/D > 0.6$ to maintain two circulation loops), Bittorf and Kresta (2003, solids cloud height), Bhattacharya et al. (2007, air entrainment, ($0.1 < S/D < 1.2$)), Khazam and Kresta (2008, floating solids ($0.1 < S/D < 1.0$))).

For mixing in pipes, the flow is more tightly constrained and the problem of fully active volume is essentially eliminated. This is also true for well-designed static mixers, micro-mixers, and confined impinging jet reactors. Bulk mixing problems can be acute in the large-scale equipment typical of world scale chemical plants and large water treatment lagoons. They can also be present in quite small equipment if the flow is highly directional and well aligned – for example a Y-tube junction in a pipe, shown in Figure 2.5a, compared to the confluence of two rivers with little macro-mixing between the streams (see the fully worked example for this geometry in Paul et al., 2004, pp. 24–38).

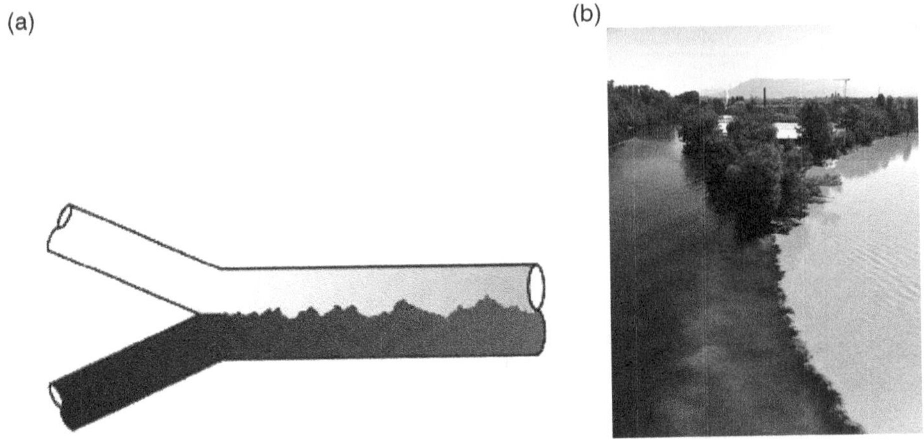

Figure 2.5 Y-tube junction where the flow is turbulent, but there is no macro-scale radial mixing. This is rare on the very small scale, but will frequently occur on the large scale, as seen in (a) a 5 cm pipe and (b) a photo of the confluence of the Rhone and Arve rivers in Geneva, Switzerland (Reprinted from http://www.istock.com, dla 29 September 2014)

This degree of macro-segregation would be the exception rather than the rule in pharmaceutical applications.

2.4 Fully Turbulent Limits and the Scaling of Turbulence

The concept of fully turbulent flow is profoundly important and quite simple to explain, but is often only loosely followed in practice. In the limit of perfectly laminar flow, many terms drop out of the equations of fluid motion, leaving only the effects of viscosity. Similarly, in fully turbulent flow, many terms drop out of the equations of fluid motion, and the flow is dominated by inertial effects due to (mass and velocity). For both of these limits, the equations can be made dimensionless and the results are general across a wide range of fluids. The most familiar example of this is the friction factor-Reynolds number curve for flow in pipes, which has a close analog in the power number curve for impellers. In transitional flow, however, both viscosity and density play an important role, all of the terms in the equations of motion must be retained, the effect of scale-up is unclear, and changing the fluid can have a significant effect on mixing. The transitional flow regime is to be avoided in process design and in scaled-down experiments wherever possible. Note that the limiting Reynolds number for fully turbulent flow depends on the geometry of the flow: for pipes it is $Re = \rho D_p V_s / \mu = 2000$, while for free round jets it is $Re = \rho D_0 V_0 / \mu = 10\,000$ (Bhattacharya and Kresta, 2006). Recent work by Machado et al. (2013), see Figure 2.6, shows that close to the impeller in a stirred tank it is about $Re = \rho N D^2 / \mu = 20\,000$, depending on the impeller, but close to the surface, the limiting Re can be as high as 300 000.

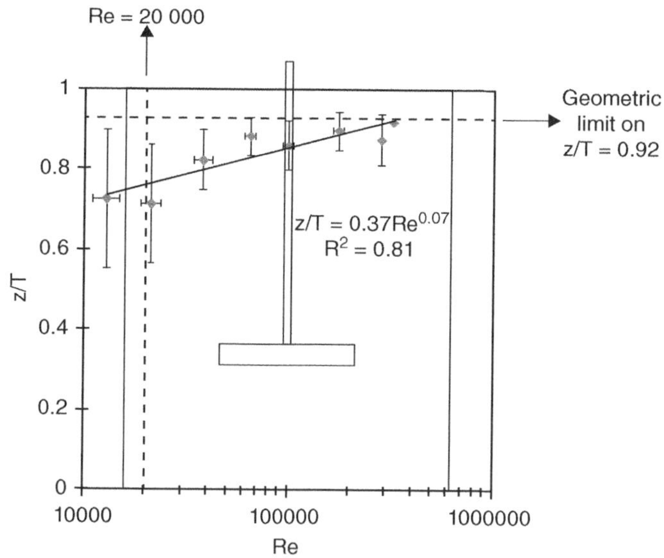

Figure 2.6 *The impeller Reynolds number required to achieve fully turbulent conditions increases as z/T increases. Re ≈ 20 000 will sustain fully turbulent flow up to z = 2/3T, but at z = 0.92T, Re = 448 000 is needed. (Reprinted with permission from* Chem. Eng Sci., *Transition from turbulent to transitional flow in the top half of a stirred tank, Machado, Márcio B., Kevin Bittorf, Vesselina Roussinova, Suzanne M. Kresta, 98, 218–230 Copyright (2013) Elsevier)*

The first test of fully turbulent flow at both the small scale and the plant scale is a power number (N_p), which is constant with increasing Reynolds number, but this characterizes only the average power draw at the impeller. The second test is self-similarity of velocity profiles, as shown in Figure 2.7. In fully turbulent flow, or completely laminar flow, the velocity profile will scale exactly with the tip speed of the impeller. Even if the rotational speed is doubled, dividing all measured velocities by (πND) or simply by (ND) will collapse the data onto a single dimensionless velocity profile. The third test is to apply this same scaling principle to the fluctuating velocity field, and the estimated local energy dissipation. This test is more severe because the fluctuating velocity is cubed to find the dissipation, so any errors or deviations from similarity are also cubed. The fourth and final test is an absolute requirement for a rigorous physicist's study of turbulence. This requires full isotropy of all of the Reynolds stresses in the flow so that there is truly no directional preference in the eddies. This test has never been successfully applied to any location in a stirred tank, so when we say that the flow is isotropic and fully turbulent, we are always making an engineering approximation. In regions close to the impeller, and for the purposes of engineering design, this is usually close enough.

The last two points needed to connect turbulence characteristics to mixing performance are, ensuring there is enough energy to meet the process requirements, and matching the scales of turbulence to the required scales of segregation. These will be covered in the last section of the chapter. Before they can be addressed, a few more elements of theory have to be introduced.

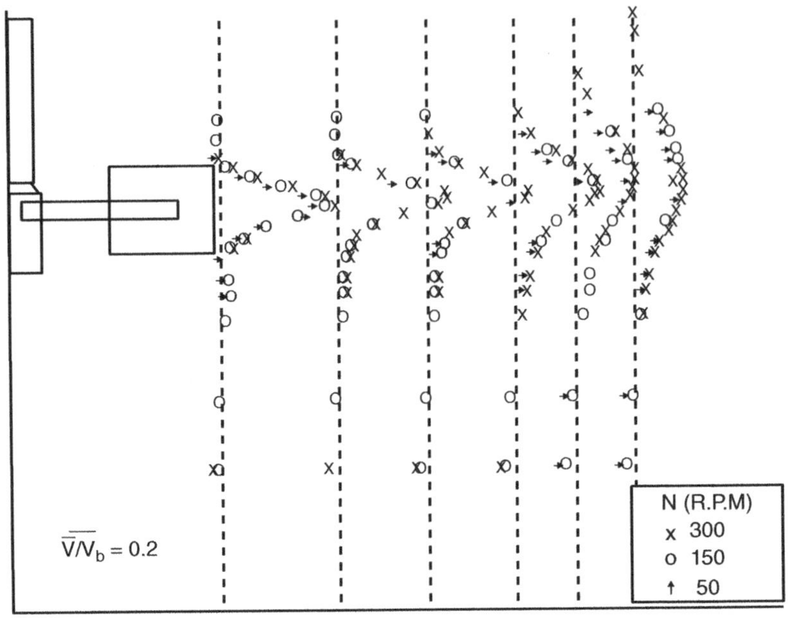

Figure 2.7 Self-similar radial velocity profiles at the tip of the Rushton turbine blade. Notice how the dimensionless velocity is the same for all Ns, even in the steepest parts of the profile (Reprinted with permission from Nouri, J.M., Whitelaw, J.H., Yianneskis, M., 1987. The Scaling of the Flow Field with Impeller Size and Rotational Speed in a Stirred Reactor, in: Turner, J., Fraser, S. (Eds.), Laser anemometry : advances and applications : 2nd International conference. Springer-Verlag, Strathclyde, Scotland)

2.5 The Spectrum of Turbulent Length Scales, Injection of a Scalar (Either Reagent or Additive) and the Macro-, Meso- and Micro-Scales of Mixing

Figure 2.8 gives three different pictures of the spectrum of turbulent length scales. Figure 2.8a shows the velocity fluctuations at a fixed point in the flow as the mean velocity carries turbulent eddies across a measurement probe. There are a number of frequencies in this signal. If the frequency spectrum of the velocity signal is calculated, the result looks like Figure 2.8b, plotted on a log-log scale. This figure is used to illustrate the relative energy in different sizes of eddies, and to identify the location of the key length scales in the spectrum. Figure 2.8c provides a conceptual sketch of the spectrum of eddies, represented as random circular cross sections of various eddies.

Above the integral scale, L_I, all motion is geometry dependent. As the eddies organize and absorb energy, coherent packets of motion form around L_I. These eddies break up, and start to propagate as smaller scales of motion. These inertially dominated eddies do not remember their origins, have no directional preference, and are not affected by viscosity. They are referred to as the universal range of eddies. They are self-similar, and independent of geometry. At the Kolmogorov scale, η, viscous and inertial forces are balanced with a local Re = 1. Viscous effects are evident for scales smaller than about 6η, with rapid viscous dissipation of energy below η.

Return for a moment to the second and third figures. The power spectrum is plotted versus 1/wavelength on the x-axis, or 1/length scale, so the smallest eddies are on the far right hand side. The large, energy containing eddies are geometry dependent and appear as a broad shoulder on the left hand side where the energy gets organized and enters the equilibrium

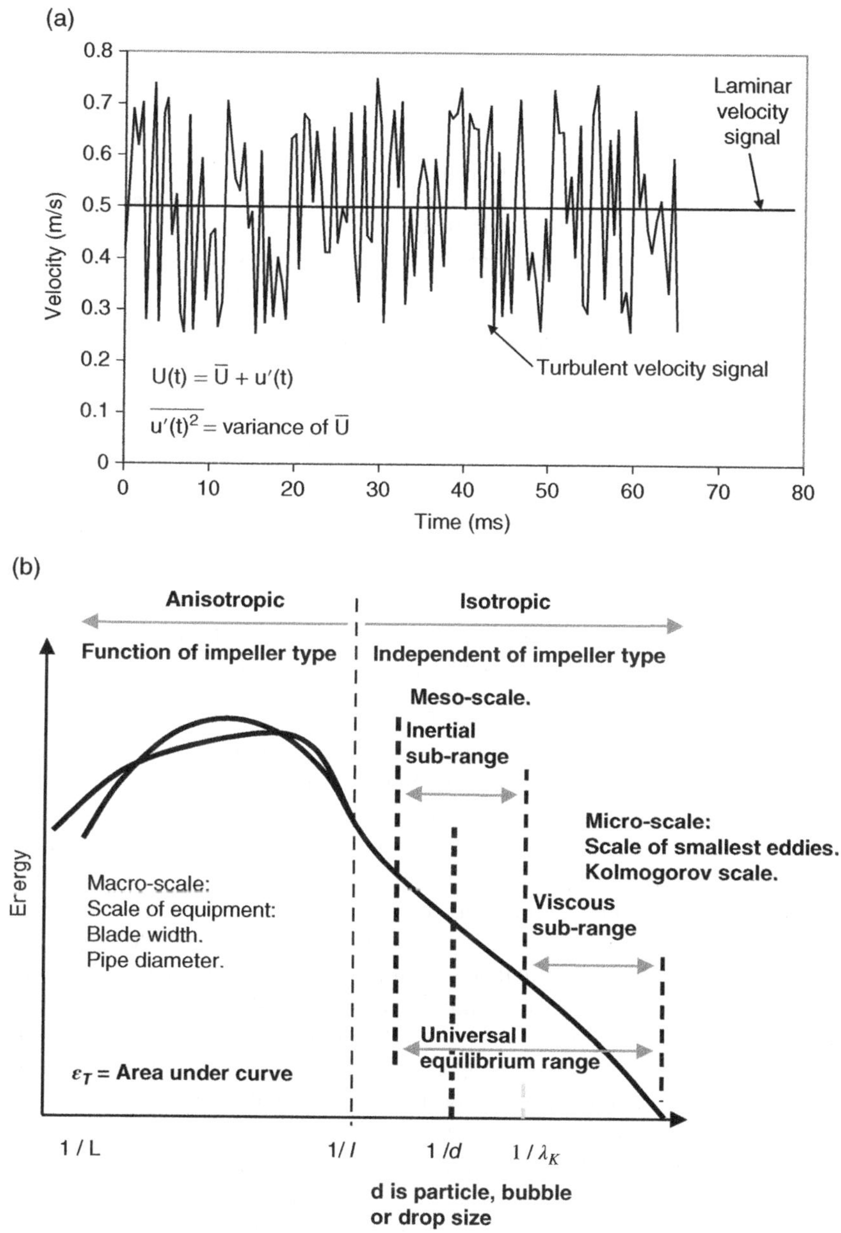

Figure 2.8 *(a) Fluctuating velocity signal, (b) power spectrum versus wave number ($2\pi/\lambda$), and (c) conceptual sketch of the eddy spectrum*

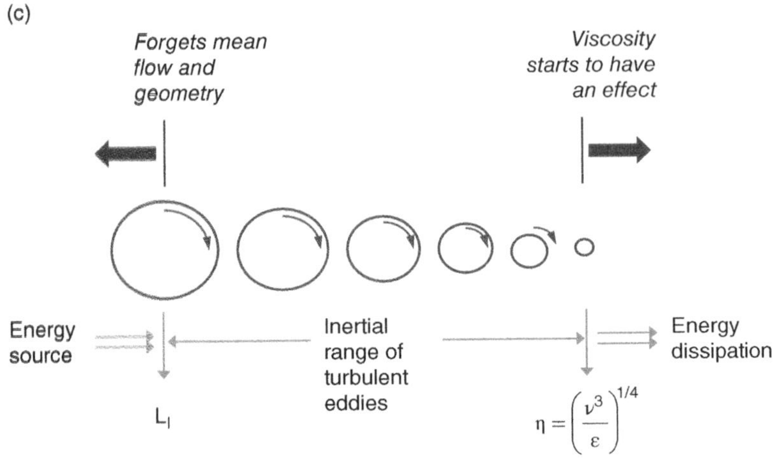

Figure 2.8 (continued)

cascade. The integral scale of turbulence appears close to the top of the inertial sub-range of turbulence, where the slope of the curve is –5/3. The slope begins to deviate from a linear –5/3 power as we approach the Kolmogorov scale, where the inertial and viscous forces come into balance and energy starts to dissipate into viscous friction at an increasing rate.

There are several models for the timescale of mixing from injection to final diffusion at the Batchelor scale. The *Corrsin mixing equation* gives the time taken for eddies to cascade down the inertial range of eddies to the Kolmogorov scale. Starting at the scale of the tank, this equation can be used to derive the blend time equation; and starting from the average eddy size, it leads to the Bourne engulfment model, which defines the micro-mixing time at the scales of the smallest eddies. The *Batchelor timescale,* $\tau_B = \tau_K = (\nu / \varepsilon)^{1/2}$, is used to identify the final timescale for diffusion across a single striation in a Kolmogorov sized eddy (Batchelor, 1959).

At the intermediate scale of a feed pipe with a slow injection of feed (either reagent or additive) the meso-mixing time can be used to identify a limiting feed rate. As long as the feed is injected more slowly than the meso-mixing limit, the turbulence surrounding the feed pipe will disperse the feed quickly enough to prevent a build-up of concentration close to the feed pipe (Bourne, 2003). A limit on feed pipe back mixing is used to ensure that the surrounding fluid does not flow back up into the feed pipe (Paul et al., 2004, p. 824).

At this point, it is useful to point out that the velocity field is not the same as the scalar field. Turbulent velocity fluctuations generate eddies that disperse additive, reagent, or some other scalar. The scalar is often easy to observe (e.g., the plume of water vapor condensing as it leaves a power plant on a cold winter day), but the underlying velocity fluctuations are quite different. The scalar fluctuations always persist to a much smaller striation thickness than the scales of the smallest eddies. The Batchelor scale (smallest striations) is related to the Kolmogorov scale (smallest eddies) through the Schmidt number as $\lambda_B = \eta / Sc^{1/2}$, where $Sc = \nu/D_{AB}$. Linking these scales (roughly) to the scales of mixing, the velocity micro-scale is in the range of η; the meso-scales cover the inertial sub-range, and the macro-scales are anything of the size of L_I and larger. Feed pipes typically fall into the meso-scale range, or just above it. Impeller blade widths are typically twice the local L_I.

At the micro-scale, molecular diffusion is slower than momentum diffusion so the Batchelor length scale is smaller than the Kolmogorov length scale. The key thing to understand about the Batchelor scale is that the time required for diffusion of the scalar is exactly equal to the time required for the energy of the eddy to dissipate (Batchelor, 1959).

At the meso-scale for the mixing equipment, but at the largest scales for the scalar, injection takes place through a feed pipe, so the integral scale of the scalar is always smaller than the scale of the equipment (e.g., tank diameter or pipe diameter). It is easiest if this largest scalar dimension falls inside the universal range of turbulent eddies, so the scalar is injected into the most predictable region of the turbulent spectrum and mixing behavior can be predicted with greater confidence.

In summary, we can approximate the different scales of mixing as follows: macro-mixing is characterized by the blend time and happens on the scale of the tank, or the pipe diameter. In the macro-mixing stage, gross segregation is smoothed out and the concentration fluctuations drop to 5% of the initial variance. At the micro-scale, molecular diffusivity of mass and momentum meets the smallest turbulent eddies and concentration striations. At this scale, the final processes of mixing reduce segregation to the molecular scale. The time scale is the micro-mixing time. The meso-scale is everything in between, but is most commonly applied to design of the feed pipe and dispersion of a second phase. At this scale, the ideal mixing situation is to have the rate of dispersion by turbulence at the feed point at least equal to (and hopefully faster than) the feed rate of additive (Bourne, 2003). A second model (interaction by exchange with the mean – IEM) is given by Villermaux and Falk (1994), which directly considers the interaction of a plume of scalar with the surrounding eddies when the injection rate is faster than the local rate of turbulent dispersion. Alternate solutions to the meso-mixing problem have been proposed by several authors, including use of a second up-pumping impeller at the surface (bringing more turbulence to feed at the surface of the liquid) and injection of reagent by a jet that provides its own mixing energy (Bhattacharya and Kresta, 2004).

2.6 Turbulence and Mixing of Solids, Liquids, and Gases

The interaction of turbulence with a second phase is an active area of research with many challenges, particularly with respect to the effects of surface forces and trace amounts of additive.

What we can say is that turbulent eddies interact with particles, drops and bubbles most strongly when the eddies are close to the same size as the particle – meaning 2–3 times bigger, or 2–3 times smaller. This is illustrated in Figure 2.9 for a liquid-liquid dispersion, and in Figure 2.10 for solids suspension. When drops are much smaller than large eddies, they are simply swept along with the flow. When the drops are much bigger than the eddies, the eddies dissipate at the interface, perhaps eroding away a small drop if the interfacial tension is very low. Drop break-up is most effective when the drops and eddies are a similar size. The same can be said for lifting individual solid particles up from the bottom of the tank, and dispersing gas bubbles into a continuous fluid.

This leads us back to the importance of fully turbulent flow and accurately capturing the integral scale and Kolmogorov scale of turbulence, along with the rate of energy dissipation, when attempting to scale-up and scale-down. There are many additional complexities due

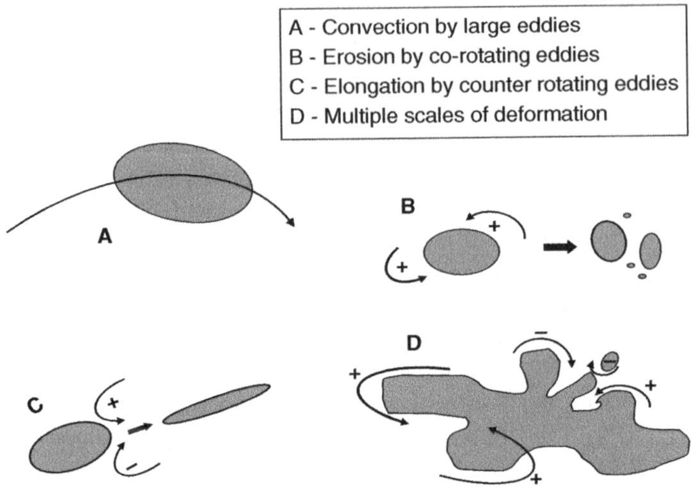

Figure 2.9 Drop break up by turbulent eddies (Reproduced with permission from Paul et al. 2004)

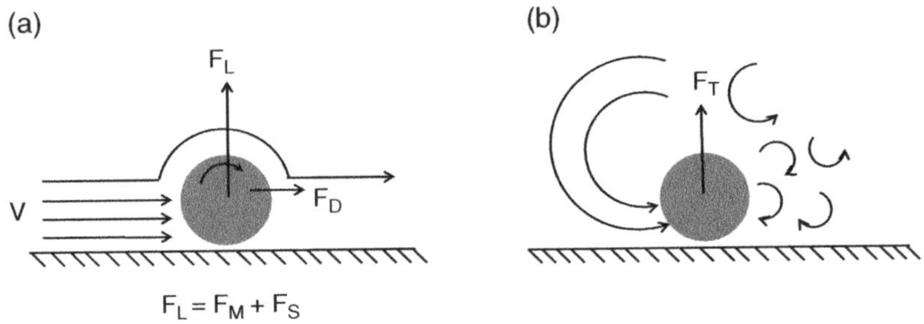

Figure 2.10 Particle suspension at the bottom of the tank due to (a) convection, which is a combination of drag and (in some cases) lift, and (b) turbulent eddies that are a similar size to the particle diameter, and which have enough energy to overcome the inertia of the particle (Reproduced with permission from Ayranci et al., 2012 Copyright (2012) Elsevier)

to fluid properties, which are considered more fully for various specialized applications in the *Handbook of Industrial Mixing* (Paul et al., 2004).

2.7 Specifying Mixing Requirements for a Process

We have now introduced the meaning of turbulence in a velocity field, and how turbulence might interact with a second phase. This fluid flow information is combined with the mixing requirements for a process:

1. the required intensity of segregation, or uniformity in concentration;
2. the scale of segregation (e.g., drop size, bubble size, particle size, or striation thickness);
3. the mixing time, or the rate at which mixing is accomplished at a particular scale in the vessel (blend time, meso-mixing, micro-mixing, Batchelor, and Kolmogorov time scales).

The intensity of segregation is usually most important at the macro-scale and is characterized by the blend time. The scale of segregation dominates for meso-scale mixing, most particularly of a second phase. The micro-mixing time is usually most critical for processes that are limited at the micro-scale, particularly mixing sensitive reactions or mass transfer. There is a large body of mixing literature that relates these mixing times to the dissipation, ε, and the average power dissipated per unit mass of fluid ($P/\rho V_{TANK}$).

2.8 Conclusions

Turbulence is a dynamic, three-dimensional, multi-scale phenomenon that contains a whole range of length scales, from L_I down to η. These scales are set by the geometry, at the large scales, and by the local dissipation, ε, and physical properties of the fluid, μ and ρ, at the smallest scales.

Mixing specifications consider homogenization of concentration, reduction of length scales, and critical rates in the process that are affected by slow mixing. Successful scale-down of processes, and successful design and operation at the large scale, both require a good understanding of turbulent flow and its impact on mixing.

Notation

Roman Characters

A	cross sectional area (m^2)
C	impeller off-bottom clearance (m)
d	scale of segregation of a dispersed phase (m)
D	impeller diameter (m)
D_{AB}	molecular diffusivity (m^2/s)
D_o	diameter of a jet at the origin (m)
D_p	pipe diameter (m)
F_D	drag force (N)
F_l	lift force (N)
F_T	force due to turbulent eddies (N)
H	liquid height (m)
l	length scale of a turbulent eddy (m)
L_I	integral length scale of turbulence (m)
N	impeller rotational speed (rps or rpm)
N_P	power number (dimensionless)
P	power (W)
Q	volumetric flow rate (m/s)
r	radial coordinate (m)
Re	Reynolds number (dimensionless)
S	impeller submergence, measured from the liquid surface (m)
Sc	Schmidt number (dimensionless)
t	blade thickness (m)

T	tank diameter (m)
U	instantaneous velocity (m/s)
$\overline{U}$	mean velocity (m/s)
u′	fluctuating velocity component (m/s)
V_o	superficial velocity of a jet at its origin (m/s)
V_s	superficial velocity in a pipe, Q/A (m/s)
V_{TANK}	tank volume (m^3)
V_{TIP}	tip speed of the impeller, πND, (m/s)
W	baffle width (m)
z	axial location in the tank, measured from the bottom (m)

Greek Characters

ε_{MAX}	the maximum local epsilon (W/kg)
ε	rate of dissipation of turbulent kinetic energy per unit mass (W/kg)
η	Kolmogorov length scale (m)
λ	turbulent length scale (m)
λ_B	Batchelor striation length scale (m)
λ_K	Kolmogorov length scale (m)
μ	kinematic viscosity (kg/ms)
ν	dynamic viscosity (m^2/s)
ρ	density (kg/m^3)
τ	time scale of a turbulent eddy (s)
τ_B	diffusion time scale of a Batchelor sized scalar striation (s)
τ_K	dissipation time scale of a Kolmogorov sized turbulent eddy (s)

References

Ayranci, I. and S.M Kresta, 2011, Design rules for suspending concentrated mixtures of solids in stirred tanks, *ChERD*, **89**, 1961–1971.

Ayranci, I., M.B. Machado, A.M. Madej, J.J. Derksen, D.S. Nobes, and S.M. Kresta, 2012, Effect of Geometry On The Mechanisms For Off-Bottom Solids Suspension In A Stirred Tank, *Chem. Eng. Sci.*, **79,** 163–176.

Batchelor, G.K., 1959, Small-scale variation of convected quantities like temperature in a turbulent fluid, *J. Fluid. Mech.*, **5**, 113–133.

Bhattacharya, S. and S.M. Kresta, 2006, Reactor performance with high velocity surface feed, *Chem. Eng. Sci.,* **61**, 3033–3043.

Bhattacharya, S. and S.M. Kresta, 2004, Surface feed with minimum by-product formation for competitive reactions, *Chem. Eng. Res. Des.*, **82**, 1153–1160.

Bhattacharya, S., D. Hebert and S.M. Kresta, 2007, Air entrainment in baffled stirred Tanks, *Chem. Eng. Res. Des.*, **85**, 654–664.

Bittorf, K.J. and S.M. Kresta, 2000, Active volume of mean circulation for stirred tanks agitated with axial impellers, *Chem. Eng. Sci.*, **55,** 1325–1336.

Bittorf, K.J. and S.M. Kresta, 2003, Prediction of cloud height for solid suspensions in stirred tanks, *Chem. Eng. Res. Des.*, **81**, 568–577.

Bourne, J.R., 2003, Mixing and the selectivity of chemical reactions, *Org Proc Res. Dev.*, **7**, 471–508.

Chapple, D., S.M. Kresta, A. Wall, and A. Afacan, 2002, The effect of impeller and tank geometry on power number for a pitched bladed turbine, *Chem. Eng. Res. Des.*, **80**, 364–372.

Khazam, O. and S.M. Kresta, 2008, Mechanisms of solids drawdown in stirred tanks, *Can. J. Chem. Eng.*, **86**(4), 622–634.

Kukukova, A., J. Aubin, and S.M. Kresta, 2009, A new definition of mixing and segregation: Three dimensions of a key process variable, *Chem. Eng. Res. Des.*, **87**, 633–647.

Machado, M., R. Nunhez, D. Nobes, and S.M. Kresta, 2012, Impeller characterization and selection: balancing efficient hydrodynamics with process mixing requirements, *AICHE Journal*, **58,** 2573–2588, doi: 10.1002/aic.12758.

Machado, M.B., K. Bittorf, V. Roussinova, and S.M. Kresta, 2013, Transition from turbulent to transitional flow in the top half of a stirred tank, *Chem. Eng. Sci.*, **98**, 218–230.

Motamedvaziri, S. and P. Armenante, 2012, Flow regimes and surface air entrainment in partially filled stirred vessels for different fill ratios, *Chem. Eng. Sci.*, **81**, 231–250.

Nouri, J.M., J.H. Whitelaw, and M. Yianneskis, 1987, The scaling of the flow field with impeller size and rotational speed in a stirred reactor, *2nd Intl Conf on Laser Anemometry, Advances and Applications*, Strathclyde, Scotland, Sept. 21–23.

Paul, E.L., V. Atiemo-Obeng, and S.M. Kresta (eds) 2004, *Handbook of Industrial Mixing*, John Wiley & Sons, Inc., Hoboken.

Rao, M.A. and R.S. Brodkey, 1972, Continuous flow stirred tank turbulence parameters in the impeller stream, *Chem. Eng. Sci.*, **27**, 137–156.

Villermaux, J. and L. Falk, 1994, A generalized mixing model for initial contacting of reactive fluids, *Chem. Eng. Sci.*, **49**, 5127–5140.

Zhou, G. and S.M. Kresta, 1996, Impact of geometry on the maximum turbulence energy dissipation rate for various impellers, *AIChE Journal*, **42**, 2476–2490.

3

Laminar Mixing Fundamentals

P.J. Cullen[1] *and N.N. Misra*[2]
[1] *School of Chemical Engineering, University of New South Wales, Australia*
[2] *School of Food Science & Environmental Health, Dublin Institute of Technology, Ireland*

3.1 Laminar Flows

Mixing of immiscible fluids involves two distinct simultaneous phenomena namely stirring and diffusion. The former process, stirring helps to increase the gradient in concentration, whereas the latter, diffusion, plays a role in decreasing this gradient in concentration at a molecular scale. The net result is an increase in the homogeneity of the system. Intuitively one can visualize the role of turbulence (Chapter 2) in mixing, conversely the orderly motion of fluid particles associated with laminar flow portrays an environment of little mixing. Indeed such steady flows are commonly found to have inferior mixing properties compared to their time-dependent counterparts (Grigoriev 2011). However, when one takes a more in-depth look, laminar mixing is found to play an important and effective role in fluid and particle mixing. The topic has been an active area of research over the past few decades with interest and developments in such areas as micro fluidics to powder blending.

The dimensionless Reynold's number is the criteria for deciding if a flow is laminar or turbulent and represents the ratio of inertial to viscous forces acting on the system. If v and l denote the characteristic velocity and length scales, and μ is the kinematic viscosity, R_e is defined as:

Pharmaceutical Blending and Mixing, First Edition. Edited by P.J. Cullen, Rodolfo J. Romañach, Nicolas Abatzoglou and Chris D. Rielly.

$$R_e = \frac{vl}{\mu} \tag{3.1}$$

The characteristic length l of the system by itself means that R_e is dependent on the geometry of the system. Laminar flows displaying an orderly flow regime are characterized by the absence of eddies, which are recognized to result in lateral mixing. It may be noted that such systems are often characterized by non-Newtonian flow behaviour.

Laminar flows are inherently characterized by a high degree of symmetry, imposed by the confining effects of either surface tension in free-surface flows or channel walls. Such symmetry leads to the existence of flow invariants (Haller and Mezic 1998) and ultimately poor mixing. The level sets of one invariant define surfaces on which the three-dimensional flow is effectively two-dimensional (Vainchtein 2011). Addition of a further invariant again reduces the flow dimensionality, i.e. a flow with two invariants is effectively one-dimensional. As flow cannot cross the invariant surface, the existence of invariants is highly undesirable in the mixing problem as their presence inhibits complete stirring of the full fluid volume by advection (Vainchtein 2011). Chaos theory states that at least three degrees of freedom is required for a dynamic system to be chaotic. Consequently, even chaotic advection may not be sufficient for good mixing, as time-dependent flows can have chaotic streamlines restricted to two-dimensional surfaces in the presence of an invariant (Vainchtein et al. 2008). Therefore, the key to achieving effective chaotic mixing in any laminar flow is to ensure that all flow invariants are destroyed (Vainchtein 2011).

3.2 Mixing in Laminar Flows

Mixing under laminar conditions may be challenging in that fluid entities tend to flow in layers and require more work to overcome the dominant viscous forces. Often practitioners consider mixing in low Reynolds number regime to be 'the worst' mixing problems (Alvarez et al. 2002). Under low speed conditions, for viscous materials, the contribution of molecular diffusion to achieving homogeneity also becomes negligible. Molecular diffusion can aid mixing in capillary tubes, but such effects are rarely of significance in scaled-up industrial-scale mixing. Therefore, under ordinary conditions, mixing in laminar flow will lead to spatial inhomogeneity. Practically, the complete laminar mixing of components or phases can only occur over very large length scales and time scales if left at the discretion of ordinary conditions, in a simple channel. However, it was established that mixing in laminar extensional flows may prove to be more effective than turbulent mixing (Erwin 1978a, b). Fortunately, there are approaches to achieve efficient mixing even with the constraints in Reynold's number. These include the introduction of 'chaos' in the fluid system, promoting diffusion resulting from shear, and the use of secondary flows. However, Szalai et al. (2004) aptly mention that at this point of time laminar mixing is an art, as the current state of understanding of the process needs a great deal of advancement. We proceed from here by reviewing the basics of dynamical chaotic systems and the contributions of the same towards laminar fluid mixing.

3.2.1 Chaos and Laminar Chaotic Mixing

Chaos in the context of laminar mixing is discussed later in this chapter. To begin it is important to identify that most chaotic mixers rely on the repetitive stretching and folding of fluid elements (see Figure 3.1). The stretching and folding increases the inter-material area leading to homogeneity. Conceptually, this can also be referred to as the 'split and recombine' scenario. An analogy of this description can be drawn from the stretching and folding of dough carried out by a baker, hence the concept is also referred to as 'Bakers Transformation.' To mix a flow, the non-diffusive stirring of the interface needs to be completed by diffusion. Naturally as the inter-material area increases, the molecular diffusion becomes prominent. This type of stretching and folding is realized by means of geometric elements of mixers, which cause periodic twisting and swirling, both in time and space. Based on the above, it is easy to visualize the formal definition of lamination as the ensemble of mechanisms generating striations within flows (Rossi et al. 2012).

An important class of mixers where periodic stretching and mixing can be practically visualized are the static (motionless) mixers, such as the Kenics mixer and its modified versions, as shown in Figure 3.2(A). The basic principle underlying its operation is the introduction of inserts inside the tube to cut, fold, twist and re-combine fluid elements (Saatdjian et al. 2012). It is evident from the figure that this leads to a good mixing with the dark and light coloured fluids turning homogeneous at the exit of the mixer, after only six passes. As the fluid passes through the mixer, the fluid elements move across the streamlines due to the twisting and swirling motions and also the addition of cross-stream flows. The design of the blades in a static mixer however, can vary depending on specific applications. For example, a helical design is more suited for high viscosity blending

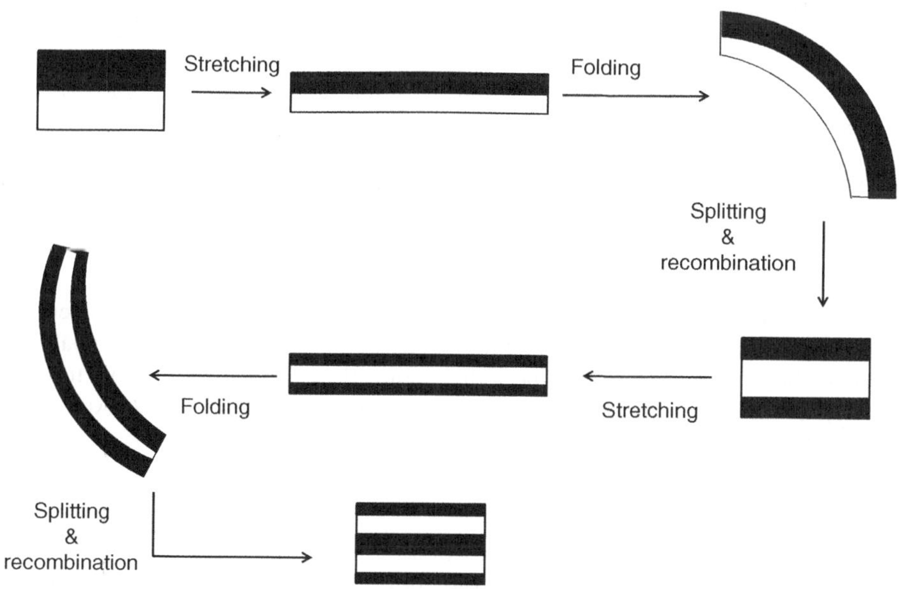

Figure 3.1 Stretching and folding of fluid elements leads to good mixing and therefore homogeneity

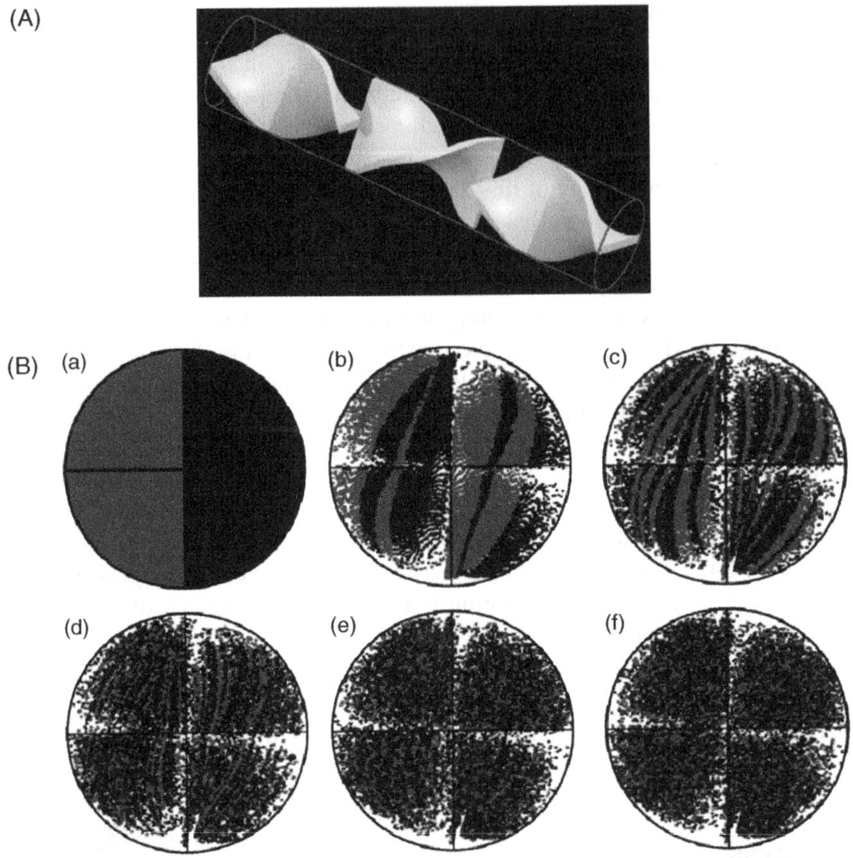

Figure 3.2 (A) The helical twisted tape inserts of a modified Kenics static mixer, where the internal elements are obtained by deforming the plates. (B) Mixing of red and blue fluid of passive particles, each one occupying half of the inlet cross section of the mixer. The particle distributions are plotted at (a) the inlet cross section and after (b) 2, (c) 4, (d) 6, (e) 8 and (f) 10 mixing elements. Adapted from Saatdjian et al. (2012), Copyright (2012) Elsevier

and/or folding applications. Laminar mixing and striations also occur in stirred tanks operating in low Reynolds number conditions (Alvarez et al. 2002). The principal notion however, is that the introduction of periodicity in a flow can cause the flow to behave chaotically, resulting in good mixing (Ottino 1989; Ottino et al. 1992; Aref and El Naschie 1995).

3.2.1.1 The Lyapunov Exponent

The theory of chaos in laminar mixing was first introduced by Aref (1984). For chaotic flows fluid elements are stretched in one direction while simultaneously compressed in another exponentially fast. In order to appreciate chaos in laminar mixing, let us track the trajectories of two (hypothetical) neighbouring passive particles (of course in a Lagrangian

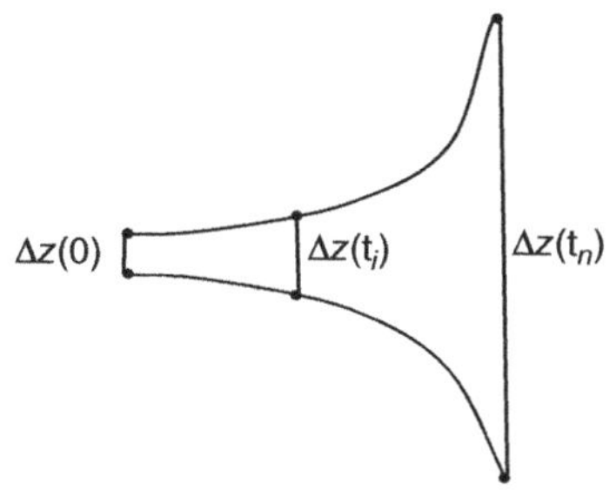

Figure 3.3 *The two Lagrangian particles of a fluid initially in close proximity move apart exponentially during the flow. The ratio of the separation of the trajectories at infinitesimally large time respective to initial separation is the Lyapunov exponent*

sense) in a chaotic laminar flow. The passive particles are considered as fluid particles or particles of a second tracer fluid; they neither perturb the flow nor diffuse themselves. When doing so, one observes an exponential divergence of the trajectories of the particles with time. If the initial distance between the two particles at time $t = 0$ is given by $\Delta z(t_0)$, and the distance at any time $t = n$ to be $\Delta z(t_n)$, then the stretching of the fluid element, λ is given by-

$$\lambda = \frac{\Delta z(t_n)}{\Delta z(t_0)} = e^{\Lambda t_n} \tag{3.2}$$

and the ratio of the separations at infinity with respect to the initial separation can be represented as-

$$\Lambda = \lim_{\substack{n\to\infty \\ |\Delta z(t_0)|\to 0}} \frac{1}{t_n} \log_e \frac{|\Delta z(t_n)|}{|\Delta z(t_0)|} \tag{3.3}$$

where, λ is defined as the maximum Lyapunov exponent. A pictorial presentation for this is shown in Figure 3.3. Mathematically, this quantity is the asymptotic limit of the stretching within the defined constraints.

The Lyapunov exponent can be taken as a measure of the degree of chaos in a flow, and it may be noted that a chaotic system must have at least a single positive Lyapunov exponent greater than 1. A direct physical consequence of the exponential divergence is the assurance (at least theoretically) that the Lagrangian particles will cover almost the entire chaotic mixing domain within the asymptotic time limit. If we are unsure of the spatial identity of the particles even by a certain degree (which is always the case), then this error will also propagate exponentially, which implies an unpredictability of the system (Soulvaiotis et al. 1995). At this point of the discussion, it is worthwhile mentioning that the hallmark feature of a chaotic system is its sensitivity to the initial condition, which per se justifies the term 'chaotic mixing.'

3.2.1.2 Poincaŕe Maps

Taking the discussion of the baker's process a step forward, the stretching and folding of the fluid elements in a chaotic system occurs under the influence of periodic points; these Lagrangian points return to their initial location after exactly n periods ($n \in I^+$). This allows the study of chaos in a dynamical system by yet another approach- the Poincaŕe map. This approach involves defining and introducing a plane (section) perpendicular to the direction of flow. When tracer particles are introduced into the flow and a few tagged particles are continuously tracked, these will cross the chosen plane at regular intervals depending on their period. In general, the nth order periodic points can be either of an elliptic, hyperbolic or parabolic nature. The superimposed distribution of the points of intersection of particles on this perpendicular plane after several periods is referred to as a Poincaŕe map (see Figure 3.4). The key advantage of the approach stems from the dimensionality reduction, that is, the initial system dimension reduces by one, without loss of vital information about the dynamics.

Note that if there are empty regions in the Poincaŕe maps, these indicate regular flow regions and that these are regions of poor mixing (see Figure 3.5). These closed curves are referred to as invariant or KAM (Kolmogorov–Arnold–Moser) surfaces and basically arise from the Hamiltonian nature of 3D laminar flows with sufficient degrees of freedom (Aref and El Naschie 1995; Ottino 1989; Harvey et al. 2000). Such regions (also called islands) are to be avoided as fluid particles are unable to cross their boundaries, except by diffusion and mixing inside the region is not efficient as the trajectories are closed and therefore not chaotic. The whole idea of good mixing is to avoid such isolated mixing regions by varying process parameters or changing mixer design.

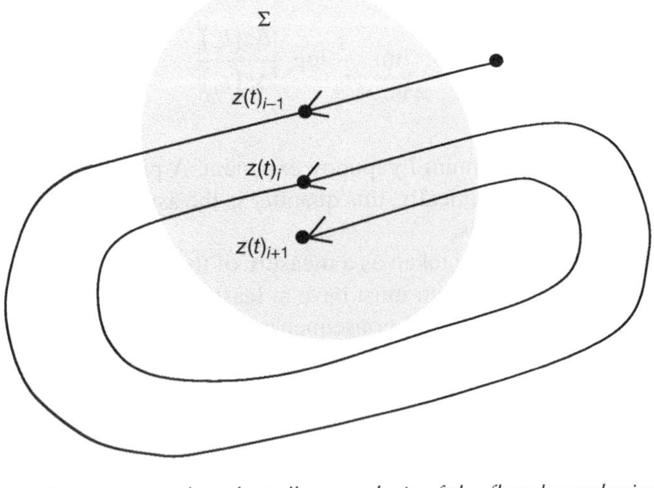

Figure 3.4 Poincaŕe maps are plots that allow analysis of the flow by reducing the number of dimensions. The intersection of points with the plane placed perpendicular to the path of flow gives the Poincaŕe map over several time periods

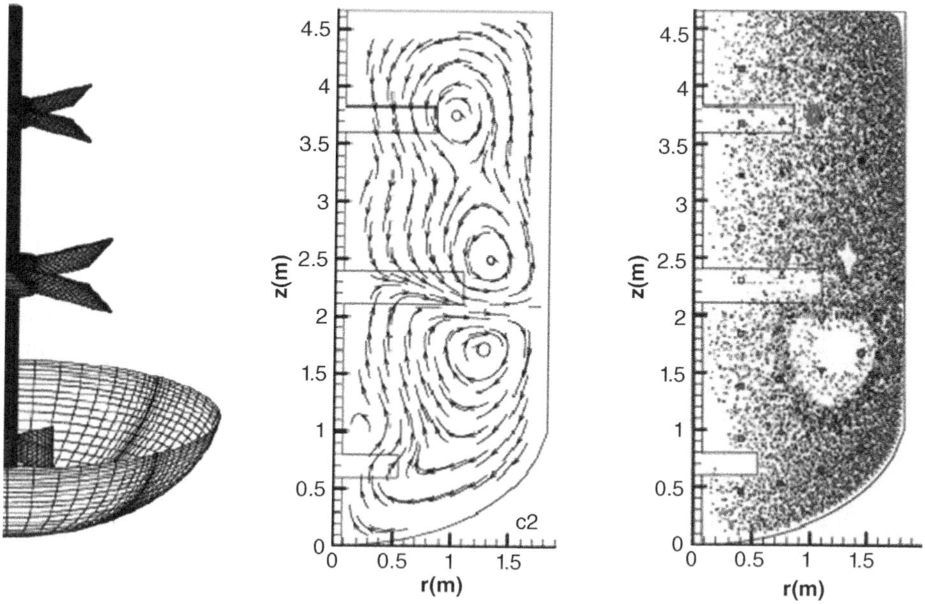

Figure 3.5 *The geometry with surface mesh, cross-flow streamlines and Poincafe map for a stirred tank reactor with three impellers. Two KAR tori can be observed- one blow the second impeller and another small one just above it. Adapted from Harvey et al. (2000) Copyright (2000) Elsevier*

3.2.1.3 Other Recent Approaches to Chaos

The stretching and folding of fluids has also been explained from a topological point of view by Boyland et al. (2000). The method relies on Thurston–Nielsen classification theorem and is a potential tool for predicting and analysing the existence and amount of chaos in stirring systems. One advantage of this method arises from the fact that it depends only on the topology of motion of boundaries and does not depend on any detailed fluid flow calculations.

Recently, Rossi and Lardeau (2011) proposed a new measure to explore lamination within flows. The authors defined the local measure of lamination, M_{lam} as the ratio of the total length of a material line within a circle centred on the material line to a circle's diameter $\varphi = \iint_{disc} \mathrm{d}l$, following which the typical local striation thickness (d) can be estimated as:

$$d = \frac{\varphi}{\left(1 + M_{lam}\right)} \tag{3.4}$$

In 3D, φ would turn out to be the diameter of an equivalent sphere. The position of the sphere will give the spatial location of the measure and the diameter of the sphere will correspond to the length-scale under consideration. The material lines correspond to small vectors attached to the particles.

3.2.2 Granular Chaotic Mixing

Granular mixing is an important unit operation in the manufacture of pharmaceutical solid dosage forms, often coupled with wetting and agglomeration. Particulate materials constitute a large group of solids that can range in size from submicron particles to large solids (e.g. study of rocks in minerals processing and mining engineering). With regards to pharmaceutical processes, we are mostly confined with granular materials with diameter below 4 mm. Rotating cylinders, partially filled with granular material are widely used for mixing, reaction, coating, and drying processes in the pharmaceutical industries (Prasad and Khakhar 2010; Perry and Green 2007). Although we discussed the concept of chaotic mixing in the context of fluid flows, these theories also extend to the mixing of granular solid materials. The underpinning idea remains the same- introduction of time-periodicity in the flow. Chaotic mixing can occur spontaneously as a result of unsteady flows in shearing layers of fine grains (Nasuno et al. 1997). The challenge however, is the lack of a proper theory for segregation in granular flows and its relationship with mixing, and is a topic of active research. The analogous of laminar fluid flow for non-cohesive granular materials is the flow of granules in rolling regime.

Unlike flow of fluids, the flow of granular materials (particles, powders or grains) has remained under researched primarily due to the complexity of such flows. Granular flows can behave like solids, liquids or gases, examples for which include a pile of sand, flow from a silo and a case of strong agitation respectively (Jop et al. 2006; Jaeger et al. 1996). This type of flow can also be visualized as a two-phase flow comprising of particulates and an interstitial fluid. When the particles are acted upon by a shearing force, they may either flow like a fluid, or behave as a solid by offering resistance to shear. Therefore, the dual nature of the flows makes them very difficult to analyse. Our primary interest in the following section lies in discussing the fluid (liquid) like behaviour. To proceed further, it is important to establish a means for classifying particulate or granular material based on their ease of flow. This is classically studied using Mohr's circle, a concept first developed in the field of soil mechanics and civil engineering.

3.2.2.1 Flow Behaviour of Granular Materials

In order to be able to predict the flow behaviour of dense granular materials, it is desirable to have a model which considers all the complexity at inter-granular scale, yet is applicable at large scales. Drawing analogies from Eulerian–Langrangian treatments of fluids, continuum approaches for studying granular flows have also developed. The continuum approach to granular material flow revolves around the fact that particles can withstand shear stresses to a certain degree before yielding and deforming. The resistance to flow emerges from the frictional forces and steric constraints. This is analogous to the plastic rheological models for non-newtonian fluids. The plot of the shear stress, τ (tangential component of force) versus the compression stress, σ (normal component) is referred to as the 'Yield Locus', Note that stress refers to force per unit 'area of contact.' The stress tensor concept following continuum approach is summarized in Figure 3.6.

Mohr diagrams are a visual way of presenting the relationship between the stresses on a granular element and its flow properties, thus aiding in establishment of a formal quantitative approach to characterize the material. In a Mohr diagram, the normal stresses are plotted

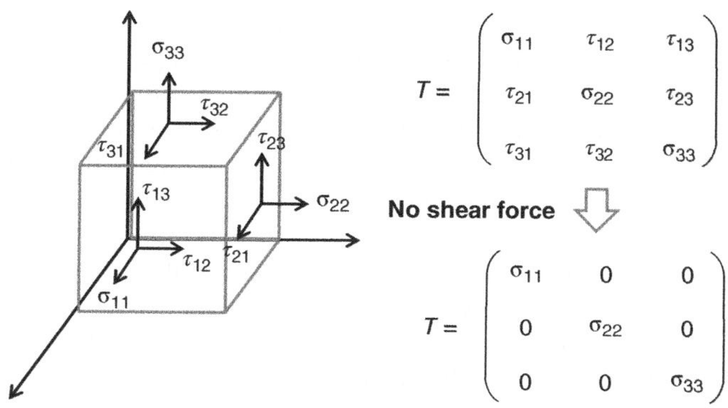

Figure 3.6 *The stress tensor notation for a cubic element of the material and the corresponding matrix. When the three perpendicular principal planes only are considered, meaning no shear stress acts, the matrix is simplified and can be represented as a tetrahedron with three principal planes*

along the abscissa axis of the coordinate system, while the shear stresses along the ordinate axis. Analysis of Mohr's circle yields the flow functions, which is used for classifying the flow behaviour of granular materials. A flow function value between: 1–2 is considered to give poor flowability (cohesive material), 2–4, moderate flowability, 4–10, good flowability, and >10, excellent flowability (free flowing). In summary, a granular material with a higher value of flow function indicates better flowability (Jenike 1964).

3.2.2.2 Analysis of Granular Mixing

From these classifications of the flow behaviour of granular materials, our interest shifts toward understanding the mixing mechanism during flow of the granular materials at low speeds. One can generalize the mechanism of mixing to be an assemblage of (1) convective movement of relatively large portions of the solid granules, (2) shear failure, which reduces the scale of segregation (i.e. the tendency to separate, discussed in Chapter 5), and (3) diffusive movement of individual particles (micromixing).

Rotating Cylinder: Circular Geometry. To help visualize the dynamics of granular materials, an example of rotary mixers operating in a laminar flow regime (i.e. low rotational speeds) is introduced. The operational speed criteria of such rotating mixers is often expressed using the dimensionless Froude number (F_r), given by:

$$F_r = \frac{\omega^2 R}{g} \tag{3.5}$$

where, R is the radius of the cylinder (more precisely, the length scale of the system) and ω is the rotational speed of the cylinder along the axis. The rotating cylinder is often maintained either horizontally or at small inclinations. At low rotational speeds (low F_r) the granules slip on the cylinder surface or flow as a series of discrete time-periodic avalanches, sometimes also referred to as slumping (Hajra and Khakhar 2005). When operated at higher speed, the mixing occurs in rolling, cascading, cataracting and/or centrifuging regimes. It is well-recognized that mixing and segregation in the rotating cylinder are predominantly confined to the superficial inclined layer of the granular bed, where the particles move, individually or collectively, from one site of the drum downhill to the opposite (Arntz et al. 2008). For the sake of simplicity, the mixing of the granules in the cylinder can be studied as the sum of mixing along the axis of the cylinder (axial mixing) and that along a cross-section of the cylinder (cross-sectional mixing). The axial mixing occurs due to the particle diffusion, while the cross-sectional due to convective mixing, in addition to diffusion. It should be noted that the diffusivity of the granules is not a material property, but rather influenced by the flow conditions and has been shown to be anisotropic (Campbell 1997). The relative contribution of the two modes of mixing is dictated by the degree of filling for the cylinder. In order to determine the self-diffusivity component (of tracer particles) in the mixing layer of a rotating cylinder, the following continuum model in two dimensional space co-ordinates has been proposed (Hajra and Khakhar 2005; Khakhar et al. 1997):

$$\frac{\partial f}{\partial t} + v_x \frac{\partial f}{\partial x} + v_y \frac{\partial f}{\partial y} = D \frac{\partial^2 f}{\partial y^2} \tag{3.6}$$

where, f is the number fraction of the tracer particles, (v_x, v_y)is the velocity field in the layer, and D is diffusivity. The authors have emphasized on the point that although the magnitude of the self-diffusivity in the flow direction is greater than that perpendicular to the flow direction, diffusion in the flow direction has little effect on mixing as transport in this direction is dominated by convection. Based on simulation studies and experiments, the authors have concluded that the mixing per pass increases with increasing particle size and decreases with rotational speed. As in the case of fluids, it should be noted here that the dependency of the diffusivity on the flow conditions is a source of chaos in the mixing process.

Non-Circular Geometry. In the former case of a rotating cylinder with circular cross-sectional geometry, if the flow in the cylinder is time-independent (steady flow), this causes the streamlines to become time invariant and the resulting structure of the steady flow is Hamiltonian with one degree of freedom. This implies that the system cannot be chaotic (Ottino 1990). However, if the cross-section is non-circular (e.g. a square, triangle or ellipse), then the superficial flowing layer would temporally shrink and grow. The frequency of these dynamics will be at least twice that of the mixer rotation. The geometric component of mixing can be appreciated from the fact that particles at different locations within a mixer will have different residence times, consequently entering the striated layers at different times. By corollary, a non-circular geometry results in introduction of time-periodicity in flows, implying the possibility of chaos in the flow. Following the same arguments as for chaotic liquid flows earlier, the non-circular geometry would therefore result in improved granular mixing. The validity of this hypothesis has been demonstrated by Khakhar et al. (1999) and Cisar et al. (2006) through experiments and simulations. Figure 3.7 presents the deformation of an initially uniformly distributed circular blob

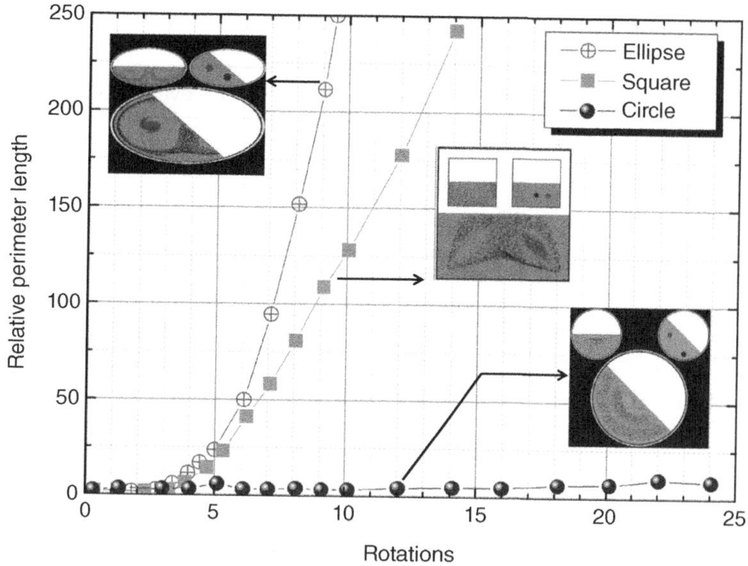

Figure 3.7 Variation of the relative perimeter length of a blob with time in the mixers obtained by computational analysis. Data adapted from Khakhar et al. (1999) Copyright (1999) AIP Publishing LLC

versus the number of rotations obtained through simulations, for different geometries of the mixer. It may be observed that the perimeter length in the circular mixer grows linearly, whereas the length in the non-circular mixers grows exponentially. Furthermore, the filaments formed from the blob repeatedly fold upon themselves in elliptic and square geometries. This type of exponential stretching and presence of a homoclinic structure being a hallmark of chaotic mixing supports the fact that a non-circular geometry is more efficient.

3.3 Recent Advances

The development of mathematical models to simulate and investigate the flow of granular materials is a topic of significant relevance to pharmaceutical process engineering. In order to develop a rigorous continuum mathematical formulation of the granular mixing, accurate estimates of the dynamic properties such as particle positions, stress, strain and void volume are highly desirable (McCarthy et al. 1996) and some successful progress in this area has been made using advanced material characterization techniques such as positron emission tomography (PET), X-ray tomography and nuclear magnetic resonance (NMR) imaging. Table 3.1 lists some studies employing these methods for granular flows along with their advantages. Techniques such as positron emission particle tracking (PEPT) and particle imaging velocimetry (PIV) give a direct visualization of the flow patterns within the bulk of powder and at the boundaries (typically the free surface), respectively.

Table 3.1 Advanced approaches to track particles and visualize mixing and segregation of granular material

Approach	Salient Feature	Relevant Studies
Magnetic Resonance Imaging	Entire powder bed can be imaged non-intrusively by doping with a MRI sensitive solution	Sommier et al. (2001), Hill et al. (1997b), Nakagawa et al. (1993), Hill et al. (1997a)
X-ray (micro) tomography	Complete spatial information can be obtained; non-intrusive method	Baxter et al. (1989), Chester et al. (1999), Fukushima (1999), Liu et al. (2013)
Positron Emission Tomography (PET) and Positron Emission Particle Tracking (PEPT)	Ability to trace within fairly thick particulate system for extended periods of time; non-intrusive method	Parker et al. (1997), Broadbent et al. (1993), Parker et al. (2002), Hiseman et al. (2002)
Particle Imaging Velocimetry (PIV)	Ability to produce 2- or 3-D velocity field simultaneously; non-intrusive method	Lueptow et al. (2000), Jain et al. (2002)

Despite these developments, the fact that stress in granular materials is principally carried in 'stress chains' (Liu et al. 1995) by itself poses a question mark over the general applicability of continuum approach treatment of granular materials. Such an approach of course overlooks the local behaviour of individual particles. Consequently, systems consisting of a small number of particles cannot be modelled with this approach (Bertrand et al. 2005). In light of this, particle based discrete element models (DEM) have gained much attention in recent years. These models although elegant in their mathematical foundation and versatile in the sense that they can be coupled to classical fluid dynamics using finite element, finite volume or Lattice–Boltzmann methods, are computationally expensive. Chapter 17 of this book provides a comprehensive discussion of the discrete element models and simulations of particle mixing using these models.

References

Alvarez MM, Zalc JM, Shinbrot T, Arratia PE, Muzzio FJ (2002) Mechanisms of mixing and creation of structure in laminar stirred tanks. *AIChE Journal* 48 (10):2135–2148. doi:10.1002/aic.690481005

Aref H (1984) Stirring by chaotic advection. *Journal of Fluid Mechanics* 143:1–21. doi:10.1017/S0022112084001233

Aref H, El Naschie M (1995) *Chaos Applied to Fluid Mixing*. Pergamon, Oxford

Arntz MMHD, den Otter WK, Briels WJ, Bussmann PJT, Beeftink HH, Boom RM (2008) Granular mixing and segregation in a horizontal rotating drum: A simulation study on the impact of rotational speed and fill level. *AIChE Journal* 54 (12):3133–3146. doi:10.1002/aic.11622

Baxter G, Behringer R, Fagert T, Johnson G (1989) Pattern formation in flowing sand. *Physical Review Letters* 62 (24):2825–2828. doi:10.1103/PhysRevLett.62.2825

Bertrand F, Leclaire LA, Levecque G (2005) DEM-based models for the mixing of granular materials. *Chemical Engineering Science* 60 (8–9):2517–2531. doi:10.1016/j.ces.2004.11.048

Boyland PL, Aref H, Stremler MA (2000) Topological fluid mechanics of stirring. *Journal of Fluid Mechanics* 403:277–304. doi:10.1017/s0022112099007107

Broadbent CJ, Bridgwater J, Parker DJ, Keningley ST, Knight P (1993) A phenomenological study of a batch mixer using a positron camera. *Powder Technology* 76 (3):317–329. doi:10.1016/S0032–5910(05)80013–0

Campbell CS (1997) Self-diffusion in granular shear flows. *Journal of Fluid Mechanics* 348:85–101. doi:10.1017/s0022112097006496

Chester AW, Kowalski JA, Coles ME, Muegge EL, Muzzio FJ, Brone D (1999) Mixing dynamics in catalyst impregnation in double-cone blenders. *Powder Technology* 102 (1):85–94. doi:10.1016/S0032–5910(98)00193–4

Cisar S, Umbanhowar P, Ottino J (2006) Radial granular segregation under chaotic flow in two-dimensional tumblers. *Physical Review E* 74 (5). doi:10.1103/PhysRevE.74.051305

Erwin L (1978a) Theory of mixing sections in single screw extruders. *Polymer Engineering & Science* 18 (7):572–576. doi:10.1002/pen.760180705

Erwin L (1978b) An upper bound on the performance of plane strain mixers. *Polymer Engineering & Science* 18 (9):738–740. doi:10.1002/pen.760180910

Fukushima E (1999) Nuclear magnetic resonance as a tool to study flow. *Annual Review of Fluid Mechanics* 31 (1):95–123. doi:10.1146/annurev.fluid.31.1.95

Hajra SK, Khakhar DV (2005) Radial mixing of granular materials in a rotating cylinder: Experimental determination of particle self-diffusivity. *Physics of Fluids* 17 (1):013101. doi:10.1063/1.1825331

Haller G, Mezic I (1998) Reduction of three-dimensional, volume-preserving flows with symmetry. *Nonlinearity* 11:319–339

Harvey AD, West DH, Tufillaro NB (2000) Evaluation of laminar mixing in stirred tanks using a discrete-time particle-mapping procedure. *Chemical Engineering Science* 55 (3):667–684. doi:10.1016/s0009–2509(99)00309–7

Hill KM, Caprihan A, Kakalios J (1997a) Axial segregation of granular media rotated in a drum mixer: Pattern evolution. *Physical Review E* 56 (4):4386–4393

Hill KM, Caprihan A, Kakalios J (1997b) Bulk segregation in rotated granular material measured by magnetic resonance imaging. *Physical Review Letters* 78 (1):50–53

Hiseman MJP, Laurent BFC, Bridgwater J, Wilson DI, Parker DJ, North N, Merrifield DR (2002) Granular flow in a planetary mixer. *Chemical Engineering Research and Design* 80 (5):432–440. doi:10.1205/026387602320224012

Jaeger HM, Nagel SR, Behringer RP (1996) Granular solids, liquids, and gases. *Reviews of Modern Physics* 68 (4):1259–1273

Jain N, Ottino JM, Lueptow RM (2002) An experimental study of the flowing granular layer in a rotating tumbler. *Physics of Fluids* 14 (2):572. doi:10.1063/1.1431244

Jenike AW (1964) Storage and flow of solids, vol 53. Bulletin no. 123, vol 26. *Bulletin of the University of Utah*, Utah

Jop P, Forterre Y, Pouliquen O (2006) A constitutive law for dense granular flows. *Nature* 441 (7094):727–730. doi:10.1038/nature04801

Khakhar DV, McCarthy JJ, Gilchrist JF, Ottino JM (1999) Chaotic mixing of granular materials in two-dimensional tumbling mixers. *Chaos* 9 (1):195–205. doi:10.1063/1.166390

Khakhar DV, McCarthy JJ, Shinbrot T, Ottino JM (1997) Transverse flow and mixing of granular materials in a rotating cylinder. *Physics of Fluids* 9 (1):31. doi:10.1063/1.869172

Liu CH, Nagel SR, Schecter DA, Coppersmith SN, Majumdar S, Narayan O, Witten TA (1995) Force fluctuations in bead packs. *Science* 269 (5223):513–515. doi:10.1126/science.269.5223.513

Liu R, Yin X, Li H, Shao Q, York P, He Y, Xiao T, Zhang J (2013) Visualization and quantitative profiling of mixing and segregation of granules using synchrotron radiation X-ray microtomography and three dimensional reconstruction. *International Journal of Pharmaceutics* 445 (1–2):125–133. doi:10.1016/j.ijpharm.2013.02.010

Lueptow RM, Akonur A, Shinbrot T (2000) PIV for granular flows. *Experiments in Fluids* 28 (2):183–186. doi:10.1007/s003480050023

McCarthy JJ, Shinbrot T, Metcalfe G, Wolf JE, Ottino JM (1996) Mixing of granular materials in slowly rotated containers. *AIChE Journal* 42 (12):3351–3363. doi:10.1002/aic.690421207

Nakagawa M, Altobelli SA, Caprihan A, Fukushima E, Jeong EK (1993) Non-invasive measurements of granular flows by magnetic resonance imaging. *Experiments in Fluids* 16 (1):54–60. doi:10.1007/BF00188507

Nasuno S, Kudrolli A, Gollub JP (1997) Friction in Granular Layers: Hysteresis and Precursors. *Physical Review Letters* 79 (5):949–952

Ottino J, Muzzio F, Tjahjadi M, Franjione J, Jana SC, Kusch H (1992) Chaos, symmetry, and self-similarity: Exploiting order and disorder in mixing processes. *Science* 257 (5071):754–760

Ottino JM (1989) *The Kinematics of Mixing: Stretching, Chaos, and Transport, Vol 3.* Cambridge University Press

Ottino JM (1990) Mixing, chaotic advection, and turbulence. *Annual Review of Fluid Mechanics* 22 (1):207–254. doi:10.1146/annurev.fl.22.010190.001231

Parker DJ, Dijkstra AE, Martin TW, Seville JPK (1997) Positron emission particle tracking studies of spherical particle motion in rotating drums. *Chemical Engineering Science* 52 (13):2011–2022. doi:10.1016/S0009–2509(97)00030–4

Parker DJ, Forster RN, Fowles P, Takhar PS (2002) Positron emission particle tracking using the new Birmingham positron camera. *Nuclear Instruments and Methods in Physics Research Section A: Accelerators, Spectrometers, Detectors and Associated Equipment* 477 (1–3):540–545. doi:10.1016/S0168–9002(01)01919–2

Perry RH, Green DW (2007) *Perry's Chemical Engineers' Handbook.* 8th edn. McGraw-Hill, New York

Prasad DVN, Khakhar DV (2010) Mixing of granular material in rotating cylinders with noncircular cross-sections. *Physics of Fluids* 22 (10):103302. doi:10.1063/1.3481779

Rossi L, Doorly D, Kustrin D (2012) Lamination and mixing in laminar flows driven by Lorentz body forces. *EPL (Europhysics Letters)* 97 (1):14006

Rossi L, Lardeau S (2011) Lamination and folding in electromagnetically driven flows of specified geometries. *Journal of Turbulence* :N6. doi:10.1080/14685248.2010.534796

Saatdjian E, Rodrigo AJS, Mota JPB (2012) On chaotic advection in a static mixer. *Chemical Engineering Journal* 187:289–298. doi:10.1016/j.cej.2012.01.122

Sommier N, Porion P, Evesque P, Leclerc B, Tchoreloff P, Couarraze G (2001) Magnetic resonance imaging investigation of the mixing-segregation process in a pharmaceutical blender. *International Journal of Pharmaceutics* 222 (2):243–258. doi:10.1016/s0378–5173(01)00718–9

Soulvaiotis A, Jana SC, Ottino JM (1995) Potentialities and limitations of mixing simulations. *AIChE Journal* 41 (7):1605–1621. doi:10.1002/aic.690410702

Szalai ES, Alvarez MM, Muzzio FJ (2004) Laminar Mixing: A Dynamical Systems Approach. In: Paul EL, Atiemo-Obeng V, Kresta SM (eds) *Handbook of Industrial Mixing: Science and Practice.* John Wiley & Sons, Inc., Hoboken, pp 89–144

Vainchtein D (2011) Resonances and mixing in near-integrable volume-preserving systems. In: Grigoriev RO (ed.) *Transport and Mixing in Laminar Flows: From Microfluidics to Oceanic Currents.* Wiley-VCH Verlag GmbH & Co. KGaA, Weinheim, Germany. doi:10.1002/9783527639748.ch1

4

Sampling and Determination of Adequacy of Mixing

Rodolfo J. Romañach
Department of Chemistry, University of Puerto Rico, Puerto Rico

4.1 Introduction, Process Understanding, and Regulations

Adequacy of mixing is a requirement of the Current Good Manufacturing Practices (CGMPs). The CGMPs indicate in 211.110 (a) that

> To assure batch uniformity and integrity of drug products, written procedures shall be established and followed that describe the in-process controls, and tests, or examinations to be conducted on appropriate samples of in-process materials of each batch. Such control procedures shall be established to monitor the output and to validate the performance of those manufacturing processes that may be responsible for causing variability in the characteristics of in-process material and the drug product.

These control procedures include the "Adequacy of mixing to assure uniformity and homogeneity."

Adequacy of mixing is more than a regulatory requirement; as it is a necessary goal to provide the desired dose to the patient. To obtain the desired dose, drug concentration and the mass of the unit dose must be controlled. The adequacy of mixing is usually evaluated only in terms of the variation in the drug content. However, blends are an intermediate step and the drug product should be prepared with ease of manufacturability and will also

Pharmaceutical Blending and Mixing, First Edition. Edited by P.J. Cullen, Rodolfo J. Romañach, Nicolas Abatzoglou and Chris D. Rielly.

require adequate dissolution and ultimately bioavailability with a suitable product appearance to inspire customer confidence. Thus, a product that shows adequacy of mixing, but provides poor dissolution results and shows significant problems during tablet compression cannot be considered a validated product. Adequacy of mixing is one of the goals required for a new formulation, and is an important requirement for formulation development efforts.

The assessment of adequacy of mixing requires sampling of blends. Thus, the formulator needs to develop an adequate sampling method at the same time that the blending process is developed. The formulator cannot take the sampling process for granted and assume that sampling problems will not occur. For example, Hwang and collaborators illustrated a systematic approach for optimizing blending and lubrication that also evaluated the sampling methods and tablet compression [1]. This systematic approach involved the use of lab scale blenders of 4 and 16 quarts, and production scale blenders of 2 and 10 ft^3. The systematic approach provided a blending profile where the %RSD of the drug content was plotted versus time to choose an optimum blending time. The use of blending profiles as shown in Figure 4.1 is common in the validation of blending processes in many pharmaceutical companies.

The CGMPs state the regulations, but do not discuss how the requirements of 211.110 (a) can be met. Two guidance documents, one in 1999 and another in 2003 have been developed to avoid inconsistencies in the way that companies evaluate blend uniformity data and their subsequent evaluation by FDA review chemists [2,3]. However, the evaluation of the blend should not be a mere checklist exercise to determine whether the requirements of the guidance are met. The process must be visualized from a holistic point of view, with key questions asked. For example, as indicated on page 23 of *Mixing in the Process Industries*: "When is a mixture well mixed? A traditional but insensitive, reply to the question is that a mixture is well mixed when it is good enough for its duty" [4]. This question should be a guiding principle for the sampling and validation of powder blends.

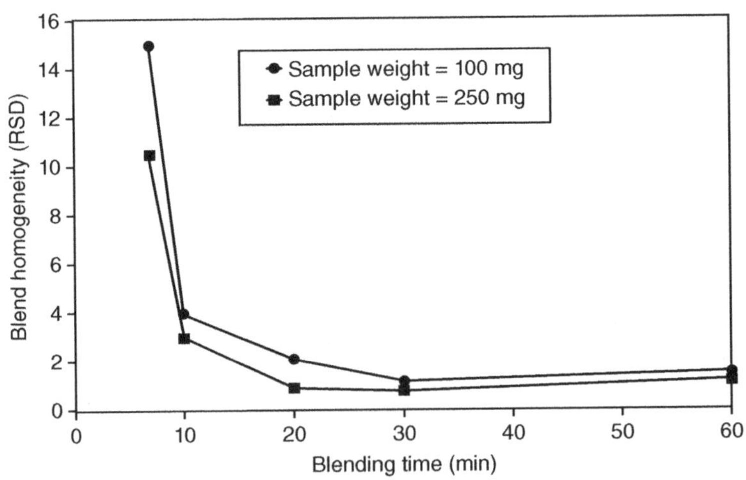

Figure 4.1 *Typical blending profile used by pharmaceutical scientists in the validation of a blending process. Adapted from reference [1]*

The blending process and its sampling should be designed to meet the requirements and expectations for the formulation.

This chapter has the ambitious goal of providing a holistic view of the sampling and validation of powder blends starting with the fundamental concepts related to the Theory of Sampling, which unfortunately have been neglected in many pharmaceutical studies. The guidance documents for the evaluation of adequacy of blending, and a number of previous studies will be discussed. However, alternative methods to define and assess adequacy of mixing will also be discussed. The FDA's Pharmaceutical CGMPs for the 21st Center and Quality by Design (QbD) initiatives are opening the door to innovative science based methods. As a result the traditional definition of quality ("product meets specifications") should shift a focus on performance as indicated by Woodcock who defined: "a high quality drug product as a product free of contamination and reproducibly delivering the therapeutic benefit promised in the label to the consumer" [5]. As the definition of quality evolves, the requirements for adequacy of mixing should also evolve. Thus, the first topic is the theory of sampling and what can be learned from efforts in other industries.

4.2 Theory of Sampling

Sampling is necessary in practically every evaluation of a process or product manufactured. However, very few analytical chemistry books provide a detailed discussion of sampling [6]. Many chapters are dedicated to instrumental methods, equilibrium calculations, significant figures and statistical comparisons, but sampling is hardly discussed [7,8]. The importance of sampling should not be underestimated since as Brittain has indicated: "*Samples* are therefore defined as the units upon which a program of testing is conducted" [9]. Nevertheless, sampling errors may be up to 1000 times greater than the analytical method bias [8,10]. Every pharmaceutical company should discuss its sampling practices in the Quality System documents.

Gy has defined sampling as "mass reduction of lot L by selection of a certain subset of units, with the purpose – not always fulfilled – of obtaining a true, reliable sample S (when the conditions of sampling correctness are respected)" [10]. Mass reductions in sampling are often 1:100,000 and 1:1,000,000 [11]. In the pharmaceutical industry it is not uncommon to work with a blend sample of 300 mg obtained from a 300 kg lot; a 1:1,000,000 sample reduction. Statistics books generally consider samples as group of objects selected from the population of all such objects [12]. Gy also emphasizes that a sample is a subset of a lot, the elements of which have been selected in the correct way, and therefore are reliable [10]. Correct means that two conditions are fulfilled simultaneously: all constituents making up the lot have an equal probability P of being selected, and the integrity of the selected constituents (increments, sample) is duly respected. Gy uses the term specimen in reference to a subset of a lot the elements of which were not selected correctly. The distinction between samples and specimens is not made in the majority of articles that address the analysis of pharmaceutical blends, and will not be used in this chapter. However, a number of other concepts described in the theory of sampling developed by Gy will be discussed throughout this chapter.

The variance that will be observed in the blends will not be solely from the variation of the mixing, as there will always be variance related to the analytical method, and related to the sampling of the mixture. Sampling errors are intimately related to the concepts of: homogeneity and heterogeneity. Homogeneous is when all the units are strictly identical to each other [10,13,14]. Thus, in the real world materials are never homogeneous, there are always some differences in materials and homogeneity is an abstract concept that does not exist. Materials are always heterogeneous showing some variations in their composition. Pharmaceutical blends consist of discrete particles and homogeneity will not be observed, the goal will to obtain an acceptable degree of heterogeneity. In lot L, component A will be present in a_L an actual but unknown decimal proportion by mass. When a sample is selected from L, a_E, there is also an actual but unknown proportion by mass of component A in the sample E. As a result, the relative sampling error may be defined as:

$$e = \frac{a_E - a_L}{a_L}$$

The error e is a random variable that may be characterized by a certain function or distribution. As a result, a random and unavoidable sampling error will occur. Heterogeneity is recognized as the sole source of this random error distribution that occurs as a_E and a_L vary. However, systematic sampling errors that introduce a bias in the results may also occur. To avoid the introduction of bias and limit errors to the random sampling error, samples should be obtained in a correct manner such that [10]:

1. All the constituent elements of the lot have an equal probability of being taken into the sample.
2. The increments and the sample are not altered in any way.

A recent study focused on how to reduce the size of any sample (lot, or primary sample) to obtain a representative sample prior to analysis [11]. The study emphasizes that secondary, tertiary sample reductions are common to obtain the adequate sample size for an analytical method once a sample is brought to the lab. Table 4.1 describes the composition of a 2 kg lot size prepared for this study, which included a trace component at 0.1% (w/w) concentration and different material properties selected to provide a system with potential for flow segregation. A total of 17 methods and devices commonly used for sample reduction were evaluated in the reduction of the 2 kg mass to obtain 100 or 125 grams of the sample. After every mass reduction, the composition of the resulting subsamples was determined, with a screening system consisting of two sieves and a bottom collecting pan, all mounted on a shaking table which collected the wheat, rape seed and glass, respectively. The particles were then separated and weighed to obtain the analytical fraction a_s. Two operators repeated

Table 4.1 *Description of 2 kg lot mass prepared before mass reductions to get either 100 or 125 g in the final sample, depending on the nature of the method or device [9]*

Sample	Concentration (%)	Avg. Density (g/cm^3)	Avg. Grain Size	Surface Properties
Wheat grains	89.9	0.75	6.0 × 3.0 mm as a "cylinder"	Slightly softer
Rape seeds	10.0	0.77	2.6 mm	Smooth
Glass spheres	0.1	2.60	1.0	Very smooth

the same mass reduction/sub-sampling/weighing procedure 20 times in blocks of 10 for all methods and devices investigated. The devices evaluated in this study included six riffler splitters, two revolving splitters, shoveling methods (spoon, alternative shoveling, fractional shoveling, and grab sampling). The study compared the representativeness of the 17 sub-sampling devices. Representativeness was defined as the sum of the mean squared error in terms of both accuracy and precision, so to a value close to zero is desirable. The methods with the highest values were the grab sampling, shoveling and spoon methods. The evaluation did not include a sample thief, the most common probe for performing grab sampling in the pharmaceutical industry. Figure 4.2 shows the schematic representation for a sample thief. The 17 methods provided a range of representativeness values that may vary from 50- to 60-fold, demonstrating the importance of proper sampling. The findings from this study apply to the evaluation of pharmaceutical powder blends, and in many other production processes where the sample obtained from a lot is much larger than that evaluated by the ultrasensitive instruments that characterize analytical laboratories.

In many industries a large sample is collected and then sub-sampling is performed for the different methods to be carried out in the lab, followed by additional sub-sampling occurs to obtain quantities suitable for analysis in a laboratory. However, in the pharmaceutical industry powder mixtures equivalent to 1–3 dose units are usually obtained directly from the powder blend. Therefore, it should be possible to analyze the sample blends in the QC laboratories without additional sub-sampling. The limit of 1–3 dose units is the consequence of *The US vs. Barr Laboratories* where Judge Wolin ruled for the government that the appropriate sample size for Blend Uniformity Analysis (BUA) is, at most, three times the weight of the final dosage unit [13]. The ruling also stated that the 3× sample provides ample material for the initial test as well as two retests. Furthermore, the ruling stated that blend samples must be collected from "places that might be problems," but

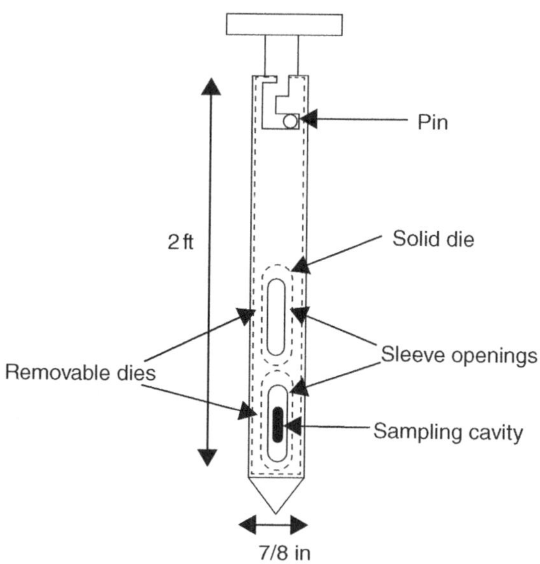

Figure 4.2 *Schematic representation of a sample thief commonly used in industry*

declined to support the government's position that the site of sampling should be restricted to the mixer. BUA in the pharmaceutical industry has been intimately tied to the Barr case and subsequent FDA guidances. One publication indicates: "Unfortunately, the thief is the only tool currently available that allows the pharmaceutical industry to comply with CDER's recommendations for BUA" [15]. This view has been maintained for many years and is the source of many of the documented BUA problems in the industry [15–21].

Allen has contributed two golden rules for powder sampling:

1. the powder should be sampled while in motion,
2. the whole of the stream should be obtained for many short increments of time in preference to part of the stream being taken for the whole of the time.

Both Allen and Gy emphasize that the whole of the stream should be sampled, as particles in the edge may be different than those in the center and particles at the top of the powder bed may be different than those at the bottom [10,22]. Allen mentions the situation that "hopper cars," which should be analogous to intermediate containers for pharmaceutical manufacturing applications should be sampled when these containers are being filled. The sampling procedure should include a receiver large enough that the largest particles can be collected. Allen explains that a free flowing powder should never be sampled when it is static because of the segregation that has "almost certainly occurred." Instead he recommends sampling the powder as the container is being filled. For example, flowing powders may be sampled systematically every 2 min. The data obtained could then be analyzed by a number of methods described by Gy to evaluate whether any tendencies or autocorrelations are observed in the data [10,23].

A sample thief violates both golden rules, but is still the main probe for grabbing powder samples the adequacy of mixing in the pharmaceutical industry [24]. Pharmaceutical manufacturing plants have procedures that indicate the order and location of the samples obtained as shown in Figure 4.3 [25]. As a result the particles in the lot do not have an equal probability for being selected. As a sample thief may disturb the powder distribution, the total number of samples is usually limited to 10–20 to avoid obtaining samples from areas that have been disturbed making it impossible to take a representative

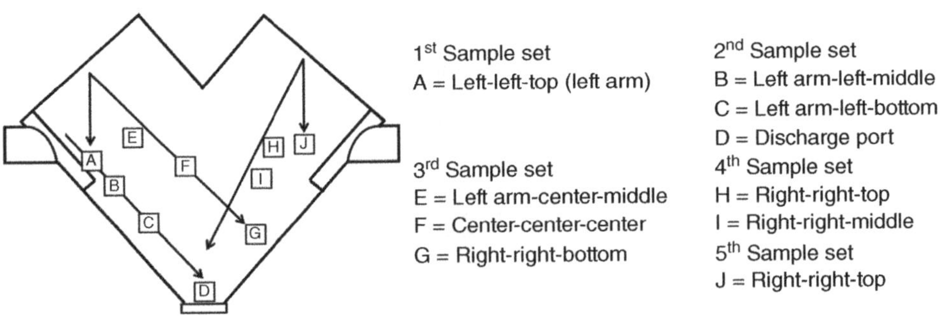

Figure 4.3 *Drawing showing how to sample a V-blender with a sample thief to minimize disturbance of a powder bed. Reprinted with permission from http://www.ikev.org/haber/bozzonemay31.pdf. Copyright (2001) Pfizer*

characterization of all regions of the blend [17]. However, in conversations with the author many manufacturing plants indicated that they have found a thief that provides acceptable results for their process.

4.3 Sampling of Pharmaceutical Powder Blends

A survey published in 2001 indicated that sample thief probes remain the preferred method for powder sampling, with 25 of the 28 respondents indicating that they used a side-compartment thief device [26]. The sample thief usually consists of two concentric tubes, one enclosing the other [27,28]. The outer tube is pointed, with matching openings in the inner and outer tubes that are maintained closed as the thief is inserted in the powder bed. Once the thief is in the desired position the powder is allowed to flow into the openings, and then the openings are closed to capture or grab the powder. Different designs have been used such as the plug thief and pocket thief [19]. The two principal types of errors associated with the sample thief have been that: the mixture is disturbed and particles of different size flow unevenly into the cavity [17].

The scientific literature includes a number of situations where tablets met content uniformity requirements while powder blends showed erroneous results. One notable example was the analysis of 343 tablet cores with results between 97% and 108% of label claim, while 92 of 93 blend samples below label claim and showed a wider variation [15]. Another study found that for locations deeper in the blender, the concentration of drug in the powder sample increased (approximately to 115–120% label claim) [19]. Since powder at the bottom of the blending container is discharged onto the tablet press first, then these first tablets should also have increased concentration. However, the trend was not observed, and the tablet content uniformity showed that the blend samples were not representative of the true blend uniformity. The concentration gradient observed from the surface to the bottom of the blender was eventually determined to be related to electrostatic charge, and increasing the grounding for the blender from 30 min to 90 h resulted in values that moved closer to the label claim.

Any thief used should be thoroughly evaluated before use. The thief might not work as expected, and could extract material even with the compartments closed [17]. If the thief extracts powders while closed, this is indicative that it obtains material from the path traveled through the powder bed, and the sample obtained is a composite instead of the composition at location of interest [17]. The fact that a thief worked well for process A, does not mean that it will work well for process B, where the formulation may have different flow or electrostatic properties. The sampling of the powder blend needs to be addressed while the formulation is being developed [1].

There are a number of examples that address alternative means of obtaining pharmaceutical powder samples. The use of stream sampling for the development of a blending process has been reported [29]. In this alternative approach the powder blend consisted of ibuprofen and spray-dried hydrous lactose which was mixed for 0.5, 1, 3, 5, 10, and 20 min in a 4-quart V-blender. After these blending times the blender was emptied and 20–25 samples were collected from the flowing stream. The blend was captured in stainless steel cups capable of sampling about 100 mg of blend. A separated blend was prepared for each of the blending times, a total of six blends. The powder captured in the cups was weighed and the ibuprofen concentration determined with a validated ultraviolet spectroscopic method. The %RSD of the ibuprofen concentration at each blending time was used to develop a blending profile.

The stream sampling approach also employed near infrared (NIR) spectroscopy. The NIR spectrum of each of the powder samples in the cups was obtained. NIR spectra may be obtained without sample preparation, in a non-invasive mode, and quickly. Absorption of radiation in the NIR region is the result of the stretching vibrations of C-H, O-H, and N-H overtones and combination bands of the vibration bands that occur in the mid-infrared region. A blending profile was developed by calculating the relative standard deviation of NIR spectra. Two profiles were developed based on the spectral changes [29]. One blending profile was based on the changes in the concentration of the active ingredient (ibuprofen), while the second profile that covered practically the entire spectrum (12,000–5000 cm^{-1}) was based on the changes in the distribution of both excipients and drug. NIR spectroscopy facilitates the development of blending profiles where changes in the concentrations of excipients are considered.

Stream sampling has been used in industry in the validation of blending processes. The cups can be designed and manufactured to limit the sample volume to 1–3 dosage units. One of the advantages of the stream sampling method is that it can be used to collect an unlimited number of samples, while the number of samples obtained with a sample thief must be limited to avoid excessive disruption of the powder bed when the thief is inserted. The stream sampling method also takes advantage of a process that always occurs, as tablet compression requires the flow of the blend from a hopper or bin located over the compressing machine. The author knows that stream sampling has been used in industry, and has been accepted by the FDA. However, the industrial data remains proprietary.

The use of rifflers is recommended in the scientific literature however, there are very few examples of their use in pharmaceutical applications [30]. Rifflers consist of a feeding system that may include a hopper and a vibratory feeder to continuously feed the powder blend into a set of containers on a revolving table. A commercially available rotary micro riffler was used in a study to assess the potential for segregation of pharmaceutical blends. The riffler was used to obtain samples of powder blends with a sample size suitable for HPLC analysis. The authors indicate that "the %RSD of the riffled samples was always low, suggesting that the riffling technique was adequate." A number of samples from a blend with a 25% (w/w) drug load showed a low 1% RSD when the riffler was used. Higher RSD values were obtained when the powder blends were subjected to conditions that lead to segregation. Differences in concentration of up to 20% were observed in the blends subjected to conditions that promoted segregation. The study clearly showed that the riffler was able to sample the segregated powder blends.

The similarities between a spinning riffler and a rotary tablet press have been discussed [31]. A compressing machine has a hopper from which the powder blend flows to a forced feeder and to a number of dies in a rotating die table. The spinning riffler also has a hopper, substituting the rotating die table with a turn table and the dies with powder reservoirs. A rotary tablet press can be visualized as a compacting spinning riffler, and its use as a sampling device for blending validation was shown.

The use of a rotary press as compacting spinning riffler is consistent with the golden rules of sampling described by Allen since the powder is sampled while in motion capturing "the whole of the stream for many short increments of time in preference to part of the stream being taken for the whole of the time" [22]. The study was conducted with a challenging blend with only 1% (w/w) drug load. After mixing in a V-blender, composite powder sample of 300 grams were obtained during the beginning, middle and end part of the unloading phase. The composite powder sample was compressed into tablets, in a 15-station press and using tooling of three different sizes that provided tablets with total weights of approximately 100, 350, and 550 mg. The powder blend was unloaded after tablet manufacture, and a total of 10 powder samples were obtained with a conventional slit thief. The powder blend mass obtained in the press was very precise, but significant variation was observed in the lower weight (120 mg) powder blends captured by the sample thief. The results with both methods were very close to the expected target level, and the relative standard deviation was less than 2.5%. The study also proposed the use of a capsule-filling machine as a sampling device for blend validation, but did not provide data for this application. In this particular formulation, excellent results were obtained with the sample thief. However, a small R&D tablet press could be used as a sampling device with blends that are problematic when a sample thief is used. Tablet compression could then occur in a similar high volume machine.

4.4 Stratified Sampling Approach

The stratified sampling approach resulted from a collaborative study involving the FDA's Center for Drug Evaluation and Research (CDER), industry, and academia. The 1999 "Guidance for Industry. ANDA's: Blend Uniformity Analysis" lead to a rather large number of industry concerns, and the eventually formation of a Blend Uniformity Working Group (BUWG) by the Product Quality Research Institute (PQRI). The BUWG conducted an industry survey, organized a workshop, provided a blend uniformity and content uniformity troubleshooting guide, and eventually using the consensus reached by participants in this workshop developed a draft recommendation: "The Use of Stratified Sampling of Blend and Dosage Units to Demonstrate Adequacy of Mix for Powder Blends" [26,32–34]. The 2003 Draft Guidance was the direct result of BUWG contributions. but it was withdrawn by the Food and Drug Administration in August 2013. It is discussed in this chapter, because of its historical importance in the development of sampling in the pharmaceutical manufacturing.

The stratified sampling approach is the process of sampling units at predefined intervals and collecting samples from specifically targeted locations in the compression or filling operation that the greatest potential for providing high or low results. Thus, the approach requires some knowledge of the blending and material transfers involved in the process, and it assumes that these targeted locations will always be equally probable to provide high or low results. The stratified sampling approach does not attempt to obtain representative samples. To obtain a truly representative sample all virtual units making up the lot must have the same probability of being selected [10,11], while in the 2003 Draft Guidance the units with the most potential of showing the greatest variation were favored. In spite of these shortcomings, the 2003 Draft Guidance will be discussed in detail since it has been widely implemented throughout the industry.

The 2003 Draft Guidance also followed the traditional approach of evaluating blend uniformity solely on the distribution of the active ingredient, where the excipients are not taken into account. This Draft Guidance first addressed the exhibit or validation batches. The stratified sampling approach recommends identifying at least 10 sampling locations in the blender where there is potential for poor mixing, collecting three replicate samples from each location. These samples should include at least two depths within the blender. In the case of ribbon blenders, the implementation of uniform volumetric sampling to include the corners and discharge area (at least 20 locations are recommended). The analysis of drug concentration for at least 10 blends from the tumble blender and 20 from the ribbon mixer in these samples should yield: (1) a relative standard deviation ≤ 5%, and (2) all individual results within 10.0% (absolute) of the mean drug concentration. The Draft Guidance provides a clear and detailed flowchart describing its application.

The second part of the stratified sampling approach is the analysis of dosage units, once again selected to include events such as hopper changeover and beginning and end of filling with the greatest potential for high or low drug concentrations. At least 20 locations should be identified and at least seven dosage units collected for a total of 140 units, and at least three of seven assayed with the results weight corrected. The results of the 60 dosage units are then evaluated to identify any trends or bimodal distributions from the process. The analyzed units are said to *readily pass* if:

- For all individual results (for each batch n ≥ 60) the RSD ≤ 4.0%.
- Each location mean is within 90.0–110.0% of target strength.
- All individual results are within the range of 75.0–125.0% of target strength.

In cases where the dosage units fail to meet the *readily pass* criteria, the guidance recommended the analysis of all the remaining dosage units (all seven units per location). The units *marginally pass* if they meet the following criteria:

- For all individual results (for one batch n ≥ 140) the RSD ≤ 6.0%.
- Each location mean is within 90.0–110.0% of target strength.
- All individual results are within the range of 75.0–125.0% of target strength.

The most important advantage of the stratified sampling approach is that it provides a way to meet the in-process testing of adequacy of mixing without additional testing and analysis during routine manufacture. The Draft Guidance first recommended a thorough evaluation of the data taking into account significant process events and their effect on in-process dosage unit and finished dosage unit quality attributes. Following this evaluation, the in-process test requirement is met by analyzing units from the locations identified as having the greatest potential of failing in commercial product manufacture. Table 4.2 describes the Draft Guidance requirements which are also addressed USP dose uniformity requirements. The Standard Criteria Method (SCM) is recommended for product that readily passed the validation. The SCM has stage 1 and stage 2 testing as shown in Table 4.2. The SCM stage 1 criteria for the commercial manufacturing the tablets the RSD for all tablets (n ≥ 10) should be ≤ 5.0%, with the mean of all results within 90.0–110.0% of target assay. The batch meets the in-process and USP dose uniformity requirements, when it meets these stage 1 requirements and then stage 2 is not needed. Stage 2 is only required when the product fails to meet stage 1 requirements.

Stage 2 of the SCM required that the remaining dosage units are analyzed and for all individual units (n ≥ 30) the RSD ≤ 5.0%, and the mean of all results is 90.0–110.0% of target assay. Products that meet these requirements are considered as adequate and stage 1

Table 4.2 *Requirements for dosage units obtained from stratified sampling locations. All results are weight corrected*

Standard Criteria Method (SCM)	
Stage	
1	n ≥ 10 and mean is 90.0–110.0% of target and RSD ≤ 5.0%,
2	n ≥ 30 and mean is 90.0–110.0% of target and RSD ≤ 6.0%,
Marginal Criteria Method (MCM)	
	n = 30 and mean is 90.0–110.0% of target and RSD ≤ 6.0%

of the SCM can be used in the next batch. However, if the batch does not comply with SCM then the Marginal Criteria Method (MCM) must be used.

The MCM was also used for products with a *marginally pass* validation. The MCM does not require additional testing; and consists of determining whether the weight corrected results of stage 2 meet the following criteria: the RSD of drug concentration is ≤ 6.0%, and the mean of all results is 90.0–110.0% of target assay. If the batch does not comply with stage 2 tests then an investigation and process improvements are required. The Draft Guidance also indicated that it is possible to switch back to the reduced testing of SCM, if five consecutive batches meet the MCM criteria and result in RSD ≤5.0%. At least one study has shown the application of the Draft Guidance to industrial blends [16].

One of the most significant advances of this Draft Guidance was that it encompassed the analysis of blends as well as tablets or dose units. The analysis of tablets may be useful in identifying post blending segregation problems [35–37], and in detecting problems associated with a sample thief. The analysis of tablets could also show better content uniformity results due to mixing in the feed frame, or difficulties with the sampling procedure.

4.5 Testing

The author's first exposure to the analysis of powder blends were the complaints of a QC laboratory supervisor regarding the high amount of solvent needed for analysis of powder samples, and how these samples were responsible for the lab exceeding the budgeted solvent expenses. Each sample was the weight of 10–20 dose units and required 500 mL of solvent for analysis. This situation was about to change with the Barr case that required the analysis of 1–3 times the dose unit mass.

Current testing for adequacy of mixing usually involves the HPLC analysis of a samples powder sample with a mass that is 1–3 times the dose unit that are usually obtained with a sample thief. The results of the analysis are usually reported in terms of percent of label claim, or mg of drug per gram of blend. The use of a sample thief eliminates the need for sub-sampling of the blend. Generally, the same HPLC procedure used for the analysis of tablets is used to analyze the powder samples. This validated procedure is considered adequate for powder blends, as the samples are similar except that they are not compacted and thus should be even easier to analyze.

One of the difficulties of working with a sample thief is releasing the powder so that it falls within the bottle or sample container sent to the lab for analysis. The bottles often have narrow openings, very similar to the diameter of the sample thief. The author while working in industry observed that a number of bottles received in the QC lab had powder adhered to their outer surface. This powder was part of the weight recorded by the analytical balance but was obviously not assayed as the solvent for the HPLC analysis was added to the powder inside the bottle. This problem was solved by using wide mouth bottles, making it much easier for operators to place the powder sample within the bottle, and improve the precision of the sample masses obtained. The larger bottles required a larger volume of solvent, up to 60 mL to contact and dissolve the active pharmaceutical ingredient dispersed throughout the bottle walls, and a number of validation tests in support of the new sample preparation procedure. However, this additional work was well worth the problems avoided. This discussion might appear to be too simplistic, but these simple details are often the source of significant manufacturing difficulties.

Discussions on testing for adequacy of mixing or blend uniformity have centered on evaluating the drug concentration and standard deviation of the samples selected. However, in recent work FDA scientists have also studied blend uniformity in the final dosage product [38]. A total of five grades of experimental tablets containing the same amounts of furosemide and microcrystalline cellulose were prepared by varying the mixing procedure to produce tablets ranging from well blended to unblended. Near infrared chemical imaging (NIR-CI) was then used to obtain over 76,000 spectra of the tablet surface and provide images showing the distribution of furosemide. Differences between the five grades of experimental tablets were easily detected through simple visual inspection of the chemical images. A quantitative assessment was also performed using partial least squares discriminant analysis (PLS-DA) to calculate the drug concentration associated with each of the spectra. The standard deviation of the calculated concentrations was about 11% for the well mixed tablets, and 240% for the unblended tablets. The NIR-CI method provided spatial information on the distribution of the drug thereby measuring intra tablet variability instead of the inter-tablet or inter-powder sample variability discussed in the majority of blend uniformity evaluations.

The intra tablet evaluation through NIR-CI detects drug aggregates in tablets that could affect dissolution. Large drug clusters could also indicate the possibility of over potent tablets, especially in potent drug formulations. These aggregates or micro-domains are not detected in HPLC, UV, or other methods where the entire contents of the dose unit are analyzed. The authors indicate that testing of the drug product complements blend analysis, and "Blend uniformity testing provides feedback to assist in the process development, while the end-product test provides assurance that the blend remained uniform during processing." However, the opinions expressed in the article are those of the authors and do not necessarily reflect the views and policies of the U.S. Food and Drug Administration (FDA).

4.6 Process Knowledge/Process Analytical Technology

The Process Analytical Technology (PAT Guidance) does present the views of FDA, although it does not indicate a new regulatory requirement [39]. The Agency has defined PAT as "a system for designing, analyzing, and controlling manufacturing through timely measurements (i.e., during processing) of critical quality and performance attributes of raw and in-process materials and processes, with the goal of ensuring final product quality." In this case the term "*analytical* in PAT is viewed broadly to include chemical, physical, microbiological, mathematical, and risk analysis conducted in an integrated manner." The main message of this guidance is that the risk of producing a poor product is reduced as process knowledge is increased [40]. The PAT Guidance marked the beginning a long term effort by FDA to increase pharmaceutical process understanding and encourage innovation in pharmaceutical manufacturing [41]. Chapter 15, authored by Nicolas Abatzoglou provides a more detailed discussion of PAT and blending.

The PAT system strongly depends on the sampling of the manufacturing process. The timely measurements during processing may involve a non-invasive spectroscopic method where the radiation interacts with a small fraction of the sample as the process involves. In a PAT system the mixing time will not be 10 min or a fixed time for every batch that is manufactured. As indicated in the Guidance: "Within the PAT framework, a process end point is not a fixed time; rather it is the achievement of the desired material attribute." The mixing time will be within a specific time period that will vary according to the physical variations of the excipients and API. The mixing time will rely on real time measurements that in turn depend on the sampling through real time spectroscopic measurements of a reduced mass of the powders.

Spectroscopic methods may be used during the development of a new manufacturing process to fully understand the dynamics of mixing and gather process understanding. These experiments may be performed in small scale blenders, and this experience may then be applied to real time monitoring of the manufacturing process. For example, in a recent application a 6 cm (tall) by 4 cm (diameter) cylinder-shaped aluminum mini-blender was constructed, with a top quartz window [42]. Once loaded, the vessel secured into a lab-scale bin blender rotated at 25 rpm. After blending for a specific time the mini-blender was removed and six chemical images were collected for each blend, the first two across the quartz window. The mixture was compressed into a compact and two imaged of the bottom part of the compact were obtained, before cutting it into two halves and obtaining two final images from the cross section. The study showed that blending profiles developed by plotting the %RSD as a function of time revealed a minimum in the variation of drug concentration after 15 min of blending but did not show that excipients were segregated in the blends. NIR chemical imaging provided insight into the distribution of the size of the domains of active ingredient and excipients through the different blending times.

Another lab scale study involved the use of NIR spectroscopy and a sample thief to determine the end point of a two-component mixture consisting of 3, 7, or 11% salicylic acid as active ingredient and lactose as excipient [43]. The blender was stopped at specific time points to allow for collection of NIR spectra, and removal of powder blend with a thief probe. A UV (ultraviolet spectroscopy) method was used to evaluate the drug concentration of the samples from the thief. Near infrared spectra of the contents of an 8-qt V-blender were obtained by installing six sapphire windows that allowed a fiber optic probe to be positioned against the sapphire windows. The salicylic acid was placed in the left side of the blender. The subsequent experiments employed the NIR, NIR-CI, and the sample thief to study of the slow migration of the SA across the vertical axis of the blender. In addition, a NIR chemical imaging system was installed with access to top surface after the lids were removed from the V-blender.

The thief collected powder samples of about 1 gram from six different locations in the powder bed. In this study the blend results were considered acceptable if all samples were between 90 and 110% of the label claim and for the RSD to be <5%. The 3% blend did not meet these requirements, even after 30 min of blending. The RSD obtained for the endpoints ranged from 3.52–4.71%. In addition, NIR spectra were obtained when the blender was stopped. The spectra corresponding to the early blending times were identified, as well as those corresponding to the blends that provided acceptable results after UV analysis. The NIR spectra were then classified as corresponding to the homogeneous blend or corresponding to the early stages of blending. The study also used a number of spectral associated with salicylic acid and lactose and used their standard deviation to develop a blending profile for each of the concentrations. The blending endpoints indicated by the NIR and UV methods were similar for the 7%, 11% A, and 11% B SA powder blends.

The advantage of the system described in this study is that it can be implemented to understand the mixing dynamics of a new formulation in a small scale lab. As such it can be a useful tool to gather the process knowledge currently describe by the ICH Q8 Pharmaceutical Development guidance [44]. Even though the NIR system discussed requires a considerable investment, it is much lower than the cost for installing and implementing a system capable of real time monitoring.

4.7 Real Time Spectroscopic Monitoring of Powder Blending

In recent years extensive research has demonstrated the applicability of near infrared spectroscopy (NIRS) for monitoring powder mixing [45–55]. High signal to noise NIR spectra may be obtained in a second or less, providing an opportunity for monitoring mixing in real time. Thus, a blending profile may be obtained without having to send samples to the lab for HPLC analysis, and minimizing the exposure of manufacturing plant operators to potential hazardous compounds. The non-invasive installation of NIR systems is also an important advantage, eliminating the possible erroneous results observed when the powder bed is disturbed with a sample thief or other grab sampling approach. Furthermore, the same NIR spectrum that is used for monitoring mixing may be used to identify the formulation, providing an additional control of pharmaceutical operations [56]. These are the principal advantages of monitoring mixing processes with NIR spectroscopy but others will become apparent throughout this section.

The use of NIR or other spectroscopic non-invasive method does not eliminate sampling. At any given time the near infrared radiation is interacting with a "reduced mass" in comparison to the mass within the blender, drier or other processing equipment. The near infrared spectrum is obtained for possibly 100–200 mg, a very reduced mass if compared to the entire mass within the blender. Mark provides a valuable discussion of the sources of error for calibrations, and these are applicable to the use of near infrared or other analytical methods in monitoring mixing [57]. Mark indicates that all measurements are subject to: (1) random error in the optical data, (2) random error in the values of the reference laboratory, and (3) Systematic error in the relationship between these two. The systematic error will often occur when the near infrared beam or other real time analyzer is interacting with 100 mg of sample, while the off-line reference method is evaluating 500 mg of sample. The systematic error occurs when the spectroscopic method is interacting with a sample that is different from that brought to the lab for analysis with the reference method. The systematic error is then a sampling error.

Sampling errors were evaluated in a recently published method for in-line monitoring of moisture content in fluid bed dryers with NIR spectroscopy [58]. In this study the ultimate goal was to determine the end point of fluid bed drying following granulation with NIR spectroscopy. Calibration models were developed relating the NIR spectra to the moisture content determined with two off-line reference methods: loss on drying (LOD) and the Karl Fischer titration. The study included a 600 L system where it was possible to obtain high signal to noise spectra with the probe directly inserted in the dryer. However, the turbulence in the 65 L and 300 L dryers made it impossible to obtain high signal to noise spectra when the probe was directly inserted into the dryer. These two dryers required the design of a sampling interface to hold the granules while the spectra were obtained and an air purge to remove the granules and avoid probe fouling. The probe was subsequently modified to allow removal of the same granules held for NIR measurements with a powder thief. The modified cup provided better results showing the importance of having similar samples measured by the spectroscopic and the off-line reference methods.

The article emphasizes that assurance that similar samples are analyzed by the real time analyzer and the reference method is not sufficient, if the sample removed for off-line analysis is not representative of the lot that is being dried. The article discusses the global estimation error:

$$\mathrm{GEE} = \frac{a_\mathrm{R} - a_\mathrm{L}}{a_\mathrm{L}}$$

where a_R represents the analytical result while a_L is the actual, unknown value of component A in lot L. The GEE is a function of both the total sampling error (TSE) and the total analytical error (TAE) [10]:

$$\mathrm{GEE} = \mathrm{TSE} + \mathrm{TAE} = \frac{a_\mathrm{S} - a_\mathrm{L}}{a_\mathrm{L}} + \frac{a_\mathrm{R} - a_\mathrm{S}}{a_\mathrm{L}}$$

These equations apply for both the spectroscopic method and the reference method; there is a GEE for the spectroscopic method and a second GEE for the laboratory reference method. Each method also has its own TSE and TAE. As a result, when similar results are obtained by the spectroscopic method and the reference method; this means that both methods have similar GEE; however, the TSE may still be substantial and the results obtained might not be representative of the lot being processed. Good agreement between the spectroscopic and the reference methods does not guarantee that the endpoint is determined correctly.

An interesting aspect of this application is that both a_R and a_L are constantly changing, because the range of measurements and the moisture content of the lot are constantly changing. During blending, the composition of the lot will also change and once again a_R and a_L will be constantly changing. The changes in a_R and a_L will be typical of processes where the materials are processed towards an endpoint and real time measurements are made. However, as the heterogeneity of the sample is reduced and an end-point is approached, then the TSE and GEE should also be reduced.

The challenges of sampling powder samples are also evident in a recent application where the in-line prediction of powder particle size distribution has been described for powder blends that are prone to segregate during flow [59]. Even though this application did not involve powder mixing it underlines the challenges associated with the sampling of powders. The novel sampling approach was designed for samples where the ratio of the diameters of the large particle to small particle-size fractions is at least 2, and developed after initial efforts provided results where the precision was not adequate for industrial applications. Instead of working against unavoidable particle size segregation, an experimental set up was developed for a system to facilitate particle size segregation. The powder is poured into a first mass flow silo. As the particles flow from the first to the second silo, the particles segregate as the larger particles tend to roll out against the wall in the second silo and the finer particles tend to aggregate in the middle section. Silo 2 is a so-called funnel flow silo and will cause the fine particles (middle section) to come out first when valve 2 is opened. The last powder particles to flow out of silo 2 will be the coarse particles, which are closest to the walls. The powder particles then flow and impact an acoustic sensor, and the resulting vibrations are converted to an electrical signal. The acoustic sensor consists of many dipoles with the same orientation, and the impact of the particles result in continuous signals (as a function of time). The continuous signals are converted to the frequency domain using the fast Fourier transform to obtain acoustic effect spectra.

The initial calibration model for particle size was then developed using the acoustic spectra as the X matrix and the particle size from sieving experiments as the Y matrix variable. The results from the calibration model showed that the prediction of particle size distributions with acoustic chemometrics was possible, but precision was 5.7–10.2%, with the best precision obtained with the smallest grain size (5.7%). This precision was not adequate for industrial application and the quality of the Y-reference values was considered to be the main source of error. The recorded signals were not representative of the powder sample, as flow segregation occurred before the particles impacted the acoustic sensor. This error, associated with flow segregation, also affected the analysis of routine samples. Even though this application involved particle size distribution, similar challenges could be observed in applications with near infrared spectrometers or other sensors used to monitor pharmaceutical blending.

The real time methods monitor at a specific time a sample volume and mass that is usually less than the unit dose currently analyzed by HPLC or UV methods in the lab. As a consequence a number of scientists have had difficulties in comparing real time and lab results. A number of NIR studies have included estimates of the sample volume from which the NIR spectrum was obtained [48,52]. The studies have considered the sample area illuminated, the depth of penetration for the radiation, and the fact that many times spectra are averaged and thus the powder flow rate is needed to calculate the sample volume. The coefficient of variation that may be expected from sampling a portion has a larger statistical variance than when the entire sample, as shown with a statistical proof and experimental study [60]. The study involved the analysis by HPLC or tablets with two active ingredients. The content uniformity test was performed for whole, half, and quarter tablets. A single tablet was the source for one half and two quarter tablets. For the first active ingredient the coefficient of variation increased from 0.7 to 2.4% when comparing whole to quarter tablets, and for the second it increased from 1.6 to 5.1%. The authors conclude that if portions of tablets or other solid oral dosage forms pass the content uniformity requirements then the individual whole tablets must pass.

Finally, the real time spectroscopic methods should be considered in light of the golden rules of sampling. The real time methods meet the first rule of sampling a powder while it is in motion unless probe fouling occurs (powder is adhered to the window of the spectrometer). However, they do not meet the second requirement: the whole of the stream should be obtained for many short increments of time in preference to part of the stream being taken for the whole of the time. In most applications, the real time methods will be sampling part of the stream for the whole of the time. Fortunately, as the movement of particles in the process increases, the sensor will interact with a greater fraction of the tablets and the effect of sampling part of the stream should be less.

4.8 Looking Forward, Recommendations

This chapter has summarized the extensive work in this area. However, an important question remains: what have we learned, what recommendations can be made to improvement pharmaceutical manufacturing.

The first recommendation is to design the formulation. The blending process for a cohesive drug at a 0.02% drug load provides an excellent example of formulation design [61]. In this case the process included a number of steps to obtain an ordered mix where the drug was distributed evenly throughout the surface of lactose particles. The formulation evaluation included the samples obtained with a thief and testing of the final product, and also the use of scanning electron microscopy to view drug distribution. Thus, the formulation design should be complemented with some type of visualization method, such as scanning electron microscopy or NIR chemical imaging that provides a picture of the final formulation. This first part should provide an understanding of whether a random mix or ordered mixed is being achieved.

The second recommendation is to evaluate the equilibrium between mixing and segregation [62]. The formulation should be subjected to testing to evaluate its propensity to segregation under various conditions that could favor segregation, and compared to results obtained under normal operating conditions [30,63].

The third recommendation is to recognize that a number of alternatives to the use of a sample thief are available, although the pharmaceutical industry has consistently favored the use of thief probes. The use of a riffler has been shown to be a good alternative for pharmaceutical samples [30], and a recent in depth study of these systems has been published [11]. A small rotary tablet press or capsule may be also be used to sample the powder. Compressing machines should be visualized as accessories for sampling powder blends. In fact, compressing machines are generally better designed than any available thief probe.

A sample thief could be used to probe a limited number of points that could be dead spots or of concern to formulators. The order in which the samples are obtained must be specified as in the example in Figure 4.3. However, the sample thief should be one that has been previously tested and known to provide limited disruption of the powder blend, and tested to make sure that material does not leak in when the compartment is closed. The sample thief may be used recognizing that it is not capable of representative sampling as all locations in the blender do not have the same probability of being sampled. Thus, the sample thief is only capable of providing an initial assessment or cursory evaluation of drug distribution in the blend.

NIR spectroscopy and other sensors are also available. These sensors could be used in more than one way. For example, NIR spectroscopy could be used to gather process knowledge in a lab scale blender as demonstrated by El-Hagrasy and Drennen [43]. The installation and validation of a real time blend uniformity system might be too high for some companies. However, the use of near infrared spectroscopy to develop a new process is not. Hopefully, we will see additional use of this technology in the future; the formulator could be a PAT scientist [64].

Regardless of the approach used to obtain samples and evaluate the powder blend, it is important that the formulator or other qualified personnel follow the entire process. A common problem in industry is that too often nobody is familiar with all the tasks involved in a process. For example, the analyst is not aware of how the samples were obtained. Thus, formulators should be familiar with the sampling process and should make sure that samples are obtained as they were specified in the validation protocol or procedures.

A fourth recommendation is the development of a more ample or holistic view of blend uniformity, in accordance with modern Quality Assurance systems and ICH Q10, as well as the CGMPs for the 21st Century initiative [65]. The use of NIR spectroscopy opens the door to a more ample definition of blend uniformity where the distribution of both drug and excipients is evaluated. Blend uniformity has been traditionally defined only in terms of the drug distribution in the blends [1]. However, excipients also play very important roles in the performance of a drug product. A number of studies have shown that NIR spectra can provide a blending profile based on changes in drug concentration as well as changes in excipient concentrations [29,42,46]. NIR chemical imaging may be used to further study drug distribution within the tablet [38]. The holistic view needs to include the fact that the amount of drug in a dose unit also depends on the weight of the dose. Die filling is affected by powder flow properties, and surprisingly feed frames have been seldom studied systematically [66].

This more ample view of blend uniformity is also necessary to facilitate the progress of continuous manufacturing. It is difficult to visualize having to stop a continuous manufacturing process to obtain a powder sample with a thief probe. The continuous manufacturing process may be monitored with NIR spectroscopy and eventually the NIR will be used to control the process [54].

Finally recognizing that tablets are samples of blends, NIR spectroscopy could be used to analyze tablets obtained throughout the lot. NIR spectroscopy could easily determine the drug concentration of 30–40 tablets per hour, a substantial time reduction in comparison with HPLC methods [67–69]. A greater number of tablets could be analyzed throughout a lot without increasing the time needed to manufacture a product, providing a greater opportunity to detect any post-blending segregation. The compressing machine could be visualized as blend sampling probe, and one that obeys the two golden rules of powder sampling. The analysis of a much greater number of tablets, coupled with in depth process understanding of the formulation and manufacturing process would provide stronger Quality Systems throughout the industry.

4.9 Conclusion

The sampling of pharmaceutical blends has been a major problem during the development and validation of pharmaceutical processes. The belief that a sample thief is the only means for acquiring samples has been one of the reasons. The methods discussed in the chapter show that many alternatives are available. Hopefully, the advent of process analytical technology and the CGMPs for the 21st Century initiative will lead to the implementation of the suggestions discussed in this chapter.

4.10 Acknowledgments

The author has been able to study this important area of research with funding received from INDUNIV (Puerto Rico Industry University Government Research Consortium), the Dane O. Kildsig NSF Center for Pharmaceutical Process Research, and the National Science Foundation, (ERC Research Grant EEC-0540855). Dr. Garnet Peck is thanked for a very insightful distribution that was very helpful to understand the historical evolution of this topic. Dr. Saly Romero, Dr. David Ely, and Dr. Ruey-Chin Hwang are also thanked for their advice. The author is especially indebted to Dr. Teresa Carvajal for very helpful discussions.

References

[1] R.C. Hwang, M.K. Gemoules, and D.S. Ramalose, A systematic approach for optimizing the blending process of a direct-compression tablet formulation, *Pharm. Technol.* **22**, (3), 158–170 (1998).
[2] Draft Guidance for Industry, *ANDAs: Blend Uniformity Analysis*, August 3, 1999. (withdrawn by FDA in May 2002).
[3] Draft Guidance for Industry: *Powder Blends and Finished Dosage Units Stratified In-Process Dosage Unit Sampling and Assessment*, October 27, 2003.
[4] N. Harby, M.F. Edwards, A.W. Nienow, Mixing in the Process Industries, Butterworth-Heinemann, Oxford, 1992.
[5] L.X. Yu, Pharmaceutical quality by design: product and process development, understanding, and control, *Pharm. Res.*, **25**, 781–791 (2008).
[6] D.T. Harvey, Modern Analytical Chemistry, McGraw-Hill, Dubuque, 1999.
[7] P.M. Gy, Introduction to the theory of sampling I. Heterogeneity of a population of uncorrelated units, *TRAC*, **14,** 67–76 (1995).
[8] L. Peterson, P. Minkkinnen, K.H. Esbensen, Representative sampling for reliable data analysis, *Chemom. Intell. Lab. Syst.*, **77**, 261–277 (2005).
[9] H.G. Brittain, Particle-size distribution ii: the problem of sampling powdered solids, *Pharm. Technol.*, **26**(7), 67–73 (2002).
[10] P. Gy, *Sampling for Analytical Purposes*, John Wiley & Sons, Ltd, Chichester, 1998.
[11] L. Peterson, C.K. Dahl, and K.H. Esbensen, Representative mass reduction in sampling – a critical survey of techniques and hardware, *Chemom. Intell. Lab. Syst.*, **74**, 95–114 (2004).
[12] J.C. Miller and J.N. Miller, *Statistics for Analytical Chemistry*, Ellis Horwood, Chichester, 1987.
[13] P. Gy, Sampling of discrete materials – a new introduction to the theory of sampling I. Qualitative approach, *Chemom. Intell. Lab. Syst.*, **74**, 7–24 (2004a).
[14] P. Gy, Sampling of discrete materials II. Quantitative Approach-sampling of zero dimensional objects, *Chemom. Intell. Lab. Syst.*, **74**, 25–38 (2004b).
[15] J. Berman, The compliance and science of blend uniformity analysis, *PDA J. Pharm. Sci. and Tech.,* **55**, 2001 (209–222).
[16] M. Howard-Sparks and A. Gawlikowski, Evaluation of blend uniformity and content uniformity based on 2003 Stratified Sampling Guidance and 1999 Blend Uniformity Analysis Guidance: Product A, *PDA J. Pharm. Sci. and Tech.*, **58**, 222–230 (2004).

[17] F.J. Muzzio, P. Robinson, and C. Wightman, D. Brone, Sampling practices in powder blending, *Int. J. Pharm*, **155**, 153–178 (1997).
[18] J. Kræmer, J.R. Svensson, and H. Melgaard, Sampling bias in blending validation and a different approach to homogeneity assessment, *Drug Dev. Ind. Pharm.*, **25**, 217–222 (1999).
[19] T. P. Garcia, S. J. Wilkinson, and J.F. Scott, The development of a blend-sampling technique to assess the uniformity of a powder mixture, *Drug Dev. Ind. Pharm.*, **27**, 297–307 (2001).
[20] F.J. Muzzio, M. Roddy, D. Brone, A.W. Alexander, and O. Sudah, An Improved powder sampling tool, *Pharm. Technol.*, **23**(4), 92–110 (1999).
[21] F.J. Muzzio, C.L. Goodridge, A. Alexander, P. Arratia, H. Yang, O. Sudah, and G. Mergen, Sampling and characterization of pharmaceutical powders and granular blends, *Int. J. Pharm*, **250**, 51 -64 (2003).
[22] T. Allen, *Powder Sampling and Particle Size Determination*, Elsevier, Amsterdam, 2003.
[23] L. Petersen and Kim H. Esbensen, Representative process sampling for reliable data analysis – a tutorial, *J. Chemometrics*, **19**, 625–647 (2005)
[24] R.C. Hwang and S.J. Wu, Challenges of blend uniformity testing for tablet formulation, *Amer. Pharm. Rev.*, **7**(1), 101–103 (2004).
[25] S. Bozzone, Solid oral dosage forms powder blending, *İkev Meeting* presentation, May **31**, 2001.
[26] G. Boehm, Report on the Industry Blend Uniformity Practices Survey, *Pharm. Technol.*, **25**(8), 20–26 (2001).
[27] H.J. Venables, Powder Sampling, *in Encyclopedia of Pharmaceutical Technology*, Marcel Dekker, New York 2007.
[28] H.J. Venables and J.I. Wells, Powder sampling, *Drug Dev. Ind. Pharm.*, **28**, 107–117 (2002).
[29] M. Popo, S. Romero-Torres, C. Conde, and R.J. Romañach, Blend uniformity analysis using stream sampling and near infrared spectroscopy, *AAPS PharmSciTech*, **3**(3), article 24 (2002).
[30] K.R. Shah, S.I. Faraq Badawi, M.M. Szemraj, D.B. Gray, and M.A. Hussain, Assessment of segregation potential of powder blends, *Pharm. Dev. Technol.*, **12**, 457–462 (2007).
[31] R.K. Chang, X. Guo, and J.W. Lai, The use of a rotary tablet press as a compacting spinning riffler for blending validation, *Pharm. Technol.*, **28**(3), 78–84 (2004).
[32] J.H. Timmermans, A report of the PQRI workshop on blend uniformity, *Pharm. Technol.*, **25**(9), 76–84 (2001).
[33] J.K, Prescott and T.P. Garcia, A solid dosage and blend content uniformity troubleshooting diagram, *Pharm. Technol.*, **25**(3), 68–79 (2001).
[34] G. Boehm, J. Clark, J. Dietrick, et al., The use of stratified sampling of blend and dosage units to demonstrate adequacy of mix for powder blends, *PDA J Pharm Sci and Tech.*, **57**, 67–74 (2003).
[35] E. D. Liss, S. L. Conway, J. A. Zega, and B. J. Glasser, Segregation of powders during gravity flow through vertical pipes, *Pharm. Technol.*, **28**(2), 78 (2004).
[36] M.J. Barajas, A. Rodriguez Cassiani, W. Vargas, C. Conde, J. Ropero, J. Figueroa, and R.J. Romañach, A near infrared spectroscopic method for real time monitoring of pharmaceutical powders during voiding, *Appl. Spectrosc.*, **61**, 490–496 (2007).
[37] C. Benedetti, N. Abatzoglou, J.S. Simard, L. McDermott , G. Léonard , L. Cartilier, Cohesive, multicomponent, dense powder flow characterization by NIR. *Int J Pharm*, **336**, 292–301 (2007).
[38] R.C. Lyon, D.S. Lester, E.N. Lewis, E. Lee, L.X. Yu, E.H. Jefferson, and A.S. Hussain, Near-infrared spectral imaging for quality assurance of pharmaceutical products: analysis of tablets to assess powder blend homogeneity, *AAPS PharmSciTech*, **3**(3), article 17 (2002).
[39] Food and Drug Administration, *PAT a Framework for Innovative Pharmaceutical Development, Manufacturing, and Quality Assurance*, September 2004.
[40] M.T. Carvajal, C. Velázquez, M. Alcalà, and R.J. Romañach, The time for process understanding, *Pharmaceutical Technology Europe*, **20**(5), 26–31 (2008)
[41] R.J. Romañach, Research initiatives to support science-based pharmaceutical manufacturing, *Pharmaceutical Technology Europe*, **19**(10), 47–51 (2007).
[42] H. Ma and C.A. Anderson, Characterization of pharmaceutical powder blends by NIR chemical imaging, *J. Pharm. Sci*, **97**, 3305–3320 (2008)

[43] A.S. El-Hagrasy, H.R. Morris, F. D'amico, R.A. Lodder and J.K. Drennen, Near-infrared spectroscopy and imaging for the monitoring of powder blend homogeneity, *J. Pharm. Sci.*, **90**, 1298–1307 (2001).

[44] International Conference on Harmonisation of Technical Requirements for Registration of Pharmaceuticals for Human Use, *ICH Harmonised Tripartite Guideline, Pharmaceutical Development Q8 (R1)*, Step 4, November 2008a.

[45] O. Berntsson, L.G. Danielsson, B. Lagerholm, and S. Folestad, Quantitative in-line monitoring of powder blending by near infrared reflection spectroscopy, *Powder Technol.*, **123**, 185–193 (2002).

[46] S. Sekulic, H.W. Ward, D.R. Brannegan , E.D. Stanley, C.L. Evans, S.T. Sciavolino, P.A. Hailey, and P.K. Aldridge, On-line monitoring of powder blend homogeneity by near-infrared spectroscopy. *Anal. Chem.*, **68**, 509–513 (1996).

[47] R.D. Maesschalck, F.C. Sánchez, D.L. Massart, P. Doherty, and P. Hailey, On-line monitoring of powder blending with near-infrared spectroscopy. *Appl. Spectrosc.* **52**, 725–732 (1998).

[48] L.J. Bellamy, A. Nordon, and D. Littlejohn, Effects of particle size and cohesive properties on mixing studied by non-contact NIR, *Int. J. Pharm.*, **361**, 87–91 (2008).

[49] Z. Shi, R.P. Cogdill, S.M. Short, and C.A. Anderson, Process characterization of powder blending by near-infrared spectroscopy: Blend end-points and beyond, *J. Pharm. Biomed. Anal.*, **47**, 738–745 (2008).

[50] A.S. El-Hagrasy, F. D'Amico, and J.K. Drennen III, A Process Analytical Technology approach to near-infrared process control of pharmaceutical powder blending. Part I: D-optimal design for characterization of powder mixing and preliminary spectral data evaluation, *J. Pharm. Sci*, **95**, 392–406 (2006a).

[51] A.S. El-Hagrasy, M. Delgado-Lopez, and J.K. Drennen III, A Process Analytical Technology approach to near-infrared process control of pharmaceutical powder blending: Part II: Qualitative near-infrared models for prediction of blend homogeneity, *J. Pharm. Sci.*, **95**, 407–421 (2006b).

[52] A.S. El-Hagrasy and J.K. Drennen III, A Process Analytical Technology approach to near-infrared process control of pharmaceutical powder blending. Part III: Quantitative near-infrared calibration for prediction of blend homogeneity and characterization of powder mixing kinetics, *J. Pharm. Sci.*, **95**, 422–434 (2006).

[53] C.V. Liew, A.D. Karande, and P.W.S. Heng, In-line quantification of drug and excipients in cohesive powder blends by near infrared spectroscopy, *Int. J. Pharm.*, **386**, 138–148 (2010).

[54] A.U. Vanarase, M. Alcalà, J.I. Jerez Rozo, F.J. Muzzio, and R.J. Romañach, Real-time monitoring of drug concentration in a continuous powder mixing process using NIR spectroscopy, *Chemical Engineering Science*, **65**(21), 5728–5733 (2010).

[55] C. Ufret and K.R. Morris, Modeling of powder blending using on-line near-infrared measurements, *Drug Dev. Ind. Pharm.*, **27,** 719–729 (2001).

[56] M. Blanco, J. Coello, A. Eustaquio, H. Iturriaga, and S. Maspoch, Development and validation of a method for the analysis of a pharmaceutical preparation by near-infrared diffuse reflectance spectroscopy, *J. Pharm. Sci.*, **88**, 551–556 (1999).

[57] H. Mark, *Principles and Practice of Spectroscopic Calibration*, John Wiley & Sons, Inc., New York, 1991.

[58] R.L. Green, G. Thurau, N.C. Pixley, A. Mateos, R.A. Reed, and J.P. Higgins, In-line monitoring of moisture content in fluid bed dryers using Near-IR spectroscopy with consideration of sampling effects on method accuracy, *Anal. Chem.*, **77**, 4515–4522 (2005).

[59] M. Halstensen and K. Esbensen, New developments in acoustic chemometric prediction of particle size distribution – the problem is the solution, *J. Chemometrics*, **14**, 463–481 (2000).

[60] T. Li, A.D. Donner, C.Y. Choi, G.P. Frunzi, and K.R. Morris, A statistical support for using spectroscopic methods to validate the content uniformity of solid dosage forms, *J. Pharm. Sci.*, **92**, 1526–1530 (2003).

[61] L.S. Wu, J. Pang, J.G. Chen, and M.A. Hussain, Dry blending process scale-up for a very low dose drug candidate, *AAPS PharmSciTech*, **1**(3), article TN2 (2000).

[62] T. Shinbrotand F.J. Muzzio, Mixing and segregation in tumbling blenders, *in Encyclopedia of Pharmaceutical Technology*, Marcel Dekker, New York, 2002.

[63] J.N. Staniforth, H.A. Ahmed, and P.J. Lockwood, Quality assurance in pharmaceutical: powder processing, *Drug Dev. Ind. Pharm.* **15**, 909–926 (1989).
[64] R.J. Romañach, PAT – A team effort, *Pharmaceutical Technology Europe*, **20**(10), 44–46 (2008).
[65] International Conference on Harmonisation of Technical Requirements for Registration of Pharmaceuticals for Human Use, *ICH Harmonised Tripartite Guideline, Pharmaceutical Quality System Q10*, Step 4, 4-June-2008b.
[66] R.A. Mendez, F. Muzzio, and C. Velazquez, Study of the effects of feed frames on powder blend properties during the filling of tablet press dies, *Powder Technol.*, **200**, 105–116 (2010).
[67] C. Peroza Meza, M.A. Santos, and R.J. Romañach, Quantitation of drug content in a low dosage formulation by transmission near infrared spectroscopy, *AAPS PharmSciTech*, **7**(1), Article 29 (2006).
[68] M. Blanco and M. Alcalà, Content uniformity and tablet hardness testing of intact pharmaceutical tablets by near infrared spectroscopy. A contribution to process analytical technologies, *Anal. Chim. Acta*, **557**, 353–359 (2006).
[69] H. Wikström, S. Romero-Torres, S. Wongweragiat, J.A. Stuart, E.R. Grant, and L.S. Taylor; On-line content uniformity determination of tablets using low-resolution Raman spectroscopy, *Appl. Spectrosc.*, **60**, 672–681 (2006).

Part II

Applications

5

Particles and Blending

Reuben D. Domike[1] *and Charles L. Cooney*[2]

[1] *Center for Biomedical Innovation, Massachusetts Institute of Technology, USA; and School of Business at the University of Prince Edward Island, Canada*

[2] *Department of Chemical Engineering, Massachusetts Institute of Technology, USA*

5.1 Introduction

Validated theoretical descriptions of powder movement or blending of powders composed of complex particles, such as those commonly found in pharmaceuticals, are not established (Metcalfe et al., 1995, Prescott and Barnum, 2000). Historically, the majority of theoretical descriptions of powder blending have been successfully applied to the mixing of spherical particles that differ only in color and do not account for variations in shape, cohesion, or interaction between the components being mixed (Wang and Fan, 1974). The results derived from theory based on such simplified systems have not been widely used for describing practical pharmaceutical powders and, as a result, most powder mixing science in use has been empirical. The empirical approaches employed have been primarily based on trial-and-error and provided limited insight into the fundamentals of powder blending or extrapolation to new powder systems (Crowder and Hickey, 2000, Hersey, 1976).

In order to fundamentally understand the macroscopic movement and blending of powders, an understanding of their discrete elements at smaller scales (individual particles and/or groups of particles; hereafter generally referred to as "particles") must be understood. The key parts of the relevant physics are the geometries of the particles and the interactions of particles with their surroundings. Particle geometry, interparticle forces and their impact on powder blending are discussed in theory and practice in this chapter.

Pharmaceutical Blending and Mixing, First Edition. Edited by P.J. Cullen, Rodolfo J. Romañach, Nicolas Abatzoglou and Chris D. Rielly.

5.2 Particle Geometry

Particle geometry includes the size and shape. Given that particles used in the production of pharmaceuticals can take on a wide range of geometries, defining measurements of geometry is useful to provide a common basis for discussion.

5.2.1 Particle Size and Size Distribution

Particle diameter is the most common metric of particle size. For non-spherical particles, multiple methods of measuring particle diameter are in use, some two-dimensional examples of which are shown in Figure 5.1 and all of which provide a different measure of "diameter" depending upon the shape of the particle. The Feret diameter is the distance between the perpendicular projections of the tangents to the extremities of the particle profile. The Martin diameter is equal to the length of a line that divides the particle profile into two equal areas. The equivalent circle diameter is the diameter of a circle that would occupy the same area that the particle occupies. Equivalent volume sphere diameter and equivalent surface-volume sphere diameter are also used when three-dimensional analysis is available. Depending upon how non-spherical the particles are, the different definitions of particle diameter may result in very different results (Alonso et al., 1991, Rhodes, 1998, Sastry et al., 1997, Snow et al., 1997).

Particle size and particle size distribution can be measured using a variety of methods. These methods include direct visualization of particles, sieving of powder to separate into groups of particles, and indirect measures.

Using direct visualization, optical microscopy can be used to measure particles as small as 5 μm in diameter. An electron microscope can be used to visualize smaller particles (Rhodes, 1998). For non-spherical particles, the diameters measured from microscopy are dependent on the profile orientation of the particles relative to the point of view (Rhodes, 1998, Snow et al., 1997). Direct visualization of small or cohesive particles can be difficult because the particles may be agglomerated or overlap one another while being visualized (Kaye, 1997). Reducing the population density of the particles (e.g., by using fewer particles and/or conditions of lower cohesion) in the field of view can reduce the overlap of particles being visualized.

Dry sieving with multiple sieves in series is a frequently employed method of determining particle size and size distribution based on the sizes of sieves being used. Dry sieving is regularly used for particles greater than 45 μm in diameter (Rhodes, 1998). With sufficient

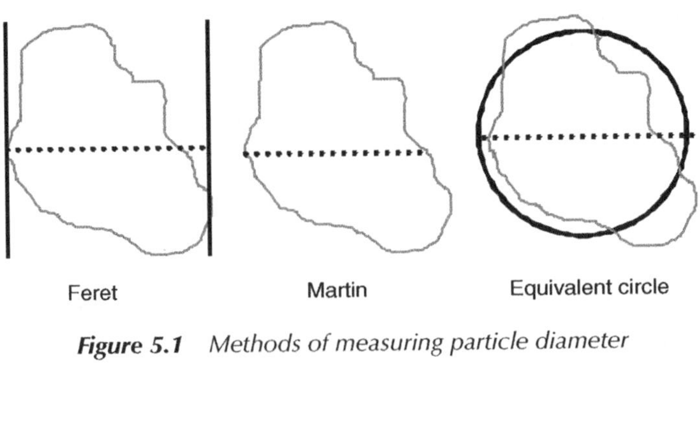

Figure 5.1 Methods of measuring particle diameter

agitation, the particles pass through sieves based on their narrowest diameter (of the diameters shown in Figure 5.1 that would be closest to the Feret diameter). Air jet sieving can reduce particle cohesion and increase agitation and has been reported to separate particle diameters down to 20 μm. Wet sieving, in which the particles are suspended in liquid, has been reported to separate particle diameters down to 5 μm (Rhodes, 1998). Two common difficulties associated with sieving are: the sieve mesh can be damaged in ways not obvious by visual inspection; and the particles must be effectively presented to the mesh, which can be difficult with cohesive particles and/or large loads of powder in which particles may not come in contact with the sieve (Snow, 1997). When these difficulties associated with sieving are overcome, then results from sieving can quantify the fraction of particles within ranges of particle size.

Other less direct methods for determining particle diameter include sedimentation, permeametry, electrozone sensing, laser diffraction, and photon correlation spectroscopy (PCS). Sedimentation of particles in a liquid relates the terminal velocity to equivalent surface-volume diameter. Permeametry relates the pressure drop of a fluid across a bed of randomly packed particles to the diameter of the particles. When non-spherical particles are used in permeametry, the calculated diameter is the equivalent surface-volume diameter. Electrozone sensing involves flowing particles through a tiny orifice that has a charge applied across it. The amplitude of the voltage pulse as a particle passes through the orifice is related to the particle volume. Laser diffraction relates the diffraction angle through a suspension of particles to the particle size yielding a "laser diameter" (Carstensen, 2001, Davies, 1997, Kaye, 1997, Rhodes, 1998). PCS is a method of determining particle sizes for small particles (nanometer to micrometer range) by monitoring their random motion due to molecular bombardment (Snow et al., 1997).

In powders, there is typically a distribution of particle sizes, which can be estimated by measuring the size of many different particles within the sample and/or dividing the sample into groups based on size (such as in sieving). Common particle size distributions that have been found empirically include arithmetic-normal (Gaussian) distribution, log-normal distribution, and Rosin–Rammler distribution (Alonso et al., 1991, Sastry et al., 1997).

5.2.2 Particle Shape and Shape Distribution

For non-spherical particles, the shapes and distribution of shapes within a sample can be diverse and difficult to describe. The most complete description of shape is to be able to view the particles in three dimensions. Simpler descriptions of shape have been developed to simplify the idea of shape into a single factor.

There are a number of different shape factors that are used to quantify particle shape and each provides slightly different descriptions of the particles. The volume shape factor is the ratio of particle volume to the particle diameter cubed. The surface shape factor is the ratio of particle surface area to the particle diameter squared. The specific surface shape factor is the ratio of surface shape factor to volume shape factor (Carstensen, 2001, Sastry et al., 1997). Sphericity, also called Carman's shape factor, is the ratio of the surface area of a sphere with the same volume as the particle to the surface area of the particle (Sastry et al., 1997, Rhodes, 1998). Circularity is the ratio of the perimeter of a circle with the same area to the perimeter of the particle.

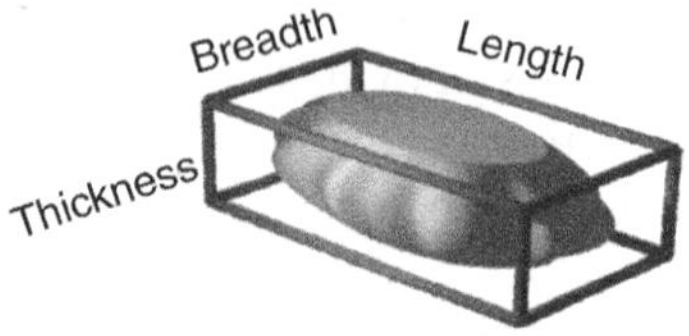

Figure 5.2 *Dimensions of a particle*

Some shape indices are also used to compare the relative lengths of the three dimensions of a particle. The thickness, the breadth, and the length of a non-spherical particle are shown in Figure 5.2. One index is the aspect ratio, or elongation, which is the maximum length of the particle profile divided by the width of the particle profile (Rhodes, 1998). The reciprocal of the aspect ratio is the chunkiness factor, which has a range from zero to one. Flakiness or flatness is the ratio of breadth to thickness. Zigg's index is the ratio of elongation to flakiness (Sastry et al., 1997).

As most particles are not smooth, descriptions of the shape of a particle can extend down from the full shape to surface features. One example metric of smoothness of the particle surface is the rugosity, which is the ratio of the particle perimeter to the perimeter of a smooth curve that circumscribes the particle perimeter. Another related metric is the surface roughness, which is the ratio of the perimeter of the particle to the perimeter of an ellipse with the same area (Gotoh, 1997). Surface features and topographies can have significant impact upon particle interactions with their surroundings.

5.3 Particle Interactions

The interactive surroundings of pharmaceutical particles typically include other particles, fluids (e.g., air, solvents), and equipment. As particles interact with these other items the particles may exert and/or experience forces of attraction and/or repulsion. Multiple types of theoretical forces may be acting simultaneously and the empirical force represents the net force by or on the particles. The theoretical forces that are commonly significant for interacting solids, and therefore relevant to particles, are described in the following sections.

5.3.1 van der Waals Forces

van der Waals forces are based on molecular attraction and decrease as the distance between particles increases. In a dry environment for powders, van der Waals forces are reported to be significant for particles less than one micron in diameter. When adsorbed liquid layers exist on the particles, then van der Waals forces have been reported to be important up to particle diameters of 100 μm (Rhodes, 1998).

Calculation of the theoretical van der Waals force between two spheres of different radii is given by Equation 5.1 (Masuda and Gotoh, 1997). In Equation 5.1, A is the Hamaker constant and depends upon the material of the particles (on the order of 10^{-19} or 10^{-20} J), l is the length between the two spheres, d_1 is the diameter of one sphere, d_2 is the diameter of the second sphere.

$$F_{vW} = \left(\frac{A}{12l^2}\right)\left(\frac{d_1 d_2}{d_1 + d_2}\right) \tag{5.1}$$

5.3.2 Electrostatic Forces

Electrostatic charging, or triboelectrification, occurs as a result of friction between particles and/or between particles and equipment. Electrons physically transfer between the different solids, and charge is accumulated (Rhodes, 1998). Electrostatic charges that build up may cause some particles to repel each other and others to attract each other. The electrostatic attraction between two spheres of equal diameter is given in Equation 5.2 (Shinohara, 1997). In Equation 5.2, q_1 is the charge of one sphere, q_2 is the charge of the second sphere, d is the diameter of the spheres, l is the distance between spheres. All else being equal, for a given type of material, the charge on a particle is approximately proportional to the surface area of the particle (Masuda and Gotoh, 1997). The charge per unit volume, or per mass, is then approximately inversely proportional to the particle diameter. A result of this is electrostatic forces are more important for smaller particles of a given type of material (Masuda and Gotoh, 1997).

$$F_e = \left(\frac{q_1 q_2}{d^2}\right)\left(1 - 2\frac{l}{d}\right) \tag{5.2}$$

The electrostatic charges and forces can be difficult to empirically quantify because they are commonly transient, irreproducible, and difficult to identify in comparison to other forces (Prescott and Barnum, 2000). However, there are some conditions that are found to influence electrostatic charges. High temperature and low humidity improve the environment for surface charges to accumulate and therefore the significance of electrostatic forces. The electrostatic forces are also increased by movement of the materials across one another (e.g., rubbing the materials together) as this increases the area of contact and can lead to charge accumulation. The surface area and the maximum charge density (specific to the type of material) limit the amount of charge that can accumulate on a particle. Different materials tend to accumulate charge with different levels of ease. Plastics, for example, tend to accumulate charge easily (Sastry et al., 1997). The interior of a plastic mixer may become coated with particles due to the accumulation of static charge.

In situations where electrostatic charges are negatively impacting powder flow, blending, or content uniformity, there are some actions that can be taken in attempt to relieve static include: (1) addition of solids with high surface to weight ratios that do not accumulate charge readily, (2) addition of liquids, (3) changing the interior material and configuration of the equipment, (4) increasing the humidity in the mixing environment, and (5) preparing the powders to reduce the accumulated charge (Sastry et al., 1997)

5.3.3 Adsorbed Liquid Layers and Liquid Bridges

When a condensable vapor is in contact with solid particles, some of the vapor will condense on the particles. The thickness of the resulting liquid layer is dependent upon the vapor pressure of the condensable vapor. Bonding forces between particles can develop if the liquid layers of the particles overlap on contact. The bond strength is dependent upon the area of overlap of the layers and the surface tension of the liquid (Rhodes, 1998).

When a large amount of condensed vapor is present in the system, then liquid bridges can form between particles. The state of the liquid bridges in a system can be categorized into four types. With increasing levels of liquid between particles, the states are referred to as pendular, funicular, capillary, and droplet. The pendular state is when there is a thin liquid bridge between particles, each bridge distinct from one another. The surface tension of the liquid draws the particles together. Capillary pressure resulting from the curvature of the liquid bridges also attracts the particles to each other. Moderately increasing the amount of liquid present reduces the likelihood of the bridges breaking and reduces the curvature of the liquid bridges. The funicular, capillary, and droplet states all correspond to increasing amounts of liquid between particles and decreased attractive forces as the bridges disappear. In the capillary and droplet states, all of the volume between particles is occupied by liquid (Rhodes, 1998).

The force between particles caused by a liquid bridge is found by summing the capillary force and the surface tension force, as shown in Equation 5.3 (Masuda and Gotoh, 1997). In Equation 5.3, r_2 is the radius of the liquid bridge, P_{LB} is the capillary pressure inside the liquid bridge, σ is the surface tension of the liquid in air (assuming that the interaction is occurring in air).

$$F_{LB} = \pi r_2^{\ 2} P_{LB} + 2\pi\sigma r_2 \tag{5.3}$$

When the liquid bridge cross section is approximated as a circular arc, as shown in Figure 5.3, the capillary pressure can be found in Equation 5.4 (Masuda and Gotoh, 1997). In Equation 5.4, r_1 is the radius of the circular arc.

$$P_{LB} = \sigma\left(1/r_1 - 1/r_2\right) \tag{5.4}$$

5.3.4 Solid Bridges

Solid bridges can either form when liquid is removed from a system, or by chemical reaction, or by solidification of melted components (Shinohara, 1997). In the cases of solid bridges formed on the removal of liquid, crystalline bridges may form upon liquid evaporation if the particle is soluble in the liquid. Alternatively, some portion of the liquid, such as a binder, may remain upon evaporation and create a liquid binder bridge. Solid bridges are typically more permanent bridges than liquid bridges as the materials are less mobile (Rhodes, 1998).

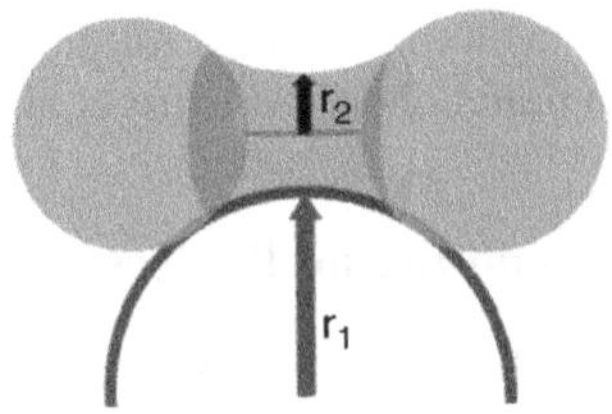

Figure 5.3 *Liquid bridge between two particles of equal diameter*

5.3.5 Use of AFM to Measure Interparticle Forces

Empirical measurement of forces between microscopic particles is non-trivial. One method that has been used to measure such forces is atomic force microscopy (AFM) by which two materials can be brought in close proximity and/or contact while measuring the force between the materials. By aligning a laser on the back of an AFM cantilever and reflecting the laser onto a photodiode, the microscopic movement of the material on the tip of the cantilever can be monitored as it is brought in contact with a second material. The cantilever is assumed to bend like a spring and the deflection of the cantilever monitored by the position of the laser reflection using the photodiode. For contact between the material on the tip and the second material in the direction normal to the second material, the force on the cantilever, F_C, is proportional to its deflection, δ_C, multiplied by its normal spring constant, k_N. This relationship is presented in Equation 5.1 (Florin et al., 1995).

$$F_C = k_N \delta_C \tag{5.5}$$

By approaching the tip to the sample surface and monitoring the change in the vertical position of the laser on the photodiode, information on any attractive or repulsive forces on approach can be obtained. Similarly, monitoring the cantilever deflection during the retraction of the tip from the sample after contact provides information on adhesion between the surfaces. An image of the cantilever with a particle adhered to the tip is shown in Figure 5.4.

Once the normal spring constant is determined, then the deflection of the cantilever can be related to relative force measurements. By completing a "force pull" (bring the particles together and then retracting them), the interparticle forces can be quantified. The quantified force from a sample force pull is presented in Figure 5.5 between two lactose particles. In this example, one lactose particle was adhered to the end of a cantilever and the second was placed on a sample disc that had been covered with double-sided tape. The force pull presented in Figure 5.5 is typical for interparticle AFM measurements. The gray shaded line (from right to left) is the force felt by the cantilever as the two particles approach one another. There is no change in force until the particles come within nanometers of one another. At this point, they are attracted to one another and "jump-to-contact" each other. This can be seen as a slight dip (attraction) in the relative force acting on the cantilever.

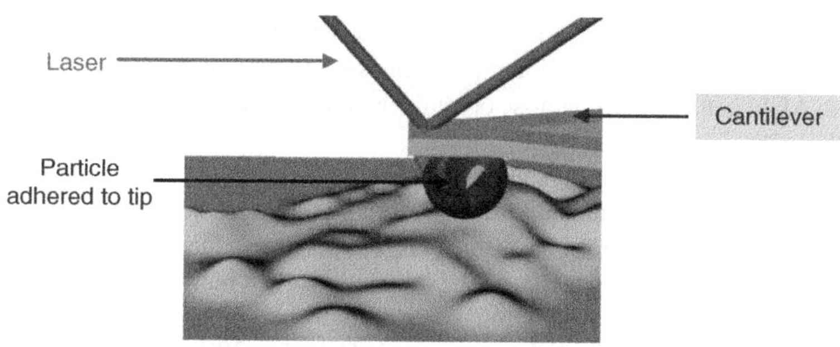

Figure 5.4 *Cantilever with adhered particle*

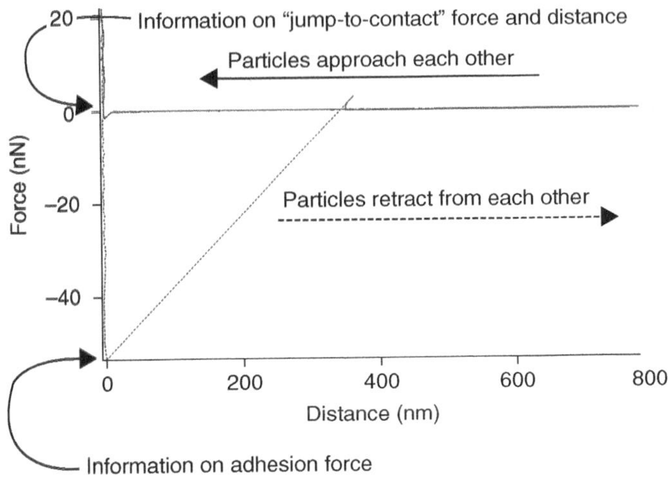

Figure 5.5 *Sample force curve between two lactose particles*

The particles are then pushed together with a predetermined amount of applied force (about 20 nN in this case) before being retracted from each other. The forces measured over the course of the retraction are presented with the dotted line. There is a relatively large force required to remove the particles from each other (labeled as "adhesion force"). After this adhesion force is overcome, then the cantilever springs back to its initial position. This spring back appears as a linear change in the force curve, but the particles are not in contact during this time, so additional information cannot be found in this part of the curve (Domike, 2004).

Forces between pharmaceutical solids have been measured with AFM previously, including some measured interactions between APIs and excipients (Berard et al., 2002, Eve et al., 2002, Price et al., 2002, Sindel and Zimmermann, 2001). For example, Berard et al. (2002) investigated the interaction between an inhalant drug crystal (zanamivir) and compacts of lactose at a range of humidities. The adhesion force ranged from 100–1000nN with significant dependence on the relative humidity. Similarly, Eve et al. (2002) investigated the rank order of adhesion between three AFM tips with micronized salbutamol particles adhered and glass, lactose, salbutamol, and polytetrafluoroethylene (PTFE). The adhesion force between the particle and both sulbutamol and PTFE was found to increase on repeated contact. This was attributed to electrostatic charging of the particles, although blunting of the tips or sample particles may have increased the contact area and total adhesion force. Price et al. (2002) investigated the adhesion of two types of drug particles, each adhered to an AFM cantilever, to lactose crystals over a range of humidities. As the humidity increased, the adhesion also increased.

The physical interface between the two materials used in the AFM methodology can have a significant impact on the measured force. For example, Sindel and Zimmerman (2001) investigated the interaction between a lactose particle adhered to the end of an AFM cantilever and a flat compact of lactose. The adhesion forces measured were between 0nN and 12nN. These values were significantly lower than the values found for adhesion between two lactose particles previously mentioned (Domike, 2004) and significantly lower than the force calculated per particle contact from macroscopic measurements of the bulk powder using a tensile strength tester and a Jenike shear cell (Schweiger and Zimmermann, 1999). The difference in these values is likely caused by the simplistic flat surface presented by the compact of lactose instead of the complex surface of a lactose particle, which may have larger contact area and topographical features that would physically bond with another lactose particle.

5.3.6 Interparticle Friction

The lateral movement of one material across a second results in a frictional resistance to the movement. In many common cases, the frictional force depends linearly on the applied load. This relationship is usually interpreted as a "boundary layer" model of friction and its development is attributed to Eyring (1935). The linear relationship between friction force and applied load is commonly called Amonton's law (9Bowden and Tabor, 1950). Physically, Amonton's law can result from the interaction of multiple plastically deformable asperities in contact. The resulting relationship between friction and applied load is theoretically independent of both contact area and sliding velocity for smooth surfaces (Muerk, 2000).

Using AFM, Hu et al. (1995) found experimentally that there was no dependence of friction force on sliding velocity for the interaction of a silicon nitride tip and mica. However, for surfaces with asperities Sundararajan et al. 2000) demonstrated that the friction coefficient will be dependent upon the applied load and velocity. The extent of these dependencies is complex and specific to the particles of interest.

A more general relationship between friction and applied force has the form presented in Equation 5.6. The friction force, f, is dependent on the sum of the applied load, L, and the adhesion, A, raised to a load index, n, and multiplied by a friction coefficient, μ. The adhesion in this way is treated as an additional applied load. The load index typically varies between two-thirds and one. A value of two-thirds corresponds to an elastic response and a value of unity corresponds to contacting of multiple asperities (Muerk, 2000). When the load index is equal to one, then the friction coefficient is constant for all applied loads.

$$f = \mu(L + A)^n \qquad (5.6)$$

Three recent works have quantified friction force between a bead adhered to the end of an AFM cantilever and flat or bead samples. Bhushan and Sundararajan (2000) investigated the friction between glass beads and surfaces of very smooth Si(100) samples. A number of different beads were used and the diameter of the beads ranged from 7.6 to 29 μm. A linear relationship between friction force and applied load was found and the coefficients of friction between the beads and the sample ranged from 0.01 to 0.15, with the larger beads demonstrating larger coefficients of friction than the smallest beads.

Meurk, et al. (2001) investigated the friction between silicon nitride beads and flat metal substrates or with other silicon nitride beads. The beads contained various amounts of poly(ethylene glycol) binder that, with increasing concentration, was found to reduce the friction coefficients. Three different beads (each with a different binder concentration) were used for friction measurements with other beads. The range of friction coefficients for these experiments was 0.06–0.07 and the load index ranged from 0.76 to 0.98.

The friction forces are specific to the particles and the environment. The environment can change over time as demonstrated by McLellan and Shand (1984) whose experiments on interactions between glass showed that the macroscopic friction coefficient of glass-glass contacts is dependent upon the cleanliness of the surfaces. Immediately after glazing, the friction coefficient was close to unity. One day after the glazing, the friction coefficient dropped to a range of 0.18–0.24.

5.4 Empirical Investigations of Particles and Blending

Many investigations into powder blending have considered variations of materials, equipment, and conditions. Significantly fewer of the historical investigations into powder blending directly consider the particle geometry and/or interactions. One key exception to this is recent simulations of powder flow that incorporate microscopic particle properties, which are discussed in Chapter 17.

A brief theoretical description of blending (further details can be found in Chapter 2) is followed by summaries of empirical investigations of particle geometry and interactions to blending.

5.4.1 Blending of Powders

There are two commonly described regimes of flow in powder tumbling blenders – avalanching and surface cascading. The avalanching flow regime is encountered at relatively low rotation speeds. In modeling the avalanching behavior, some investigators have described the process by a single constant angle of avalanche, which has been experimentally demonstrated to be dependent upon the container geometry and the powder properties (McCarthy, 1996, Peratt and Yorke, 1996, Schwedes, 2000). Alternatively, some researchers have found that there is a distribution of avalanche angle and that the state of a system within a tumble mixer undergoing avalanching is determined by chaotic dynamics with complex periodicity (Crowder and Hickey, 2000).

The mixing of identical particles (perhaps with variations only in color) within an avalanche has been modeled as a random map consisting of two parts, as shown in Figure 5.6. The radial mixing is described by a uniform random distribution and the axial mixing is described by a cross-sectionally averaged diffusion equation leading to a Gaussian random distribution (McCarthy, 1996). Non-identical particles may have other mixing patterns within an avalanche.

Another regime of powder flow encountered at higher speeds of rotation within a tumbling mixer is the surface cascading regime. The speed corresponding to the

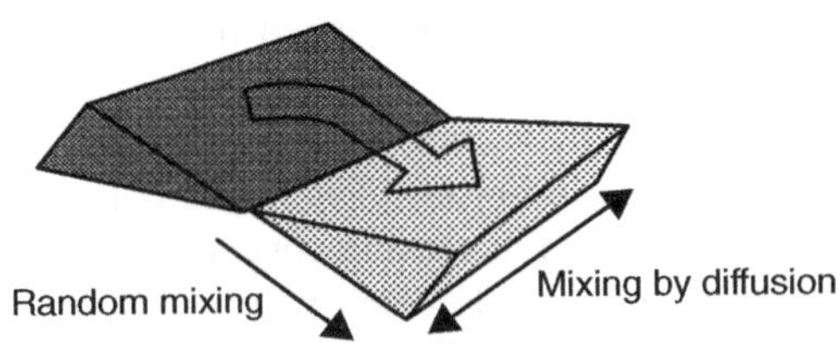

Figure 5.6 Ideal avalanching behavior

transition between the two regimes of flow in the tumble mixer is dependent upon the powders being mixed, the shape of the mixer, and upon the material of the mixer wall. The surface cascading regime is characterized by an approximately constant slope of powder surface and a thin layer of powder flowing down the surface (Carley-Macauly and Donald, 1964).

5.4.1.1 Mechanisms of Powder Mixing

The mechanisms of powder mixing in tumble mixers have been described as convective, shear, and diffusive (Muzzio et al., 2000). The dominant mechanism as the mixing proceeds changes from convective to shear to diffusive as the blend is mixed. An example plot of heterogeneity or unmixedness, σ, as the mixing proceeds is shown in Figure 5.7 (Hogg et al., 1966, Muzzio et al., 2000). Three sections are commonly found in the characteristic curve. The first section (I) is dominated by convection, the second section (II) has less convective and more shear, and the third section (III) is dominated by diffusion (Miyanami, 1997).

Convective Mixing. Convection is the transfer of a group of adjacent particles from one location to another in the mixture. Away from the axial center of the mixer, convection is initially much faster than the slower diffusion mechanism. As the mixing process proceeds and homogeneity is approached, the length-scale associated with heterogeneity becomes relatively small and diffusion becomes the primary mechanism for mixing throughout the mixer (Wang and Fan, 1974).

Shear Mixing. The shear mechanism has been defined as "the change in the configuration of the components via the setting up of slipping planes within the mixture" (Bridgwater, 1976, Wang and Fan, 1974). These slipping planes are common in the narrow region below a cascading surface. This region is characterized by high shear and density gradients as the "shear" region.

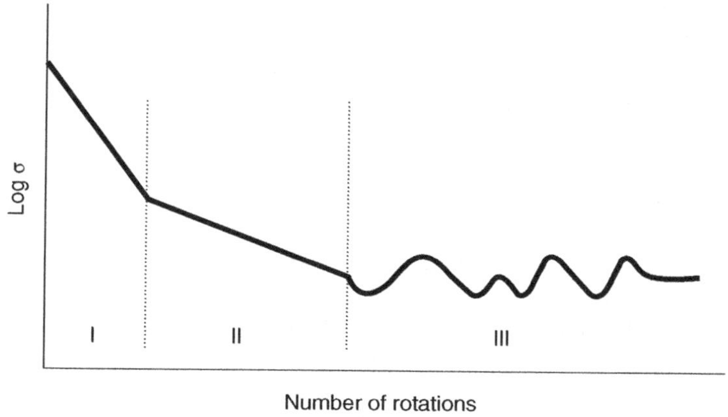

Figure 5.7 *Characteristic curve of mixing*

Diffusive Mixing. The diffusion mechanism is due to the random motion of the particles on the powder surface as the mixer rotates and agitates the particles. Diffusion is slow relative to the other mixing mechanisms. Blenders with axial symmetry, such as the bin blender and the tube blender, usually have diffusive mixing across the plane of symmetry (Muzzio, 2000).

5.4.1.2 Completion of Blending

During the blending of non-segregating powders, the blend will approach a steady state level of mixedness as described in detail in Chapter 2. Once the measurement of mixedness is relatively constant, the mixing process can be considered complete. For powders that are found to segregate on further blending, an optimum blend time may exist, above and below which the blend is less well mixed.

Mixtures that are completely mixed may be random or ordered in their distribution of particles. For any system not composed of particles with identical physical properties, the random state is not empirically expected due to tendencies for bias of movement (Bridgwater, 1976). In powder mixtures, ordered systems occur when an identical number of one type of particle (such as small particles) adhere to each particle of another type of particle (such as large particles) (Domike, 2004).

5.4.2 Impact of Particle Geometry on Blending

Powders containing groups of particles with different physical properties have been demonstrated to have a tendency to segregate. When a powder mixture is perturbed in such a way as to cause movement, rearrangement of the particle packing can take place. Gaps between particles may form, into which particles may fall. Smaller particles are more likely to fall down into gaps than large particles. As a result, the propensity to segregate is reported as being most common in non-cohesive powders with particles that differ greatly in size. This can lead to segregation of the powder mixture based on particle size. The regions consisting of smaller particles may form and be better packed than the rest of the powder mixture and may resist the action of the mixer (Bridgwater, 1976, Rhodes, 1998).

The size of the particles has been found to have a significant effect on the blend homogeneity of a mixture (Hwang et al., 1998, Johanson, 1978, Williams, 1976). Williams states that all available evidence demonstrates that the most important factor in segregation is differences in particle sizes of the mixture components. Williams investigated the mixing in an inclined drum of identical particles with mean diameters between 100 and 500 μm and found that segregation decreased as mean particle diameter decreased (Williams, 1976). Marinelli and Carson (1992) attribute reduced segregation for smaller particles to greater cohesive strength of finer particles.

When non-identical particles are mixed, segregation based on sifting can occur. Sifting of smaller particles to the bottom has been found to occur even when the large particles have higher density than the small particles (Williams, 1976, Zhou et al., 2002). For mixtures of particles all of the same size but with different densities, no segregation was found (Williams, 1976). One experiment using glass beads found that the percolation of small particles to the bottom of the mixture occurred for beads of equal density provided that the ratio of diameters of the different types of beads exceeded a value of two (Williams, 1976).

When one particle type was denser and smaller than the second particle type, a diameter ratio of 1.7 was sufficient to cause segregation, showing that differences in density may have an effect on percolation due to size differences (Williams, 1976).

Work by Bridgwater (1976) suggests that the motion of small spheres through a randomly packed bed of large spheres can occur spontaneously, without strain applied to the system, under some conditions. A radial Peclet number was used to describe the extent of dispersion in these systems. The rate of particle sifting due to size differences has been described in terms of diffusion (Williams, 1976).

Johanson (2000) suggests that when the small particles are more numerous than required to fill all of the voids between large particles or if the fines are too cohesive to flow into the voids, then segregation by sifting will not occur. Alonso et al. (1991) suggest that when particles are sufficiently small, the particle-particle cohesive forces may overcome the force of gravity acting on the body and hinder downward sifting. For comparison, segregation is reported as being seldom found when all particles in a powder mixture are less than about 50 μm. In such fine powders, forces holding the powders together, as described in Section 5.3, are large relative to the gravitational and inertial forces (Kaye, 1997, Rhodes, 1998). The particles stick to one another and are not free to move independently.

Marinelli and Carson (1992) state that particle shape is less important than particle size in flow properties and that irregularly shaped particles have more difficulty flowing than regularly shaped particles. Bridgwater (1976) found that powders with wide shape distributions formed relatively strong agglomerates. The same study suggests that the role of particle shape on segregation needs further examination (1976).

5.4.3 Impact of Interparticle Forces on Blending

When agglomeration does occur, the agglomerates are susceptible to the mixing and segregation mechanisms. Cohesive effects are described as having the potential to alter the sifting mechanism because the cohesive solid may form a thick sliding layer that does not allow percolation (Johanson, 1978). The agglomerates may be broken up or built up during blending and thereby may decrease or increase segregation. Where agglomerates are significant and need to be broken up, high-shear mixers can be used to facilitate the breaking up of agglomerates (Johanson, 2000).

5.4.3.1 Impact of Humidity

High levels of humidity may increase cohesion between particles. Liquid bridges of water have been visually found at the microscopic level for relative humidities greater than 65% (Masuda and Gotoh, 1997). The increase in cohesion is reported as more pronounced for coarse particles than fine particles (Shinohara, 1997). High humidity may also reduce electrostatic interaction among particles.

Capillary forces between lactose particles at high humidity have been reported as significant by Podczeck et al. (1996, 1997) with adhesion force measured using a centrifugal technique and, in separate work, by Berard et al. (2002) using AFM. In their studies, the force required to remove lactose particles from themselves in a bulk measurement was nearly independent of humidity below values of 75%. Above this threshold, the adhesion force required increased. In the centrifugal experiments, the adhesion force increased dramatically (three-fold increase in adhesion for humidity change from 30 to 90%). In the AFM experiments by Berard et al. (2002), the adhesion between lactose crystals increased about 50% as the relative humidity increased from 30 to 80%.

One study by Forsyth et al. (2002) has investigated the effect of relative humidity on both adhesion between a glass bead on an atomic force microscopy (AFM) cantilever and a glass slide and flow of glass beads in a rotating apparatus. At the microscopic level, the force between the bead and plate showed no change for humidities less than 40%. Above 40% relative humidity, the maximum adhesion force increased significantly with increasing humidity. At 90% RH, the maximum cohesion is 70% higher than the maximum cohesion at 40% RH. At the macroscopic level, the flow of glass beads was found to change from free-flow behavior to avalanching behavior at a critical relative humidity. The value of the critical relative humidity was dependent upon the size of the glass beads (larger glass beads had a higher critical relative humidity). The adhesion force measured with AFM was only done with the smallest glass beads in the experiments (16 μm diameter) and the adhesion force as measured by AFM increased for all relative humidity values (there was not a consistent critical humidity found for both microscopic and macroscopic experiments).

In a separate set of experiments, the same study calculated the theoretical interparticle force at which the flow transition occurred for iron spheres in a magnetic field [20]. Three sets of particles with particle diameters from 250–1600 μm and the flow transition occurred at a Bond number, shown in Equation 5.7, of about 9 in all cases. The Bond number quantifies the ratio of interparticle force to gravitational force and provides an estimation of the relative importance of microscopic interparticle forces.

$$\mathrm{Bo} = \frac{\text{Adhesion Force}}{\text{Gravitational Force}} = \frac{F_A}{F_G} \tag{5.7}$$

Beyond just relative humidity changes, Williams (1976) completed experiments of adding small quantities of water to powder mixtures and monitoring segregation. After adding 2% water by weight to free-flowing sand, segregation was dramatically reduced in a rotating drum. This trend was found in a tumbling mixer as well.

5.4.3.2 *Impact of Lubricants*

A small amount of lubricants are typically used to improve the flowability or blending of a mixture. The lubricants may alter the arrangement of particles or discharge electrostatic charge (Kaye, 1997, Masuda and Gotoh, 1997). Taylor et al. (2000) found amorphous fumed silica and/or magnesium stearate with a weight fraction ranging from 0.001 to 0.015 improved the flow of their pharmaceutical mixtures.

5.4.3.3 *Angle of Repose Differences*

The angle of repose of a pile of powder is commonly used as a metric of powder flowability dependent upon the particle geometry and interparticle forces. When materials with different angles of repose are mixed or poured, the material with the steeper angle tends to concentrate in the center of the pile or mixer (Johanson, 1978). Segregation by the angle of repose mechanism has been described as accentuating segregation due to size differences because fines are usually found to have a higher angle of repose than coarse particles (Johanson, 1978, 2000). From the center of the powder pile, the small particles would percolate down through the pile. A powder mixture that is cohesive will be less likely to segregate based on differences in angle of repose. The importance of angle of repose extends to blending as angles of repose differences has been described as the primary mechanism of segregation in tumble mixers (Johanson, 2000)

5.4.4 Impact of Blender Conditions on Blending

Blend performance or segregation for a set of particles depends upon the blending conditions. Experiments related to the material of construction of the interior of the container, blender rotation speed, and loading fraction in the blender are summarized in the following sections.

5.4.4.1 Impact of Material of Construction of the Container Wall

Certain particles within the mixture may be preferentially attracted to the wall, either by shape, size, moisture content, or electrostatic charge. The area near the container wall can be prone to have relatively high electrostatic charge, which can lead to cohesive agglomeration of particles. When the particle diameter is larger than 1/20 of the tube diameter in flow through a tube, significant wall effects have been found. Additionally, a container with a rough wall has been shown to be less conducive to free flow than a similar container with a smooth wall (Bridgwater et al., 1968, Carstensen, 2001).

5.4.4.2 Impact of Mixer Rotation Speed

Two differing empirical results of the impact of mixer speed have been reported. In one study, the effect of speed of rotation in a horizontal cylinder tumbler upon the mixing kinetics was found to have no general effect but perhaps a complex secondary effect (Carley-Macauly and Donald, 1964). In a separate study, it is concluded that the mixer speed has a large effect upon the pattern of powder segregation. At low mixer speed, formation of a core of segregated particles occurred and bands of segregated particles also formed. Increasing the mixer speed first reduces the number of bands, and then their intensity, and then the central core is eliminated (Rogers and Clements, 1971).

5.4.4.3 Impact of Loading Fraction

The impact of loading fraction upon mixing is dependent on the mixer type studied. For fill levels above one-half in most bin blender designs, a central core of material can form that will never avalanche and will not participate in the mixing process. The loading fraction in a tumbling mixer is described by Carley-Macauly and Donald (1964) as having the most outstanding impact of any variables upon the mixing kinetics. In their experimental work, the fastest mixing appears to occur at small load fractions.

5.5 Simulation Techniques

A number of different types of models of powder movement have been investigated by previous researchers. Three types of models are presented in the following sections.

5.5.1 Full Physics Models Using Discrete Element Modeling

Discrete element models that simulate particle movement, every particle collision, and track the forces on each particle through every time simulated time point are in use. Modelling of this type is described in greater detail in Chapter 17. The equations of motion are integrated over time to determine the position and velocity of every particle. At each time step, any contacts between neighboring particles are determined, the forces from the contacts are evaluated, and the equations of motion are integrated for all particles.

The primary advantage to this model is that it is physically rigorous and accounts for every particle as opposed to a continuum approach. Additionally, in theory, the particle geometries and interparticle forces incorporated into the model can be based on experimentally measured values and thereby incorporate all relevant physics.

The primary disadvantage to this model is that it is computationally intensive. It may not be feasible to run this simulation long enough to determine whether segregation of different particles will occur. Particle geometries more complex than spheres require increased amount of computation time. To limit computation time required, simplifications of geometries and/or forces are employed that have the potential to reduce the accuracy of the results. For example, in modelling blending, Ottino and McCarthy (1998) suggest simulating the bulk of the material in the mixer as stagnant and only calculating interactions near the powder surface to reduce computation time. They found that this method decreased the computation time by an order of magnitude for the two tumbler systems investigated.

DEM simulations have been applied to applications similar to the flow and blending of pharmaceutical powders. By varying the interparticle friction coefficient and modelling all particles as non-cohesive spheres, a coefficient of friction can be found that accurately predicts the macroscopic flow pattern measured experimentally (Moakher et al., 2001, Stewart et al., 2001, Zhou et al., 2002). However, in a detailed analysis, Stewart et al. (2001) found that different areas of the simulated mixer required different coefficients of friction to correctly predict the flow. This apparently nonphysical result highlights the importance of complete and correct particle geometries and forces.

The incorporation of cohesion can significantly improve accuracy of the modelling as demonstrated by Nase et al. (2001) in completing a two-dimensional DEM simulation of round particles, with diameters between 0.5 and 10 mm, which included cohesion from theoretical liquid-liquid bridges. The simulation results compared well with experimental studies of a similar system composed of spherical glass beads with water added (2001).

5.5.1.1 Modeling Particle Interactions

The most common method of modelling pharmaceutical particles where interactions are important is to use a "soft" particle model. The soft particle model allows for contacts of finite time between particles. This is achieved by allowing colliding particles to overlap slightly. A particle may collide with more than one other particle at a given time. Each contact exerts a force and a moment, which are summed for each particle and used to determine the trajectory of the particle. The description of collisions of the particles contains three basic components (Campbell et al., 1997):

1. A normal force at the point of contact that pushes the particles apart.
2. Energy dissipating during collision
3. Frictional interaction that acts tangential to the area of particle contact.

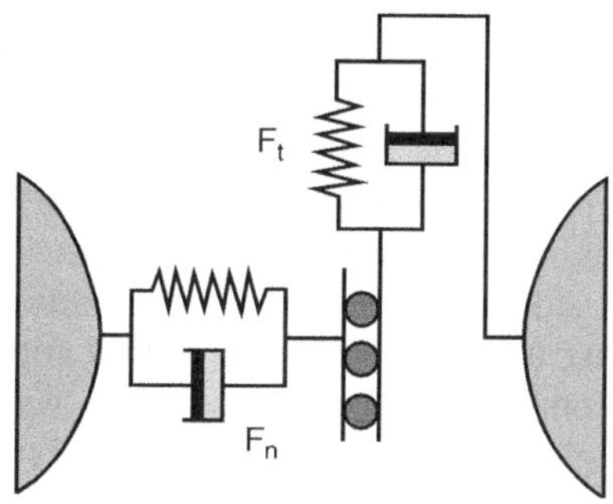

Figure 5.8 *Spring and dashpot model of particle collisions. Reprinted with permission from ref. [10]. Copyright (2001) Elsevier*

Typically, a spring is used to model elastic deformation of the contacting surfaces and a dashpot is used to model plastic deformation. The tangential forces acting on the particles are limited by friction, represented by the discs in Figure 5.8 (Cleary, 2001). The equations of the normal, F_n, and tangential forces, F_t, acting on a particle are given in Equations 5.8 and 5.9. The normal force is dependent upon the particle overlap, Δx, the spring constant, k, the normal velocity, v_n and the damping coefficient, C. The tangential force is usually linearly proportional to the normal force. The proportionality constant is the friction coefficient, μ.

$$F_n = -k \cdot \Delta x + C \cdot v_n \tag{5.8}$$

$$F_t = \min\left\{\mu \cdot F_n, \int k \cdot v_t \cdot dt + C \cdot v_t\right\} \tag{5.9}$$

In addition to the geometric inputs for use in the simulation, typical inputs that depend on the powder properties include coefficients of restitution for particles, coefficients for the springs, particle-particle friction coefficients, and particle-wall friction coefficients (Cleary and Hoyer, 2001, Nase et al., 2001). The difficulty of measuring some these input parameters are was discussed in Sections 5.3.5 and 5.3.6. The input parameters can be constant for all particles, or varied for different particles within the mixture.

5.5.2 Continuum Models

Continuum models of powder movement treat the powder similarly to a fluid. Continuity equations that conserve both mass and momentum are commonly used. The properties of the powder are continuous functions and the discrete nature of individual particles is not considered. Some continuum models include microstructural parameters that improve the predictive power of the model (Moakher et al., 2000). Continuum models have been demonstrated to be somewhat successful in applications related to soil mechanics where cohesion between particles is usually not important. Continuum models have not been demonstrated to be successful with pharmaceutical powders (Thomson, 1997).

5.5.3 Cellular Automata

The cellular automata discrete method applies deterministic rules to particle motion. One cellular automata model of a tumbling mixer that has been developed by Muzzio et al. (2001) assumes that particle rearrangements only occur in the surface layer of the powder. The surface layer is further assumed to be a plane. The plane is broken up into gridpoints, at which particles may be located. The different types of particles in the mixture have different probabilities of moving to a new gridpoint. With a correctly chosen set of model parameters, the cellular automata model compared well with experimental studies of tumbling mixers filled with glass beads but is not likely to be applicable to new systems (Muzzio et al., 2001).

References

Alonso, M., Satoh, M., and Miyanami, K. "Optimum combination of size ratio, density ratio and concentration to minimize free surface segregation," *Powder Technology*, 68, pp. 145–152 (1991).

Berard, V., Lesniewska, E., Andres, C., Pertuy, D., Laroche, C., and Pourcelot, Y. "Affinity scale between a carrier and a drug in DPI studied by atomic force microscopy," *Intl. J. of Pharmaceutics*, 247 (1–2), pp. 127–137 (2002).

Bowden, F.P. and Tabor, D. *The Friction and Lubrication of Solids*, Oxford University Press, London, 1950.

Bridgwater, J., "Fundamental powder mixing mechanisms," *Powder Technology*, 15, pp. 215–236 (1976).

Bridgwater, J., Bagster, D.F., Chen, S.F., and Hallam, J.H. "Geometric and dynamic similarity in particle mixing," *Powder Technology*, 2, pp. 198–206 (1968.

Campbell, C.S., Potapov, A.V., and Tsuji, Y. "Simulation," in Gotoh, K., Masuda, H., and Higashitani, K. (eds), *Powder Technology Handbook*, Marcel Dekker, New York, pp. 777–815, (1997).

Carley-Macauly, K.W., and Donald, M.B. "The mixing of solids in tumbling mixers-II," *Chemical Engineering Science*, 19, pp. 191–199 (1964).

Carstensen, J.T., *Advanced Pharmaceutical Solids*, Marcel Dekker, Inc., New York (2001).

Cleary, P.W., "Charge behaviour and power consumption in ball mills: sensitivity to mill operating conditions, linear geometry and charge composition," *International Journal of Mineral Processing*, 63, pp. 79–114 (2001).

Cleary, P.W. and Hoyer, D. "Centrifugal mill charge motion and power draw: comparison of DEM predictions with experiment," *International Journal of Mineral Processing*, 59, pp. 131–148 (2000).

Crowder, T.M. and Hickey, A.J. "The physics of powder flow applied to pharmaceutical solids," *Pharmaceutical Technology*, Feb., pp. 50–58 (2000).

Davies, R., "Size measurement," in Gotoh, K., Masuda, H., and Higashitani, K. (eds), *Powder Technology Handbook*, Marcel Dekker, New York, pp.15–42 (1997).

Domike, R.D., *Pharmaceutical Powders in Experiment and Simulation: Towards a Fundamental Understanding*, Massachusetts Institute of Technology, Cambridge, MA, USA, (2004).

Egermann, H. and Orr, N.A. "Ordered mixtures – interactive mixtures," *Powder Technology*, 36, pp. 117–118 (1983).

Eve, J.K, Patel, N., Luk, S.Y., Ebbens, S.J., and Roberts, C.J. "A study of single drug particle adhesion interactions using atomic force microscopy," *Intl. J. of Pharmaceutics*, 238, pp. 17–27 (2002).

Eyring, H. "The activated complex in chemical reactions" *J. Chem. Phys.* 3. pp. 107–115 (1935).

Florin, E.-L., Rief, M, Lehmann, H., Ludwig, M., Dornmair, C., Moy, V.T., and Gaub, H.E. "Sensing specific molecular interactions with the atomic force microscope," *Biosensors & Bioelectronics*, 10, pp. 895–901 (1995).

Forsyth, A.J., Hutton, S., and Rhodes, M.J. "Effect of cohesive interparticle force on the flow characteristics of granular material," *Powder Tech.*, 126 pp. 150–154 (2002).

Gotoh, K., "Particle shape characterization," in Gotoh, K., Masuda, H., and Higashitani. K. (eds), *Powder Technology Handbook*, Marcel Dekker, New York, 1997, pp. 43–56.
Hersey, J.A., "Powder mixing: theory and practice in pharmacy," *Powder Technology*, 15, pp. 149–153 (1976).
Hogg, R., Cahn, D.S., Healy, T.W., and Fuerstenau, D.W., "Diffusional mixing in an ideal system," *Chemical Engineering Science*, 21, pp. 1025–1038 (1966).
Hu, J., Xiao, X.-d., Ogletree, D.F., and Salmeron, M. "Atomic scale friction and wear of mica," *Surface Science*, 327, pp. 358–370 (1995).
Hwang, R., Gemoules, M.K., Ramlose, D.S., and Thomasson, C.E. "A systematic formulation optimization process for a generic pharmaceutical tablet," *Pharmaceutical Technology,* May pp. 48–64 (1998).
Johanson, J.R., "Particle segregation … and what to do about it," *Chemical Engineering,* May 8, pp. 183–188 (1978).
Johanson, J.R., "Smooth out solids blending problems," *Chemical Engineering Progress*, Apr. pp. 21–37 (2000).
Kaye, B., "Mixing of powders," in Fayed, M.E., and Otten, L. (eds), *Handbook of Powder Science & Technology*, Chapman & Hall, New York, 1997, pp. 568–585.
Kaye, B., "Particle shape characterization," in Fayed, M.E., and L. Otten (eds), *Handbook of Powder Science & Technology*, Chapman & Hall, New York, 1997, pp. 35–52.
Kaye, B., "Particle size characterization," in Fayed, M.E., and Otten, L. (eds), *Handbook of Powder Science & Technology*, Chapman & Hall, New York, 1997, pp. 1–34.
Kaye, B., *Powder Mixing*, Chapman and Hall, London 1997.
Marnelli, J., and Carson, J.W. "Solve solids flow problems in bins, hoppers, and feeders," *Chemical Engineering Progress*, May, pp. 22–28 (1992).
Masuda, H., and Gotoh, K. "Adhesive force of a single particle," in Gotoh, K., Masuda, H., and Higashitani, K. (eds), *Powder Technology Handbook*, Marcel Dekker, New York, 1997, pp. 133–142.
McCarthy, J.J., Shinbrot, T., Metcalfe, G., Eduardo Wolf, J., and Ottino, J.M. "Mixing of granular materials in slowly rotated containers," *AIChE Journal*, 42, 12 (1996).
McLellan, G.W., and Shand, E.B. *Glass Engineering Handbook*, 3rd edn McGraw-Hill, New York, 1984.
Metcalfe, G., Shinbrot, T., McCarthy, J.J., and Ottino, J.M. "Avalanche mixing of granular solids," *Nature*, 374, Mar. 2, (1995).
Meurk, A., Yanez, J., and Bergstrom, L. "Silicon nitride granule friction measurements with an atomic force microscope: effect of humidity and binder concentration," *Powder Technology*, 119, pp. 241–249 (2001).
Miyanami, K., "Mixing," in Gotoh, K., Masuda, H., and Higashitani, K. (eds), *Powder Technology Handbook*, Marcel Dekker, New York, 1997, pp. 609–626.
Moakher, M., T. Shinbrot, and Muzzio, F.J. "Experimentally validated computations of flow, mixing and segregation of non-cohesive grains in 3D tumbling blenders," *Powder Technology*, 109, pp. 58–71 (2000).
Muerk, A., "Force measurements using scanning probe microscopy," thesis, Institute for Surface Chemistry, Stockholm (2000).
Muzzio, F.J., Moakher, M., and Shinbrot, T. "Experimentally validated computations of flow, mixing and segregation of non-cohesive grains in 3D tumbling blenders," *Powder Technology*, 109, pp. 58–71 (2000).
Muzzio, F.J., Shinbrot, T., and Zeggio, M. "Computational approaches to granular segregation in tumbling blenders," *Powder Technology*, 116, pp. 224–231 (2001).
Muzzio, F.J., Wightman, C., Moakher, M., and O. Walton, "Simulation of flow and mixing of particles in a rotating and rocking cylinder," *AIChE Journal,* 44, 6 (1998).
Nase, S.T., Vargas, W.T., Abatan, A.A., and McCarthy, J.J. "Discrete characterization tools for cohesive granular material," *Powder Technology*, 116, pp. 214–223 (2001).
Ottino, J.M., and McCarthy, J.J. "Particle dynamics simulation: a hybrid technique applied to granular mixing," *Powder Technology*, 97, pp. 91–99 (1998).
Peratt, B.A., and Yorke, J.A. "Continuous avalanche mixing of granular solids in a rotating drum," *Eurphysics Letters*, 35 (1), pp. 31–35 (1996).

Podczeck, F., Newton, J.M., and James, M.B. "Influence of relative humidity of storage air on the adhesion and autoadhesion of micronized particles to particulate and compacted powder surfaces," *J. Colloid and Interface Sci.*, 187 pp, 484–491 (1997).

Podczeck, F., Newton, J.M., and James, M.B. "The influence of constant and changing relative humidity of the air on the autoadhesion force between pharmaceutical powder particles," *Intl. J. of Pharmaceutics*, 145, pp. 221–229 (1996).

Prescott, J.K., and Barnum, R.A. "On powder flowability," *Pharmaceutical Technology*, Oct, pp. 60–84 (2000).

Price, R., Young, P.M., Edge, S., and Staniforth, J.N. "The influence of relative humidity on particulate interactions in carrier-based dry powder inhaler formulations," *Intl. J. of Pharmaceutics*, 246, pp. 47–59 (2002).

Rhodes, M., *Introduction to Particle Technology*, John Wiley & Sons, Ltd, Chichester, 1998.

Rogers, A.R., and Clements, J.A. "The examination of segregation of granular materials in a tumbling mixer," *Powder Technology*, 5, pp. 167–178 (1971).

Sastry, K.V.S., Cooper, H., Hogg, R.H., Jespen, T.L.P., Knoll, F., Parekh, B., Rajamani, R.K., Sorenson, T., and Wechsler, I. "Solid-solid operations and equipment," in Perry, R.H., and D.W. Green (eds), *Perry's Chemical Engineers' Handbook*, 7th edn, McGraw-Hill, New York, 1997.

Schwedes, J., "Testers for measuring flow properties of particulate solids," *Powder Handling & Processing*, 12, 4 (2000).

Schweiger, A., and Zimmermann, I. "A new approach for the measurement of the tensile strength of powders," *Powder Technology*, 101, pp. 7–15 (1999).

Shinohara, K., "Fundamental and rheological properties of powders," in Fayed, M.E., and Otten, L. (eds), *Handbook of Powder Science & Technology*, Chapman & Hall, New York, 1997, pp. 96–145.

Sindel, U., and Zimmermann, I. "Measurement of interaction forces between individual powder particles using an atomic force microscopy," *Powder Technology*, 117, pp. 247–254 (2001).

Snow, R.H., Allen, T., Ennis, B.J., and Litster, J.D. "Size reduction and size enlargement," in Perry, R.H., and Green, D.W. (eds), *Perry's Chemical Engineers' Handbook*, 7th edn, McGraw-Hill, New York, 1997.

Stewart, R.L., Bridgwater, J., Zhou, Y.C, and Yu, A.B. "Simulated and measured flow of granules in a bladed mixer – a detailed comparison," *Chemical Engineering Science*, 56, pp. 5457–5471 (2001).

Sundararajan, S., and Bhushan, B. "Topography-induced contributions of friction forces measured using an atomic force/friction force microscope," *J. Appl. Physics*, 88 (8), pp. 4825–4831 (2000).

Taylor, M.K., Ginsburg, J., Hickey, A.J., and Gheyas, F. "Composite method to quantify powder flow as a screening method in early tablet or capsule formulation development," *AAPS PharmSciTech*, 1, 3 (2000).

Thomson, F.M., "Storage and flow of particulate solids," in Fayed, M.E., and Otten, L. (eds), *Handbook of Powder Science & Technology*, Chapman & Hall, New York, 1997, pp. 389–486.

Wang, R.H., and Fan, L.T. "Methods for scaling-up tumbling mixers," *Chemical Engineering*, May 27, 1974, pp. 88–94.

Williams, J.C., "The segregation of particulate materials. A review," *Powder Technology*, 15, pp. 245–251 (1976).

Zhou, Y.C., Xu, B.H., Yu, A.B., and Zulli, P., "An experimental and numerical study of the angle of repose of coarse spheres," *Powder Technology*, 125, pp. 45–54 (2002).

6

Continuous Powder Mixing

Juan G. Osorio[1], Aditya U. Vanarase[2], Rodolfo J. Romañach[3], and Fernando J. Muzzio[1]
[1] Department of Chemical and Biochemical Engineering, Rutgers, The State University of New Jersey, USA
[2] Bristol-Myers Squibb Co., USA
[3] Department of Chemistry, University of Puerto Rico, Puerto Rico

6.1 Introduction

Continuous powder mixing has been the subject of much research in the past few years since it offers several advantages over the conventional batch mixing methods still used in the pharmaceutical industry [1–9]. These advantages include the opportunity for meaningful process analytical technologies (PAT) and modeling techniques to be implemented for automated process control leading to finished products with improved quality. With continuous manufacturing, the same equipment used for process development can often be used in manufacturing. Therefore, product scale up is eliminated or reduced, accelerating the introduction of new products to the market. The advantages also include significant reductions in equipment size and the ability for integration with other continuous processes already in use (such as tableting, capsule filling, roller compaction, hot melt extrusion, etc.). Integration with an intrinsically continuous process such as tableting would yield higher production efficiency and minimize segregation of the mixed materials. Moreover, because a continuous process can achieve a desired set point after transient of just a few minutes, entire sets of designed experiments can often be explored in a matter of just a few days, with great savings in materials and time. Overall, these advantages can significantly reduce

Pharmaceutical Blending and Mixing, First Edition. Edited by P.J. Cullen, Rodolfo J. Romañach, Nicolas Abatzoglou and Chris D. Rielly.

costs during development and manufacturing of pharmaceuticals. This chapter provides an overview of continuous powder mixing and its mechanisms. Theoretical and experimental characterization, modeling, and process control efforts are described. Recommendations for future directions both in research and within industry are explained in detail.

6.2 Overview

Most continuous powder mixers are fixed cylindrical chambers with diameters and lengths averaging 3.5–20 cm and 25–75 cm, respectively. Their capacities range from ~10 kg hr^{-1} up to ~500 kg hr^{-1} [10]. At one end of the cylindrical chamber, there is a vertical inlet allowing gravimetric feeding of ingredients into the blender. At the other end, another opening allows the blended powder to exit the blender and enter the next unit operation (Figure 6.1). The cylindrical chamber contains a motor-driven impeller along its entire length. The impeller typically used is a bladed, ribbon, or ribbon-bladed impeller that directs flow by means of convection in the axial direction. The motion of the impeller and the blades also encourage inter-particle collisions, causing shearing and dispersion of the materials being mixed. Hence, the same mechanisms of particle motion and mixing (convection, dispersion, and shearing) found in batch mixing are encountered in continuous powder mixing.

Continuous mixing is governed by raw material properties as well as process and design parameters. These affect powder flow behavior in the blender, final blend properties, and overall blend homogeneity (Figure 6.1). Raw material properties include, but are not limited to, particle size distribution, flow properties and electro static behavior. The process parameters for a continuous mixer include total flow rate and impeller rotation rate. The

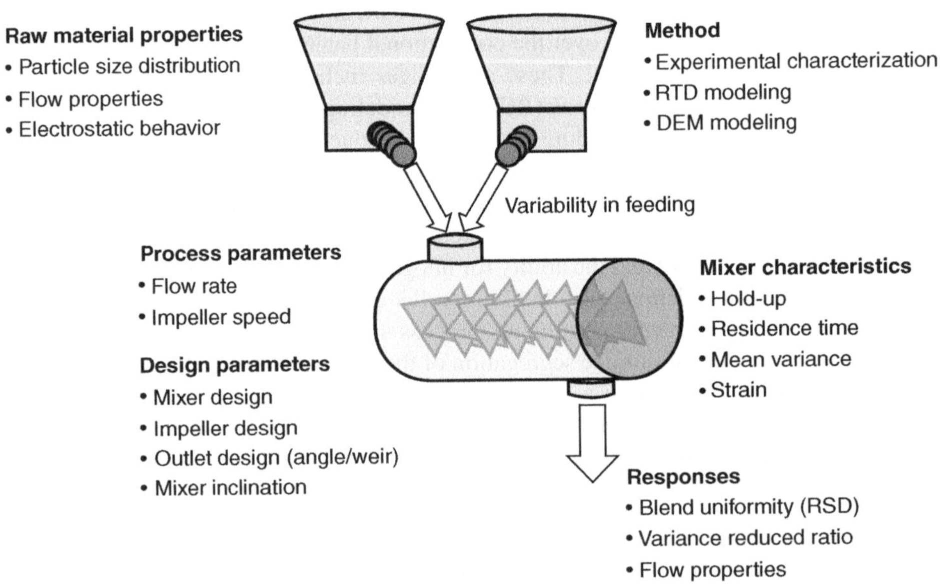

Figure 6.1 *Feeder/mixer suite. Important process parameters and characterization techniques*

design parameters of a continuous mixer include the diameter and length of the blender (volume), impeller design, outlet design, and, in some cases, mixer inclination. Several designs of continuous blenders are available, and while they are all fairly similar in basic design, some variation in design parameters is common.

Because of the blender geometry, mixing dynamics can be categorized in terms of radial (mainly micro-mixing) and axial (mainly macro-mixing) homogenization (Figure 6.2). An important aspect of a continuous mixer is to homogenize in the radial direction powders that enter the blender at different positions of the inlet. This is accomplished by shearing the powder with the impeller. Even more importantly, a continuous mixer main function is to homogenize by axial dispersion the composition fluctuations caused by the feeders. This is accomplished by the residence time distribution (RTD) (Figure 6.3). Particles follow different trajectories through the blender, and consequently spend variable amounts of time in it. This causes axial mixing.

Axial mixing and recirculation are important to achieve a consistent degree of homogenization. Due to the intrinsic cohesion of most powders of practical interest, accurate feeding is a difficult, sometimes unattainable, task. As a result, the instantaneous composition fed to a mixer by multiple gravimetric feeders exhibits fluctuations in time. This becomes more challenging, resulting in higher feeding variability, at low concentrations of critical ingredients. Moreover, available gravimetric feeding technologies present accuracy limitations at low flow rates. Axial mixing minimizes the effect of such feeding variations of different ingredients. The RTD spreads such fluctuations along the axis of the mixer, decreasing their intensity. In fact, the axial mixing rate, quantified in terms of the dispersion coefficient and the residence time, determines the capability of the continuous blender to filter out fluctuations coming from the feeders (Figure 6.3). Consequently, the axial mixing capacity of a continuous blender can be quantified, and modeled, in terms of the RTD response of an instantaneous pulse at the inlet. Once the RTD is known, mixing performance can be modeled by decomposing the feeding stream into a series of instantaneous pulses. Thus, to achieve an effective design, continuous powder blending should not be examined by itself, but rather as a component of a larger process that also includes the feeders [11]. In fact, the determination of the maximum acceptable feed rate variability depends on the installed downstream mixing capability, or, conversely, the homogenization capability needed in a manufacturing line depends on the intensity of feed rate variability. Integrated examination of feeders and mixers is an essential design strategy in order to develop effective continuous blending systems [12].

Gravimetric feeding is the most common technology used for the feeding of granular materials. A wide range of loss-in-weight feeders is available. Volumetric feeding has also been used, but has been found to be less reliable to feed powders due to the fluctuations in density typically displayed by cohesive powders [1]. A loss-in-weight feeder consists of a

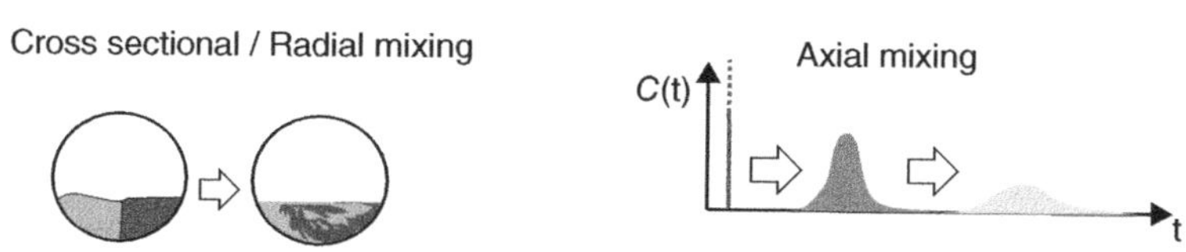

Figure 6.2 Radial and axial mixing representation

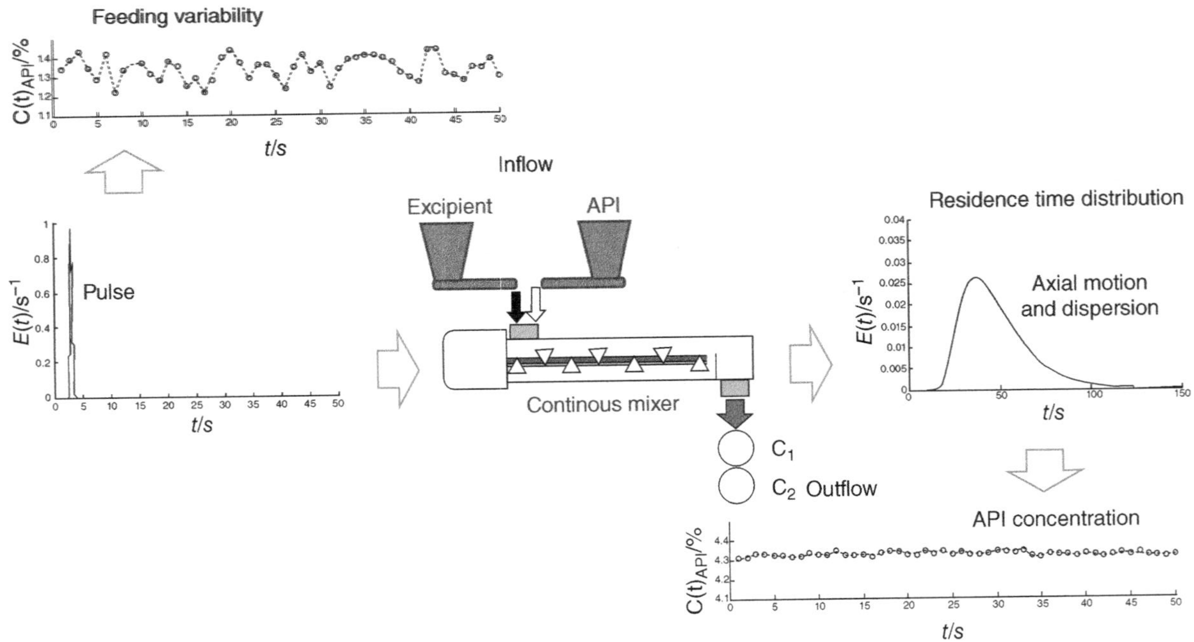

Figure 6.3 *Feeding variability filtered by both radial and axial mixing. Residence time distribution representation characterized by an instantaneous pulse response*

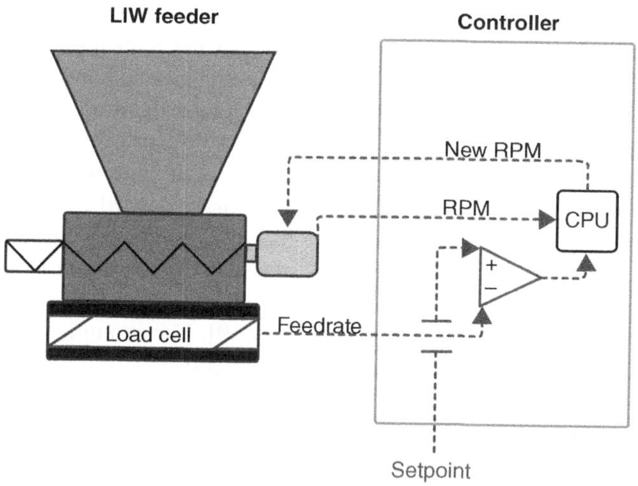

Figure 6.4 *Loss-in-weight (LIW) feeder control mechanism*

hopper with an agitator around the inside diameter or at the bottom to break up any bridging. At the bottom of the hopper, a screw or screws inside a nozzle direct and control the amount of powder being fed. These feeders have a feedback control mechanism that uses a high frequency load cell to record the mass being fed, continuously correcting for its loss (Figure 6.4). A feed factor correlates volumetric feeding of the powder to the actual mass of the powder being fed. This feed factor controls the rotation rate of the screw or screws while accounting for the loss of mass in the feeder.

Loss-in-weight feeders have been developed in a wide range of sizes to overcome challenges in feeding powders for many target concentrations and flow rates. In addition, replaceable tooling with various nozzle sizes, screw sizes and types, and agitator types have been developed to be able to feed ingredients with large variations in material properties. Although manufacturers of loss-in-weight feeders have recommendations for feeding powders with specific bulk densities, feeding optimization should be performed for each constituent in a pharmaceutical blend. Materials with similar bulk densities can and do behave differently due to varying material properties such as electrostatic behavior, moisture uptake, and particle shape.

As previously mentioned, the dynamic behavior and mixing efficiency of a continuous blender are a function of the design and operational parameters of the blender itself as well as the material properties of each of the materials being mixed, and the properties of the resulting blend. The throughput capacity of a continuous blender is typically a function of the length and diameter (volume) of the mixing chamber, and the bulk density of the constituents and the final blend. Other important design parameters found in all cylindrical continuous blenders include the impeller type, the number of blades, the size of the blades, and their orientation with respect to the axial flow. The angle of the blender with respect to the horizontal position, the weir angle, and the angle of the outlet are also design parameters that affect the amount of powder retained by the blender (hold-up) and degree of powder recirculation within the mixer. Operation parameters include the total flow rate of materials through the blender and the rotational speed of the impeller.

To understand how the blender design affects mixing in the radial and axial directions, it is helpful to visualize what happens to a portion of powder after it enters the blender. For moderate agitation rates, once steady flow is reached, an agitated powder bed is established on the bottom of the blender. As the impeller blades rotate, the motion of the blades drags powder in the angular direction, turning over portions of the powder bed, leading to radial mixing. Typically, the blades in the impeller are at an angle with respect to the horizontal plane of the impeller. This induces either forward or backward motion of the powder, depending on the blade angle. Alternatively, a blade perpendicular either parallel or perpendicular to the shaft will hinder the axial flow of powder. The extent to which the impeller regulates forward versus backward movement of the powder determines the rate of axial mixing, hold-up and recirculation in the blender [8, 9]. For example, if all of the blades "pump forward," such a configuration will have the fastest flow through, the smallest hold-up, and the least amount of axial mixing. Alternatively, if most blades are angled to produce backward flow; the blender will be easily clogged. Clearly, an optimum design exists that combines the right degrees of forward flow and recirculation. While we have not demonstrated this rigorously, our experience indicates that such an optimum configuration depends on powder cohesion as well as overall system size. Determining the optimum blender geometry remains an open question.

If the homogeneity of the final blend was the only design goal, then finding the optimum design of a blender would be relatively straightforward. Such a mixer would have a large volume, with many blades that would maximize residence time and axial mixing. However, the addition of too much mechanical strain on a powder blend can change powder material properties, which can lead to process and product failures. Moreover, too large a holdup, and consequently too long a residence time would make a continuous system very sluggish, and perhaps unstable, from a control perspective. In fact, we want to maximize homogeneity and controllability. Thus, optimum design of an online mixer requires careful analysis of the interplay of design and operational parameters and material properties of the constituents and the final blend, and might have multiple design goals regarding effectiveness, efficiency, and controllability.

To this end, theoretical and experimental principles originally developed to describe the efficiency of continuous fluid mixing systems and their bulk dynamic behavior have been adapted for continuous powder processes. These techniques include measurements of the variance reduction ratio, hold-up, RTD, mean residence time, and mean centered variance (or its reciprocal, the dispersion coefficient). The mixing efficiency, as in any batch mixing process, is also characterized by statistical quantification of the total variability in the composition of the desired material or materials in the final blend. Typically, the concentration of the active pharmaceutical ingredient (API) is quantified for a set of samples, or in some cases, for multiple *in-situ* measurements. However, the established practice of characterizing only the homogeneity of API can be insufficient; often, achieving a homogeneous blend of other constituents can also be important. In our experience, variability in the concentration of lubricants, surfactants, and disintegrants can have a profound effect on dissolution and hardness attributes of the finished product. However, identification of those ingredients whose homogeneity is critical to product quality often requires substantial amount of work, and such work is often performed only after product failures make this issue unavoidable.

In continuous powder mixing, powder behavior can be affected by the process in a readily observable manner. Thus, product formulation and process design are intimately linked. In order to create blends with the desired attributes, one must often examine multiple grades of excipients and particle size of actives. This can entail a large amount of experimental work, due to the widely varying physical properties of powders. Moreover, ingredients always exhibit lot-related variability; and sometimes powder properties are also affected by age, environmental conditions, and so on. Quality by Design can be advantageously applied to study such situations, which also offer ample opportunity for the meaningful application of PAT tools, such as Near-Infrared (NIR) spectroscopy for in-line monitoring and in-process control. Proper models can be developed to enable the use of process parameters to counteract material property variability. The development of models and correlations from raw material and final blend properties, such as powder flow properties, particle size, and electrostatic behavior, with continuous mixing performance and powder phenomena characteristics as a function of design and operational parameters allows superior controllability of the process and its integration with other intrinsically continuous processes such as roller compaction, hot melt extrusion, tableting, and capsule filling.

6.3 Theoretical Characterization

6.3.1 Residence Time Distribution (RTD) Modeling

Powder mixing processes are governed by intrinsic powder flow mechanisms such as convection, shear, and dispersion [3]. These mechanisms induce fluid-like behavior on powders while mixing in a continuous flow system. Therefore, powder dynamics in continuous mixing can be characterized by the RTD originally developed to describe fluid systems [13]. The RTD is used to characterize macroscopic flow behavior in non-ideal reactors [14]. Various methods have been identified for modeling RTDs. The fractional tubularity model [5], a delay and a dead volume model, and dispersion models [14, 15] are commonly used in the evaluation of RTDs. One of the common RTD models used is the axial dispersion model, which describes mixing in the axial direction.

The axial dispersion model (Eq. 6.1) is a classical approach to model axial mixing in both continuous and batch mixers. The one-dimensional diffusion equation used to describe mixing in the axial direction is given by

$$\frac{\partial C}{\partial t} + v_z \frac{\partial C}{\partial z} = E_z \frac{\partial^2 C}{\partial z^2} \tag{6.1}$$

where C is the concentration of the pulse, t is time, v_z is the axial velocity, z is the direction of the axial flow, and E_z is the dispersion coefficient of the system.

The dispersion equation can be transformed into the Fokker–Plank equation. This equation describes the time evolution of the distribution of particles of each component inside a continuous system using actual physical and measurable properties [2]. The Fokker–Plank equation is described in Eq. (6.2).

$$\frac{\partial C}{\partial \theta} + \frac{\partial C}{\partial \varepsilon} = \frac{1}{Pe} \frac{\partial^2 C}{\partial \varepsilon^2}, \tag{6.2}$$

where $\varepsilon = \frac{z}{l}$ and $\theta = \frac{t}{\tau}$ are the dimensionless relative location and time in the continuous mixing system with l and τ representing the total length of the continuous mixer and the mean residence time, respectively. The Peclet number ($P_e = \frac{v_z l}{E_z}$, where v_z and E_z are the axial velocity and the dispersion coefficient of the system) is the ratio of the rate of advection caused by bulk flow to cross-sectional dispersion.

One common solution of this equation, known as the Taylor dispersion model [16] (Eq. 6.3), calculates RTD [$E(t)$] obtained from experimental data by estimating the concentration as a function of dimensionless location (ε) and dimensionless time (θ) with known and measured parameters.

$$C(\varepsilon,\theta) = \frac{C_o Pe^{1/2}}{(4\pi\theta)^{1/2}} e^{-P_e(\varepsilon-\theta)^2/4\theta} \tag{6.3}$$

for which C_o represents the initial concentration of the pulse when it enters the blender. Usually, the RTD is determined at the outlet of the blender, where $z = l$, therefore the dimensionless relative location, ε, is set to equal 1.

6.3.2 Variance Reduction Ratio

Early work described the variance reduction ratio (VRR) as the overall performance of continuous and semi-continuous blenders [17]. The VRR (Eq. 6.4) is defined as the ratio of the input variance (s_i^2) to the output variance (s_o^2). The VRR can also be used to determine the overall efficiency of continuous powder mixing.

$$VRR = \frac{s_i^2}{s_o^2} \tag{6.4}$$

A general relationship between the VRR and the RTD [$E(t)$] (Eq. 6.5) was developed for continuous powder blenders [4] given by

$$\frac{1}{VRR} = 2\int_{r=0}^{\infty} E(t)E(t+r)R(r)d\tau + \frac{s_{o,ideal}^2}{s_i^2} \tag{6.5}$$

where $R(r) = \frac{\delta_i(t')\delta_i(t'-r)}{\sigma_i^2}$ is the autocorrelation function of $C_i(t)$ for the time interval r. $s_{o,ideal}^2$ is the variance of the ideal random powder mixture. This theoretical approach can be used to predict the VRR using the RTD or *vice versa*.

6.4 Experimental Characterization

The dynamic behavior and mixing performance of continuous powder blenders has been characterized using various metrics previously developed for continuous fluid systems. These metrics can be measured experimentally. Some have also been modeled using theoretical correlations such as the RTD and variance reduction ratio introduced in section 6.3. The dynamic flow behavior in a continuous mixer can be described by the powder hold-up and the RTD. The mixing performance can be quantified by the variance reduction ratio and the blend homogeneity. Next, a description of each of these metrics is given along with its physical significance.

6.4.1 Hold-Up

The hold-up (Eq. 6.6) is the amount of material in the continuous blender at any given time. When flow is initiated, the hold-up initially increases until it reaches a plateau when the powder flow through the blender reaches steady state. The steady state hold-up is important because it determines the average residence time (Eq. 6.7). This, in turn, determines the total amount of mechanical energy experienced by the blend as it flows through the mixer.

$$Hold\text{-}up = accumulation = mass_{in} - mass_{out} \tag{6.6}$$

$$Bulk\,residence\,time = \frac{hold\text{-}up}{\dot{m}} \tag{6.7}$$

The hold-up can be measured non-invasively by monitoring the amount of powder being fed into the blender and exiting the blender from start-up until the flow has reached steady state, or simply by mounting the mixer on a load cell. A high hold-up indicates that the average time that the powder as a bulk spends in the blender is longer, having more time to mix. A high hold-up also indicates that the powder will experience more energy as it travels through the mixer, which can sometimes lead to adverse effects such as dusting, attrition of granulations, and over-lubrication. Moreover, as mentioned, a larger hold up makes the system more sluggish from a dynamical point of view, hindering controllability. Thus, an optimum hold-up is desired to reach acceptable blend homogeneity without affecting the blend adversely, and without impairing controllability.

6.4.2 Residence Time Distribution (RTD) Measurements

The RTD is defined as a probability distribution that determines the amount of time that powder components spend inside the mixer. The RTD in a continuous mixer can be measured by the response to an instantaneous pulse of a tracer material added to the inlet stream. The concentration of the pulse material [$C(t)$] is measured as a function of time at the outlet of the blender. The RTD [$E(t)$] function is calculated as shown in Eq. (6.8). From the RTD measurement, the mean residence (*MRT*, τ) is calculated (Eq. 6.9). The MRT, as its name indicates, is the average time that a portion of the powder will spend inside a continuous blender. The mean centered variance (*MCV*, σ_τ^2) (Eq. 6.10) is also obtained from the RTD function. The MCV is the spread of the RTD function.

Residence time distribution [$E(t)$, RTD]:

$$E(t) = \frac{C(t)}{\int_0^\infty C(t)dt} \tag{6.8}$$

Mean residence time [τ, MRT]:

$$\tau = \int_0^{\infty} tE(t)\,dt \tag{6.9}$$

Mean centered variance [σ_τ^2, MCV]:

$$\sigma_\tau^2 = \frac{\int_0^{\infty} (t-\tau)^2 E(t)\,dt}{\tau^2} \tag{6.10}$$

A large mean residence time indicates that the bulk powder spends a longer time in the blender, both allowing the materials to have more time to blend, and also experiencing more shear. A high mean residence time is also able to filter lower frequency fluctuations from the feeders. The mean centered variance is an efficiency indicator of a continuous blender at the specific operating conditions. The MCV always has a value between 0 and 1. For a perfectly mixed system (i.e., an ideal continuous stirred-tank reactor, CSTR), the MCV is equal to 1, and for a perfectly unmixed system (i.e., plug-flow reactor, PFR), the MCV is equal to 0. The higher the MCV is, the higher the axial mixing efficiency of the blender. The inverse of the MCV yields the theoretical number of CSTRs in series represented by a continuous mixer. The mean residence time and the mean centered variance fully describe axial mixing in a continuous flow system [18].

6.4.3 Mean Strain

In a continuous mixer, the energy input is provided by the impeller rotation. This energy is dissipated in the convective transport of the powder through the random fluctuations of the velocity of the particles (granular temperature), friction between the impeller and the powder, and the mean strain (velocity gradients in the powder). Since the impeller rotation rate has an effect on the mean residence time, the strain, which is proportional to the product of the shear rate (ω) and the mean residence time (τ), can be calculated in terms of the number of blade passes (N_p) as shown in Eq. (6.11).

$$N_p = \omega \cdot \tau \tag{6.11}$$

6.5 Continuous Mixing Efficiency

6.5.1 Variance Reduction Ratio

The variance reduction ratio (VRR) of the critical component(s) (usually the API) can be measured experimentally. The input variance is determined by the feeding variability of the critical component. Likewise, the output variance is determined by the blend uniformity of the critical component. The VRR equation was defined in section 6.3 (Eq. 6.4) as the ratio of the input variance to the output variance. A higher VRR value represents better mixing performance in a continuous blender. Rarely discussed, but nonetheless important, is the fact that practical quantification of both the input and output variance require the definition of a scale of examination (i.e., a "sample size"). Selecting the appropriate scale of examination depends on the purpose of quantifying mixing. For a product quality application, the scale of examination should be the unit of material that is most relevant to product quality, which is usually the unit dose. However, from the perspective of understanding and optimizing the process, consideration should be given both to system dynamics (characterization frequency should be at least 10 times higher than the typical characteristic response time of the system under examination) as well as the accuracy of the measurement system. For example, for NIR blend monitoring, multiple measurements should often be averaged so that the amount of powder examined in the measurement is large enough to make individual measurements reasonably accurate, so that measurement error does not dominate the measurement.

6.5.2 Blend Homogeneity

The blend homogeneity of the critical component is characterized using the same basic statistical relations used in batch mixing (Eq. 6.12). In batch mixing, blend homogeneity is often determined by sampling at a specific blending time at multiple positions within the blender. In continuous mixing, samples are taken as a function of time after powder flow has reached steady state and various mean residence times have passed. Typically, feeders are designated to a specific ingredient. Each feeder and its configuration must be optimized to feed a desired flow rate of each material with minimum variability. Due to the intrinsic behavior of powders, there is always some variability in feed rate, which, for a properly designed mixer, is largely eliminated by axial mixing in the blender. The effectiveness of the axial mixing process can be quantified by calculating the relative standard deviation of a set of composition measurements. In Eq. (6.12), $\bar{C}$ is the average concentration of the total number of samples (N) and C_i is the concentration of each sample. s is the standard deviation calculated using sample concentrations. A low RSD value is indicative of better mixing. Regulatory agencies have different standards on what the RSD value should be. This value typically must be <5%. However, and importantly, we should note that in batch mixing, the RSD is usually calculated based on a small number of measurements, typically no more than 20. This leads to RSD estimates with poor reliability. A significant advantage of continuous mixers equipped with PAT sensors is that the RSD measurements can be calculated based on a much larger set of measurements, thus leading to much more reliable estimates of the effectiveness of the mixing processes.

$$RSD = \frac{s}{\bar{C}} = \frac{\sqrt{\frac{\sum_1^N \left(C_i - \bar{C}\right)^2}{N-1}}}{\frac{1}{N}\sum_1^N C_i} \tag{6.12}$$

6.6 Effects of Process Parameters on Mixing Behavior and Performance

All continuous mixing process attributes described previously are a function of the design and operational parameters of the blender and the material properties of the pure ingredients and the blend. The optimum operating condition of a continuous blender is determined by studying all these characteristics. These determine the final blend attributes. Continuous processes can achieve mixture quality comparable or better than those obtained from batch mixing. However, since continuous mixing can be monitored more thoroughly, the quality of the final blend can be controlled continuously.

As a comprehensive example, the following section presents results and correlations obtained using a Gericke GCM-250 (Figure 6.5a) with a diameter of 10 cm and a length of 30 cm containing 12 blades along the impeller (Figure 6.5b). This specific blender has a weir at the outlet (Figure 6.5c). This blender has been previously characterized and documented elsewhere [19, 20]. The capacity of the blender ranges from 10–500 kg hr^{-1}. The capacity of the continuous blender depends on the properties of the materials being blended and the process parameters being used [10]. The bulk behavior and mixing performance of other cylindrical continuous powder blenders follow similar trends. However, final mixing

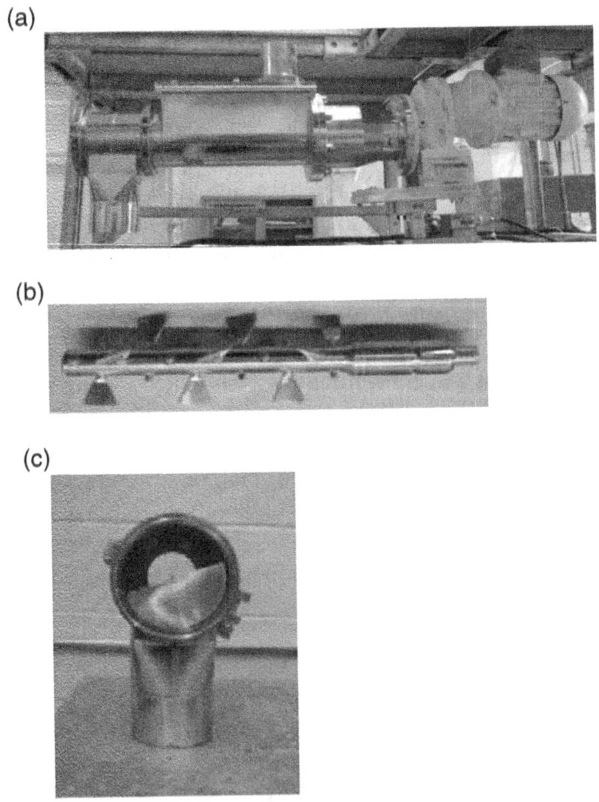

Figure 6.5 Continuous mixer and design used as reference in chapter. (a) Continuous mixer (Gerick GCM-250). (b) Impeller with 12 triangular blades. (c) Outlet weir angled at 20°

performance and specific correlations between performance, material properties, and operating parameters are dependent on the blender design.

6.6.1 Hold-Up

The hold-up is correlated to the process and design parameters. The blade configuration and weir angle have an effect on hold-up. The impeller blade configuration can be modified to vary hold-up and recirculation in the blender. For example, all blades can be positioned to push the powder forward (F), which leads to lower hold-up. An alternating blade configuration (A) where half of the blades push forward and the other half push back, or a combination of blade configurations can be used. The angle of the blade with respect to the impeller axis, or the size and/or shape of the blade, can also be varied. The blade configuration and weir angle (or no weir) control the amount of back-mixing and recirculation inside the blender. Interestingly, while our work clearly shows that the blade geometry has a large effect on holdup and other important variables, almost no work has been performed to optimize blade design in continuous mixers.

In the GCM-250, the hold-up decreases as the rotation rate increases (Figure 6.6a and b). The hold-up is higher for the alternating blade configurations when compared to the all-forward blade configuration, as expected. The hold-up is higher for the 20° angle blade orientation than for the 45° angle along the axis of the impeller. The hold-up is also higher for a 20° and 45° weir angles when compared to having 0° angle on the weir position (or the configuration with no weir) (Figure 6.6c). The effect of the blade configuration and weir angle on the hold-up becomes less significant at higher impeller rotation rates. This means that the rotation rate is predominant in controlling the hold-up and the recirculation within the blender. The powder in the blender also becomes fluidized at higher rotation rates creating a transition to a different mixing regime.

The effect of total flow rate on hold-up has also been studied. The hold-up increases with increasing flow rate through the system (Figure 6.7a). The bulk residence time decreases with increasing flow rate for lower rotation rates (Figure 6.7b). The effect of total flow rate on bulk residence time diminishes at higher rotation rates. This indicates that the mixing performance should not be affected by throughput at higher rotation rates [19].

6.6.2 RTD Measurements

RTD experiments are useful to further study the flow behavior and mixing performance of continuous blenders. RTDs are studied as a function of design and process parameters [19, 21]. For instance, the effect of rotation rate on RTDs for the all-forward blade configuration is shown in Figure 6.8. A higher rotation rate results in sharper and narrower distributions. This means that the material spends less time inside the blender at higher rotation rates.

RTDs have been measured at various rotation rates and compared for 30 and 45 kg hr^{-1} (Figure 6.9). The distributions are substantially different at lower rotation rates. As the rotation rate increases, the difference in the RTDs diminishes. At higher rotation rates, RTDs do not vary with varying total flow rate. The mean residence time, the mean centered variance, and the number of blade passes are easily calculated to quantify the effect of design and process parameters from the RTDs.

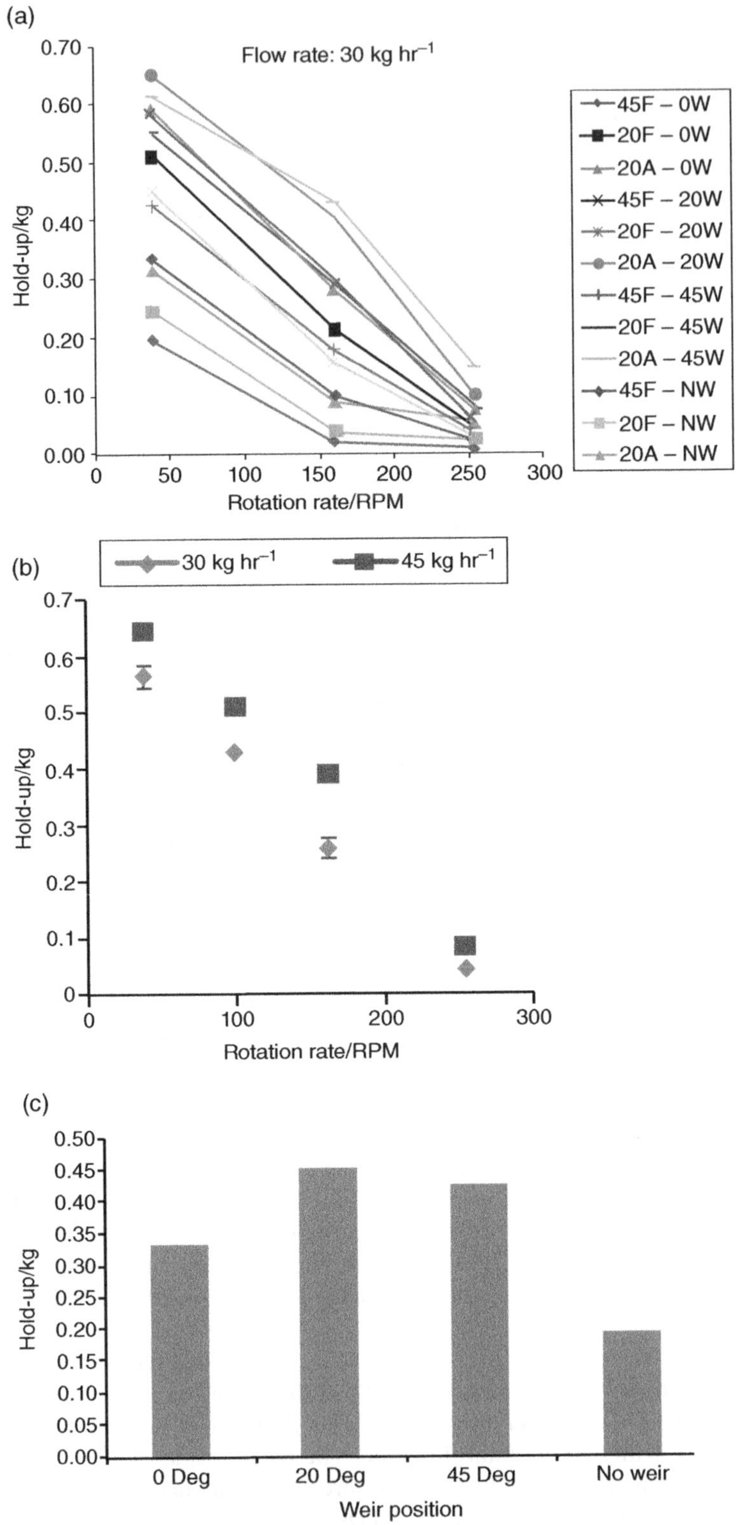

Figure 6.6 *Hold-up. (a) Hold-up as a function of rotation rate for various blade configurations and weir angles. (b) Hold-up as a function of rotation rate for 30 and 45 kg hr^{-1} total flow rate. Blade configuration: all forward. Weir position: 20° (c) Hold-up as a function of weir position (angle). Flow rate: 30 kg hr^{-1}. Blade configuration: all forward*

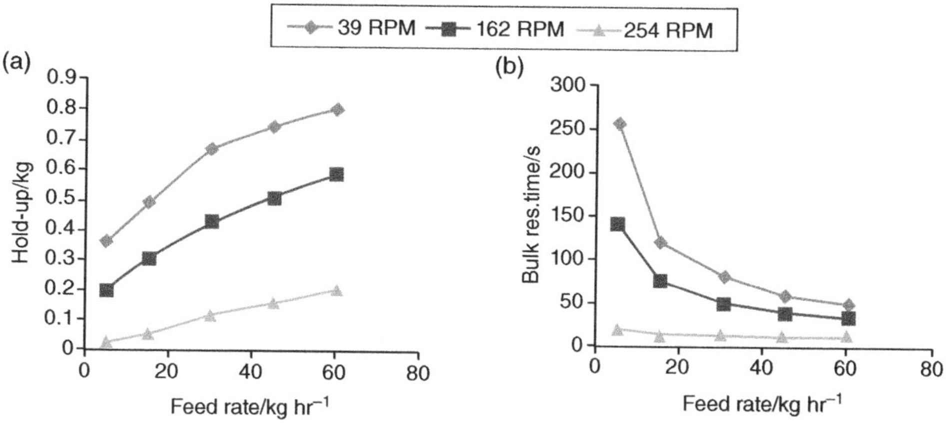

Figure 6.7 *(a) Hold-up as a function of total feed rate at various impeller rotation rates. (b) Bulk residence time as a function of feed rate at various impeller rotation rates. Note: all figures presented from here were using a 20° weir position*

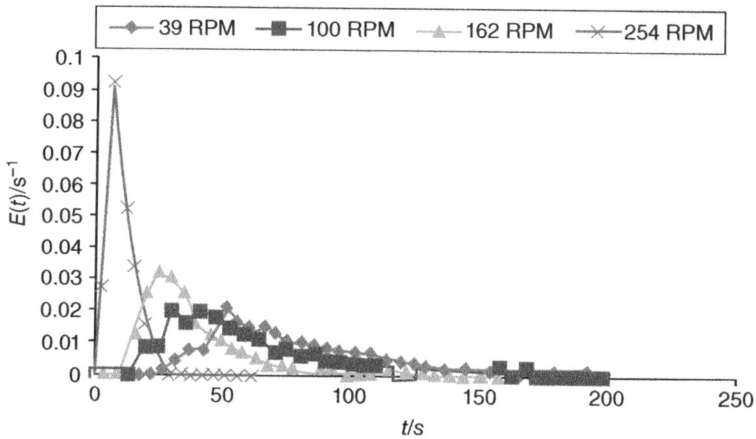

Figure 6.8 *Residence time distribution for various rotation rates at 30 kg hr^{-1} total flow rate. Blade configuration: all forward*

The mean residence time (MRT, τ) decreases with increasing rotation rate (Figure 6.10a). The mean centered variance (MCV, σ_τ^2) increases as the rotation rate increases (Figure 6.10b). The mean residence time is higher for the lower flow rates at low rotation rates. This difference is small at higher rotation rates. This effect was anticipated from the RTD measurements from which the MRT was calculated. Furthermore, the reciprocal of the MCV gives the number of theoretical CSTRs needed to obtain a similar RTD. The number of CSTRs represents the degree of dispersion of the pulse for each condition. In this case, fewer CSTRs are an indication of faster dispersion, meaning more efficient axial mixing. The MRT at high rotation rates is low while the MCV is high indicating that an intermediate rotation rate would give rise to better mixing.

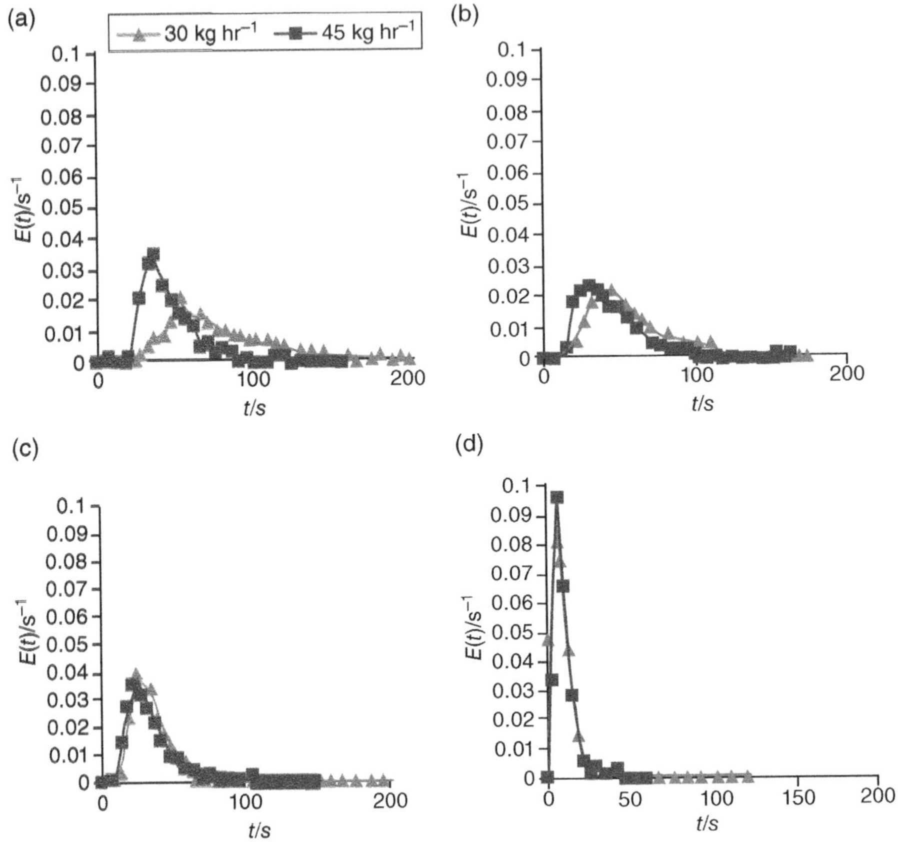

Figure 6.9 Residence time distribution for 30 and 45 kg hr⁻¹ total flow rate at impeller rotation rates (a) 39 RPM, (b) 100 RPM, (c) 162 RPM and (d) 254 RPM. Blade configuration: all forward

Since the impeller rotation rate has an effect on the MRT, the strain, which is proportional to the product of the shear rate (ω) and the mean residence time, can be estimated. In order to approximate the amount of strain that the powder experiences in the blender, the number of blade passes (N_p) is calculated as shown in Eq. (6.11). The number of blade passes is maximum at intermediate rotation rates (100–162 RPM) indicating that maximum strain is experienced (Figure 6.10c). This correlation between the mean strain and the rotation rate can be used qualitatively to estimate the values of parameters that would yield the "best" mixing performance. Finally, as it was shown for all other measurements, the difference between the number of blade passes for the two flow rates (30 and 45 kg hr^{-1}) diminishes as the rotation rate increases.

The effects of process parameters, flow rate, and rotation rate, on powder mixing behavior were just described. In addition, as mentioned, it is also important to understand the effects of design parameters such as the blade configuration. Hold-up measurements showed that the blade configuration was a significant factor. Similarly, RTDs for two blade

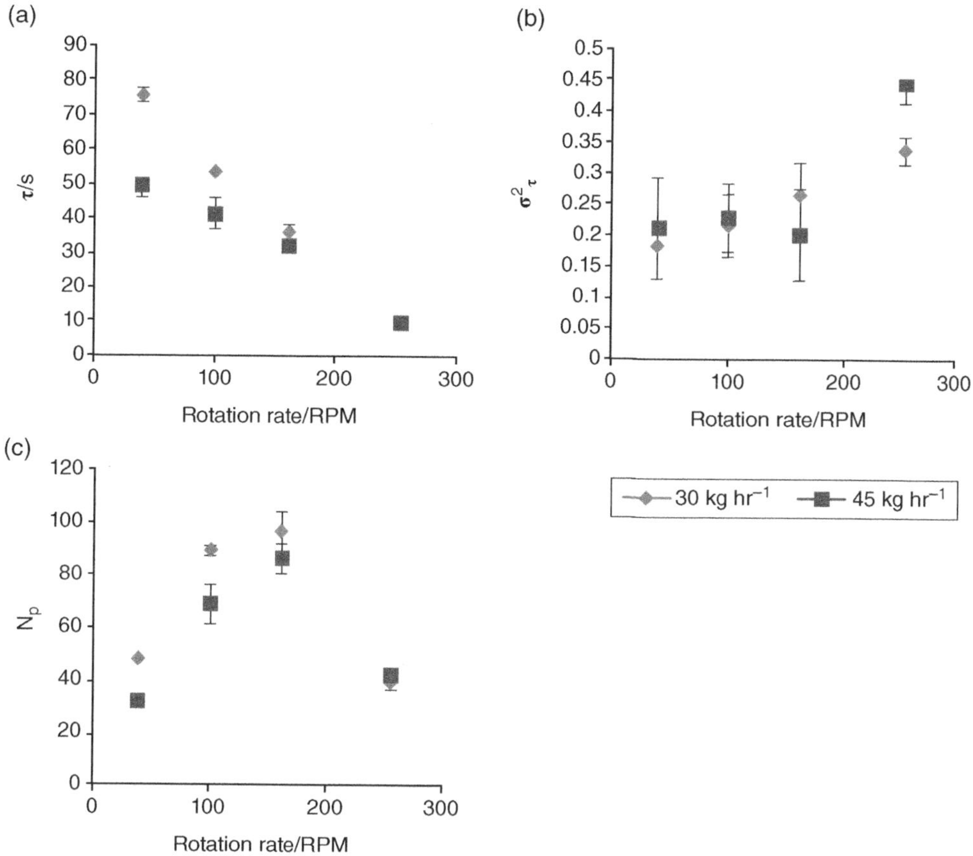

Figure 6.10 *(a) Mean residence time as a function of impeller rotation rate, (b) Mean centered variance, and (c) Number of blade passes for 30 and 45 kg hr^{-1}. Blade configuration: all forward*

configurations were measured at various rotation rates (Figure 6.11). The two blade configurations were the "all forward" and "alternate" with the blades at a 20° angle with respect to the axis of the impeller. The RTD results obtained at lower rotation rates (40 and 100 RPM) were not significantly different. At higher rotation rates, the RTD curves start to differentiate. This can be caused by the amount of recirculation that the blade configuration creates. At higher rotation rates, the effect of the blade configuration is significant, inducing more recirculation for the alternate blade configuration.

The mean residence time, the mean centered variance and the number of blade passes (Figure 6.12) were calculated from the RTD measurements. The mean residence time is higher for the alternate blade configuration (Figure 6.12a). This difference is more noticeable at higher rotation rates. The mean centered variance is also higher for the alternate blade configuration with this difference being more noticeable at higher rotation rates (Figure 6.12b). This is also the case for the number of blade passes. The number of blade passes is higher for the alternate blade configuration, especially at higher rotation rates

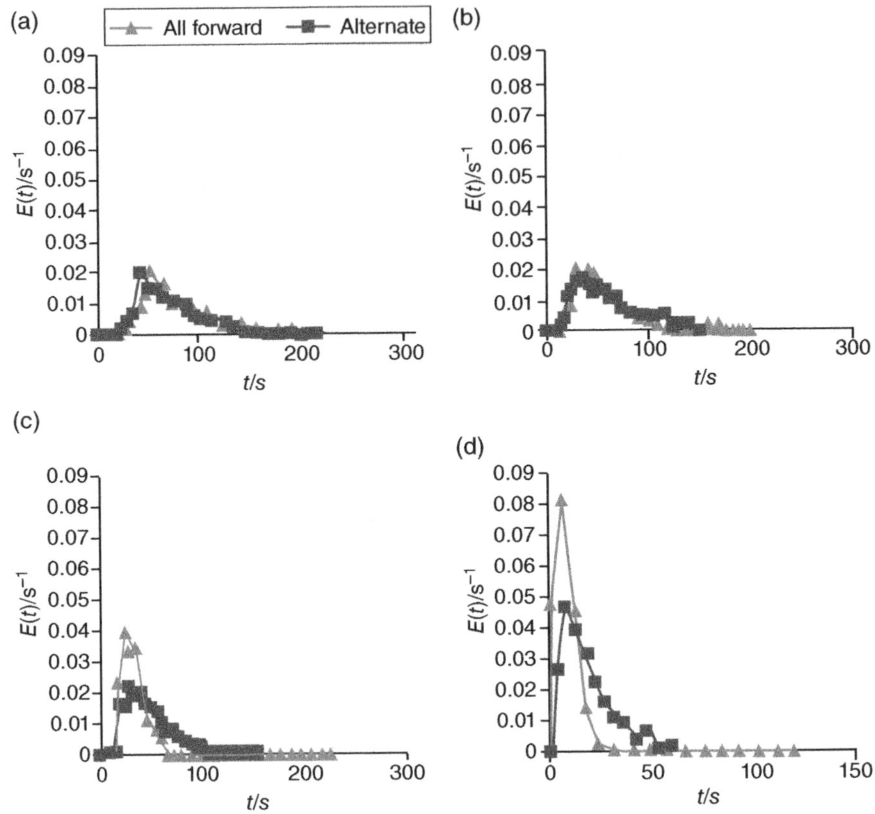

Figure 6.11 *Residence time distribution blade configuration comparison – all forward and alternate at impeller rotation rates. (a) 39 RPM, (b) 100 RPM, (c) 162 RPM, and (d) 254 RPM*

(Figure 6.12c). The number of blade passes for the alternate blade configuration follows the same trend as the all-forward blade configuration, having a maximum at intermediate rotation rates.

6.7 Mixing Performance

Previous measurements such as the mean centered variance and the mean strain (number of blade passes) described to some extent the mixing performance of a continuous blender. However, to measure directly the mixing performance, the variance reduction ratio (VRR) and the relative standard deviation (RSD) are measured for various process and design parameters. A higher VRR or a low RSD are indicative of higher mixing efficiency. VRRs obtained from experimental work have shown maximum values at intermediate rotation rates (Figure 6.13a). The same trend is obtained for the RSD, which is lowest at intermediate rotation rates (Figure 6.13b). This is in agreement with the maximum strain that the powder experiences at the intermediate rotation rates. The VRR results from 30 and 45 kg hr^{-1} are

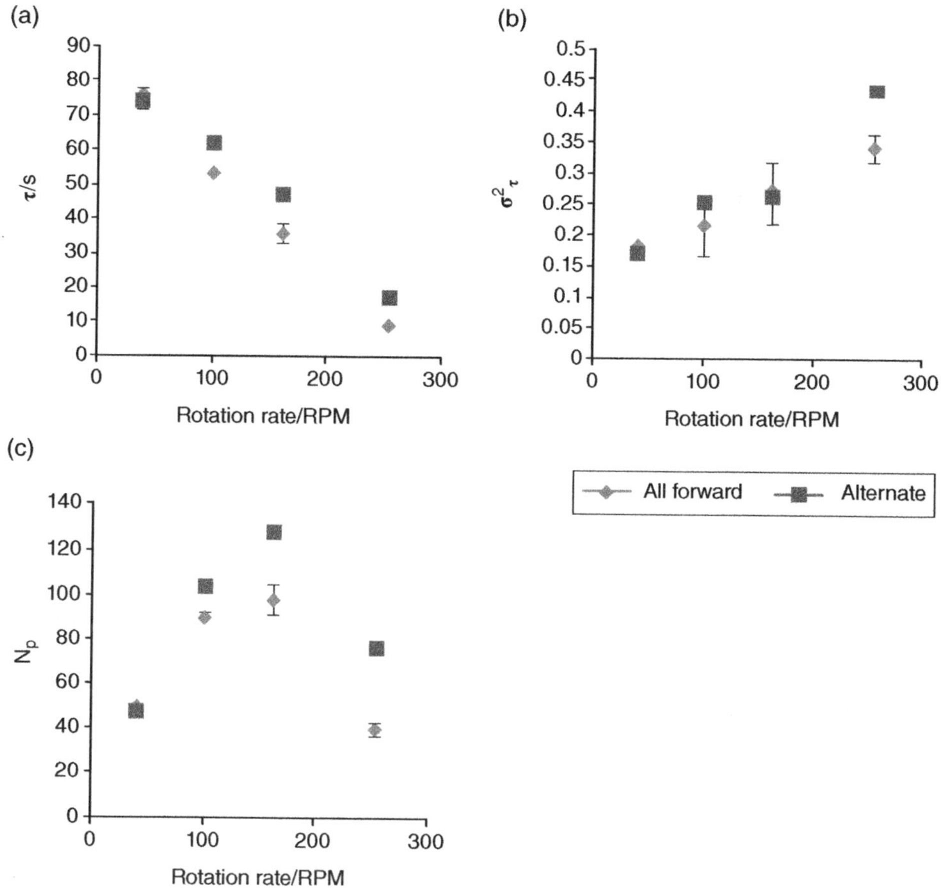

Figure 6.12 Blade configuration comparison – all forward and alternate as a function of impeller rotation rates. (a) Mean residence time, (b) Mean centered variance, (c) Number of blade passes

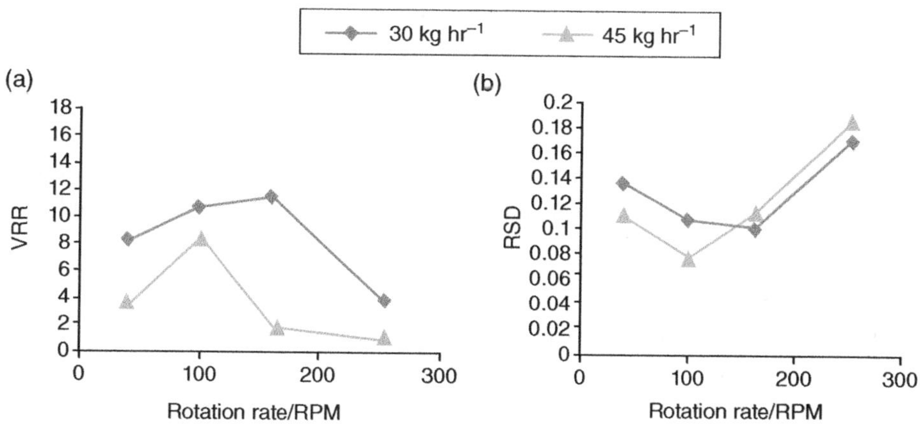

Figure 6.13 Mixing efficiency as a function of impeller rotation rate for 30 and 45 kg hr^{-1}. (a) Variance reduction ratio and (b) Relative standard deviation

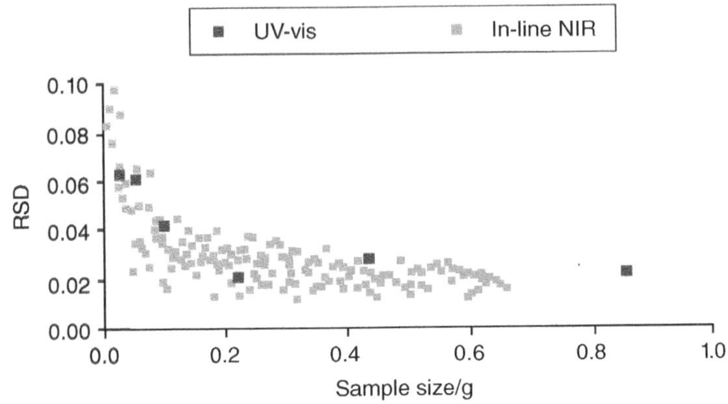

Figure 6.14 *Relative standard deviation as a function of sample size. Comparison between measurements with UV-vis and in-line NIR using fiber optic probes. Flow rate: 30 kg hr^{-1}. Blade configuration: alternate*

also compared. The VRR is higher for lower flow rates. This can be explained by the higher bulk mean residence time the powder spends in the blender allowing the powder to mix for more time. The RSD at the two feed rates is only significantly different at lower rotation rates. This can be explained by the difference in RTDs at lower rotation rates.

This work with a cohesive API (acetaminophen) [19] yielded high RSD results (8–20%). The high RSDs obtained can be explained by high variability when feeding acetaminophen, the fact that only 20 samples were used, and that NIR was used as the quantification method. NIR is only able to see a small sample of ~10–20 mg. Lower RSDs (<5%) have been obtained when using in-line NIR and other quantification techniques such as ultraviolet visible spectroscopy (UV-vis). Also the RSD as a function of sample size has been studied (Figure 6.14). RSDs can also be reduced by high shear mixing (milling) of the main excipients and the cohesive API before going into a continuous blender [22].

When the mill was used as a low residence time high-shear blender, it was demonstrated to eliminate any lumps in the cohesive API. Once in the continuous blender, high frequency fluctuations obtained from feeding are filtered along the axis of the blender. A schematic of this process with the mill placed between the feeders and the continuous mixer is shown in Figure 6.15a. Sample results are shown in Figure 6.15b. Clearly, the RSDs are lower when this process is used for low API concentrations. In the case of higher API concentrations, this technique will help in breaking API lumps that the shear in the continuous mixer will not. Therefore, in any scenario, this method guarantees a more homogeneous blend.

6.7.1 Modeling

Several modeling techniques have been used to describe and predict powder mixing behavior and its efficiency. Specific models for continuous powder mixing are categorized into data-based statistical models [8, 23, 24], RTD models [12, 25], discrete element method (DEM) based models [26–31], and population balance models (PBM) [32–34]. Hybrid models using both DEM and PBM have also been recently studied [35]. Hybrid models that include two or more processes in a continuous fashion are referred to as

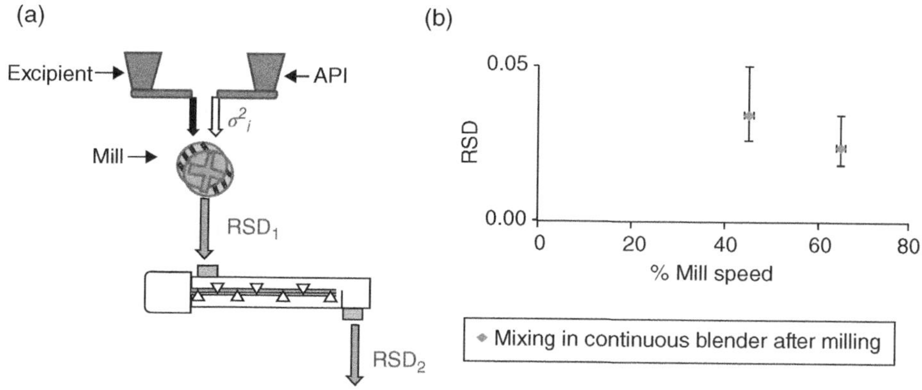

Figure 6.15 *Improvement of mixing efficient using a mill as a high shear mixer before the continuous mixer. (a) Experimental set: feeders, co-mill and continuous mixer. (b) Relative standard deviation measurements at two mill speeds at 30 kg hr*$^{-1}$*. RSD is reduced by using this set-up when compared to results in Figure 6.13. Blade configuration: alternate*

flowsheet modeling in other industries (i.e., petrochemical) and have been recently introduced in the pharmaceutical industry.

These modeling techniques generate potential uses for design, optimization, and control of the continuous blending process. Specifically, DEM models can be used for design purposes and faster statistical and RTD models can be used for control and dynamic optimization. Brief descriptions of some of the continuous mixing models in the literature with their potential engineering applications and main findings are given here. More detail on the modeling procedures and techniques can be found in the literature presented.

One of the most important modeling techniques used in continuous mixing was presented in Section 6.2, the RTD. The RTD describes the bulk flow dynamics and the efficiency of a continuous blender. The RTD in continuous mixing has been modeled using various techniques such as the Taylor dispersion model [25]. Other modeling techniques such as the Markov Chain [6, 36] and population balance models to describe the RTD [32, 33, 37] have been used. RTD modeling allows the prediction of the continuous mixing performance in various ways. RTD metrics such as the mean residence time, the mean centered variance and the dispersion coefficient can be obtained. All of these metrics determine the ability of a continuous mixer to filter out variability from feeding even before a material is fed. Furthermore, correlations with actual RTD data enable the prediction of the mixing performance (blend homogeneity) as measured by the RSD. This modeling technique is useful in predicting behavior from upstream processes (feeding) to the final blend homogeneity. Further studies correlating RTD metrics and the powder flow properties of final blends should be considered in order to be able to predict the performance of downstream processes.

Experimental powder methods often lack the capability to measure important variables and to resolve some of the powder phenomena occurring in the blender (most notably, the flow field and the forces between particles are often unknown in experimental studies). Therefore, one approach is to use DEM methods [38] to further understand particle-to-particle interactions, particle positions and trajectories, velocities and accelerations; shear rates, stress and strain histories, and bulk flow behavior among several others. DEM is a numerical technique able to simulate the behavior of granular materials by tracking single particles in the system of interest (Chapter 17). DEM models the forces acting on each simulated particle. These forces are categorized into two types: contact forces due to interactions with other particles and boundary conditions, and external forces such as gravity. The forces acting on each particle are calculated by solving Newton's equations of linear and rotational motion

DEM has been used to study the mixing dynamics in continuous blenders. Dubey *et al.* concluded that the same flow behavior described by experimental studies was achieved by using DEM in continuous mixing [28]. In addition, the velocity profiles and diffusion coefficients were obtained as a function of the mixing parameters and compared to theoretical characterization obtained from experiments. Gao [29, 30] and Sarkar [26, 27, 31] used periodic section modeling to study the effect of rotation rate and blade configuration on the dispersion coefficient, axial velocity profiles and mixing efficiency. The results from periodic section modeling with DEM concluded that similar mixing behavior is obtained and this technique can save large amounts of computational time. In all cases, DEM was proven to be a good tool for the simulation of continuous mixing. Thus it can be used to design a more effective blade configuration or more effective mixers as a whole.

The use of DEM coupled with PBM has created hybrid modeling techniques. These hybrid models have been proven to be useful to simulate and understand continuous mixing, as well as upstream and downstream processes. Sen used a DEM-PBM flow sheet model to study crystallization, filtering and drying of the API coupled with continuous mixing [35]. Coupling crystallization with continuous mixing can be useful in cases where the API is produced in-house. This hybrid model demonstrates the usefulness of flow sheet modeling in pharmaceutical continuous manufacturing. Boukouvala studied different manufacturing scenarios using hybrid flowsheet modeling [37]. In this case, population balance and data-based models were used. Scenarios such as continuous direct compression (feeding, mixing, and tableting) were considered. Singh also demonstrated the use of these hybrid models including modeling of control mechanisms in a continuous pharmaceutical manufacturing line with dry granulation (roller compaction) [39].

The unification of modeling techniques with control strategies takes the perspective of continuous pharmaceutical processing to a new level. In all examples shown, the use of modeling techniques in continuous mixing, and other processes, upstream and downstream, have demonstrated them to be powerful tools. These models can be used to predict and optimize the behavior of each unit operation separately and as a one continuous manufacturing process. The implementation of flowsheet modeling with control strategies up to now has been theoretical. Therefore, experimental tests in actual continuous manufacturing plants must be performed. Once all these methodologies are proven and fully integrated closed-loop controls are in place, the reality of continuous pharmaceutical manufacturing would reach a whole new level.

6.7.2 PAT, QbD, and Control

The advantages of using continuous powder mixing over batch have been previously described at the beginning of this chapter. Although these advantages are clear, the transition from batch to continuous will require time to develop, validate, and implement these new methods.

Pharmaceutical companies and research programs have recently started to implement process analytical technologies (PAT) to further understand both batch and continuous processes (Chapter 15). Scientifically understanding any process takes into account the quality by design (QbD) efforts. QbD in batch processes is useful in optimizing the process as a whole, but is not deterministic enough for real-time control of the process being monitored.

QbD can be applied to continuous processes using various PAT tools available to monitor the operating point. Whenever an offset from the operating point is perceived, the process would dynamically adjust to yield a high quality blend. The ultimate goal in continuous mixing is to use closed-loop control integrated with feeders and consecutive processes such as tableting. Therefore, it is critical to choose the right PAT tool to monitor continuous powder mixing. One of the most used PAT tools in the pharmaceutical industry is near-infrared (NIR) spectroscopy [40].

Recent research has shown that NIR can be used to quantify the concentration and variability of the key components of the final blend in continuous powder mixing [41, 42]. In-line NIR spectroscopy has been proven suitable for monitoring the blend concentration and homogeneity after the powder exits a continuous blender. Although NIR has been shown to monitor continuous powder mixing as well as other pharmaceutical processes, further development of NIR sensors and research to optimize its use and integration with control systems is being conducted. NIR can be used as a PAT tool along with adequate continuous mixing models to control and dynamically optimize the process. Powder blending never yields the finished product, therefore control systems for processes upstream (feeding) and downstream (i.e., tableting or granulation) have to be coupled with one another.

In batch mixing, blend uniformity is often determined by physical sampling throughout the whole blender volume. Sampling can introduce bias in the determination of the final blend concentration. This is different than continuous mixing, where no physical sampling along the blender length or depth is needed (or even practical) to determine blend uniformity. Only the powder exiting the blender to the next unit operation is considered. This generates a logical choice on where to place the NIR for determination of final blend concentration.

NIR is also useful in matching the scale of scrutiny (sample size) to that of the final dosage form. Since the powder is in motion (flowing) when it comes out of the blender, the sample size scan by the NIR can be approximated to match that of a tablet or capsule. The sample size is approximated by the velocity of the powder passing through the NIR probe, its bulk density, and the penetration depth, the diameter of the beam and the sampling (scanning) frequency of the NIR. The only two controllable variables are the velocity of the powder that can be adjusted depending on the set-up used, and the scanning frequency of the NIR. The blend uniformity can then be determined using typical statistics. The scanning frequency (acquisition time) must be suitable with regard to the mixing dynamics of the continuous blender. For example, if the mean residence time is 30 s then the RSD must be calculated from samples taken within that time frame to ensure steady operation.

Although flowing powder out of the mixer is beneficially used to approximate the required sample size (e.g., one unit dose) while using NIR measurements, this can also introduce noise in the spectral measurements because of powder density fluctuations. Therefore the design of the flowing powder-NIR interface might be carefully done. Typically, an interface with an optical window may be used to measure the flowing powder after it exits the blender. The powder will fall across the optical window while the NIR spectrometer is scanning. The in-line NIR probe can also be mounted on top of the blend, where no optical window is necessary. The study of these interfaces designs is the subject of on-going work. This work will determine the optimum interface designs for a variety of material properties and process parameters.

Although the logical choice to place the NIR probe or probes is at the outlet of the continuous blender, the question still remains of how many measurements are necessary to monitor the final blend concentration and homogeneity of the powder stream. In batch, after a blend is finished, representative samples of the full volume of the blender can be considered (with some well-known limitations). Typically, a few samples are used to describe the final blend uniformity, and regulatory agencies have developed standard statistical criteria for this situation. In continuous mixing, the powder is constantly flowing and the final blend concentration and uniformity may vary with time. In continuous mixing, the composition of the blend is constantly measured, yielding thousands of measurements. Regulatory statistical criteria for evaluating mixing uniformity in this situation remain to be developed. Moreover, some new physics might be at issue. The powder coming out of the blender is in a dilated state, and depending on the flow properties, expands to a certain degree when it falls onto the interface. Since the NIR beam is only a few millimeters in diameter, using a single point probe will only monitor a small portion of the powder across the whole flow stream coming out of the blender. For this purpose, the concept of using multi-point NIR probes commonly used in other industries (i.e., paper) has been studied [43].

The use of NIR spectroscopy with high acquisition frequency and multi-point probes as a PAT tool can improve monitoring of continuous powder mixing. These PAT tools make sampling across the stream possible in continuous manufacturing. Such methods are excellent for research purposes, but they might not be required in all manufacturing processes. Another issue is that the while the NIR beam penetrates several millimeters as evidenced in transmission measurements, the radiation received by a diffuse reflectance detector is mostly from the top 0.5–2.0 mm of the powder bed [44, 45]. Therefore, critical studies must be performed in order to determine if the NIR sampling technique is deterministic enough when it only samples the outer layer of a powder blend.

Once the right PAT tools and control and predictive models are in place, continuous mixing must be coupled with feeding and consecutive processes. As previously shown in Sections 6.2 and 6.5, several modeling techniques can help describe and predict continuous mixing behavior. As mentioned, the most recently developed approach uses dynamic flowsheet modeling and sensitivity analysis [34, 39]. This approach uses population balances, RTD, and performance-based models to simulate continuous powder blending, with feeding, and consecutive processes. Models for feeding, and real-time concatenation of processes must also be in place to have a fully operational and controllable system. This flowsheet modeling has already been tested theoretically. The next step is to test the models with a full continuous manufacturing line. Flowsheet modeling is a start in the effort to control an integrated continuous manufacturing process.

6.8 Conclusions and Continuing Efforts

This chapter has touched upon the main topics involving continuous mixing and pharmaceutical manufacturing. However, continuous mixing is just one important part of the overall manufacturing process. Continuous pharmaceutical manufacturing have several advantages over traditional batch processing. Therefore, over the last decade, we have witnessed a very large increase in interest to study these processes. Several research institutions and pharmaceutical companies have made advances that place continuous manufacturing as the "new" manufacturing platform in the pharmaceutical industry.

In general, the characterization of these technologies in terms of unit operations has proven useful. For example, continuous direct compression has been proven to perform at least as good, and often better, than its batch equivalent and it is now the chosen platform by several companies currently developing commercial processes. However, there is still much work needed in order to fully understand continuous pharmaceutical manufacturing. In addition, there is still the need to further develop, understand and implement PAT and modeling tools for control purposes.

Continuous manufacturing will also require further development of predictive testing methods in order to support real-time release of the finished products. The combination of PAT tools and models to control the manufacturing process have started to trace a good path for this. In this effort, research has already started to study a series of techniques that would serve as a surrogate to the typical dissolution testing required by regulatory agencies.

While predictions are often risky, the authors of this chapter believe that in the next few years, continuous manufacturing will spread from brand to generic and from in-house to contract manufacturing, until it becomes a standard tool in the pharmaceutical manufacturing toolbox. More importantly, since continuous manufacturing is an ideal platform to develop predictive control methodologies and to achieve a higher standard of process understanding, we expect that the lessons learned while implementing continuous manufacturing processes will make significant contributions to the design and optimization of batch processes. All the more reason to develop them with enthusiasm.

References

[1] Harwood, C.F., et al., *The performance of continuous mixers for dry powders.* Powder Technology, 1975. **11**(3): p. 289–296.

[2] Kehlenbeck, V. and K. Sommer, *Modeling of the mixing process of very fine powders in a continuous dynamic mixer.* Fourth International Conference on Conveying and Handling of Particulate Solids, 2003: p. 9.26–9.31.

[3] Pernenkil, L. and C.L. Cooney, *A review on the continuous blending of powders.* Chemical Engineering Science, 2006. **61**(2): p. 720–742.

[4] Weinekotter, R. and L. Reh, *Continuous mixing of fine particles.* Particle & Particle Systems Characterization, 1995. **12**(1): p. 46–53.

[5] Ziegler, G.R. and C.A. Aguilar, *Residence time distribution in a co-rotating, twin-screw continuous mixer by the step change method.* Journal of Food Engineering, 2003. **59**(2–3): p. 161–167.

[6] K. Marikh, H.B., V. Mizonov, E. Barantseva, D. Ponomarev, *Flow analysis and Markov chain modelling to quantify the agitation effect in a continuous powder mixer.* Chemical Engineering Research and Design, 2006. **84**(11): p. 1059–1074.

[7] Berthiaux, H., K. Marikh, and C. Gatumel, *Continuous mixing of powder mixtures with pharmaceutical process constraints.* Chemical Engineering and Processing, 2008. **47**(12): p. 2315–2322.

[8] Portillo, P.M., M.G. Ierapetritou, and F.J. Muzzio, *Effects of rotation rate, mixing angle, and cohesion in two continuous powder mixers - A statistical approach.* Powder Technology, 2009. **194**: p. 217–227.

[9] Portillo, P.M., M.G. Ierapetritou, and F.J. Muzzio, *Characterization of continuous powder mixing processes*. Powder Technology, 2008. **182**: p. 368–378.

[10] Weinekotter, R., *Compact and efficient continuous mixing processes for production of food and pharmaceutical powders*. Trends in Food Science & Technology, 2009. **20**: p. S48–S50.

[11] Engisch, W.E. and F.J. Muzzio, *Method for characterization of loss-in-weight feeder equipment*. Powder Tech., 2012. **228**: p. 395–403.

[12] Gao, Y., F. Muzzio, and M. Ierapetritou, *Characterization of feeder effects on continuous solid mixing using fourier series analysis*. AIChE Journal, 2010. **57**(5): p. 1144–1153.

[13] Danckwerts, P.V., *The definition and measurement of some characteristics of mixtures*. Appl. Sci. Res., 1952. **3**: p. 279–296.

[14] Fogler, H.S., Elements of chemical reaction engineering. 4th edn. Prentice Hall PTR International Series in the Physical and Chemical Engineering Sciences, 2006, Upper Saddle River, NJ: Prentice Hall PTR. xxxii, 1080 p.

[15] Whittles, D.N., et al., *An investigation into the parameters affecting mass flow rate of ore material through a microwave continuous feed system*. Advanced Powder Technology, 2005. **16**(6): p. 585–609.

[16] Harris, A.T., J.F. Davidson, and R.B. Thorpe, *The influence of the riser exit on the particle residence time distribution in a circulating fluidised bed riser*. Chemical Engineering Science, 2003. **58**(16): p. 3669–3680.

[17] Beaudry, J.P., *Blender efficiency*. Chemical Engineering, 1948. **55**: p. 2.

[18] Nauman, E.B., *Residence time theory*. Industrial & Engineering Chemistry Research, 2008. **47**(10): p. 3752–3766.

[19] Vanarase, A.U. and F.J. Muzzio, *Effect of operating conditions and design parameters in a continuous powder mixer*. Powder Technology, 2011. **208**(1): p. 26–36.

[20] Vanarase, A.U. and Rutgers University. Graduate School--New Brunswick., *Design, modeling and real-time monitoring of continuous powder mixing processes,* 2011. p. ix, 159 p.

[21] Mizonov, V., et al., *Influence of crosswise non-homogeneity of particulate flow on residence time distribution in a continuous mixer*. Powder Technology, 2009. **190**(1–2): p. 6–9.

[22] Vanarase, A.U., J.G. Osorio, and F.J. Muzzio, *Effects of powder flow properties and shear environment on the performance of continuous mixing of pharmaceutical powders*. Powder Tech., 2013. Volume **246**, 63–72

[23] Boukouvala, F., F.J. Muzzio, and M. Ierapetritou, *Predictive modeling of pharmaceutical processes with missing and noisy data*. AIChE Journal, 2010. **56**(11): p. 2860–2872.

[24] Boukouvala, F., F.J. Muzzio, and M. Ierapetritou, *Design space of pharmaceutical processes using data-driven-based methods*. Journal of Pharmaceutical Innovation, 2010. **5**: p. 119–137.

[25] Gao, Y., et al., *Characterizing continuous powder mixing using residence time distribution*. Chemical Engineering Science, 2011. **66**(3): p. 417–425.

[26] Sarkar, A. and C. Wassgren, *Continuous blending of cohesive granular material*. Chemical Engineering Science, 2010. **65**(21): p. 5687–5698.

[27] Sarkar, A. and C. Wassgren, *Simulation of a continuous granular mixer: Effect of operating conditions on flow and mixing*. Chemical Engineering Science, 2009. **64**(11): p. 2672–2682.

[28] Dubey, A., et al., *Computational approaches for studying the granular dynamics of continuous blending processes, 1-DEM based methods*. Macromolecular Materials and Engineering, 2011. **296**(3–4): p. 290–307.

[29] Gao, Y., M. Ierapetritou, and F. Muzzio, *Investigation on the effect of blade patterns on continuous solid mixing performance*. The Canadian Journal of Chemical Engineering, 2011. **89**(5): p. 969–984.

[30] Gao, Y., M. Ierapetritou, and F. Muzzio, *Periodic section modeling of convective continuous powder mixing processes*. AIChE Journal, 2012. **58**: p. 69–78.

[31] Sarkar, A. and C.R. Wassgren, *Comparison of flow microdynamics for a continuous granular mixer with predictions from periodic slice DEM simulations*. Powder Technology, 2012. **221**: p. 325–336.

[32] Sen, M., et al., *Multi-dimensional population balance modeling and experimental validation of continuous powder mixing processes*. Chem. Eng. Sci., 2012. **80**: p. 349–360.

[33] Sen, M. and R. Ramachandran, *A multi-dimensional population balance model approach to continuous powder mixing processes*. Advanced Powder Tech., 2013. **24**: p. 51–59.

[34] Boukouvala, F., et al., *An integrated approach for dynamic flowsheet modeling and sensitivity analysis of a continuous tablet manufacturing process*. Computers & Chemical Engineering, 2012. **42**: p. 30–47.

[35] Sen, M., et al., *Multi-scale flowsheet simulation of an integrated continuous purification-downstream pharmaceutical manufacturing process*. Inter. J. Pharm., 2013. **445**: p. 29–38.

[36] Mizonov, V., et al., *Modeling continuous powder mixing by means of the theory of Markov chains*. Particulate Science and Technology, 2004. **22**(4): p. 379–389.

[37] Boukouvala, F., et al., *Computational approaches for studying the granular dynamics of continuous blending processes, 2-population balance and data-based methods*. Macromolecular Materials and Engineering, 2012. **297**(1): p. 9–19.

[38] Bharadwaj, R., *Using DEM to solve bulk maerial handling problems,* in *Chemical Engineering Progress*2012, AIChE. p. 54–57.

[39] Singh, R., M. Ierapetritou, and R. Ramachandran, *An engineering study on the enhanced control and operation of continuous manufacturing of pharmaceutical tablets via roller compaction*. Int. J. Pharm., 2012. **438**: p. 307–326.

[40] Roggo, Y., et al., *A review of near infrared spectroscopy and chemometrics in pharmaceutical technologies*. Journal of Pharmaceutical and Biomedical Analysis, 2007. **44**(3): p. 638–700.

[41] Kehlenbeck, V., Use of near infrared spectroscopy for in- and off-line performance determination of continuous and batch powder mixers: opportunities & challenges. 11th International Congress on Engineering and Food (ICEF11), 2011. **1**: p. 2015–2022.

[42] Vanarase, A.U., et al., *Real-time monitoring of drug concentration in a continuous powder mixing process using NIR spectroscopy*. Chemical Engineering Science, 2010. **65**(21): p. 5728–5733.

[43] Vanarase, A.U., et al., *Development of a methodology to estimate error in the on-line measurements of blend uniformity in a continuous powder mixing process*. Powder Tech., 2013. **241**: p. 263–271.

[44] Bellamy, L.J., A. Nordon, and D. Littlejohn, *Real-time monitoring of powder mixing in a convective blender using non-invasive reflectance NIR spectroscopy*. The Analyst, 2007. **133**: p. 58–64.

[45] Popo, M., et al., *Blend uniformity analysis using stream sampling and Near Infrared spectroscopy*. AAPS PharmSciTech., 2002. **3**(3): p. Article 24.

7

Dispersion of Fine Powders in Liquids: Particle Incorporation and Size Reduction

Gül N. Özcan-Taşkın
BHR Group (trading name for VirtualPiE Ltd), UK

This chapter will discuss the challenges and approaches relating to mixing powders into liquids. When fine (micron or sub-micron size) powders are added in a liquid, they tend to form macroscale clusters, containing air and dry powder, thereby forming a hierarchy of structures. The ultimate aim of the process is to prepare a homogenous, fine dispersion that is stable with a narrow size distribution. The first requirement is therefore to achieve a suspension with particles incorporated into the liquid phase without settling. This pre-dispersion can then be processed further to reduce the size of the agglomerates and achieve a fine dispersion. These two main processes of interest, powder incorporation and deagglomeration or size reduction, are discussed in this chapter.

7.1 Particle Incorporation into Liquids

The ease at which powder incorporation will be achieved depends on both the physical properties of the solid and liquid phases, presence of additives that can affect these and the hydrodynamic conditions in the process device. The process device commonly used for

Pharmaceutical Blending and Mixing, First Edition. Edited by P.J. Cullen, Rodolfo J. Romañach, Nicolas Abatzoglou and Chris D. Rielly.

this purpose is the stirred tank as this can also act as the holding tank for the intermediate product or as the feed tank prior to passing the pre-dispersion to a more power intensive device to achieve break up. In-line devices that can be used for this purpose as well are briefly presented at the end of this section.

Incorporation of a powder into a liquid will be spontaneous if the added powder has a density higher than the liquid phase, the liquid phase wets the powder easily and any clusters formed are not strongly bonded (Etchells, 2001a,b). This is often not the case and whilst the density of the powder may be higher than the liquid phase, poor wettability as well as the low bulk density due to the air trapped in these clusters result in the powder floating at the liquid surface. The first step of the dispersion process is therefore to ensure that wetting is achieved to be able to incorporate the solid phase into the liquid.

7.1.1 Wetting

When fine powder clusters are added to the liquid surface, the liquid phase begins to penetrate into the clusters to make it clusters, which results in clusters being engulfed. Through penetration of the liquid phase replacing the air within the cluster, the density of the cluster increases until it detaches and is incorporated into the liquid phase. The Young–Dupré equation is used to describe the different stages of wetting:

$$\gamma_{s/V} = \gamma_{s/L} + \gamma_{L/V} \cos\theta \tag{7.1}$$

where $\gamma_{s/v}$, $\gamma_{s/L}$, $\gamma_{L/v}$ are the interfacial free energies at the solid-vapour, solid-liquid and liquid-vapour interfaces, respectively, and θ is the contact angle.

The three stages of wetting have been defined (Parfitt and Barnes, 1997) as shown in Figure 7.1. The work required for *adhesional wetting*, W_a, is related to the contacting of the solid with a liquid and expressed as follows:

$$W_a = \gamma_{s/L} - (\gamma_{L/v} + \gamma_{s/v}) = -\gamma_{L/v}(\cos\theta + 1) \tag{7.2}$$

Positive W_a means work is required to achieve adhesional wetting whereas for $\theta < 180°$, W_a is negative and therefore adhesional wetting is spontaneous.

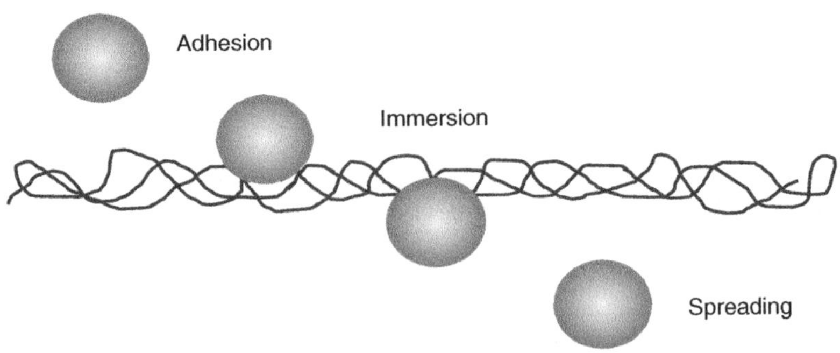

Figure 7.1 *Different stages of wetting: adhesional, immersional and spreading wetting*

The energy exchange for completely immersing the solid into a liquid is described by the work for *immersion*, W_i:

$$W_i = 4\gamma_{s/L} - 4\gamma_{s/v} = -4\gamma_{L/v}\cos\theta \quad (7.3)$$

If $\theta < 90°$, W_i is negative and therefore immersional wetting is spontaneous.

Work for *spreading* liquid over the surface if a solid, W_s, is expressed as:

$$W_s = (\gamma_{s/L} + \gamma_{L/v}) - \gamma_{s/v}) = -\gamma_{L/v}(\cos\theta - 1) \quad (7.4)$$

W_s is negative only if $\theta = 0°$. These calculations allow one to identify which stage of the wetting process is spontaneous or which is retarding the overall process. The overall work that needs to be expended for the whole process can be predicted from the sum of these:

$$\sum W = W_a + W_i + W_s = 6\gamma_{s/L} - 6\gamma_{s/v} = -6\gamma_{L/v}\cos\theta \quad (7.5)$$

Whilst the contact angle for liquids over smooth surfaces can be determined, this is a challenging task for clusters of very fine powders due to the roughness of the surface and the porous nature.

In addition to determining the work required for wetting, the rate of wetting or rate of penetration of liquid into the interstices of particle clusters is also of importance. For this, a simple case consideration (horizontal capillaries, i.e. where gravity can be neglected) has led to the Washburn equation:

$$l = \sqrt{\frac{rt\gamma_{L/v}\cos\theta}{2\mu}} \quad (7.6)$$

where l is the depth of penetration in time t and μ is liquid viscosity.

For a packed bed of particles, the radius has been replaced by a size factor, K, which contains the radius for the bed and turtuosity factor that takes into account the complex path formed by the channels between the particles and aggregates:

$$l^2 = \frac{Kt\gamma_{L/v}\cos\theta}{2\mu} \quad (7.7)$$

To achieve quick penetration, $\gamma_{L/v}$ should be high and so should K (i.e. loosely packed powder), θ and μ low.

It is worth noting that whilst high $\gamma_{L/v}$ and low θ will give the fastest penetration, these two are incompatible (Parfitt and Barnes, 1997). A contact angle of 90° means that the liquid is relatively non-wetting; 5° means that it is relatively wetting (Nelson, 1988). Surfactants are used to alter these properties to promote the wetting process.

Whilst the ease at which particles will be incorporated into the liquid phase can be predicted from these calculations, in industrial practice, the choice of the process equipment, operating conditions and the resulting hydrodynamics also determine the incorporation time or the rate of incorporation if the process is continuous. The following sections are related to process equipment.

7.1.2 Stirred Tanks for Particle Incorporation

Stirred tanks are commonly used to incorporate the dry powders into a liquid and maintain them in suspension to generate a crude dispersion prior to feeding this into a 'high intensity' device (Figure 7.2).

Powder additions are typically made at the liquid surface. The study of flow conditions close to the liquid surface in a stirred tank presents several difficulties in terms of both experimental and computational techniques available. The liquid surface is invariably rough due to waves, stable or intermittent vortices: the latter also introducing air bubbles, hence another phase. This prevents the measurement of velocities sufficiently close to the surface to be carried out using optical techniques and also poses challenges for the use of computational methods. Based on experimental studies, progress could be made in terms of the importance of equipment choice, operating conditions and scale up.

For particles that float at the liquid surface due to density difference, we determine 'just draw down speed,' N_{JD} and corresponding power consumption, P_{JD}. In most cases, it is sufficient to operate at a speed that ensures draw down. The corresponding speed determines the gear box size and power, motor size and operating costs. N_{JD} is defined as the speed at which no solids remain at the liquid surface for more than 2–4 s. It is worth pointing out that other definitions have also been used by researchers, such as 1–2s as the criterion or no solids remain stationary at the surface.

For fine powders that can float although they are of a higher density than the liquid phase, we determine the time required to incorporate at a given speed and hence power consumption. References are made to both cases in the paragraphs that follow.

The only *correlation* relating to particle incorporation is an empirical one and is specific to a given geometry where a single baffle of a width of $0.2T$ immersed at the top of the liquid to a wetted depth of $0.3T$ was used (Joosten et al., 1977). Joosten's correlation relates the Froude number ($Fr = N^2D/g$) for draw down to D/T and $\Delta\rho/\rho_L$:

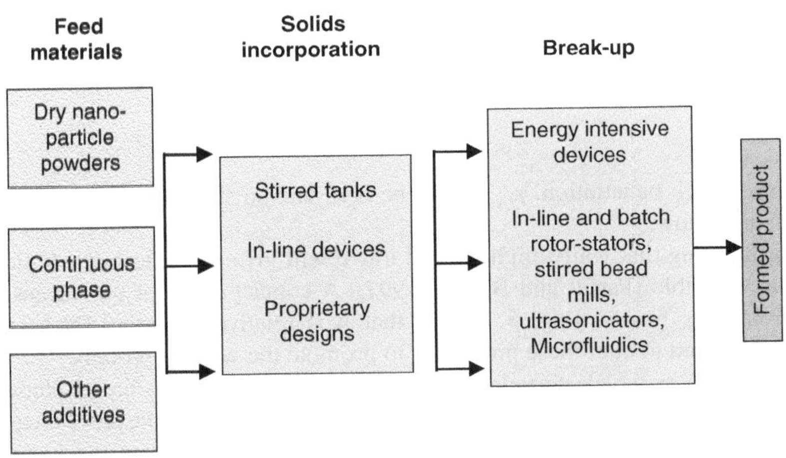

Figure 7.2 Different process devices used for particle incorporation and deagglomeration (break up) of fine particle clusters

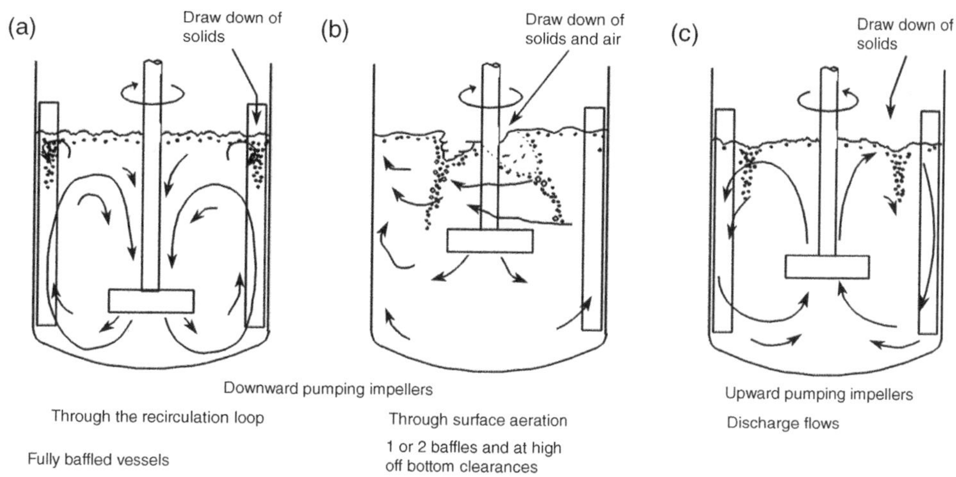

Figure 7.3 *Draw down modes with up and down pumping impellers (Őzcan-Taşkin and Wei, 2003; Őzcan-Taşkin, 2006). Reprinted with permission from* Chem. Eng. Sci.*, The effect of impeller-to-tank diameter ratio on draw down of solids by Gül Özcan-Taşkin, Hongyuan Wei, 58, 10, 2011–2022. Copyright (2003) Elsevier*

$$\mathrm{Fr}_{\mathrm{JD}} = k\left(\frac{D}{T}\right)^{-3.65}\left(\frac{\Delta\rho}{\rho_L}\right)^{0.42} \tag{7.8}$$

for the following conditions:

$0.27 \leq T \leq 1.8$ m; $0.29 \leq D/T \leq 0.60$; $0.1 \leq (\Delta \rho/\rho_L) \leq 0.76$; $0.11 \leq C/T \leq 0.33$;
$2 \leq d_p \leq 13$ mm; $\mu = 1 \times 10^{-3}$ Pa s; $\rho_L = 1000$ kg m^{-3}.

Values of k were different for different impeller types: 3.3×10^{-2} for a six-bladed inclined paddle; 3.6×10^{-2} for a four-bladed inclined paddle; 7.4×10^{-2} for a two-bladed inclined paddle and 19.6×10^{-2} for a three-bladed marine propeller.

Further studies have shown that draw down is not only affected by the type of impeller but also its position, pumping mode as well as presence and number of baffles in the tank. Three different *mechanisms of draw down* could be identified as shown in Figure 7.3 (Őzcan-Taşkin and McGrath, 2001; Őzcan-Taşkin and Wei, 2003; Őzcan-Taşkin, 2006). In a fully baffled tank using a down pumping impeller, floating particles are drawn down into regions close to the tank walls through the recirculation loops (Figure 7.3a). It has for long been assumed that the formation of air ingesting vortices need to be generated to entrain floating particles from the surface. This is indeed possible in un-baffled or partially baffled tanks, when the impeller is mounted close to the surface (Figure 7.3b). Standard impeller submergence (C_s) is 2/3–3/4 tank diameter and submergences smaller than half the tank diameter result in the formation of surface vortices also depending on the liquid viscosity. This is, however, an undesirable condition as the overall flow pattern is predominantly in the tangential direction, that is, with little top-to-bottom mixing, impairing homogeneity. In addition, the formation of unstable vortices, the waviness of the liquid surface can result in shaft vibrations, torque instabilities and fouling of vessel walls. The presence air bubbles may not be desirable for certain products. When, on the other hand, an upward pumping impeller is used, the flows heading away from the impeller are directed towards the liquid surface where the particles float, entraining the particles (Figure 7.3c). Floating particles can be drawn down into the liquid without the formation of a vortex; the liquid surface is reported to be less wavy with minimal splashing. This mode of operation has also shown to be advantageous for particle incorporation in terms of power requirement as detailed in the following paragraphs.

7.1.2.1 Importance of Operating Conditions on Particle Incorporation and Scale Up

The way in which floating particles are incorporated from the surface has an effect on the speed and power required for draw down. As Figure 7.4 shows, with up pumping impellers the power requirement is lower in comparison to down pumping impellers. This is because the impeller discharge, that is, the zone of high liquid velocities and turbulence, is directed towards the liquid surface as described previously.

It is worth noting the differences in up and down pumping modes in terms of the effect of impeller submergence (C_s). As the distance between the impeller and liquid surface, that is, impeller submergence, decreases, the power required using an up pumping impeller decreases. In the case of a down pumping impeller, at high submergences, that is, when the impeller is closer to the tank base, floating particles are drawn down through the recirculation loop as shown in Figure 7.3a. As the distance between the impeller and liquid surface decreases, the power requirement increases and once surface aeration starts with vortices entraining both air and floating particles (Figure 7.3b), a drop in power demand is noted (Figure 7.4).

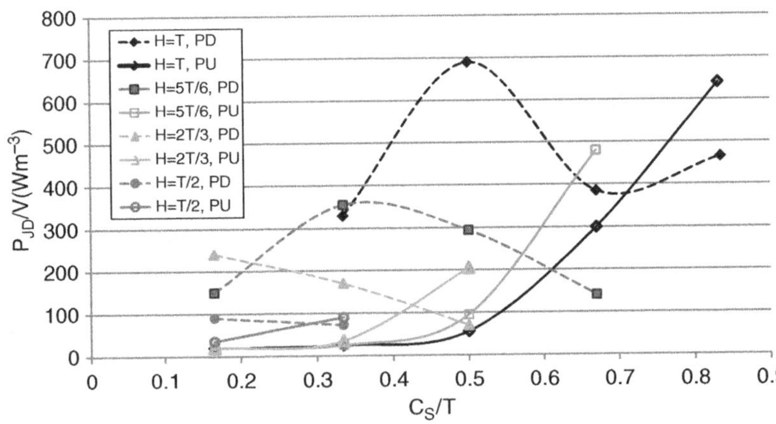

Figure 7.4 *Effect of pumping mode, impeller position and liquid height on draw down power. The impeller used a pitched blade turbine (PBT) of D = T/3 in a fully baffled tank of T = 2.67 m. 1% polyethylene particles (904 kg/m³) in water were used (Őzcan-Taşkin, 2006). Reprinted with permission from* Chem. Eng. Sci., *Effect of scale on the draw down of floating solids by Gül Özcan-Taşkin, 61, 9, 2871–2879 Copyright (2006) Elsevier*

For scale up, maintaining specific power input constant is reported to be the most appropriate criterion with up-pumping impellers (Őzcan-Taşkin, 2006) in the absence of air entrainment. With downward pumping impellers, whilst due to the complicated dependence on a range of operating conditions resulting in changes in the way solids are entrained from the surface, it was not possible to obtain a given scale-up criterion, keeping the Froude number constant meant that draw down speed could be estimated within ±30%.

7.1.2.2 Choice of Impeller Type and Diameter

An assessment of the performance of different impeller types on the basis of specific power input has shown that impellers that pump radially outwards towards the vessel walls are the least efficient (Őzcan-Taşkin and McGrath, 2001) as would be expected. This is also the case for saw tooth impellers that are known to generate high levels of turbulence in the vicinity of the teeth. Axial flow impellers have therefore received more attention for processes requiring particle incorporation from the surface. In the case of fine particles that tend to form clusters and need deagglomerating after incorporation, the saw tooth impeller as an additional impeller can prove to be useful as discussed later in this chapter.

A comparison of axial flow impellers of a *diameter* of 1/3 and 1/2 the tank diameter has shown that with the smaller diameter, D = T/3, impeller, the axial flow is more predominant resulting in a lower power demand to achieve just draw down conditions except when solid are drawn down via surface vortices that also entrain air as shown in Figure 7.5 (Őzcan-Taşkin and Wei, 2003). It could be shown through LDA measurements and CFD predictions that with the larger impeller, the discharge flows had an important radial

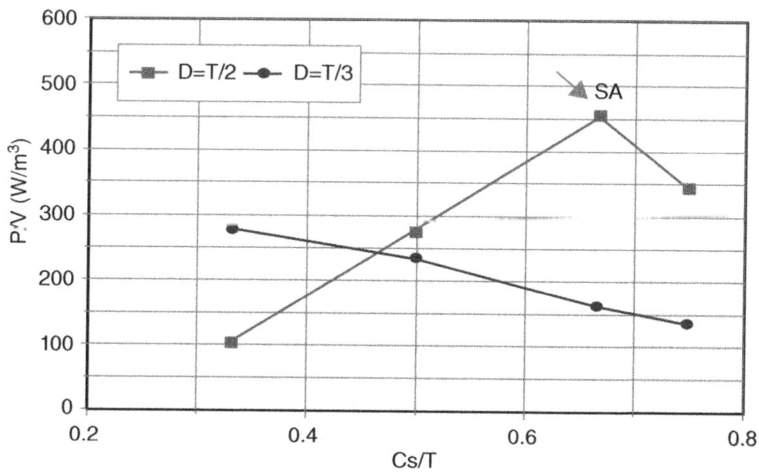

Figure 7.5 *Importance of impeller diameter on specific power (P\V)jd required to draw down solids with down-pumping PBTs. Polyethylene particles at 1% w:w in water (Őzcan-Taşkin and Wei, 2003). Reprinted with permission from* Chem. Eng. Sci.*, The effect of impeller-to-tank diameter ratio on draw down of solids by Gül Özcan-Taşkin, Hongyuan Wei, 58, 10, 2011–2022. Copyright (2003) Elsevier*

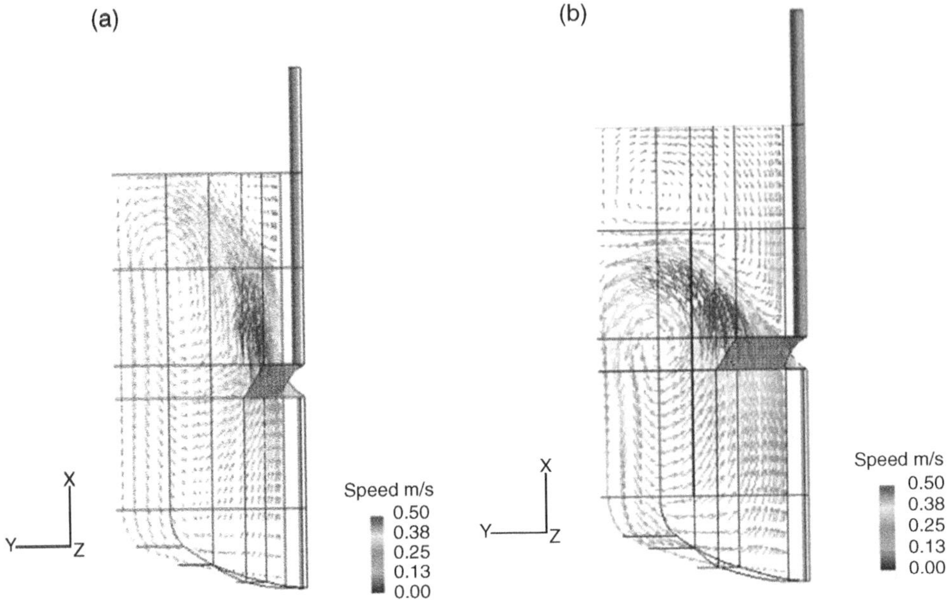

Figure 7.6 *Flow patterns with (a) D = T/3 and (b) D = T/2 PBT pumping up (Őzcan-Taşkin and Wei, 2003). Reprinted with permission from* Chem. Eng. Sci., *The effect of impeller-to-tank diameter ratio on draw down of solids by Gül Özcan-Taşkin, Hongyuan Wei, 58, 10, 2011–2022. Copyright (2003) Elsevier*

component resulting in the flow being at an angle thereby requiring a higher power consumption to achieve drawdown from the surface. Figure 7.6 shows CFD predictions of the effect of impeller diameter on the flow patterns generated with an up pumping impeller.

7.1.2.3 Incorporation of Fine Powders and Rate of Draw Down

Findings reported here are for relatively large particles (of the order of some mm in size) that float at the liquid surface due to density difference. Further work with fine powders, for example clusters of nanoscale particles, were also in agreement in terms of overall findings and it could be shown that, with up pumping axial flow impellers, powder incorporation can be achieved much faster under given conditions. As explained previously, such materials are often of a higher density than the liquid phase and can be incorporated into the liquid phase over a wide range of conditions (N and P); different from the case of light particles for which a certain speed has to be exceeded. Hence, it is how quickly they will be incorporated, that is, the rate of incorporation that is relevant for fine powders.

Figure 7.7 shows the comparative performance of different types of impellers for incorporating clusters of nanoscale hydrophilic silica powder (Aerosil 200V) into water. In line with findings for larger particles that float due to density difference, an up-pumping hydrofoil (LE-20) close to the liquid surface achieves incorporation faster than others (Őzcan-Taşkin et al., 2006; Xie et al., 2007).

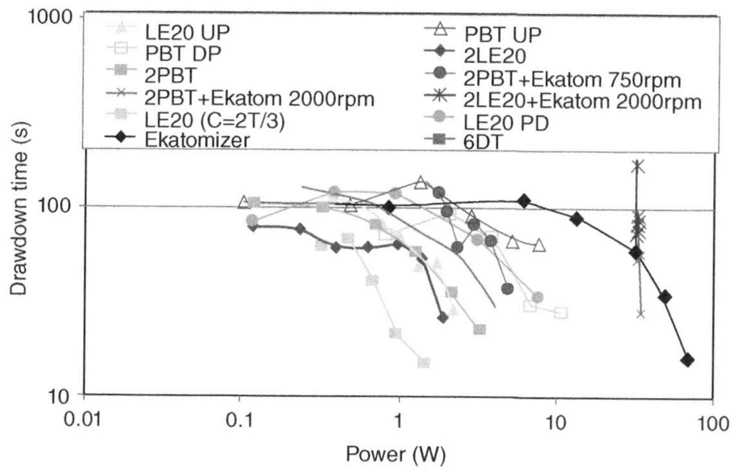

Figure 7.7 *Time required to incorporate 1% w:w of clusters of nanoscale hydrophilic silica powder (Aerosil 200V) into water using a range of impellers: axial flow hydrofoil, LE20; mixed flow pitched blade turbine and the sawtooth impeller Ekatomizer (Őzcan-Taşkin et al., 2006; Xie et al., 2007). Reprinted with permission from* Chem. Eng. Res. Des., *85, 5, 676–684. Copyright (2007) Elsevier*

The effect of power input on incorporation time can also be seen in Figure 7.7: whilst this is not prominent at low speeds, incorporation becomes faster as the speed, hence power input is increased.

It is worth noting though that although the power input by the different types of impellers is very different, the incorporation time is of the order of a few minutes in all cases for this given specific type of particle, and the energy input ($E = P \times t$) is determined primarily by the power input. Differences due to the choice of impeller type and operating conditions become obvious when the particle concentration is higher than a few per cent by weight, which often requires the introduction of the powder over a period. In industrial practice, a simple rule-of-thumb is sometimes followed and the powder is introduced at a rate of 1% per minute. This may well work at low concentrations but once it exceeds 3–5%, incorporation time increases steeply as shown in Figure 7.8 (Őzcan-Taşkin et al., 2006). This is also consistent with findings using larger particles that float due to density difference: Edwards and Ellis (1984) and Thring and Edwards (1990) reported that the effect of solid concentration is negligible covering solid mass ratios less than 3.75%. The consequence of this would be the powder accumulation at the surface as shown in Figure 7.9. It is therefore important to have a prior knowledge of the operating window over which 1% per minute will hold and either increase the speed once a critical concentration is exceeded, or wait longer.

7.1.2.4 *Proprietary Designs*

Recent publications on a proprietary design, the Ytron Y Jet, have highlighted some of its advantages, in particular for increasing powder concentrations (Őzcan-Taşkin, 2012; 2013). The design includes a down pumping axial flow impeller placed in a short, baffled

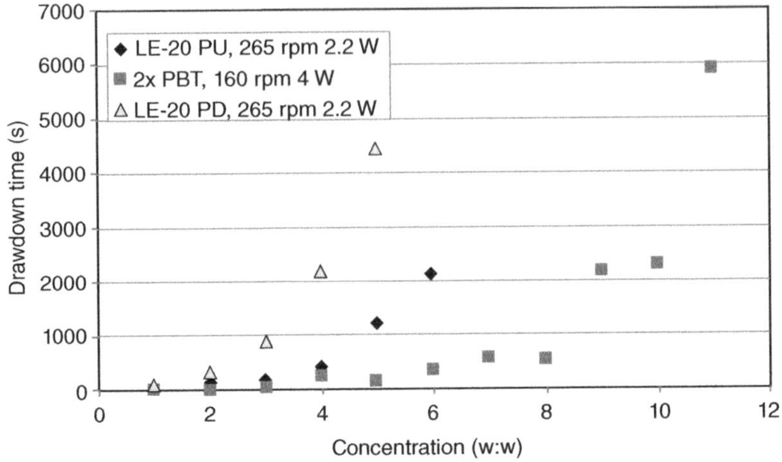

Figure 7.8 *Importance of powder concentration on incorporation time with different types of impellers. Additions of nanoscale hydrophilic silica (Aerosil 200V) are made into water at increments of 1% w:w and values on the x-axis are cumulative; incorporation time is for each increment (Őzcan-Taşkin et al., 2006). Reprinted with permission from* Chem. Eng. Sci. *61, 9, 2871–2879. Copyright (2006) Elsevier*

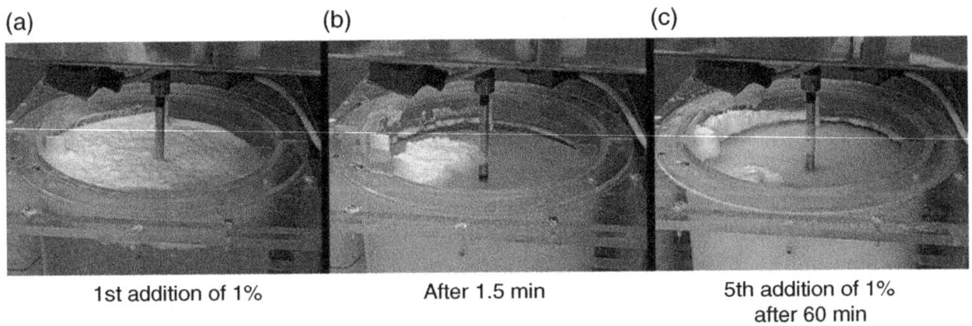

Figure 7.9 *Effect of increasing concentration of particle addition-additions of Aerosil 200V made at increments of 1% w:w: the incorporation of the first 1% addition can be completed within a few min; the fifth addition requires over an hour*

draft tube (Figure 7.10a). Due to the close clearance of the impeller and the typically high speed of operation (thousands of rpm), this is also referred to as the 'rotor-stator.' A feed tube, which is part of the design, is used to introduce the particles directly into the impeller region through suction generated by the rotating impeller. The feed tube can be connected to either a hose, the other end of which is inserted into the powder bag (Figure 7.10b), thereby preventing any dust being raised in the working environment or to a funnel where the powder is charged (Figure 7.10c). Large units make use of a hopper.

A comparison of this design with conventional configurations, adding the powder at the liquid surface, has shown that at a given specific power input it is comparable to the

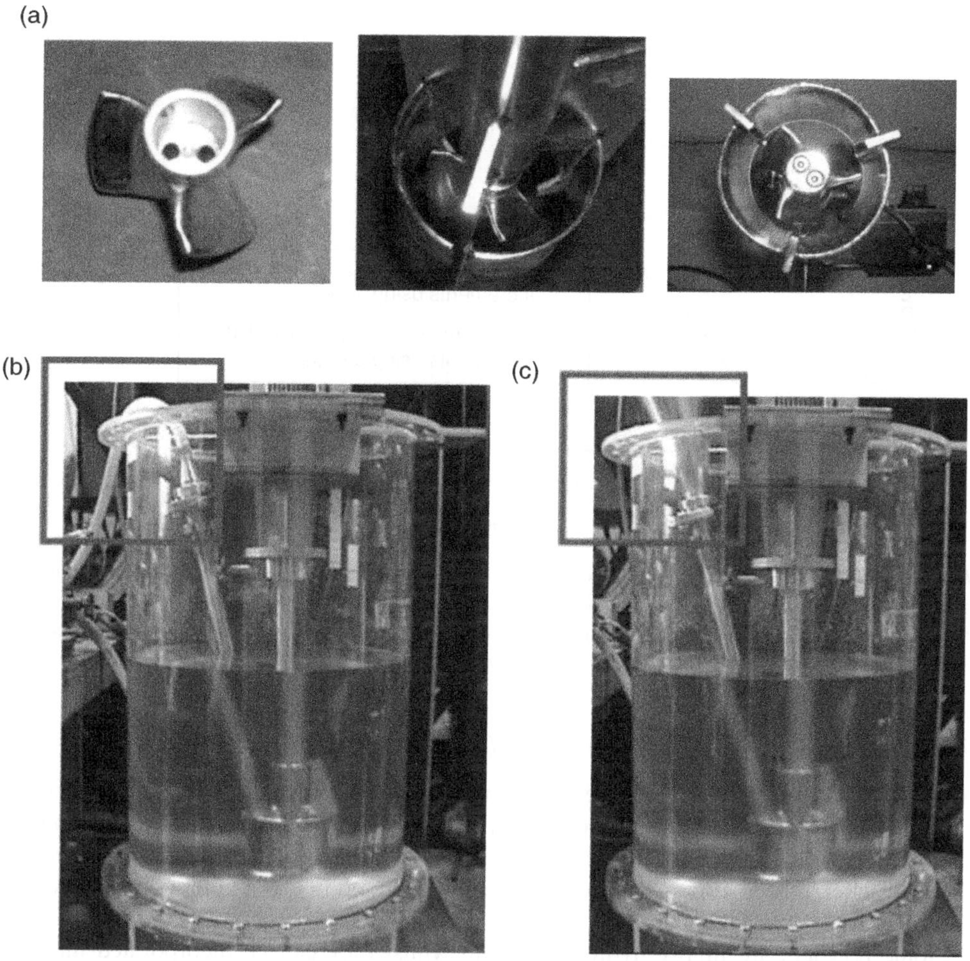

Figure 7.10 Ytron Y Jet design: (a) down pumping axial flow impeller placed in a baffled stator is placed off-centre in a tank (b) and (c). Powder feed tube can be connected to a hose which can be inserted into the powder bag (b) or (c) a funnel where particles are charged (Őzcan-Taşkin, 2012; 2013). Reprinted with permission from Chem. Eng. Res. Des., Incorporation of nanoparticle clusters into a liquid using a proprietary design mixer, Ytron Y Jet by N. Gül Özcan-Taşkın, 91, 11, 2243–2249. Copyright (2013) Elsevier

performance of a down pumping pitched blade turbine (Őzcan-Taşkin, 2012; 2013). On the other hand, when the feed pipe is used allowing the introduction of the powder into the impeller region, the drawdown rate could be maintained constant across a range of concentrations as shown in Figure 7.11 (Őzcan-Taşkin, 2013). Incorporation rate started to decrease only when a high concentration resulting in a non-Newtonian dispersion rheology was reached. The ability to make powder additions into the impeller region is the main advantage of this design.

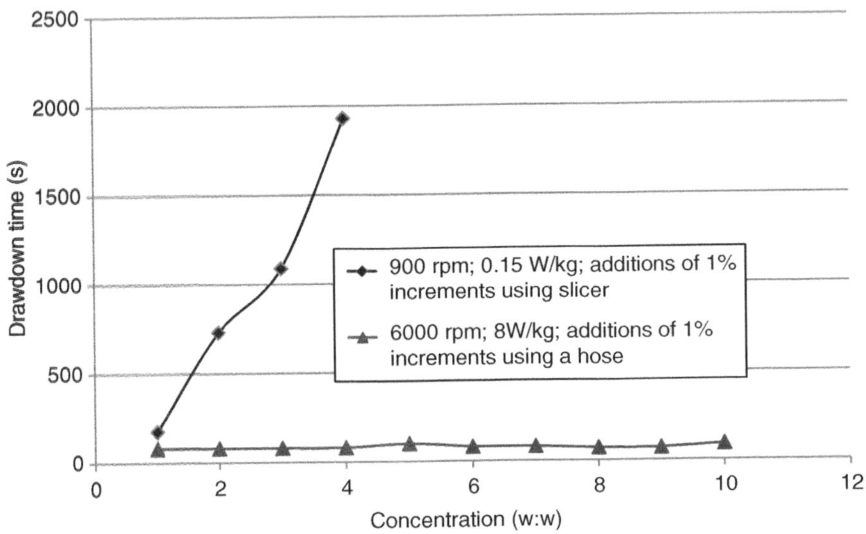

Figure 7.11 *Effect of powder concentration on the performance of Ytron Y Jet for surface additions and additions made via the feed tube (Őzcan-Taşkin, 2013). Reprinted with permission from* Chem. Eng. Res. Des., *Incorporation of nanoparticle clusters into a liquid using a proprietary design mixer, Ytron Y Jet by N. Gül Özcan-Taşkın, 91, 11, 2243–2249. Copyright (2013) Elsevier*

7.1.2.5 Final Remarks Relating to Stirred Tanks

Apart from incorporation the process may have other requirements. For example, heavy particles, once incorporated into the liquid phase, may require additional power input to maintain them in suspension. In such cases, to prevent settling at the vessel base, a second axial impeller, placed close to the vessel base and operated in down pumping mode would bring improvements.

Some powders are highly hydrophobic and whilst they can be incorporated into the liquid phase, it may not be possible to maintain them in suspension unless a certain degree of break up is achieved. With certain materials, inter-particle bridges become stronger as the proportion of liquid between particles increases when they are in contact with a liquid, and the clusters become more cohesive and more difficult to incorporate (Parfitt and Barnes, 1997). For those cases, the design should be such that incorporation and deagglomeration are achieved simultaneously.

Other recommendations include the use of a vacuum chamber to add low viscosity liquids to the powder (Nelson, 1988). Mixing high viscosity liquids require high power input. In addition, the removal of air in these liquids is much slower. Making an initial dispersion in a low viscosity liquid and subsequently evaporation may provide a solution (Nelson, 1988).

7.1.3 In-Line Devices Used for Particle Incorporation

Several in-line devices for particle incorporation are also available on the market. Some of these are shown in Figures 7.12, 7.13, and 7.14, which were downloaded from manufacturers' websites.

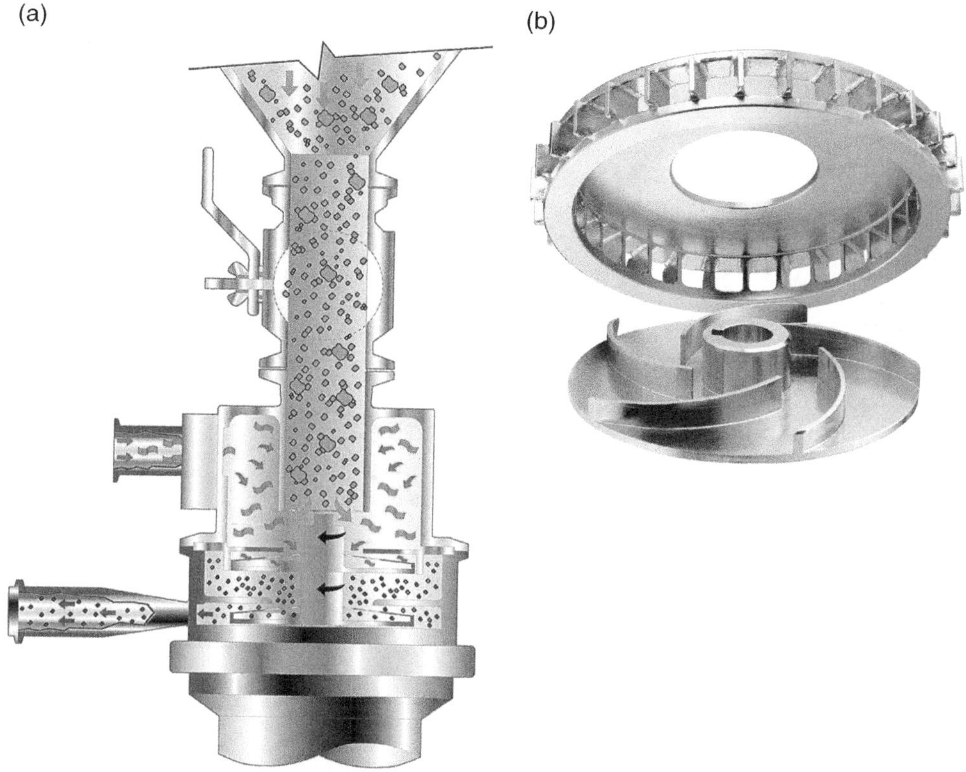

Figure 7.12 (a) Ytron XC schematic representation; (b) Ytron XC Powder Disperser Head. Copyright (2006) Ytron-Quadro (UK) Ltd

Ytron XC Powder Disperser, shown in Figure 7.12 is an example in-line rotor-stator. It is a two stage reactor. Firstly, a strong vacuum draws powders into the reactor. After contact with the liquid, the 'pre-mix' is impelled against the chamber plates, where the powder is absorbed into the liquid phase. In the second stage a homogenous wetted product is discharged.

Manufacturers recommend the use of Ytron ZC for powders that are difficult to wet. This device includes a close tolerance high shear slotted rotor-stator design. The rotor creates a liquid ring and thus a vacuum, which draws the powder into the reactor head where it is sheared into the liquid before hydration.

The Tri-blender consists of a centrifugal pump head and impeller mounted so that the suction port or inlet is pointed upwards (see www.csidesigns.com). The centrifugal pump head, rotated horizontally, sucks the powder from the hopper through the diffuser tube. The liquid phase is directed into the impeller via the outer tube. Splashing is prevented by introducing the liquid into the chamber in the same direction as the impeller so that the inlet tube can be kept dry during operation without plugging up. Vacucam® Ejector Mixer from Semi-Bulk Systems In-Line Ejector is an eductor type of mixer (see www.semi-bulk.com). Liquid phase is pumped through a nozzle, creating a converging cone of liquid. In

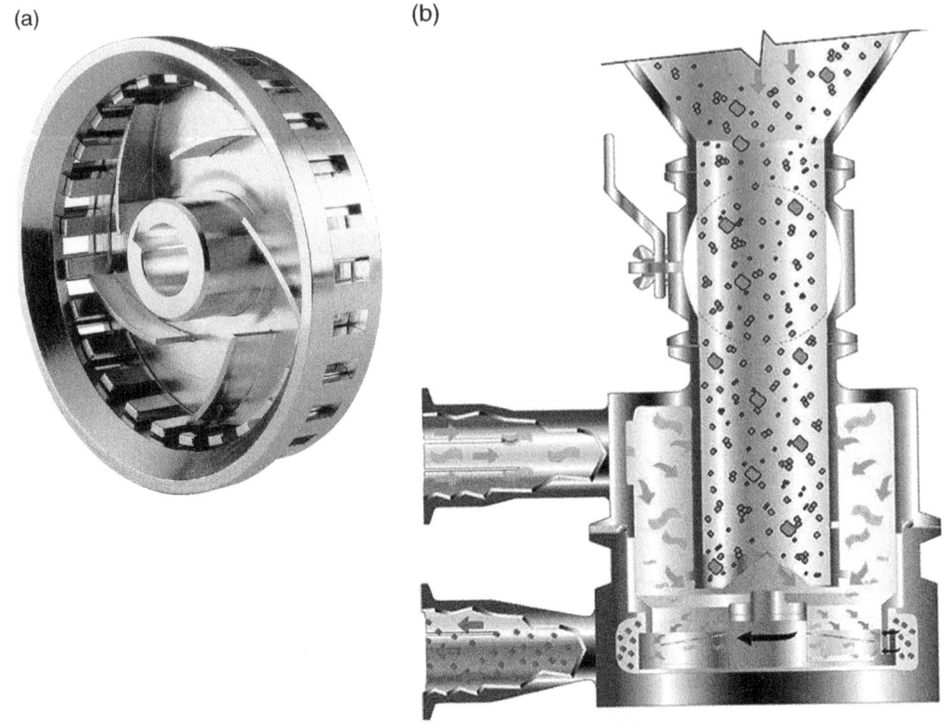

Figure 7.13 (a) Ytron ZC; (b) Ytron ZC Powder Disperser Head. Copyright (2006) Ytron-Quadro (UK) Ltd

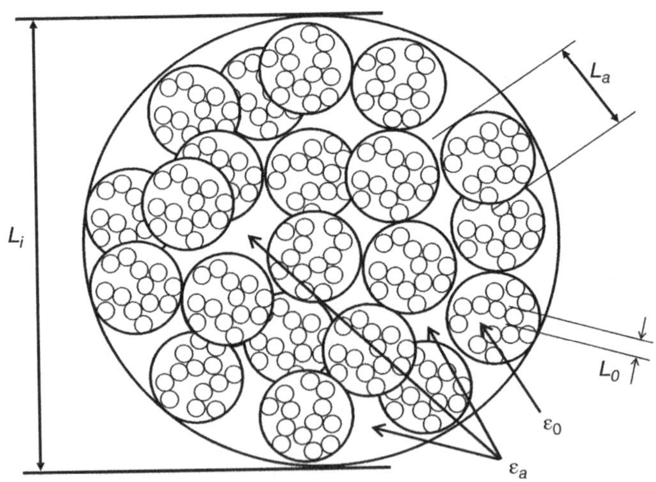

Figure 7.14 Schematic representation of a large agglomerate. Baldyga et al. (2008)

a separate stream, solids are fluidized with air to separate particles and this stream is introduced into the centre of the cone. The solid phase is thus introduced as individual particles resulting in a dispersion. Independent research evaluating the performance of these devices is typically conducted in-house for a specific product and not available in open literature.

7.2 Break Up of Fine Powder Clusters in Liquids

Once incorporated into the liquid phase, the next step is to reduce the size of the particle clusters to achieve as fine a dispersion as possible with a narrow particle size distribution. The terminology relating to these clusters can differ in different textbooks. Loosely bonded clusters of particles attached at the edges and corners are referred as agglomerates in this chapter. Aggregates, on the other hand, are held together with much stronger bonds, with particles attached on the surfaces as shown in Figures 7.14 and 7.15. Whilst the surface area of an agglomerate is not significantly different from the sum of the areas of its components, an aggregate has a much smaller surface area compared to the sum of the areas of the primary particles it consists of. It is possible to break up agglomerates in a process device, but not aggregates that have much stronger bonds. Therefore, whilst the target of the process is to reduce the size down to the primary particle size, the finest dispersion often contains aggregates. A great deal of improvement can be achieved during processing through the knowledge of the mechanism of break up and the performance of the process device used, which are discussed in the following sections.

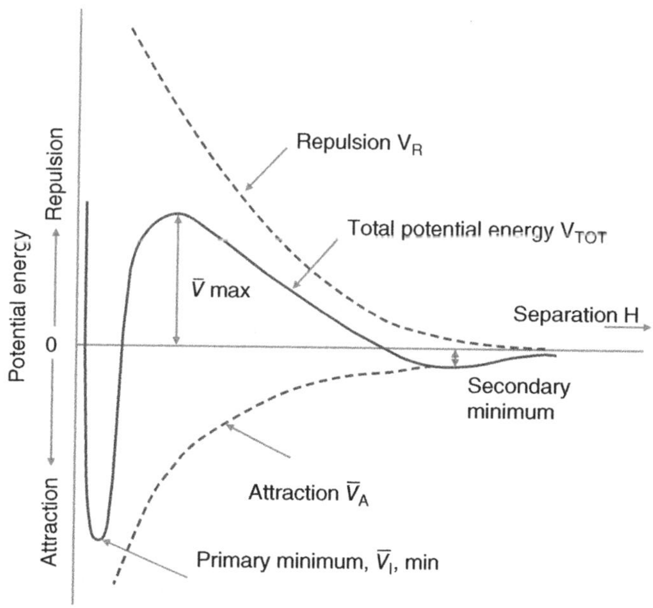

Figure 7.15 *Potential energy for two charged particles in an aqueous medium*

Break up will occur if the forces present in a processing environment are sufficiently high to overcome the physicochemical forces that bind a cluster. Three major inter-particle interactions are:

1. the London-van der Waals' attractive forces,
2. the Coulombic force, which can be attractive or repulsive, associated with charged particles, and
3. the repulsive force due to the interaction between adsorbed layers of polymer on the particle surfaces.

In addition, hydrophobic forces may play a role. DLVO theory (named after the two groups of researchers Derjagui and Landau and Verwey and Overbeek) describes the physicochemical forces (1 and 2 in the previous list) between colloidal particles. The DLVO theory predicts the potential between two spherical particles of equal radii. In reality, particles or particle clusters are hardly spherical and of the same size, but this classical theory has commonly been used as a fundamental basis. The total potential energy of the system, V_{TOT}, is calculated by the potential energy of attraction, V_A, and repulsion, V_R, $V_{TOT} = V_A + V_R$. Figure 7.15 shows the typical potential energy plot for a dispersion in aqueous media. V_R decreases exponentially depending on the thickness of the electric double layer. V_A has an inverse relationship with the square of the distance. The shape of the V_{TOT} curve is primarily determined by V_R. Of the two minima, the primary minimum is related to the particles that are in close contact and are difficult to disperse. The second minimum characterizes particles that are loosely attached and can therefore be broken up. Following on from the classical DLVO theory, the total force, F_{TOT}, is:

$$F_{TOT} = \frac{dV_{TOT}}{dH} = -\frac{dV_A}{dH} = \frac{dV_R}{dH} \tag{7.9}$$

Attractive, F_A, and repulsive forces, F_R, can be calculated as follows (Rumpf, 1962; Baldyga et al., 2006, 2007a and 2007b):

$$F_A = -\frac{HaR}{24H^2} \tag{7.10}$$

$$F_R = \frac{16\pi\chi R k_B T^2}{e^2 z^2 H}\left\{\frac{\exp\left[{}^{ze\psi_0}\!/\!_{(2k_BT)}\right]-1}{\exp\left[{}^{ze\psi_0}\!/\!_{(2k_BT)}\right]+1}\right\}^2 \exp(-\kappa H) \tag{7.11}$$

where Ha is the Hamaker constant;

R the radius and
H the distance between particles in a cluster;
χ is the static permittivity;
k_B is the Boltzmann constant;
ψ_0 the surface potential due to the surface charge on the particle (which can be taken as the zetapotential) and
κ is the reciprocal of the double layer thickness.

The total force is then calculated as: $F_{TOT} = F_A + F_R$.

Different experimental methods have been used to determine the strength of the particle clusters (e.g. tensile testing of compact pellets, notched bending of compacted beams and compression testing of compacted beds by penetration of a conical testing). These measure different properties and therefore different values will be obtained for a given agglomerate/aggregate. The expression that is commonly used to calculate the tensile strength of agglomerates, σ_T, (Rumpf, 1962; Baldyga et al., 2006, 2007a and 2007b) incorporates F_{TOT} as follows:

$$\sigma_T = 1.1\frac{(1-\varepsilon_a)}{\varepsilon_a}\frac{F_{TOT}}{L_a^2} \tag{7.12}$$

where $\varepsilon_a(L)$ is the porosity of the clusters and L_a the aggregate size, as shown in Figure 7.16.

The average volume fractions of aggregates ($\bar{\varphi}$) and porosity (ε_a) are related as follows:

$$\bar{\varphi} = 1-\varepsilon_a \tag{7.13}$$

Considering fractal geometry, this can be expressed as:

$$\bar{\varphi} = \frac{\theta_a^{\frac{D_f}{3}}\delta_a^{\frac{D_f}{3}-1}}{\delta_0^{\frac{D_f}{3}-1}}\left[\frac{Li}{L_a}\right]^{D_f-3} \tag{7.14}$$

This gives an average value. If erosion is the dominant break up mechanism, this will occur on the periphery of the agglomerate and therefore it is the local value of volume fraction on the external layer ($\phi(L)$) that would be of interest. This can be written using fractal geometry (Baldyga, 2007):

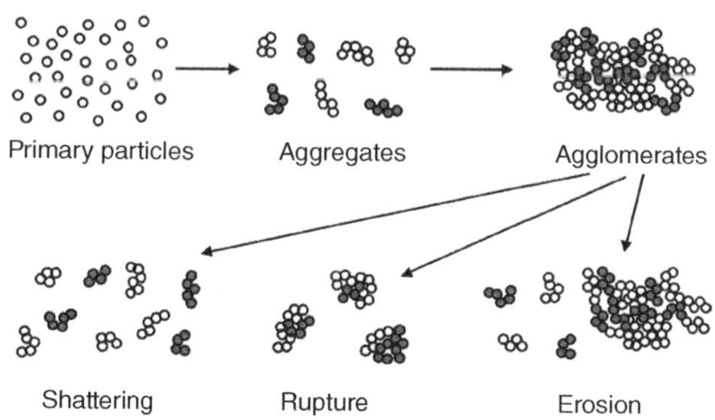

Figure 7.16 *Schematic representation of particle clusters and their breakage through erosion, rupture and shattering. Reprinted with permission from* Chem. Eng. Res. Des., *Effect of particle type on the mechanisms of break up of nanoscale particle clusters by N. Gül Özcan-Taşkin, Gustavo Padron, Adam Voelkel, 87, 4, 468–473. Copyright (2009) Elsevier*

$$\varphi(L)=\frac{D_f}{3}\bar{\varphi}=\frac{D_f}{3}\frac{\theta_a^{\frac{D_f}{3}}\delta_a^{\frac{D_f}{3}-1}}{\delta_0^{\frac{D_f}{3}-1}}\left[\frac{L_i}{L_a}\right]^{D_f-3} \tag{7.15}$$

and the external porosity is

$$\varepsilon_a(L)=1-\phi(L) \tag{7.16}$$

Under laminar conditions, break up occurs if shear and extensional stresses (τ)

$$\tau=\mu\dot{\gamma} \tag{7.17}$$

are sufficiently high to overcome the tensile strength.

Under turbulent conditions, this is achieved by turbulent stresses acting on agglomerates. If $l \gg L_i \gg \lambda_k$, l being macroscale of turbulence and λ_k Kolmogorov microscale, break up occurs through eddies in the inertial subrange of turbulence:

$$\tau \propto \rho\varepsilon^{2\backslash 3}L_i^{2\backslash 3} \tag{7.18}$$

ε being the local energy dissipation rate per unit mass of liquid. If $L_i < \lambda_{k,}$ break up occurs through viscous subrange eddies. According to Shinnar (1961):

$$\tau \propto \rho\varepsilon L_i^2\nu^{-1} \tag{7.19}$$

The theoretical basis of this approach was critiqued by Bourne and Baldyga (1993) as it involves both viscous and inertial effects. Baldyga and Bourne (1999) proposed the following:

$$\tau \propto \mu\left(\frac{\varepsilon}{\nu}\right)^{1/2}=\rho\nu^{1/2}\varepsilon^{1/2} \tag{7.20}$$

ν being the kinematic viscosity of the liquid.

Under laminar conditions, extensional and shear stresses cause the fragmentation of an agglomerate.

7.2.1 Mechanisms of Break Up

Break up occurs through different mechanisms and equally if not more importantly the kinetics of break up can be very different depending on both the material properties and the forces acting on agglomerates.

Broadly, two main mechanisms of break up were described (Rwei et al., 1990; 1991; Ottino et al., 2000), as schematically shown in Figure 7.16, along with shattering, which is a very fast break up process:

- *rupture* occurs when a large agglomerate is broken up into several agglomerates of comparable size (equisized fragments) or different sizes (uniform breakage); which are subsequently broken up further;

- *erosion* when small fragments are gradually sheared off from these large clusters or agglomerates. The resulting smaller fragments are either aggregates that cannot be broken up further under the effect of hydrodynamic stresses or primary particles; and
- *shattering* results in an agglomerate breaking up in a large number of smaller fragments in a single event.

Some similarities can be drawn between these and the break up processes in immiscible liquids: erosion is analogous to tip streaming, rupture to necking and shattering to capillary break up (Ottino, 2000).

Depending on the mechanism of break up, particle size distribution evolves differently in time during the break up process (Őzcan-Taşkin, 2009). This is schematically shown in Figure 7.17. Bi-modal size distributions are obtained if the predominant mechanism is erosion or shattering. When the smallest size fragments – aggregates or primary particles – are eroded off the surface of an agglomerate, the volume and size of coarse material decreases in time, both shifting the peak for coarse materials to the left and reducing in size whilst increasing the volume of sub-micron size material around the same mean value. When an agglomerate shatters into its finest size fragment, this also increases the volume of sub-micron material, but that for coarse material simply decreases whilst remaining around the same mean value. Where break up occurs through rupture, size distribution shifts to the left.

In addition to the mechanism of break up, knowledge of the kinetics can prove to be most useful in process design. While doing so, it is important to differentiate between fine and coarse material where bi-modal particle size distributions are obtained rather than using a mean diameter for the whole distribution. Figure 7.18 compares the evolution of the mean diameter of fines, coarse material for two dispersions. In the case of Aeroxide Alu C-in-water, break up occurs through shattering giving a practically flat profile in terms of the coarse material mean diameter, whereas with Aerosil 200V-in-water with which an erosive breakage is observed, mean diameter for coarse material decreases (Figure 7.18a). It is also worth noting the differences in the evolution of the fine volume fraction (Figure 7.18b) for these two materials.

This example illustrates differences due to material properties. For a given formulation, the rate of break up rate also depends on the processing environment defined by the choice of equipment and operating conditions.

7.2.2 Process Devices for Deagglomeration\Size Reduction of Agglomerates

Compared to powder incorporation and pre-dispersion preparation, more power intensive devices are required for deagglomeration and typically rotor-stators, ultrasonicators, high pressure devices and stirred bead mills have been used for this purpose.

Deagglomeration using an ultrasonic disperser occurs through the collapse of cavitational bubbles, which form during a low (rarefaction) pressure cycle as the sound waves propagate into the liquid. When these vacuum bubbles reach a volume at which they can no longer absorb energy, they implode during a high (compression) pressure cycle. The ultrasonic disperser is typically used for small scale for product formulation although recently larger scale productions units are also made available on the market.

In-line rotor-stators on the other hand are typically used at intermediate (pilot) and industrial scale. Their characteristic feature is a high-speed rotor in close proximity (usually

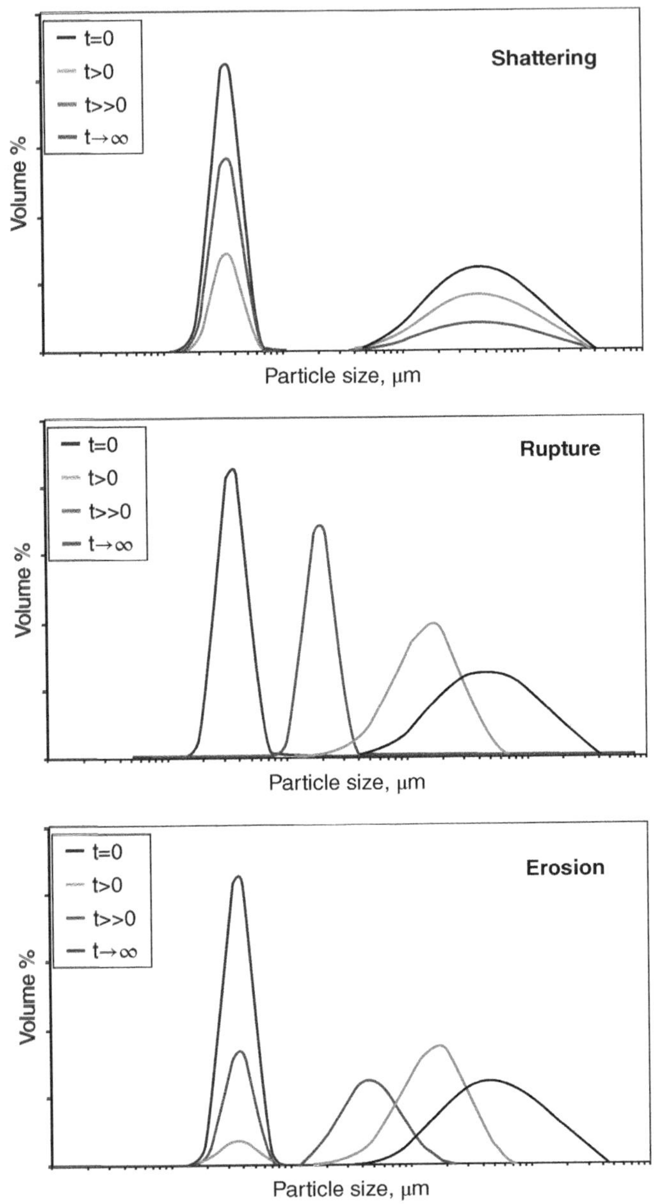

Figure 7.17 *Schematic representation of distributions that will be obtained through different mechanisms of break up. Reprinted with permission from* Chem. Eng. Res. Des., *Effect of particle type on the mechanisms of break up of nanoscale particle clusters by N. Gül Özcan-Taşkin, Gustavo Padron, Adam Voelkel, 87, 4, 468–473. Copyright (2009) Elsevier*

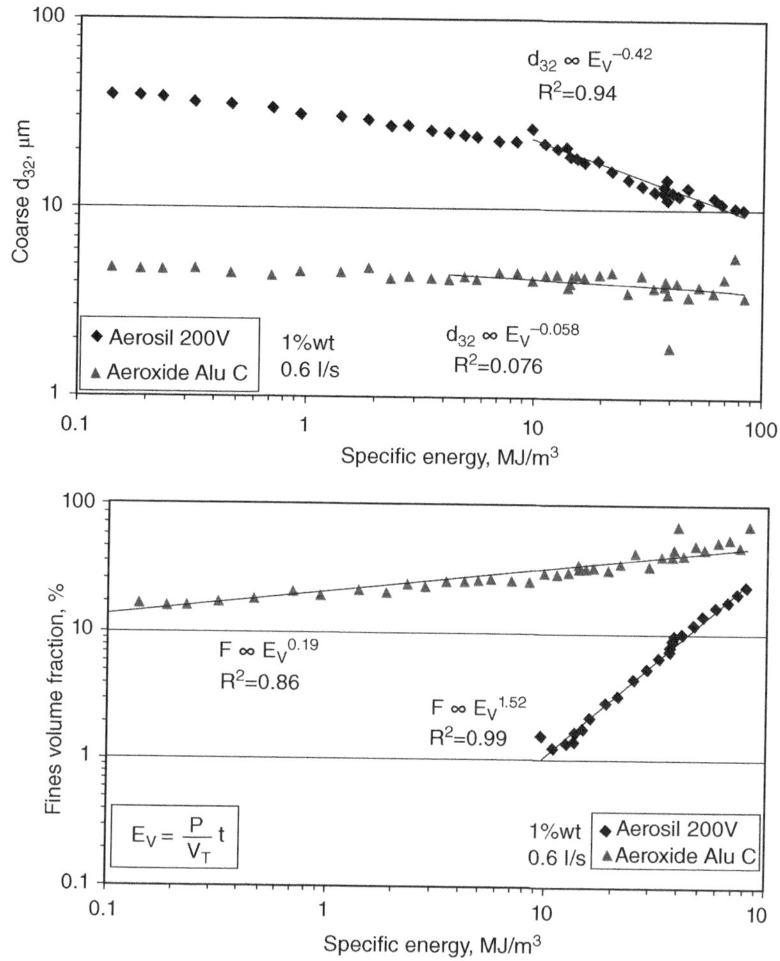

Figure 7.18 *Evolution of Sauter mean diameter of (a) coarse material (b) fines of two aqueous dispersions: 1% w:w Aerosil 200V which breaks up through erosion and 1% w:w Aeroxide AluC which breaks up through shattering (Özcan-Taşkin, 2009). Reprinted with permission from* Chem. Eng. Res. Des., *Effect of particle type on the mechanisms of break up of nanoscale particle clusters by N. Gül Özcan-Taşkin, Gustavo Padron, Adam Voelkel, 87, 4, 468–473. Copyright (2009) Elsevier*

less than 1 mm) to a fixed stator. High local shear rates are generated within the small gap between rotor and stator and the local energy dissipation rates are typically orders of magnitude greater than those obtained with conventional stirred tanks.

Several different types of process equipment exist that rely on high pressure such as high pressure jets, valve homogenizers. High pressure jets consist of a high pressure pump and a nozzle (typically of a diameter of 80–200 μm) creating pressures of several thousand bars. Elongational flow generated in the capillary and subsequently the turbulent jet at the outlet characterized with high Reynolds stresses act on particle clusters and cause break up.

Stirred bead mills have widely been used for size reduction with new recent designs on the market developed to ensure better distribution within the milling chamber, which is filled with beads. The rotating elements (called accelerators or pegs or discs, which are essentially impellers of different design) ensure the movement of beads within the chamber typically at a concentration of 50–85%. Bead collisions result in the breakup of agglomerates in the product. A combination of factors affect the performance of a stirred bead mill among which are the operating conditions such as the bead diameter and fill ratio, mill speed, flow rate. Whilst contamination of the product due to bead collisions can occur, the use of high quality beads and renewal of beads can overcome this problem. This device is particularly suited to high concentration dispersions (about 20% and above) to maximize the breakup of particle clusters and minimize bead-bead collisions, which can result in wear and contamination.

References

Baldyga, J.; Bourne, J.R. (1993) 'Drop breakup and intermittent turbulence'. *Journal of Chemical Engineering of Japan*, **26**(6): p: 738–741.

Baldyga, J.; Bourne, JR. (1999) *Turbulent Mixing and Chemical Reactions*. John Wiley & Sons, Ltd, Chichester.

Baldyga, J.; Orciuch, W.; Makowski, L.; Özcan-Taşkin N.G.; Eagles, W. (2006) 'Break up of nanoparticle clusters using an in-line rotor-stator- CFD results' *AIChE Meeting 11–15 November 2006*, San Francisco, USA.

Baldyga J.; Orciuch W.; Makowski L.; Ozcan-Taskin G.; Eagles W.; Padron G. (2007a) 'Break up of nanoparticle agglomerates in a rotor-stator device' *Inzynieria Materialowa*, **3–4**, p: 236–241.

Baldyga J.; Orciuch W.; Makowski L.; Ozcan-Taskin G.; Eagles W.; Padron G. (2007b) 'Break up of nanoparticle agglomerates in a rotor-stator device' *18th Physical Metallurgy and Material Science Conference: Advanced Materials and Technologies, 18–21 June 2007*, Warsaw, Poland.

Baldyga, J.; Orciuch, W.; Makowski, L.; Malik, K.; Őzcan-Taşkin, G.; Eagles, W.; Padron, G. (2008) "Dispersion of nanoparticles in a rotor-stator mixer" *Ind. Eng. Chem. Res.*, **47**(10), 3652–3663. DOI 10.1021/ie070899u.

Bourne, J.R.; Baldyga, J. (1993) "Drop breakup in the viscous subrange: a source of possible confusion" *Chem. Eng. Sci.* Vol.**49**, p: 1077–1078.

Edwards M.F.; Ellis D.I. (1984) 'The draw down of floating solids into mechanically agitated vessels', *Fluid Mixing II, IChemE Symposium Series*, **89**, p: 1–13.

Etchells A.W. (2001a) 'Mixing of floating solids' *Plenary lecture ISMIP4, 14–16 May 2001*, Toulouse, France.

Etchells, A.W. (2001b) 'Mixing of floating solids' *NAMF August 2001*, Poconos, USA.

Joosten G.E.H.; Schilder J.G.M. and Broere A.M. (1977) 'The suspension of floating solids in stirred vessels', *Trans. IChemE*, **55**, p: 220–222.

Nelson, R.D. (1988) *Dispersing Powders in Liquids*. Elsevier.

Ottino J.M.; DeRoussel P.; Hansel S.; Khakar D.V. (2000) 'Mixing and dispersion of viscous liquids and powdered solids', *Advances in Chemical Engineering*, **25**, p: 105–204.

Özcan-Taşkin N.G.; McGrath G. (2001) 'Draw down of light particles in stirred tanks', *Trans. IChemE*, **79**, Part A, p: 789–794.

Özcan-Taşkin N.G.; Wei H. (2003) 'The effect of impeller-to-tank diameter ratio on draw down of solids', *Chem. Eng. Sci.*, **58**, p: 201–2022.

Özcan-Taşkin N.G. (2006) 'Effect of scale on the draw down of floating solids', *Chem. Eng. Sci.*, **61**, p: 2871–2879.

Özcan-Taşkin N.G.; Eagles W.P.; Xie L.; Rielly C.D. (2006) 'Suspension of nanoparticle agglomerates in a liquid', *12th European Conference on Mixing, 27–30 June 2006*, Bologna, Italy; p: 287–294.

Özcan-Taşkin N.G.; Padron G.; Voelkel A. (2009) 'Effect of particle type on the mechanisms of break up of nanoscale particle clusters', *Chem. Eng. Res. Des.*, **87**(4), p: 468–473, (DOI 10.1016/j.cherd.2008.12.012)

Özcan-Taşkin N.G. (2012) 'Incorporation of nanoparticle clusters into liquids using a proprietary design mixer: Ytron Y Jet: particle concentration, addition method, power input, liquid height and scale' *14th European Conference on Mixing, 10–13 September*, Warsaw, Poland.

Özcan-Taşkin N.G. (2013) 'Incorporation of nanoparticle clusters into liquids using a proprietary design mixer: Ytron Y Jet: particle concentration, addition method, power input, liquid height and scale', *Chem. Eng. Res. Des.*, DOI: 10.1016/j.cherd.2013.03.019.

Parfitt G.D.; Barnes H.A. (1997) 'The dispersion of fine powders in liquid media' in *Mixing in the Process Industries* (eds Harnby N.; Edwards M.F.; Nienow A.W., 2nd Edn, Butterworth/Heinemann), p: 99–117.

Rwei S.P.; Manas-Zloczower I.; Feke D. (1990) 'Observation of carbon black agglomerate dispersion in simple shear flows', *Polym. Eng. Sci.*, **30**, p: 701–706.

Rwei S.P.; Manas-Zloczower I.; Feke D. (1991) 'Analysis of the dispersion of carbon black in polymeric melts and its effect on compound properties', *Polym. Eng. Sci.*, **32**, p: 130–135.

Rumpf, H. (1962) The strength of granules and agglomerate, in *Agglomeration* (ed. W.A. Knepper, John Wiley & Sons, Inc., New York), p: 379–418.

Shinnar, R. (1961) "On the behaviour of liquid dispersions in mixing vessels" *J. Fluid Mech.* **10**, p: 259–275.

Thring R.W.; Edwards, M.F. (1990) 'An experimental investigation into complete suspension of solids in an agitated tank', *Ind. Eng. Chem. Res.*, **29**, p: 676–682.

Xie L.; Rielly C.D.; Eagles W.; Özcan-Taşkin,G. (2006) 'Deagglomeration of pre-wetted nanoparticles using mixed flow and high shear impellers', *12th European Conference on Mixing, 27–30 June 2006*, Bologna, Italy; p: 209–216.

Xie L.; Rielly C.D.; Eagles W.P.; Őzcan-Taşkin N.G. (2007) 'Dispersion of nanoparticle clusters using mixed flow and high shear impellers in stirred tanks', *Chem. Eng. Res. Des. Part A, Chem. Eng. Research and Design*, **85**(A5), p: 676–684, DOI: 10.1205/cherd06195

8

Wet Granulation and Mixing

Karen P. Hapgood[1] *and Rachel M. Smith*[2]
[1]*Monash Advanced Particle Engineering Laboratory, Department of Chemical Engineering, Monash University, Australia*
[2]*Chemical and Biological Engineering, Sheffield University, UK*

8.1 Introduction

Granulation is a size enlargement process in which mixtures of fine powders are combined into larger agglomerates or granules. In wet granulation, a liquid (usually water, or an ethanol-water mixture) and a binder material (usually a polymer such as hydroxy-propyl cellulose (HPC), polyvinyl pyrillidone (PVP) or hydroxyl methyl propyl cellulose (HMPC)) are added to an agitated powder bed to form granules. Common types of wet granulation equipment used in the pharmaceutical industry include mixer granulators where the powder is agitated by a large impeller at the base of the mixer bowl, or fluid bed granulators where air is blown upwards through the powder to agitate and fluidize the particles. Drying of the granules drives off the liquid (usually water) but a network of solid bridges and polymeric chains give strength and cohesion to the new granules. Granulation improves flow and dust handling properties, reduces segregation, and provides the powders in a suitable form for compressing into tablets and oral dosage forms.

Granulation minimizes but does not eliminate size based segregation potential. In multi-component granulation, the composition of granules in each size fraction can vary. If the drug is concentrated in a particular size fraction, usually either the finest or the coarsest particles, then any segregation of the granules that may occur during processing and handling can result in uneven drug concentration throughout the pharmaceutical batch. For example, suppose the drug was to concentrate in the coarsest fraction of the granules in a

Pharmaceutical Blending and Mixing, First Edition. Edited by P.J. Cullen, Rodolfo J. Romañach, Nicolas Abatzoglou and Chris D. Rielly.

pharmaceutical granulation. If during hopper loading and subsequent discharge the finest material tended to exit the hopper first and the coarsest material last, then tablets compressed from this material would initially be deficient in drug and eventually would be drug enriched. If the tablet assay variation is large, the batch may not meet the quality requirements and be rejected. However, uneven drug distribution will only cause a problem in production if segregation also occurs. If a narrow particle size distribution can be obtained, or if the material is cohesive, segregation can be avoided.

A simple method to analyse the extent of blending and mixing of the drug after wet granulation is to conduct a 'sieve fraction assay', where the granules are sieved into size fractions and each size fraction is assayed for drug content. Drug depletion or enrichment can occur in each size fraction depending on the size fraction of granules measured. Several groups have studied drug distribution in wet granulation using fluid bed or high shear mixing equipment (Lachman and Sylwestrowicz 1964; Higashide *et al.* 1985; Wan *et al.* 1992; Zhang and Johnson 1997; Miyamoto *et al.* 1998; Vromans *et al.* 1999; Kato *et al.* 2001; Oostra *et al.* 2002; van den Dries *et al.* 2003; Nguyen *et al.* 2010). However, many results are difficult to interpret as the target granule size distribution frequently overlaps with the initial particle sizes of the excipients. Pharmaceutical excipients ranging in size up to 100 μm are commonly used in a formulation where the median particle size target may only be approximately 200 μm. However, studies of drug distribution in wet granulation almost always report that the coarse granules tend to be enriched with drug (Lachman and Sylwestrowicz 1964; Higashide *et al.* 1985; Wan *et al.* 1992; Zhang and Johnson 1997; Miyamoto *et al.* 1998; Vromans *et al.* 1999; Kato *et al.* 2001; Oostra *et al.* 2002; van den Dries *et al.* 2003; Nguyen *et al.* 2010). The common results are striking given the diversity of drugs and formulations used in these studies. The excipients are also non-uniformly distributed, although this is less frequently investigated (Higashide *et al.* 1985; Plank *et al.* 2001; Oostra *et al.* 2002).

There are three main stages in granulation (Iveson *et al.* 2001) (refer to Figure 8.1):

1. Nucleation and wetting: formation of the initial granules ('nuclei') as the fluid is dispersed through the powder.
2. Growth and consolidation: the agitation of the powder results in collisions between the granules, particles and equipment, which results in larger and/or denser granules.
3. Breakage and attrition: the powder agitation forces exceed the granule strength and the granule fractures into several large pieces or the outer layer of particles is attritted from the granule.

All three mechanisms can potentially affect the degree of mixing between the drug and the excipients. Each mechanism is discussed in more detail in Figure 8.1.

8.2 Nucleation

Nucleation is the process of distributing the liquid through the powder, usually by spraying onto the moving powder bed, to form the initial granules or 'nuclei'. Poor initial liquid distribution is directly reflected in the nuclei properties. Nuclei formed by poor liquid distribution will have a broad distribution of size, porosity and saturation (Knight *et al.* 1998). This in turn will lead to different growth and breakage rates for each granule. Controlling nucleation is the first step towards a well-designed and robust granulation process.

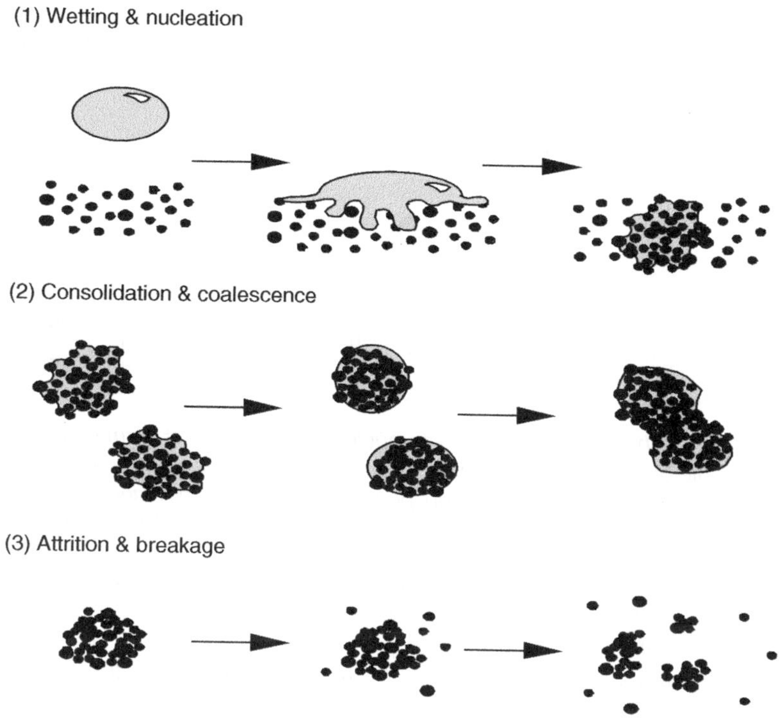

Figure 8.1 *Rate processes in granulation (1) wetting and nucleation; (2) consolidation and growth; (3) breakage and attrition. Reprinted with permission from* Powder Technology, *Nucleation, growth and breakage phenomena in agitated wet granulation processes: a review, Iveson, S.M., J.D. Litster, K.P. Hapgood and B.J. Ennis, 117, 1–2, 3–39. Copyright (2001) Elsevier*

Immersion nucleation is a process where a relatively large drop wets into a bed of fine powder to form a nucleus (Schæfer and Mathiesen 1996; Schæfer and Mathiesen 1996; Scott *et al.* 1999). There are five steps in immersion nucleation (Hapgood *et al.* 2003; Hapgood *et al.* 2009) as shown in Figure 8.2. Initially, the nozzle needs to atomize the fluid to form droplets. When the drop lands on the powder surface, the drop may shatter and break into fragments, as shown experimentally (Chouk *et al.* 2009). The drop may also coalesce with another drop already at the surface of the powder. Once the drop lands on the powder surface capillary action may cause the fluid to penetrate into the powder bed (step 4 in Figure 8.2). If the penetration time is long compared to the residence time of the drop on the powder surface, mechanical agitation and shear will be required to disperse the fluid through the powder.

Distribution nucleation (Schæfer and Mathiesen 1996; Schæfer and Mathiesen 1996; Scott *et al.* 1999) can occur in fluid beds operated with very fine drops of the same size or smaller than the particle size. Equivalent steps have been defined for drops in a fluidized powder (Schaafsma *et al.* 2006) although the mechanisms of distribution nucleation are less well understood (Boerefijn and Hounslow 2005).

Immersion nucleation can be described by two parameters – the drop penetration time and the dimensionless spray flux (Litster *et al.* 2001; Hapgood *et al.* 2002). These parameters

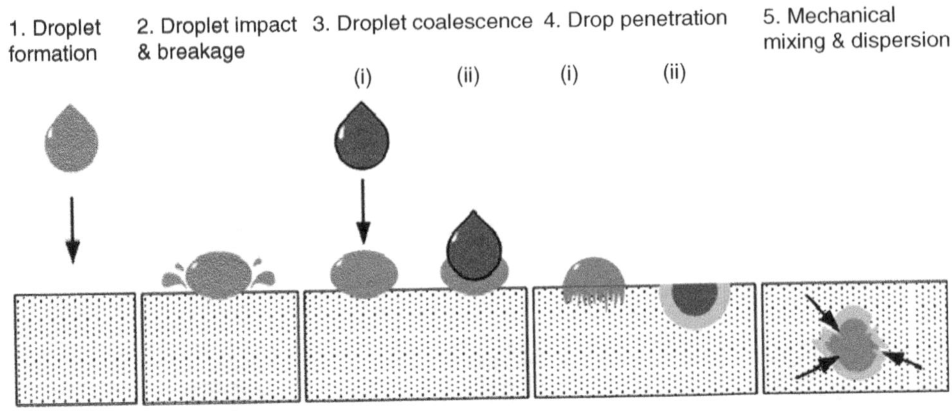

Figure 8.2 *Five possible steps in immersion nucleation (1) Droplet formation; (2) Droplet impact and possible breakage on the powder bed; (3) Droplet coalescence upon contact with other droplets at high spray flux; (4) Drop penetration into the powder bed (i) to form a nucleus granule (ii); (5) Mechanical mixing and dispersion of the liquid and powder. Reprinted with permission from* Journal of Colloid and Interface Science, *Drop penetration into porous powder beds, Karen P. Hapgood, James D. Litster, Simon R. Biggs, Tony Howes, 253, 2, 353–366. Copyright (2002) Elsevier and Reprinted with permission from* AIChE Journal, *Rewetting effects and droplet motion on partially wetted powder surfaces, Karen P. Hapgood, Thanh H. Nguyen, Sunarko Hauw, Simon M. Iveson, Wei Shen, 1402–1415. Copyright (2002) AIChE*

have been combined to form a nucleation regime map (Hapgood *et al.* 2003) and can be used for scale-up (Litster *et al.* 2002) and to quantitatively model the nuclei size distribution (Hapgood *et al.* 2004; Wildeboer *et al.* 2005; Hapgood *et al.* 2009).

8.2.1 Drop Penetration Time

As the powder moves beneath the spray zone, the small droplets will land on the powder surface and begin to mix with the powder (see Figure 8.2). The wettability of the powder, measured via the contact angle of the fluid on the powder, is an important parameter (e.g. see Zhang *et al.* 2002). When the powder is hydrophilic, that is, the effective contact angle between the powder and fluid is less than 90°, penetration of the fluid into the powder pores will begin to occur. The time required for a single drop of fluid to penetrate into a static powder bed is given by the drop penetration time t_p (Hapgood *et al.* 2002):

$$t_p = 1.35 \frac{V_d^{2/3}}{\varepsilon_{eff}^{\ 2} R_{eff}} \frac{\mu}{\gamma_{lv} \cos\theta} \tag{8.1}$$

Where V_d is the drop volume, μ is the fluid viscosity, γ_{lv} is the liquid surface tension and θ is the contact angle between the liquid and powder. This equation applies to systems with a contact angle less than 90°, otherwise the fluid will not penetrate into the pores at all. The porosity of the powder bed, ε, and the pore size, R_{pore}, need to be adjusted to account for the heterogeneous pore structure that occurs in loosely packed or agitated powder beds. This is done by using effective voidage ε_{eff} and the effective pore size R_{eff} that are defined as follows:

$$\varepsilon_{eff} = \varepsilon_{tap}\left(1-\varepsilon+\varepsilon_{tap}\right). \tag{8.2}$$

$$R_{eff} = \frac{\varphi d_{32}}{3}\frac{\varepsilon_{eff}}{1-\varepsilon_{eff}}, \tag{8.3}$$

Where ε_{tap}//I// is tap porosity, φ is the shape factor, and d_{32} is the volume-surface (Sauter) mean particle size. The effective porosity and effective pore size are estimates of the amount of pore space that is actually available for capillary driven flow. Equation (8.1) can be used to estimate the drop penetration time, and works best for particles 100 μm or larger (Hapgood *et al.* 2002). Equation (8.1) can also be used to account for differences in drop size between the experiment and the actual manufacturing process (Ax *et al.* 2008)

The drop penetration time reflects the nucleation kinetics. For a given powder, the drop penetration time is proportional to the liquid properties group $\mu/\gamma_{lv}\cos\theta$. The fluid viscosity can vary over several orders of magnitude (Hapgood *et al.* 2002). For example, the fluid may be low viscosity ~1 mPas fluid such as water or ethanol, or a viscous 7% HPC solution (~100 mPa s. Figure 8.3 shows a water drop penetrating into a lactose powder bed (contact angle of ~30°: Lerk *et al.* 1976) in ~2 s. In contrast, a similar drop of 7% HPC takes approximately 2 minutes to penetrate into the powder bed (Hapgood *et al.* 2002). This timescale for drop penetration is clearly much longer than the time scale for liquid dispersion (a few seconds at most), and implies that mechanical dispersion of the fluid (see step 5 in Figure 8.2) will dominate the nucleation process.

For a given fluid, as the powder becomes finer (i.e. the d_{32} particle size decreases) the drop penetration time increases, primarily due to a decrease in packing efficiency, which creates a higher proportion of macrovoids (Hapgood *et al.* 2002).

The second major effect on the drop penetration time is the powder wetting behaviour, represented by the contact angle. Figure 8.4 shows the dramatic increase in drop penetration time for a droplet of water from 2 s to 25 min (Nguyen *et al.* 2009) when as little as 7 wt% of hydrophobic salicylic acid (contact angle with water θ = 103°) is added to the lactose powder system shown previously in Figure 8.3. A plot of drop penetration time versus the composition of the powder bed shows a dramatic increase in drop penetration time, and

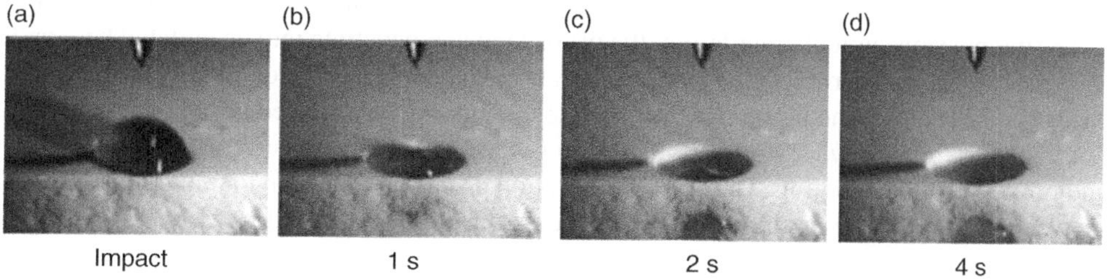

Figure 8.3 *Water droplet penetrating into lactose powder. Reprinted with permission from* Chem. Eng. Sci., *Drop penetration time in heterogeneous powder beds, Nguyen, T., W. Shen and K. Hapgood, 64(24), 5210–5221. Copyright (2009) Elsevier*

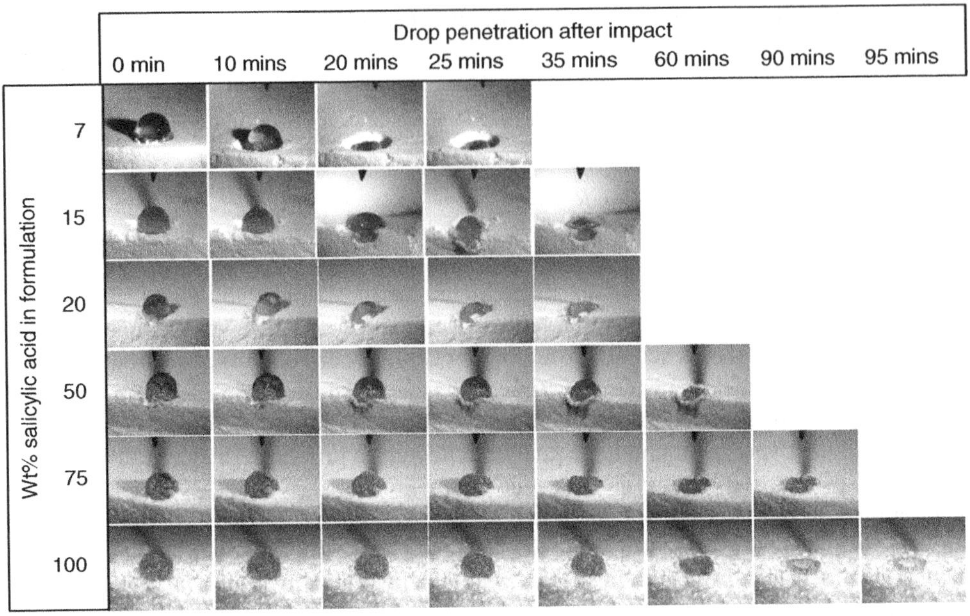

Figure 8.4 *Penetration of a drop water into various mixtures of lactose and salicylic acid. Reprinted with permission from* Chem. Eng. Sci., *Drop penetration time in heterogeneous powder beds, Nguyen, T., W. Shen and K. Hapgood, 64(24), 5210–5221. Copyright (2009) Elsevier*

that there is a critical threshold concentration of non-wetting powder, p_c, above which the bed becomes effectively hydrophobic. The changes in drop penetration time were also reflected in changes in nuclei structure, and in the uniformity of the drug distribution in the final granules. Once the concentration of the non-wetting powder exceeds the critical threshold of p_c the distribution of the drug in the granules is adversely affected. The drop penetration time can also be used as a quick screening test during formulation design to determine whether problems with blend uniformity can be expected.

On the other hand, drop penetration time tends to decrease if the powder is already partially wet (Hapgood 2000; Hapgood *et al.* 2009), and the effect is more pronounced for viscous fluids with long penetration times (Hapgood *et al.* 2009). Drops with long penetration times that land overlapping a wet section of powder will tend to penetrate into the pre-existing wet section, making uniform distribution of viscous fluids even more difficult.

During pharmaceutical granulation, the drops land and penetrate into an agitated bed, and therefore slightly different wetting and penetration behaviour occurs compared to the static cases here. However, the liquid penetration into the moving powder bed is still observed (Ax *et al.* 2008; Chouk *et al.* 2009) and is used in several companies to aid formulation design and process troubleshooting. The following section discusses the behaviour and interactions between multiple drops in the spray zone beneath the atomizing nozzle.

8.2.2 Dimensionless Spray Flux

Dimensionless spray flux Ψ_a||*I*|| describes the density of drops in the spray zone as the droplets land on the moving powder surface (Litster *et al.* 2001). The derivation compares the wetted area created by the incoming droplets to the total area of dry powder passing through the spray zone (Litster *et al.* 2001):

$$\Psi_a = \frac{\dot{a}}{\dot{A}} = \frac{3Q}{2\dot{A}d_d} \tag{8.4}$$

where $\dot{a}$ is the combined area of the spray droplets that land on the powder surface each second (m^2/s), $\dot{A}$ is the area flux of the powder (m^2/s), Q is the volumetric spray rate, and d_d is the drop diameter (usually the d_{32} Sauter mean diameter). For a mixer granulator, the area flux of powder passing through the spray zone can be calculated by:

$$\dot{A} = vw \tag{8.5}$$

where v is the powder velocity beneath the nozzle and w is the width of the spray perpendicular to the powder velocity. The powder flux $\dot{A}$ is a dynamic quantity of the area of powder passing beneath the nozzle per second (m^2/s) and cannot be replaced with the static spray area footprint, A (m^2).

Spray flux $\Psi_a \geq 1$ means that the incoming droplets will theoretically cover 100% of the dry powder passing beneath the nozzle, assuming no drop overlap occurs (Litster *et al.* 2001). The derivation is not intended to be equipment specific, although it has been most easily and frequently applied to mixer granulation.

At low spray flux ($\Psi_a \sim 0.1$) drop footprints will not overlap and each drop will form a separate nucleus with a narrow size distribution that is proportional to the drop size distribution (Waldie 1991; Hapgood *et al.* 2002). As Ψ_a increases, although the relationship becomes non-linear, the fraction powder wetted also increases. The drops begin to overlap more frequently and the nuclei distribution broadens as agglomerates begin to form. At high spray flux ($\Psi_a \sim 1$) the spray rate is too high compared to the rate of dry powder entering the spray zone and the drops significantly overlap each other as they land on the powder bed. Nuclei are then formed by the fragmentation of this wet sheet of powder and will not be linked to the original drop size distribution. Good granulation can still be achieved provided that the shear forces during granulation are large enough and uniform enough to be effective.

The impact of Ψ_a on nuclei formation has been studied in both mixer granulators (Litster *et al.* 2002; Plank *et al.* 2003; Ax *et al.* 2008; Chouk *et al.* 2009; Hapgood *et al.* 2009) and externally on a simplified moving power bed (Litster *et al.* 2001; Wildeboer *et al.* 2007). As the granulation proceeds, the material entering the spray zone will be a mixture of dry powder and previously formed wet granules that will be rewetted. The rewetting can affect the final granule size distribution for some fluids (Hapgood *et al.* 2009).

Wildeboer *et al.* (2005) extended the theory and modelling to account for the effects of drop size distribution, non-uniform spray density and for the size difference between the nucleus and the drop. The probability of a single drop forming a single nucleus is therefore related to the dimensionless nucleation number, Ψ_n (Wildeboer *et al.* 2005):

$$\Psi_n = K_a \frac{3Q}{2wvd_d} \tag{8.6}$$

The dimensionless nucleation number Ψ_n differs from the original spray flux Ψ_a by the nucleation ratio K_a, which accounts for the nucleus spreading, and is defined as the ratio of the projected area of the drop (a_d) to the area of the nucleus granule (a_n) (Wildeboer *et al.* 2005). At a given value of the dimensionless nuclei number Ψn, the density and size distribution of the nuclei formed on the surface is constant, that is, the final value of Ψ_n is the sole determinant of the final nuclei size distribution.

The fraction surface coverage and the nuclei size distribution can be predicted by combining dimensionless spray flux with the Poisson distribution. The fraction of the surface covered by drops in a single pass through the spray zone is given by (Hapgood *et al.* 2004):

$$f_{covered} = 1 - exp\left(-\Psi_a\right), \tag{8.7}$$

The fraction of nuclei formed from n drops is given by:

$$f_n = \exp\left(-4\Psi_a\right)\left(\frac{\left(4\Psi_a\right)^{n-1}}{(n-1)!}\right), \tag{8.8}$$

The fraction of drops landing without touching any other drops, f_{single}, can be calculated by using $n = 1$ in equation (8.8) that simplifies to:

$$f_{single} = exp\left(-4\Psi_a\right) \tag{8.9}$$

Using a similar procedure, at low spray flux, the entire nuclei size distribution can be calculated using equation (8.8) to determine the number of nuclei formed from n drops (Hapgood *et al.* 2009).

8.2.3 Nucleation Regime Map

The nucleation regime map is based on a dimensionless drop penetration time and the dimensionless spray flux, and describes two different regimes for liquid dispersion and nucleation (Hapgood *et al.* 2003).

The 'drop controlled nucleation' regime occurs at low drop penetration time and low dimensionless spray flux (Hapgood *et al.* 2003). When the drop penetration time is short, the fluid will quickly wet into the powder bed to form a nucleus. If the dimensionless spray flux is also low, no other drops will land or touch the drop and a single nucleus granule will be formed with a size proportional to the drop volume. This results in a nuclei size distribution that is directly proportional to the original drop size distribution. Spray flux needs to be less than $\Psi_a < 0.1$ for approximately 2/3 of the nuclei to be formed from a single drop (see equation 8.9).

In the 'mechanical dispersion' nucleation regime, the liquid is dispersed due to powder agitation and shear, rather than by fluid flow and wetting (Hapgood *et al.* 2003). This regime dominates when the spray flux and/or drop penetration time is high. At spray flux $\Psi_a > 0.1$, the spray density will be high and most drops will overlap and coalesce with other drops at the powder surface. A continuous sheet of 'caked' wet powder will be formed and subsequently broken and dispersed throughout the granulator. Alternatively, if the drop penetration time is too long, the liquid will remain on the surface of the powder and will either coalesce with other unpenetrated droplets (see step 3 in Figure 8.2), form rivulets in the powder depressions (Wildeboer *et al.* 2007), or penetrate into a pre-wetted powder section (Hapgood *et al.* 2009). In all three cases, the liquid will need to be dispersed throughout the powder via powder agitation (step 5 in Figure 8.2). The mechanical dispersion regime means that efficient mixing and agitation of the powder is required to achieve effective liquid dispersion, and does not mean that liquid distribution is always inefficient. Most mixer granulation processes operate in the mechanical dispersion regime, unless the process has been designed to achieve drop controlled nucleation.

These two regimes of nucleation can be summarized using a nucleation regime map (Figure 8.5). The axes of the map are the dimensionless spray flux Ψ_a and the dimensionless penetration time τ_p:

$$\tau_p = \frac{t_p}{t_c} \tag{8.10}$$

where t_c is the circulation time for the droplet or nuclei to return to the spray zone. Insufficient information on powder flow and circulation patterns during granulation have so far prevented t_c from being quantified (Hapgood *et al.* 2003). Since the circulation time can be presumed to be constant for the same granulator operating under the same agitation conditions, Figure 8.5 can be used by assuming the dimensionless penetration time τ_p is directly proportional to the measured penetration time t_p.

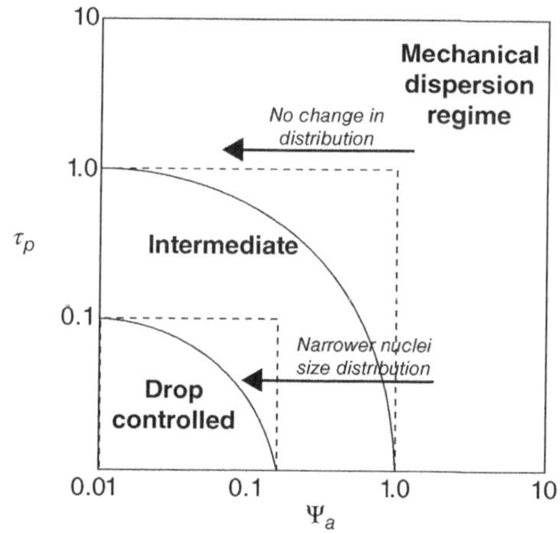

Figure 8.5 *Nucleation regime map with adjusted boundaries incorporating the drop migration due to rewetting of powder during multiple passes through the spray zone. Reprinted with permission from AIChE Journal, Nucleation regime map for liquid bound granules, Hapgood, K.P., Litster, J.D., and Smith, R., 49, 2, 350–361. Copyright (2003) AIChE. Dotted lines represent original regime boundaries. Reprinted with permission from AIChE Journal, Rewetting effects and droplet motion on partially wetted powder surfaces, Karen P. Hapgood, Thanh H. Nguyen, Sunarko Hauw, Simon M. Iveson, Wei Shen, 1402–1415. Copyright (2002) AIChE*

The nucleation regime map can be used to select the optimal conditions for liquid dispersion during process development, and for scale-up and troubleshooting at manufacturing scale. For formulations with a short drop penetration time, the spray flux can be optimized by lowering the fluid flow-rate, increasing the spray width, or increasing the powder velocity in the spray zone. These changes will be directly reflected in the initial size distribution (Litster *et al.* 2001; Litster *et al.* 2002). In contrast, optimizing the spray parameters to reduce spray flux will have little effect on formulations with long drop penetration times, as the liquid will form a 'puddle' due to the slowly penetrating drops and/or high spray density. Instead, improving the powder agitation and shear will result in more effective binder dispersion. Increasing the impeller speed will improve the powder agitation but may not be possible due to equipment or process limitations (e.g. fixed speed impellers in mixers) or due to negative side effects such as reduced granule porosity and/or changes in the growth behaviour (see Section 8.3). One way to improve mechanical dispersion is to position the spray nozzle over a highly agitated region of the granulator, For example, mixer granulators typically have a second small blade mounted on the side or top of the powder bed that rotates at 1000–3000 rpm, known as the 'chopper'. This is a localized zone of intense turbulent powder mixing, and can be used to quickly distribute viscous binder fluids (Holm *et al.* 1983).

8.3 Consolidation and Growth

Granule consolidation and growth are both functions of the granule structure and the stresses experienced by the granule in the granulator. The two key granule structure parameters are the granule saturation and the overall porosity of the granules. The granule growth regime map summarizes why different formulations and process conditions result in different growth and consolidation behaviour. Granule consolidation and the different types of granule growth are explained next, followed by an explanation of the granule growth regime map.

8.3.1 Granule Consolidation

Consolidation is defined as the reduction in granule porosity that occurs as the primary particles move closer to each other as a result of collisions and impact forces occurring to the wet granules. The granule porosity often plays an important role in determining the dissolution rate of the final granules or tablets (Ohno *et al.* 2007). The rate and extent of consolidation is affected by the primary particle size, fluid viscosity and the impeller speed or fluidizing velocity (Zoglio and Cartensen 1983; Iveson *et al.* 1996; Iveson and Litster 1998).

Despite the availability of advanced measurement techniques that can analyse pore size distributions within a granule such as mercury porosimetry (Zoglio and Cartensen 1983; Jægerskou *et al.* 1984; Berggren and Alderborn 2001) and XRT (Farber *et al.* 2003; Ansari and Štěpánek 2006; Ansari and Štěpánek 2006; Ohno *et al.* 2007), the average granule porosity (ε ||*I*||the volume fraction of air within a granule) has been found to be a very powerful parameter within granulation. The granule porosity is a very different parameter to the bulk voidage of granules, which is a measure of the packing density of granules, and is affected by the space between granules. Granule porosity is usually quite high early in a

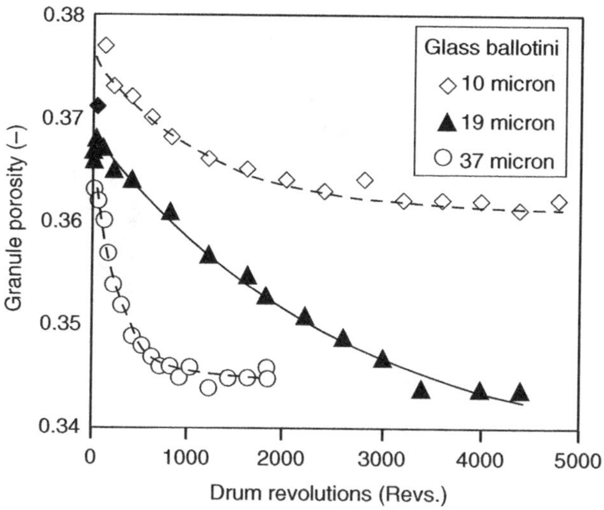

Figure 8.6 *Exponential decay in granule porosity as granulation proceeds. Reprinted with permission from* Powder Technology, *Fundamental studies of granule consolidation: Part 2: Quantifying the effects of particle and binder properties, S.M. Iveson, J.D. Litser, 99, 3, 243–250. Copyright (1998) Elsevier*

granulation process (around 50–60%), and reduces exponentially as the granulation continues and the granules consolidate (Iveson and Litster 1998). Eventually, the granules reach a minimum porosity, ε_{min}||I||, as shown in Figure 8.6. Granule consolidation and densification occurs as the granule collides within the granulator, resulting in deformation of the granule and rearrangement of the constituent particles. Iveson and Litster (1998) demonstrated that rapid densification is promoted by large particle size, low particle roughness, and lower viscosity liquid binder fluid, however, many other parameters may also affect the rate of granule densification. Low porosity granules are often produced in mixer granulation, due to the mechanical agitation and potentially high forces and velocities used in these types of equipment.

Granule saturation, s, is the fraction of the pore volume occupied by liquid, and is therefore closely related to granule porosity (see equation 8.11).

$$s = \frac{w\rho_s(1-\varepsilon)}{\rho_l \varepsilon} \tag{8.11}$$

where ε ||I||is the average granule porosity, w is the mass fraction liquid, ρ_l||I|| is the density of liquid and ρ_s||I|| is the true density of the solid particles.

Wet granules can be classified into three states based on the saturation value: pendular ($s < 25\%$), funicular ($25\% < s < 80\%$), and capillary ($s > 80\%$) (Figure 8.7) (Kristensen and Schæfer 1987). Granule saturation can be increased by either increasing the amount of binder added during the granulation, or by consolidating the granules to reduce the total pore volume (Iveson 1997; Mort 2005). Both of these processes will usually occur simultaneously during liquid addition in a granulation process. In some instances, granule

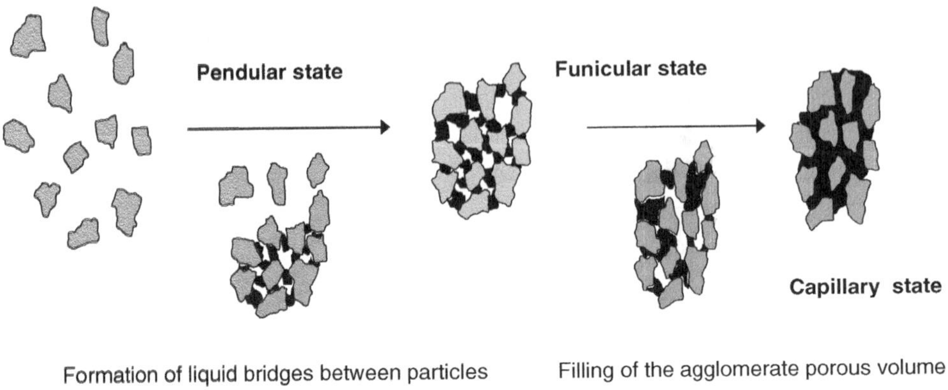

Figure 8.7 *Granule saturation has three common states as the liquid content is increased as shown here (adapted from Goldszal and Bousquet, 2001) or as the porosity decreases. Reprinted with permission from* Powder Technology, *Wet agglomeration of powders: from physics toward process optimization, Alexandre Goldszal, Jacques Bousquet, 117, 3. Copyright (2001) Elsevier*

consolidation will continue as far as the droplet state, resulting in the squeezing of liquid binder from the interior of the granule to the surface (Iveson and Litster 1998; Iveson *et al.* 2001; Wauters *et al.* 2002; Wauters *et al.* 2002; Tu *et al.* 2008). Liquid at the granule surface provides potential bonding sites for other granules, and rapid and uncontrolled coalescence and growth is often seen in these instances (Hoornaert *et al.* 1998; Iveson and Litster 1998; Wauters *et al.* 2002).

Different powder/binder combinations can produce widely varying granule consolidation rates. (Iveson *et al.* 1996; Iveson and Litster 1998). Inter-particle friction hinders consolidation, with larger particles forming more rapidly consolidating granules (see Figure 8.6). Reducing particle size increases surface area and number of inter-particle contacts, which increases the inter-particle friction and creates more resistance to consolidation (Iveson *et al.* 1996; Iveson and Litster 1998; Mackaplow *et al.* 2000). Binder fluid also has an effect on consolidation rate. The liquid can lubricate and aid particle movement and increasing liquid content will increase consolidation rate. Viscous binders will however resist flow during deformation, and will reduce the rate of consolidation

8.3.2 Granule Growth Behaviour

There are two main types of granule growth behaviour – steady growth and induction growth (Figure 8.8). 'Steady growth' occurs when the rate of growth is constant (at a given liquid level). On a plot of granule size versus granulation time, steady growth behaviour produces a linear trend. This type of growth occurs in formulations where the granules are easily deformed by the forces in the granulator, and tends to occur when using coarse powders and low viscosity fluids (Iveson and Litster 1998).

In contrast, 'Induction growth' occurs when the initial nuclei remain at a constant size for a long period, before very rapid granule growth occurs, resulting in a sudden increase in granule size (Figure 8.8). During the induction period, the granules consolidate and approach some minimum porosity (e.g. see Figure 8.6 for example data) but do not grow in size.

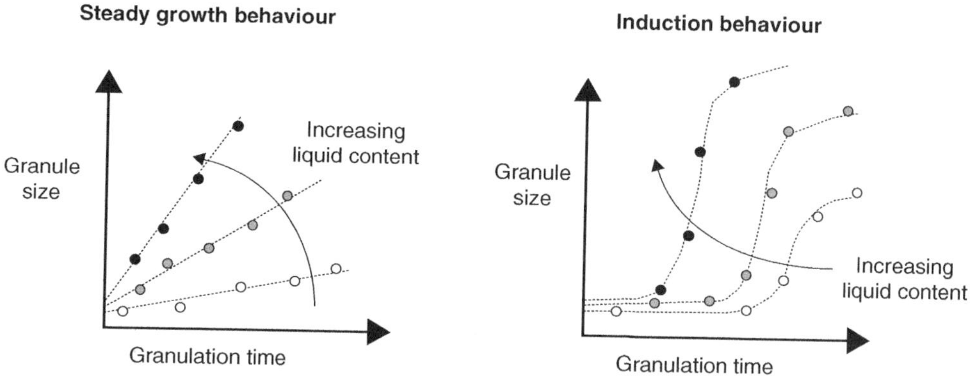

Figure 8.8 Two main types of granule growth behaviour. Reprinted with permission from AIChE Journal, *Growth regime map for liquid-bound granules*, S.M. Iveson, J.D. Litster, 44, 7, 1510–1518. Copyright (1998) AIChE

Eventually, the granule porosity can be reduced enough to squeeze liquid to the surface. This excess free liquid on the granules causes sudden rapid coalescence of many granules, and results in the rapid increase in granule size characteristic of an induction formulation.

8.3.3 Granule Growth Regime Map

Different formulations show different granulation behaviour and the same formulation may behave differently in a different granulator design. The granule growth regime map (Iveson and Litster 1998), shown in Figure 8.9, presents the often complex effects of the formulation properties, liquid level and granulator forces in a coherent framework. The granule saturation s forms the x-axis of the regime map. Saturation is a function of the amount of granulating liquid w and the granule porosity ε (see equation 8.1)).

The Stokes' deformation number, St_{def}, appears on the vertical axis of the growth regime map. The Stokes' deformation number is defined as the ratio of the kinetic energy experienced by the granules during granulation (due to collisions with the impeller, wall and other granules) compared to the deformation behaviour or strength of the granules, expressed as a yield stress (Iveson and Litster 1998):

$$St_{def} = \frac{\rho_g U_c^2}{2\sigma_p} \tag{8.12}$$

where ρ_g||I|| is the apparent granule density, U_c is the collision velocity, and σ_p||I|| is the yield strength of the granule. As there will be a distribution of all of these values during granulation, typical or average values are used in equation (8.12). The yield stress of the granule increases as the granule gradually consolidates and the porosity decreases, and is usually evaluated at the minimum porosity ε_{min}||I|| (see Figure 8.6). The collision velocity is not usually known but can usually be estimated from the impeller speed, minimum fluidization velocity (Litster and Ennis 2004).

$$s_{\max} = w\rho_s\left(1-\varepsilon_{\min}\right)/\rho_l\varepsilon_{\min}$$

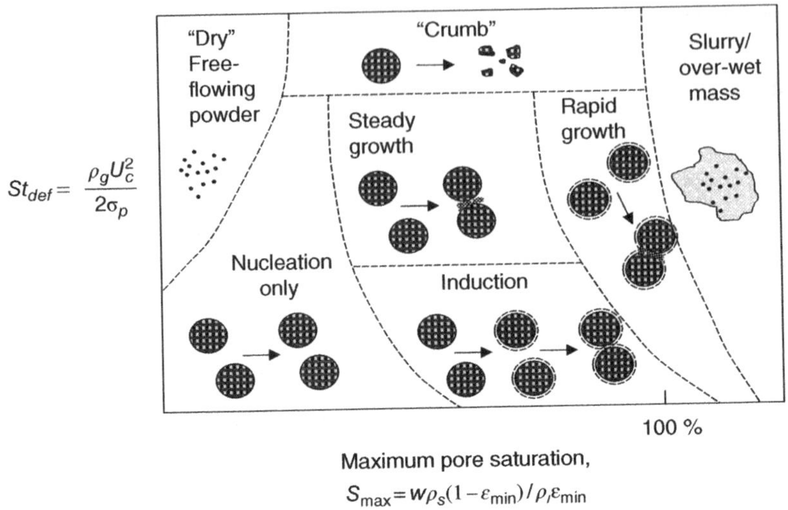

Figure 8.9 *Granule growth regime map, summarizing the different types of granule growth and the conditions that they will occur. Reprinted with permission from* Powder Technology, *Nucleation, growth and breakage phenomena in agitated wet granulation processes: a review, Iveson, S.M., J.D. Litster, K.P. Hapgood and B.J. Ennis, 117, 1–2, 3–39. Copyright (2001) Elsevier and Reprinted with permission from* AIChE Journal, *Growth regime map for liquid-bound granules, S.M. Iveson, J.D. Litster, 44, 7, 1510–1518. Copyright (1998) AIChE*

To understand the granule growth map of Figure 8.9, consider a very weak formulation such as very coarse lactose granulated with water, which would have a low granule yield strength s_p and a high St_{def}. Initially, the granule saturation s is very low. Since the granules are also very weak, the process operates in the free flowing powder section of the regime map, in the upper left hand corner. As more fluid is added to the process, the saturation increases and the process moves into the 'crumb' region. Since the granules are still very weak, the forces and collisions in the granulator are able to easily fragment and disintegrate the granules, forming a mixture similar to damp sand. The powders will be well-mixed (Bouwman *et al.* 2006) but not suitable for use in pharmaceutical manufacturing. If more liquid is added, the formulation will turn into a slurry, shown in the upper right hand corner of the map.

If the granule yield strength is increased by either decreasing the particle size, or by using a more viscous binder (e.g. HPC) the value of the granule yield strength would increase, and cause a corresponding decrease in St_{def}. Take an example where St_{def} is approximately 2/3 up the St_{def} axis. Initially, the system will be in the nucleation only regime due to the low saturation of the granules. In the nucleation only growth regime, growth is limited by the amount of water present. Nuclei granules form as the liquid is added but the saturation is too low to allow any granule growth. As more fluid is added, the saturation increases further and the system enters the 'steady growth' regime as described in Section 8.3.2. The granules here deform easily and grow steadily with time. If liquid addition is continued, the growth rate will accelerate as the saturation increases, until the 'rapid growth' regime is reached. This is usually undesirable. In extreme cases where liquid addition is continued even further, a slurry will be formed.

If a highly viscous binder or a very fine powder is used, the granules will be very strong with a high yield stress σ_p ||I||and a low St_{def}. At low saturation, the system will again begin in the nucleation only regime but as more fluid is added, it will cross into the induction regime (as described in Section 8.3.2). If the granulation time is long enough, the granule porosity will reduce and will eventually reach ε_{min}, squeezing the excess liquid to the granule surface, causing runaway growth.

Importantly, the growth regime map can be used to design a robust granulation system (usually for steady growth) by adjusting the formulation or processing parameters. For example, if a formulation is currently exhibiting induction growth, the system can be driven towards steady growth behaviour by reducing the binder fluid viscosity, increasing the particle size of the formulation, or decreasing the impeller speed. The map has been validated experimentally on several different formulations and granulators (Iveson *et al.* 2001; Bouwman *et al.* 2006; Tu *et al.* 2009) and can also be used for troubleshooting and for selecting a suitable approach to endpoint control (see Section 8.5).

8.4 Breakage

Pharmaceutical granulation mainly occurs in the nucleation, steady growth and induction regimes, as the final desired granule size is often only 2–4 times the size of the original particles in the formulation. A typical target granule diameter would be 200–400 μm, and the typical size of the particles in the formulation ranges between 50–200 μm. Granules much larger than this are commonly formed during the process (Hapgood *et al.* 2010) and hence breakage of these granules is generally desirable to control the particle size.

While significant progress has been made in the understanding of granule nucleation and growth, wet granule breakage remains poorly understood, and despite active research in the area, there is no regime map for granule breakage. Wet granule breakage is particularly relevant for mixer granulators, where mechanical agitation creates potentially high in-granulator forces and velocities.

There are two main challenges in granule breakage research: understanding the way wet granules deform and break under varying stress conditions, and understanding the stress conditions within the granulator. Research into wet granule breakage can be classified into two approaches: the study of the strength and deformation breakage of single wet granules or pellets under stress, and the study of bulk granule breakage and powder motion in granulators. Both areas are important in developing a full picture of granule breakage. Wet granules deform very differently to dry granules and the research here cannot be applied to dry granule breakage or dry milling processes.

8.4.1 Single Granule Strength and Deformation

In the study of wet granule breakage, much can be gained from studying the deformation of single granules or pellets. The study of wet granule pellets (small wet powder compacts) can be particularly helpful, as critical granule properties such as size, porosity and liquid content can be controlled, and heterogeneities within the pellets can be minimized. All these properties can be very hard to control in granules made through tradition granulation processes.

Pellet deformation has been studied experimentally by compressing granular pellets under varying strain rates (Iveson *et al.* 2002; Iveson and Page 2004; Iveson and Page 2005; Smith 2008; Smith and Litster 2012), and has been shown to vary from plastic deformation to semi-brittle fracture (Iveson and Page 2004; Smith and Litster 2012). This wide range in granule deformation type complicates the study of breakage.

In several of these experiments (Iveson *et al.* 2002; Iveson and Page 2004; Iveson and Page 2005; Smith 2008) the pellets are compressed with varying strain rates in a load frame, and the normal force is recorded with time. The normal force is converted into stress, and the peak flow stress σ_{pk}||I|| indicates the point of pellet failure. The peak flow stress can be converted to the dimensionless peak flow stress *Str** (Iveson *et al.* 2002).

$$Str^* = \frac{\sigma_{pk} d_p}{\gamma_{LV} \cos\theta} \tag{8.13}$$

The *Str** data for the experiments was plotted against the Capillary number *Ca,* which is the ratio of viscous forces to surface tension forces, and is proportional to the strain rate $\dot{\varepsilon}$:

$$Ca = \frac{\mu d_p \dot{\varepsilon}}{\gamma_{LV} \cos\theta} \tag{8.14}$$

A single line can be formed with two distinct regimes, as shown in Figure 8.10. (Iveson *et al.* 2002; Iveson and Page 2004; Iveson and Page 2005). In region 1, the strain rate is low (low *Ca*) and the peak flow stress is independent of strain rate. It is hypothesized that inter-particle friction is the dominant force in this region. In region 2, the peak flow stress is proportional to the strain rate, and viscous resistance forces begin to dominate. A critical result from this work is the observations regarding the mode of deformation: in region 1, semi-brittle fracture is the dominant mechanism for breakage, while in region 2, the pellets tended to fail plastically.

This work has been extended by Smith (2008) to include the effect of particle shape, porosity and saturation. A new empirical correlation was developed to describe pellet strength as a function of pellet saturation *s*, porosity ε, particle aspect ratio *AR* and dimensionless particle size distribution span S_p. (equation 8.15). In this equation S_p is defined as $(d_{90}-d_{10})/d_{50}$, where d_{90} is the 90th percentile of particle size, d_{10} is the tenth percentile of particle size, and d_{50} is the median particle size. Particle shape and liquid saturation were found to have a strong effect on granule strength.

$$Str^* = 4345.8 Ca^{0.401} s^{1.577} \varepsilon^{2.059} AR^{-2.250} S_p^{0.799} \tag{8.15}$$

In addition to strength measurement, pellets are very useful in studying the mode of wet granule failure. The way granules fail will affect all mechanisms of granulation, and will have an impact on the final granule properties. Wet granule failure ranges from semi-brittle fracture, characterized by a major catastrophic crack through the centre of the pellet, to plastic deformation, where the pellets compress between the platens without any crack formation (Smith and Litster 2012). Examples of these two extremes of pellet deformation are shown in Figure 8.11. The mode of failure is dependent on the formulation properties and stress conditions. Plastically deforming granules will tend to elongate and smear in the

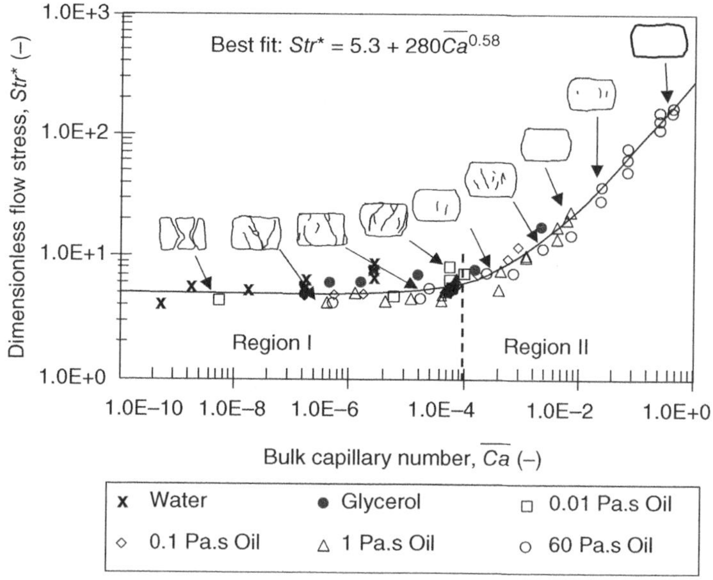

Figure 8.10 *Dimensionless flow stress versus capillary number (Iveson and Page 2004). In region 1, the stress is independent of flow rate. At higher strain rates (region 2), viscous forces dominate and the stress is proportional to the strain rate. Reprinted with permission from* Journal of Applied Mechanics, *Brittle to plastic transition in the dynamic mechanical behavior of partially saturated granular materials, S.M. Iveson, N.W. Page, 71, 4, 470–475. Copyright (2004) ASME*

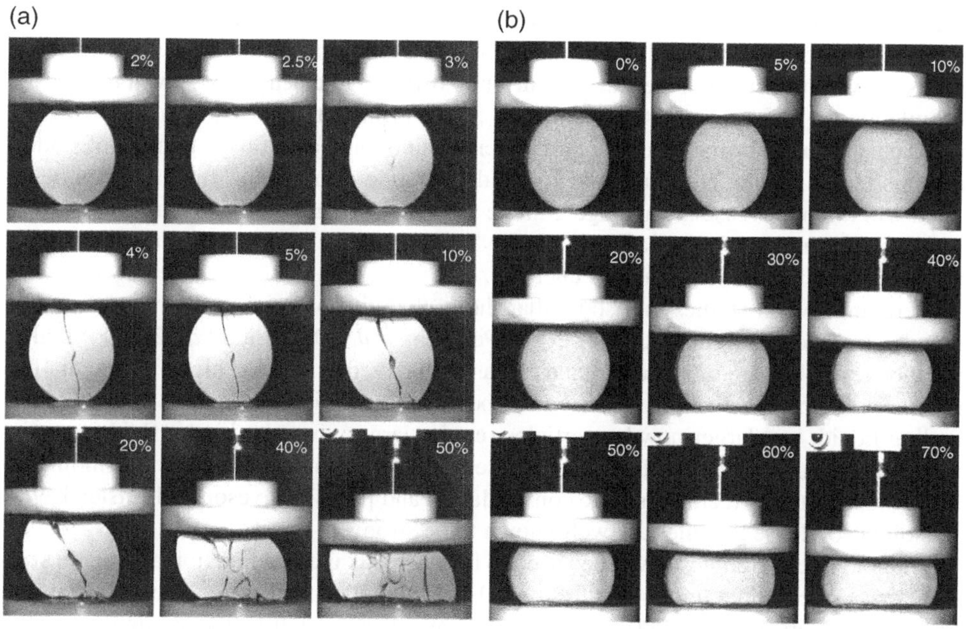

Figure 8.11 *The two modes of pellet failure (a) Semi-brittle fracture (b) Plastic deformation (Smith and Litster 2012). Percentage strains are shown in each image. Reprinted with permission from* Powder Technology, *Examining the failure modes of wet granular materials using dynamic diametrical compression, Rachel M. Smith, James D. Litster, 224, 189–195. Copyright (2012) Elsevier*

granulator when stressed beyond their yield point, whereas semi-brittle granules will fracture into discrete fragments and fines. Smith and Litster (2012) diametrically compressed pellets of wet granular material and formed criteria to define the mode of breakage. Pellets that exhibited a peak flow stress at strains less than 5% tended to fail through semi-brittle fracture, whereas pellets that did not show a peak flow stress, or had a peak flow stress at strains greater than 5% generally failed plastically.

Another approach to studying single granule deformation is to use the Stokes deformation number (see equation 8.12). Tardos *et al.* (1997) sheared granules in a fluidized bed Couette device, which applied a well-controlled shear field to the granules. Experimentally, the authors found deformation of the granule increased as the St_{def} increased, until the Stokes number reached the critical value of approximately 0.2, at which all granules broke. This critical value for St_{def} was further supported by other researchers using bulk granulation experiments (Liu *et al.* 2008) and by modelling work (Talu *et al.* 2000). Other groups studying breakage in granulators found the same overall trend, but reported much lower critical values of St_{def}~0.01 (van den Dries *et al.* 2003) and St_{def}~0.02 (Smith *et al.* 2010). Breakage was found to be size selective, that is, breakage is more likely to occur to large granules than to small granules (Tardos *et al.* 1997). The shearing method used by Tardos *et al.* (1997) is in contrast to the compressive methods discussed earlier. It is still unclear whether granules deform primarily as a result of high shear forces within zones of the granulator, or impact with the impeller, walls and granules in the granulator.

8.4.2 In-Granulator Breakage Studies

The relationship between granulation operating conditions – for example, impeller speed or fluidizing air velocity – and the collision rates and strain rates experienced by the granules is not well understood. Hence, it is currently difficult to calculate St_{def} even for a given formulation, at a fixed operating condition in well characterized equipment. However, breakage appears to be more common in mixer granulation, based on the number of studies in this style of equipment compared to fluid bed style granulators. Increasing impeller speed will often decrease the average granule size, indicating increased breakage is occurring (Vonk *et al.* 1997; Ramaker *et al.* 1998; Knight *et al.* 2000), presumably due to increased collision velocities and/or energies.

There are several studies that show that the probability of breakage is proportional to granule size. (Johansen and Schæfer 2001; Pearson *et al.* 2001; Liu *et al.* 2009). Smaller granules resist breakage (Johansen and Schæfer 2001), due to their higher strength. The granule strength for a given formulation can be increased by increasing the viscosity of the binding liquid, and larger powder particles require larger viscosity binder fluids to resist breakage (Johansen and Schæfer 2001). These findings are in line with Iveson's finding on the key parameters affecting granule consolidation and porosity (Iveson and Litster 1998). Consolidated, dense granules are well known to be stronger.

Coloured tracer granules have been used to follow breakage as a function of granule size. Three sizes of coloured tracer granules (~200, 500 and 1000 μm) were added to a running granulator (Pearson *et al.* 2001). Samples were taken as a function of time, and the proportion of coloured material in each size fraction was analysed. Tracer granules were granulated for different times before being removed and added to the running granulator. Younger, newly formed tracer granules broke at a faster rate than tracer granules that had been granulated for a longer period, allowing plenty of time for granule consolidation (Pearson *et al.* 2001). In some tracer granulation studies, the colour distribution of the granules became almost uniform within approximately 2 min (Vonk *et al.* 1997; Pearson *et al.* 2001; van den Dries *et al.* 2003) although this will not be true for all formulations or all granulation conditions.

A new approach to studying granule breakage involves using high shear mixer granulators with non-granulating powder mixtures to create realistic mixer flow conditions to test granule breakage. This system is known as a 'Breakage Only Granulator'. These experiments isolate the breakage mechanism only (i.e. there is no simultaneous nucleation or growth), simplifying the study of granule breakage. Liu *et al.* (2009) studied breakage by placing pellets of controlled size and saturation into a Breakage Only Granulator and following the survival rate of the pellets. Breakage decreased as the binder viscosity and/or surface tension increased, and as the primary particle size decreased, similar to the findings for consolidation. More saturated pellets were also found to be less likely to break. The authors developed a new expression for granule yield strength (equation 8.16) based on Rumpf's expression for static granule tensile strength (Rumpf 1962), the relationship for dimensionless peak flow stress found by Iveson *et al.* (2002) (equation 8.13) and the correlation of Smith (2008) (equation 8.15). The critical Stokes deformation number for breakage was found to occur at $St_{def^*} = 0.2$ (Figure 8.12).

$$\sigma_p = AR^{-4.3} s \left(6 \frac{1-\varepsilon}{\varepsilon} \frac{\gamma_{LV} \cos\theta}{d_{32}} \frac{9}{8} \frac{(1-\varepsilon)^2}{\varepsilon^2} \frac{9\pi\mu v_p}{16 d_{32}} \right) \tag{8.16}$$

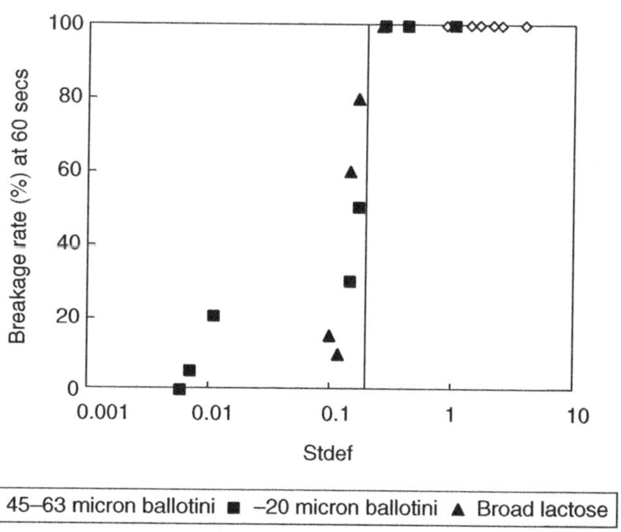

Figure 8.12 *Breakage of pellets for several different formulations in a breakage only granulator occurs at Stdef ~0.2. Reprinted with permission from* Powder Technology, *Wet granule breakage in a breakage only high-shear mixer: Effect of formulation properties on breakage behaviour, Liu, L. X., Smith, R., & Litster, J. D, 189, 2, 158–164. Copyright (2009) Elsevier*

where v_p is the relative velocity of the moving particle inside a granule after impact. v_p is a difficult parameter to measure; Liu *et al.* (2009) used a value of 15% of the tip speed, citing particle velocity values obtained by Tran (2012) using Positron Emission Particle Tracking (PEPT) as justification for this value.

Smith *et al.* (2010) used the Breakage Only Granulator to study the breakage of drop nucleated granules. This work focussed on the effect of process parameters such as impeller shape and impeller speed. Drop nucleated granules were placed into the Breakage Only Granulator, and the breakage results were compared directly to the measured peak flow stress of pellets of the same formulations. Increasing impeller speed increased the extent of breakage. The impeller shape was shown to have a considerable effect on granule breakage, with a flat plate impeller generating little to no granule breakage, and a two-blade bevelled edge impeller producing significant breakage. This result demonstrates the significance of impeller geometry. The measured peak flow stress was found to be a reasonable predictor for granule breakage.

8.4.3 Aiding Controlled Granulation via Breakage

Breakage may be advantageous in some systems, particularly in pharmaceutical granulation where large granules are undesirable and often require milling. Breakage of large granules can be a size limiting process, and help to control the final granule size distribution. Currently, it is unclear how dominant the breakage mechanism is during pharmaceutical operation. This is complicated by the presence of the 'chopper' that rotates at high speed (e.g. 200–3000 rpm) and generates high intensity mixing in a very localized area where breakage is expected to dominate. The chopper is generally used to break up large granules; however a few studies (Holm *et al.* 1983; Holm *et al.* 1984; Jægerskou *et al.* 1984; Holm 1987) find that the effect of the chopper is quite modest, most likely due to the small volume affected. Breakage still appears to be dominated by granule saturation and the overall powder flow field generated by the impeller.

Most newly-formed nuclei are porous and weak, and are more susceptible to breakage than older, denser granules (Pearson *et al.* 2001). If the granulation is operating in the mechanical dispersion nucleation regime (see Section 8.2.3), breakage of the large nuclei will help to distribute the binder fluid throughout the powder bed. Vonk *et al.* (1997) have defined a mechanism of liquid dispersion via breakage of nuclei as 'destructive nucleation' (Figure 8.13). Newly formed nuclei (i.e. the granules formed when liquid first comes into contact with the powder) have a saturation gradient – the inner core of the granule is usually highly saturated, and the liquid saturation decreases radially from the centre to the granule surface. Stronger secondary nuclei are formed when the weak primary nuclei break. The secondary nuclei go on to coalesce and grow (Vonk *et al.* 1997). Tracer studies using a coloured liquid binder have shown that increasing impeller speed reduces the proportion of primary nuclei that survive (Vonk *et al.* 1997; van den Dries *et al.* 2003), resulting in a more uniform distribution of coloured liquid tracer throughout the powder bed and within granules. This is likely to be most applicable to high shear granulation, where mechanical agitation provides high mixing forces within the granulator. In the final stage of destructive nucleation a balance between coalescence and breakage is achieved, which should lead to a stable maximum granule size. Michaels *et al.* (2009) successfully applied this (along with other work) to create a granulation system with a well-controlled granule size, where the only parameter required for scale-up was the impeller speed.

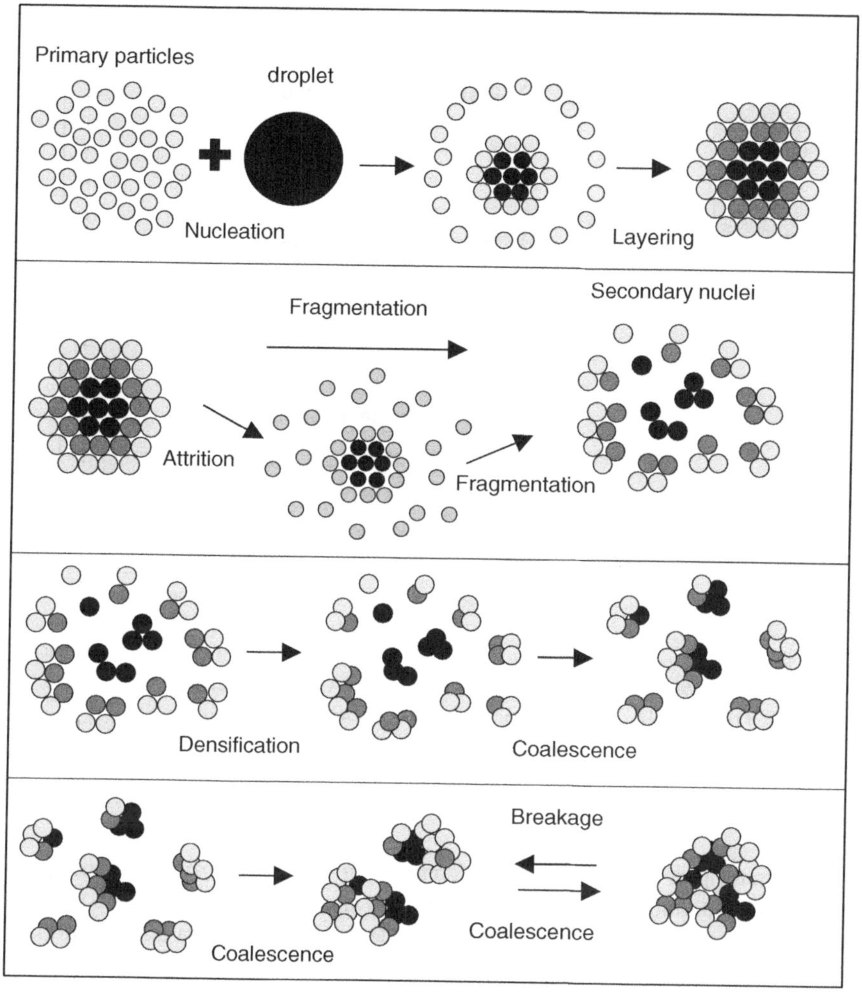

Figure 8.13 'Destructive nucleation' where nuclei undergo breakage. Reprinted with permission from International Journal of Pharmaceutics, *Growth mechanisms of high-shear pelletisation, P. Vonk, C.P.F. Guillaume, J.S. Ramaker, H. Vromans, N.W.F. Kossen, 157, 93–102. Copyright (1997) Elsevier*

Bouwman *et al.* (2006) also looked at the mixing of tracer granules and defined three mechanisms of material exchange due to breakage: disintegration where the granules are crushed completely; deformation where coalescence and deformation results in gradual mixing of the tracers; and distribution, which is similar to induction growth. They related the three mechanisms to the Stokes Deformation number (equation 8.12) and to the granule growth regime map (see Figure 8.14).

$$s_{\max} = w\rho_s\left(1-\varepsilon_{\min}\right)/\,\rho_l\varepsilon_{\min}$$

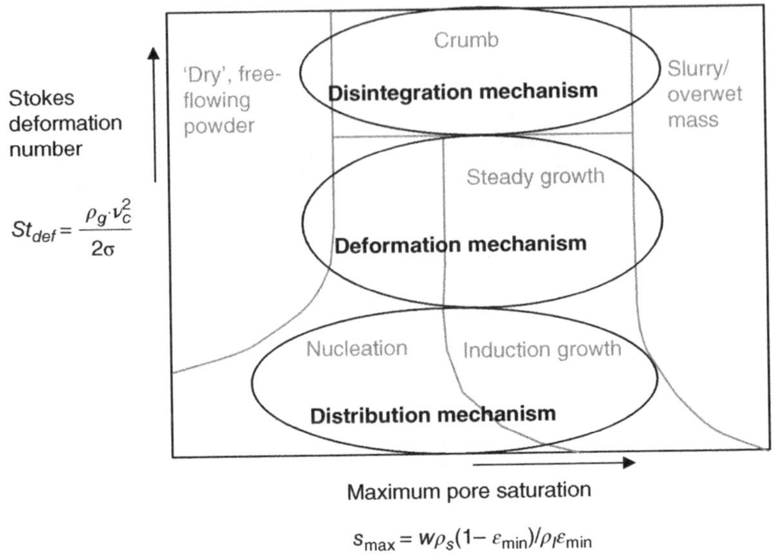

Figure 8.14 *Relationship between granule breakage mechanisms and the granule growth regime map. Reprinted with permission from* International Journal of Pharmaceutics, *The use of Stokes deformation number as a predictive tool for material exchange behaviour of granules in the 'equilibrium phase' in high shear granulation, A.M. Bouwman, M.R. Visser, G.M.H. Meesters, H.W. Frijlink, 318, 1–2, 78–85. Copyright (2006) Elsevier*

8.5 Endpoint Control

The most difficult part of granulation is determining when the desired granule properties have been achieved, and when to stop the process (Leuenberger *et al.* 2009). The aim of endpoint control is to ensure consistent granule density and uniform composition, usually by obtaining a similar granule size distribution, although all three parameters are interlinked and cannot be manipulated or optimized independently. This is often complicated by changes in equipment design and scale, as the product moves through process development and into manufacturing plants. Despite decades of research, all existing methods for determining the endpoint are still formulation and/or equipment dependent. In addition, the success or failure of the granulation process is judged by the success or failure of the final tablet or capsule, which adds several intervening processing steps, all of which may affect the final product performance. Key granule attributes and a general guide to their potential consequences on final product are summarized in Table 8.1.

The formulation is usually fixed quite early during the initial stages of product development, which leaves only binder solution concentration, solution delivery rate, impeller speed(s) and chopper speed(s) to manipulate. Some degree of fine tuning may be possible by adjusting spray nozzle design, spray flux, granulator fill level, impeller blade design, order of addition of ingredients and so on. In practice, the endpoint is determined by running multiple batches, analysing the granule and tablet properties, and finding a design window that represents the set(s) of operating conditions where the final product

Table 8.1 *Summary of granule attributes*

Granule attribute	Problem	Potential Consequences
Granule size distribution	Too many fine granules	Poor powder flow Poor blending Poor weight uniformity in tablets Risk of segregation
	Too many coarse granules	Blockage of pneumatic transfer lines Extended drying times Difficulty in achieving uniform moisture content during drying Heat build-up in dry mill, which in extreme cases causes melting/extrusion, or drug stability problems. Excessive dust generated during dry milling
Granule density	Increased density	Reduced tablet thickness Changes in tablet hardness (usually an increase) Slower tablet dissolution
	Reduced density	Fragile granules that break and attrit easily Reduced tablet hardness Faster tablet dissolution
Drug distribution in each granule size fraction	Non-uniform distribution	Risk of segregation of different sized granules, leading to segregation of drug within the batch Content uniformity problems.

performance is acceptable. The issue then becomes how to ensure that every subsequent batch is stopped at a point within this operating window.

There are four general approaches to granulation endpoint control:

1. Granulation time
2. Impeller power consumption or impeller torque
3. Online measurement of granule size
4. NIR and other spectral methods.

Each method is discussed in more detail next.

8.5.1 Granulation Time

This is the simplest and probably most common method of controlling the granulation endpoint. The solution delivery flow rate, impeller speed and chopper speed are set, and each stage of the granulation process (dry mixing, solution delivery, wet massing) runs for a predetermined time. The time steps are usually determined by the performance of several experimental batches combined with experience. Time-based endpoints are sufficient for many products in the steady growth regime (see Figure 8.8 and Figure 8.9) where the granule growth rate is linearly proportional with time, and the granules reach a constant density quite early in the process (Iveson and Litster 1998). These processes tend to behave in a well predicted and robust manner, without a tendency to suddenly over granulate, and thus are easily controlled using a time-based endpoint with only a small amount of optimization for scale-up. However, this is a poor approach for formulations that exhibit induction growth behaviour.

8.5.2 Impeller Power Consumption

Changes in the granule properties – particularly the granule size distribution and the degree of cohesion of the wet mass – are reflected in the impeller power consumption. As the cohesion increases, the resistance of the wet mass during powder flow increases and more energy must be supplied to the impeller to maintain the fixed rotation speed. Generally, impeller power is correlated with changes in granule size (Mackaplow *et al.* 2000; Holm *et al.* 2001) and/or density. Most modern pharmaceutical mixers provide impeller power consumption information although the reading may be presented as power (kW), amps (A), volts (V) or as an undefined '% load'. Impeller torque is more directly related to the wet mass cohesion (Bouwman *et al.* 2005), but is far more difficult to measure and is rarely found on pharmaceutical mixers. For a more detailed review, see Faure *et al.* (2001) or Mort (2007).

Power consumption endpoints are most useful for products that operate in the induction growth regime (see Figure 8.9), as the sudden increase in granule size when liquid is squeezed to the granule surface dramatically increases the cohesion of the wet mass. This is immediately reflected in a rapid increase in power consumption (Bouwman *et al.* 2005). For induction systems the power endpoint can be defined as a power value in kW, or based on the first derivative of the power signal, which will highlight the point where the power begins to increase rapidly. In contrast, power profiles for products operating in the steady growth regime show a gradual rise in impeller power, and setting a power endpoint criterion is difficult.

Power consumption can also be used to scale-up or transfer a granulation process from one mixer to another. A series of dimensionless groups are used to relate the power draw of the mixer to the flow pattern and mixing characteristics of the wet mass (Landin *et al.* 1996; Faure *et al.* 1999a,b; Landin *et al.* 1999; Faure *et al.* 2001). This technique has been successfully applied in several different mixer designs, and can be used to adjust for differences in mixer geometry. However, anecdotal experiences suggest that although the technique will help estimate the power endpoint, some additional work to refine the appropriate power endpoint in the new mixer is usually required. The dimensionless design groups do not currently account for changes in impeller blade design (Holm *et al.* 2001). This is still preferable to relying solely on trial and error. One common downfall is that many older mixers have only two fixed speeds, which straddle the target power endpoint.

8.5.3 Online Measurement of Granule Size

In recent years, there has been a concerted effort to develop more sophisticated granulation monitoring tools. Real-time measurement of granule size is now possible and is likely to become increasingly common in pharmaceutical manufacturing in future, given the current interest in PAT and Quality by Design. The ability to measure granule size during the granulation would be extremely useful for products in any of the typical growth regimes used in pharmaceutical manufacturing – nucleation, steady growth or induction growth.

Optical images of the granules as they move around the granulator can be taken and analysed in real time via image analysis. An early example was the 'image eye' probe (Watano and Miyanami 1995; Watano 2001) used for fluid bed granulation. Using a CCD camera mounted in a custom probe, the image eye produces real time information on the granule size distribution, average granule size as well as some granule shape information.

An alternate method of granule size analysis is Focussed Beam Reflectance Measurement (FBRM), where a probe is inserted into the powder bed, and a laser beam rotating at very high speed measures the chord length of the granules as they move past the probe. The technique is applied in a wide range of applications outside of pharmaceutical manufacturing (Sistare *et al.* 2005), and there are several reports of the use of FBRM in fluid bed granulation (Hu *et al.* 2008; Tok *et al.* 2008; Huang *et al.* 2010). The chord length correlates qualitatively with traditional particle size but is extremely difficult to convert to true particle size (Yu and Erickson 2008). However, this is not a problem in practical granulation applications where the chord length can be matched directly.

The main drawback of both optical techniques is the need to keep the camera or probe window clean, as any wet material fouling the lens will obscure the flowing granules and distort the results. The image eye has been designed to partially self-clean the window but has been used mostly in fluid bed granulation (Watano and Miyanami 1995; Watano 2001), where the granules tend to be drier. The FBRM has also been used mostly in fluid bed granulation for the same reason, but an at-line technique can be used during mixer granulation process development by removing a sample from the granulator and analysing it immediately in a small beaker (Michaels *et al.* 2009). Newer probes have a self-cleaning scraping mechanism to address this problem (Huang *et al.* 2010). Probe position is also important to ensure that the probe 'sees' the full distribution of particles (Huang *et al.* 2010).

8.5.4 NIR and Other Spectral Methods

Near infra-red spectroscopy (NIR) is a particularly interesting approach to detecting the granulation endpoint, because it offers simultaneous measurement of granule moisture and size (Frake *et al.* 1997; Findlay *et al.* 2005; Tok *et al.* 2008). Once again, this has so far been restricted to fluid bed granulation, partly because of the common use of NIR for detecting drying endpoint, and presumably partly due to the need to minimize fouling on the probe surface. The response of specific wavelengths of the spectra, plus the baseline movement, have been shown to correlate with the granule moisture content and the average particle size (Frake *et al.* 1997; Findlay *et al.* 2005).

Raman spectroscopy has also been used to determine the changes in granule density in the bed, which is correlated with average particle size (Walker *et al.* 2007; 2009). The spectra can determine the concentration and chemical composition of particles every 10 s (Walker *et al.* 2009).

The great hope for spectroscopic endpoint determination is the promise of being able to simultaneously measure the granule size distribution, moisture content, and chemical composition of the granules using different wavelengths of the spectra. These could then be used for real-time process control and feedback of several important granule properties listed in Table 8.1, in keeping with the current drive towards science-based process understanding and control.

References

Ansari, M.A. and F. Štěpánek (2006). 'Design of granule structure: Computational methods and experimental realization'. *AIChE Journal* **52**(11): 3762–3774.

Ansari, M.A. and F. Štěpánek (2006). 'Formation of hollow core granules by fluid bed in situ melt granulation: Modelling and experiments'. *International Journal of Pharmaceutics* **321**(1–2): 108–116.

Ax, K., H. Feise, R. Sochon, M. Hounslow and A. Salman (2008). 'Influence of liquid binder dispersion on agglomeration in an intensive mixer'. *Powder Technology* **179**(3): 190–194.

Berggren, J. and G. Alderborn (2001). 'Effect of drying rate on porosity and tabletting behaviour of cellulose pellets'. *International Journal of Pharmaceutics* **227**: 81–96.

Boerefijn, R. and M.J. Hounslow (2005). 'Studies of fluid bed granulation in an industrial R&D context'. *Chemical Engineering Science* **60**(14): 3879–3890.

Bouwman, A.M., M.J. Henstra, J. Hegge, Z. Zhang, A. Ingram, J.P.K. Seville and H.W. Frijlink (2005). 'The relation between granule size, granule stickiness, and torque in the high-shear granulation process'. *Pharmaceutical Research* **22**(2): 270–275.

Bouwman, A.M., M.R. Visser, G.M.H. Meesters and H.W. Frijlink (2006). 'The use of Stokes deformation number as a predictive tool for material exchange behaviour of granules in the 'equilibrium phase' in high shear granulation'. *International Journal of Pharmaceutics* **318**(1–2): 78–85.

Chouk, V., G. Reynolds, M. Hounslow and A. Salman (2009). 'Single drop behaviour in a high shear granulator'. *Powder Technology* **189**(2): 357–364.

Farber, L., G. Tardos and J.N. Michaels (2003). 'Use of X-ray tomography to study the porosity and morphology of granules'. *Powder Technology* **132**(1): 57–63.

Faure, A., I.M. Grimsey, R.C. Rowe, P. York and M.J. Cliff (1999a). 'Applicability of a scale-up method for wet granulation processes in Collette Gral high shear mixer-granulators'. *European Journal of Pharmaceutical Sciences* **8**: 85–93.

Faure, A., I.M. Grimsey, R.C. Rowe, P. York and M.J. Cliff (1999b). 'Process control in a high shear mixer-granulator using wet mass consistency: effect of formulation variables'. *Journal of Pharmaceutical Sciences* **88**(2): 191–195.

Faure, A., P. York and R.C. Rowe (2001). 'Process control and scale-up of pharmaceutical wet granulation processes: a review'. *European Journal of Pharmaceutics and Biopharmaceutics* **52**(3): 269–277.

Findlay, W.P., G.R. Peck and K.R. Morris (2005). 'Determination of fluidized bed granulation end point using near-infrared spectroscopy and phenomenological analysis'. *Journal of Pharmaceutical Sciences* **94**(3): 604–612.

Frake, P., D. Greenhalgh, S.M. Griersona, J.M. Hempenstalla and D.R. Rudda (1997). 'Process control and end-point determination of a fluid bed granulation by application of near infra-red spectroscopy'. *International Journal of Pharmaceutics* **151**: 75–80.

Goldszal, A. and J. Bousquet (2001). 'Wet agglomeration of powders: from physics toward process optimization'. *Powder Technology* **117**(3): 221–231.

Hapgood, K.P. (2000). *Nucleation and Binder Dispersion in Wet Granulation*. Brisbane, Australia, PhD thesis, Department of Chemical Engineering, University of Queensland. **PhD**.

Hapgood, K.P., R. Amelia, M.B. Zaman, B.K. Merrett and P. Leslie (2009). Improving liquid distribution by reducing dimensionless spray flux in wet granulation - a pharmaceutical manufacturing case study. *9th International Symposium on Agglomeration*, Sheffield University, Sheffield, UK.

Hapgood, K.P., R. Amelia, M.B. Zaman, B.K. Merrett and P. Leslie (2010). 'Improving liquid distribution by reducing dimensionless spray flux in wet granulation - a pharmaceutical manufacturing case study'. *Chemical Engineering Science*: accepted 9 May 2010.

Hapgood, K.P., J.D. Litster, S.R. biggs and T. Howes (2002). 'drop penetration into porous powder beds'. *Journal of Colloid and Interface Science* **253**(2): 353–366.

Hapgood, K.P., J.D. Litster and R. Smith (2003). 'Nucleation regime map for liquid bound granules'. *AIChE Journal* **49**(2): 350–361.

Hapgood, K.P., J.D. Litster, E.T. White, P.R. Mort and D.G. Jones (2004). 'Dimensionless spray flux in wet granulation: Monte-Carlo simulations and experimental validation'. *Powder Technology* **141**(1–2): 20–30.

Hapgood, K.P., T.H. Nguyen, S. Hauw, S.M. Iveson and W. Shen (2009). 'Rewetting effects and droplet motion on partially wetted powder surfaces'. *AIChE Journal* **55**(6): 1402–1415.

Hapgood, K.P., M.X.L. Tan and D.W.Y. Chow (2009). 'A method to predict nuclei size distributions for use in models of wet granulation'. *Advanced Powder Technology* **20**(4): 293–297.

Higashide, F., Y. Miki, Y. Nozawa and K. Ishibashi (1985). 'Dependence of drug content uniformity on particle sizes in fluidized bed granulation'.*Pharmazeutische-Industrie* **47**(11): 1202–1205.

Holm, P. (1987). 'Effect of impeller and chopper design on granulation in a high speed mixer'. *Drug Development and Industrial Pharmacy* **13**(9–11): 1675–1701.

Holm, P., O. Jungersen, T. Schæfer and H.G. Kristensen (1983). 'Granulation in High Speed Mixers. Part 1. Effects of process variables during kneading'. *Pharm. Ind.* **45**(8): 806–811.

Holm, P., O. Jungersen, T. Schæfer and H.G. Kristensen (1984). 'Granulation in high speed mixers. Part 2. Effects of process variables during kneading'. *Pharm. Ind.* **46**(1): 97–101.

Holm, P., T. Schaefer and C. Larsen (2001). 'End-point detection in a wet granulation process'. *Pharmaceutical Development and Technology* **6**(2): 181–192.

Hoornaert, F., P.A.L. Wauters, G.M.H. Meesters and S.E. Pratsinis (1998). 'Agglomeration behaviour of powders in a Lödige mixer granulator'. *Powder Technology* **96**: 116–128.

Hu, X., J.C. Cunningham and D. Winstead (2008). 'Study growth kinetics in fluidized bed granulation with at-line FBRM'. *International Journal of Pharmaceutics* **347**(1–2): 54–61.

Huang, J., G. Kaul, J. Utz, P. Hernandez, V. Wong, D. Bradley, A. Nagi and D. O'grady (2010). 'A PAT approach to improve process understanding of high shear wet granulation through in-line particle measurement using FBRM C35'. *Journal of Pharmaceutical Sciences* **99**(7): 3205–3212.

Iveson, S.M. (1997). Fundamental Studies of Granulation: Granule Deformation and Consolidation, University of Queensland.

Iveson, S.M., J.A. Beathe and N.W. Page (2002). 'The dynamic strength of partially saturated powder compacts: the effect of liquid properties'. *Powder Technology* **127**: 149–161.

Iveson, S.M. and J.D. Litster (1998). 'Fundamental studies of granule consolidation. Part 2: Quantifying the effects of particle and binder properties'. *Powder Technology* **99**: 243–250.

Iveson, S.M. and J.D. Litster (1998). 'Growth regime map for liquid-bound granules'. *AIChE Journal* **44**(7): 1510–1518.

Iveson, S.M., J.D. Litster and B.J. Ennis (1996). 'Fundamental studies of granule consolidation. Part 1: Effects of binder content and binder viscosity'. *Powder Technology* **88**: 15–20.

Iveson, S.M., J.D. Litster, K.P. Hapgood and B.J. Ennis (2001a). 'Nucleation, growth and breakage phenomena in agitated wet granulation processes: a review'. *Powder Technology* **117**(1–2): 3–39.

Iveson, S.M. and N. Page (2004). 'Brittle to plastic transition in the dynamic mechanical behavior of partially saturated granular materials'. *Journal of Applied Mechanics* **71**: 470–475.

Iveson, S.M. and N. Page (2005). 'Dynamic strength of liquid-bound granular materials: The effect of particle size and shape'. *Powder Technology* **152**: 79–89.

Iveson, S.M., P.A.L. Wauters, S. Forrest, J.D. Litster, G.M.H. Meesters and B. Scarlett (2001). 'Growth regime map for liquid-bound granules: further development and experimental validation'. *Powder Technology* **117**: 83–97.

Jægerskou, A., P. Holm and T. Schæfer (1984). 'Granulation in High Speed Mixers. Part 3: Effects of process variables on the intragranular porosity'. *Pharm. Ind.* **46**(3): 310–314.

Johansen, A. and T. Schæfer (2001). 'Effects of interactions between powder particle size and binder viscosity on agglomerate growth mechanisms in a high shear mixer'. *European Journal of Pharmaceutical Sciences* **12**: 297–309.

Kato, Y., K. Moroshima, M. Hashizume, H. Ando and M. Dfurukawa (2001). 'Further observation of content uniformity of d-a-tocopheryl acetate as an oily drug in granules obtained by wet granulation with a high shear mixer.' *Drug Development and Industrial Pharmacy* **27**(8): 781–787.

Knight, P.C., T. Instone, J.M.K. Pearson and M.J. Hounslow (1998). 'An investigation into the kinetics of liquid distribution and growth in high shear mixer agglomeration'. *Powder Technology* **97**: 246–257.

Knight, P.C., A. Johansen, H.G. Kristensen, T. Schæfer and J.P.K. Seville (2000). 'An investigation of the effects on agglomeration of changing the speed of a mechanical mixer'. *Powder Technology* **110**: 204–209.

Kristensen, H.G. and T. Schæfer (1987). 'Granulation. A review of pharmaceutical wet-granulation'. *Drug Development and Industrial Pharmacy* **13**(4&5): 803–872.
Lachman, L. and Sylwestrowicz (1964). 'Experiences with unit-to-unit variations in tablets'. *Journal of Pharmaceutical Sciences* **53**(10): 1234–1242.
Landin, M., P. York, M.J. Cliff and R.C. Rowe (1999). 'Scaleup of a pharmaceutical granulation in planetary mixers'. *Pharmaceutical Development and Technology* **4**(2): 145–150.
Landin, M., P. York, M.J. Cliff, R.C. Rowe and A.J. Wigmore (1996). 'Scale-up of pharmaceutical granulation in fixed bowl mixer-granulation'. *International Journal of Pharmaceutics* **133**: 127–131.
Lerk, C.F., A.J.M. Schoonen and J.T. Fell (1976). 'Contact angles and wetting of pharmaceutical powders'. *Journal of Pharmaceutical Sciences* **65**(6): 843–847.
Leuenberger, H., M. Puchkov, E. Krausbauer and G. Betz (2009). 'Manufacturing pharmaceutical granules: Is the granulation end-point a myth?' *Powder Technology* **189**(2): 141–148.
Litster, J.D. and B.J. Ennis (2004). *The Science and Engineering and Granulation Processes.* Dordrecht, Kluwer Academic Publishers.
Litster, J.D., K.P. Hapgood, J.N. Michaels, A. Sims, M. Roberts and S.K. Kameneni (2002). 'Scale-up of mixer granulators for effective liquid distribution'. *Powder Technology* **124**(3): 272–280.
Litster, J.D., K.P. Hapgood, J.N. Michaels, A. Sims, M. Roberts, S.K. Kameneni and T. Hsu (2001). 'Liquid distribution in wet granulation: dimensionless spray flux'. *Powder Technology* **114**(1–3): 32–39.
Liu, L.X., I. Marziano, A.C. Bentham, J.D. Litster, E.T. White and T. Howes (2008). 'Effect of particle properties on the flowability of ibuprofen powders'. *International Journal of Pharmaceutics* **362**(1–2): 109–117.
Liu, L.X., R. Smith and J.D. Litster (2009). 'Wet granule breakage in a breakage only high-shear mixer: Effect of formulation properties on breakage behaviour'. *Powder Technology* **189**(2): 158–164.
Mackaplow, M.B., L.A. Rosen and J.N. Michaels (2000). 'Effect of primary particle size on granule growth and endpoint determination in high-shear wet granulation'. *Powder Technology* **108**(1): 32–45.
Michaels, J.N., L. Farber, G.S. Wong, K. Hapgood, S.J. Heidel, J. Farabaugh, J.H. Chou and G.I. Tardos (2009). 'Steady states in granulation of pharmaceutical powders with application to scale-up'. *Powder Technology* **189**(2): 295–303.
Miyamoto, Y., A. Ryu, S. Sugawara, M. Miyajima, S. Ogawa, M. Matsui, K. Takayama and T. Nagai (1998). 'Simultaneous optimization of wet granulation process involving factor of drug content dependency on granule size'. *Drug Development and Industrial Pharmacy* **24**(11): 1055–1065.
Mort, P. (2007). Chapter 19, 'Scale-up of high-shear binder-agglomeration processes'. In *Handbook of Powder Technology*. M.J.H.A.D. Salman and J.P.K. Seville (eds), Elsevier Science B.V. **Volume 11: pp.** 853–896.
Mort, P.R. (2005). 'Scale-up of binder agglomeration processes'. *Powder Technology* **150**(2): 86–103.
Nguyen, T., W. Shen and K. Hapgood (2009). 'Drop penetration time in heterogeneous powder beds'. *Chemical Engineering Science* **64**(24): 5210–5221.
Nguyen, T.H., W. Shen and K.P. Hapgood (2010). 'Effect of formulation hydrophobicity on drug distribution in wet granulation'. *Chemical Engineering Science* **64**(24): 5210–5221.
Ohno, I., S. Hasegawa, S. Yada, A. Kusai, K. Moribe and K. Yamamoto (2007). 'Importance of evaluating the consolidation of granules manufactured by high shear mixer'. *International Journal of Pharmaceutics* **338**(1–2): 79–86.
Oostra, W., O. De Vegt, H. Vromans and K. Van Den Dries (2002). A study of the influence of process parameters of a high shear granulation process on the composition of the resulting granules. *World Congress Particle Technology* 4, Sydney Australia.
Pearson, J.K.M., M.J. Hounslow and T. Instone (2001). 'Tracer Studies of high-shear granulation I: Experimental Results'. *AIChE* **47**(9): 1978–1983.
Plank, R., B. Diehl, H. Grinstead and J. Zega (2003). 'Quantifying liquid coverage and powder flux in high-shear granulators'. *Powder Technology* **134**(3): 223–234.
Plank, R., J. Zega and L. Wai (2001). *Granule Content as a Function of Size Studied for Wet Granulation of a 3-Component System.* AIChE Annual Meeting.
Ramaker, J.S., M.A. Jelgersma, P. Vonk and N.W.F. Kossen (1998). 'Scale-down of a high shear pelletisation process: Flow profile and growth kinetics'. *International Journal of Pharmaceutics* **166**: 89–97.

Rumpf, H. (1962). 'The strength of granules and agglomerates'. In *Agglomeration*. W. Knepper (ed.). John Wiley & Sons, Inc., New York, pp. 379–418.

Schaafsma, S.H., P. Vonk, N.W.F. Kossen and A.C. Hoffmann (2006). 'A model for the spray zone in early-stage fluidized bed granulation'. *AIChE Journal* **52**(8): 2736–2741.

Schæfer, T. and C. Mathiesen (1996). 'Melt pelletization in a high shear mixer IX. Effects of binder particle size'. *International Journal of Pharmaceutics* **139**: 139–148.

Schæfer, T. and C. Mathiesen (1996). 'Melt pelletization in a high shear mixer VIII. Effects of binder viscosity'. *International Journal of Pharmaceutics* **139**: 125–128.

Scott, A.C., M.J. Hounslow and T. Instone (1999). 'Direct evidence of heterogeneity during high-shear granulation'. *Powder Technology* **113**: 215–213.

Sistare, F., L.S.P. Berry and C.A. Mojica (2005). 'Process analytical technology: An investment in process knowledge'. *Organic Process Research & Development* **9**(3): 332–336.

Smith, R. (2008). *Wet granule breakage in high shear mixer granulators. PhD Thesis*. Brisbane, Australia, Department of Chemical Engineering, University of Queensland.

Smith, R.M. and J.D. Litster (2012). 'Examining the failure modes of wet granular materials using dynamic diametrical compression'. *Powder Technology* **224**: 189–195.

Smith, R.M., L.X. Liu and J.D. Litster (2010). 'Breakage of drop nucleated granules in a breakage only high shear mixer'. *Chemical Engineering Science* **65**(21): 5651–5657, **doi:10.1016/j.ces.2010.06.037**.

Talu, I., G.I. Tardos and M.I. Khan (2000). 'Computer simulation of wet granulation'. *Powder Technology* **110**: 59–75.

Tardos, G.I., M.I. Khan and P.R. Mort (1997). 'Critical parameters and limiting conditions in binder granulation of fine powders'. *Powder Technology* **94**: 245–258.

Tok, A., X.P. Goh, W. Ng and R. Tan (2008). 'Monitoring granulation rate processes using three PAT tools in a pilot-scale fluidized bed'. *AAPS PharmSciTech* **9**(4): 1083–1091.

Tran, A. (2012). Powder Flow Properties in Vertical High Shear Mixers. PhD Thesis, Department of Chemical Engineering. Queensland, Australia, The University of Queensland.

Tu, W.-D., S.-S. Hsiau, A. Ingram and J. Seville (2008). 'The effect of powder size on induction behaviour and binder distribution during high shear melt agglomeration of calcium carbonate'. *Powder Technology* **184**(3): 298–312.

Tu, W.D., A. Ingram, J. Seville and S.S. Hsiau (2009). 'Exploring the regime map for high-shear mixer granulation'. *Chemical Engineering Journal* **145**(3): 505–513.

Van Den Dries, K., O.M.D. Vegt, V. Girard and H. Vromans (2003). 'Granule breakage phenomena in a high shear mixer; influence of process and formulation variables and consequences on granule homogeneity.' *Powder Technology* **113**: 228–236.

Vonk, P., C.P.F. Guillaume, J.S. Ramaker, H. Vromans and N.W.F. Kossen (1997). 'Growth mechanisms of high-shear pelletisation'. *International Journal of Pharmaceutics* **157**: 93–102.

Vromans, H., H.G.M. Poels-Janssen and H. Egermann (1999). 'Effects of high-shear granulation on granulate homogeneity'. *Pharmaceutical Development and Technology* **4**(3): 297–303.

Waldie, B. (1991). 'Growth mechanism and the dependence of granule size on drop size in fluidised bed granulation'. *Chemical Engineering Science* **46**(11): 2781–2785.

Walker, G., S.E.J. Bell, M. Vann, D.S. Jones and G. Andrews (2007). 'Fluidised bed characterisation using Raman spectroscopy: Applications to pharmaceutical processing'. *Chemical Engineering Science* **62**(14): 3832–3838.

Walker, G.M., S.E.J. Bell, K. Greene, D.S. Jones and G.P. Andrews (2009). 'Characterisation of fluidised bed granulation processes using in-situ Raman spectroscopy'. *Chemical Engineering Science* **64**(1): 91–98.

Wan, L.S.C., P.W.S. Heng and G. Muhuri (1992). 'Incorporation and distribution of a low dose drug in granules'. *International Journal of Pharmaceutics* **88**: 159–163.

Watano, S. (2001). 'Direct control of wet granulation processes by image processing system'. *Powder Technology* **117**(1–2): 163–172.

Watano, S. and K. Miyanami (1995). 'Image processing for on-line monitoring of granule size distribution and shape in fluidized bed granulation'. *Powder Technology* **83**(1): 55–60.

Wauters, P.A.L., R.B. Jakobsen, J.D. Litster, G.M.H. Meesters and B. Scarlett (2002a). 'Liquid distribution as a means to describing the granule growth mechanism'. *Powder Technology* **123**: 166–177.

Wauters, P.A.L., R. Van De Water, J.D. Litster, G.M.H. Meesters and B. Scarlett (2002b). 'Growth and compaction behaviour of copper concentrate granules in a rotating drum'. *Powder Technology* **124**(3): 230–237.

Wildeboer, W.J., E. Koppendraaier, J.D. Litster, T. Howes and G. Meesters (2007). 'A novel nucleation apparatus for regime separated granulation'. *Powder Technology* **171**(2): 96–105.

Wildeboer, W.J., J.D. Litster and I.T. Cameron (2005). 'Modelling nucleation in wet granulation'. *Chemical Engineering Science* **60**(14): 3751–3761.

Yu, W. and K. Erickson (2008). 'Chord length characterization using focused beam reflectance measurement probe – methodologies and pitfalls'. *Powder Technology* **185**(1): 24–30.

Zhang, D., J.H. Flory, S. Panmai, U. Batra and M.J. Kaufman (2002). 'Wettability of pharmaceutical solids: its measurement and influence on wet granulation'. *Colloids and Surfaces A: Physicochemical and Engineering Aspects* **206**(1–3): 547–554.

Zhang, Y. and K.C. Johnson (1997). 'Effect of drug particle size on content uniformity of low dose solid dosage forms'. *International Journal of Pharmaceutics* **154**: 179–183.

Zoglio, M.A. and J.T. Cartensen (1983). 'Physical aspects of wet granulation III. Effect of wet granulation on granule porosity'. *Drug Development and Industrial Pharmacy* **9**(8): 1417–1434.

9

Emulsions

Andrzej W. Pacek

School of Chemical Engineering, University of Birmingham, UK

9.1 Introduction

The mixing of two immiscible or partially miscible liquids frequently leads to formation of a dispersed system in which one of the liquids forms drops (dispersed phase) suspended in the second liquid (continuous phase). Such systems have large surface energy; therefore, in general, they are thermodynamically unstable and tend to separate into two layers where the surface energy reaches a minimum. Liquid/liquid dispersed systems can be stabilized by continuous addition of energy, and, depending on the size of drops and the form of energy used for stabilization it is possible to distinguish between dispersions and emulsions. The term *dispersions* is used to describe two-phase liquid/liquid systems in which one phase forms drops of the order of tens/hundreds of microns stabilized by continuous addition of mechanical energy. Dispersions are typically produced in stirred vessels, static mixers or bubble columns and are common in extraction processes as they separate relatively quickly into two layers after the addition of energy ceases (Godfrey and Slater, 1994). The term *emulsions* is used to describe liquid/liquid two phase systems containing surface active agents with drops of the order of a few microns stabilized by surface energy. Typically, emulsions are produced from dispersions by addition of mechanical energy and surfactants (also called emulsifiers), and they remain stable for days/months but they can also separate into two layers when surface energy/activity of surfactant reduces below certain critical values. Emulsions are characterized by very small drops and a large specific surface area that

Pharmaceutical Blending and Mixing, First Edition. Edited by P.J. Cullen, Rodolfo J. Romañach, Nicolas Abatzoglou and Chris D. Rielly.

allows creation of product specific microstructures and functionality; therefore, they have found wide ranging applications in several industries such as food (McClements, 2005), pharmaceuticals (Nielloud and Marti-Mestres, 2000, Davies *et al.*, 1985), cosmetics, agriculture (Becker, 1985).

In the pharmaceutical industry, water-in-oil (W/O) emulsions are used as very effective adjuvants and they represent one of the best delivery systems for vaccine antigens (Jansen *et al.*, 2005). They also can be used as controlled release systems for hydrophilic drugs (Bjerregaard *et al.*, 1999). Semi-solid W/O emulsions are frequently used as oily creams in dermatology as they frequently increase drug permeation (Nielloud and Marti-Mestres, 2000). O/W emulsions are commonly used as parenteral fat emulsions for nutrition and as carriers of drugs sensitive to hydrolysis that are insoluble in water. Artificial blood is also an O/W emulsion of perfluorized hydrocarbons dispersed in the aqueous phase (Davies *et al.*, 1985) as the combination of a large specific interfacial area of emulsion with a high solubility of oxygen and carbon dioxide in perfluorized hydrocarbons ensures very high mass transfer rates. Semi solid O/W emulsions are used in dermatology as non-oily creams (Nielloud and Marti-Mestres, 2000). Multiple W/O/W emulsions are used to enhance chemotherapeutic effects in cancer treatment, to treat drug overdose (Okochi and Nakano, 2000) and also for oral administration of insulin (Silva-Cunha *et al.*, 1998) whilst O/W/O emulsions are used as prolonged drug delivery systems (Mishra and Pandit, 1989).

Emulsions used as drug carriers should be biocompatible, biodegradable and stable and they should have a uniform drops, or at least a very narrow, drop size distribution. The first two properties depend mainly on the type of oil, composition of the aqueous phase and the type of surfactant, whilst stability and drop size are also strongly affected by the method employed to produce emulsions. The selection of oils that can be used in emulsions in human drugs is practically limited to vegetable oils (sunflower, soya bean, cottonseed) but in some applications purified paraffin oils or perfluorochemicals can also be used (Davies *et al.*, 1985). Selection of surfactants (emulsifiers) depends on the type of oil and both natural and synthetic surface active agents (emulsifiers) are used in pharmaceutical formulations. Natural surface active agents, such as different types of lecithins, are frequently used in intravenous fat emulsions (Davies *et al.*, 1985, Nielloud and Marti-Mestres, 2000), whereas synthetic anionic surfactants are used in oral, topical and perenteral emulsions (Nielloud and Marti-Mestres, 2000). The composition of the aqueous phase depends on the application of emulsions and in parenteral emulsions the aqueous phase might contain surfactants, glycerol, vitamins, drugs or electrolytes (Davies *et al.*, 1985, Cuéllar *et al.*, 2005).

Because of the wide variety of formulations used in pharmaceutical industry as well as very strict regulations governing manufacturing and composition of many products, emulsification processes are frequently based on experience and tradition rather than on scientific principles. Such an approach is not suitable for development of new products.

Modern methods of emulsion production are based on the concept of formulation engineering. Within this concept, the effect of bulk properties of aqueous and organic phases, the conditions at the liquid/liquid interface and the intensity of hydrodynamic conditions in an emulsifying device on quality of emulsions are considered. Successful applications of such methods require good understanding of the effect of all these properties on drop size, stability and rheology of emulsions, as well as the mechanisms of breakage and coalescence in different emulsifying devices. All these aspects of formulation engineering related to the manufacturing of emulsions and the equipment used in industrial emulsification processes are discussed in this chapter.

9.2 Properties of Emulsions

There are three interconnected properties of emulsions strongly affecting the quality and performance of emulsion based products: structure, rheology and stability. To simplify the description of those properties it is commonly assumed that emulsion consists of two phases (oil phase and aqueous phase) and that surfactants/stabilizers are completely soluble in one of these two phases.

Rheology of emulsions depends mainly on the volume fraction of dispersed phase and rheology of continuous phase. At a high volume fraction of dispersed phase it also depends on surface properties/surface forces and the viscosity of dispersed phase. Several models relating apparent viscosity of emulsion to viscosity of the continuous phase and the volume fraction of dispersed phase are discussed later in this section.

Stability of emulsions depends on the properties of the interface, surface forces, density difference, rheology of continuous phase and volume fraction of dispersed phase. As the properties of the interface are determined by the type and concentration of surfactant used as a stabilizer, calculation of surfaces forces is frequently system specific. Therefore, only the fundamental interactions between surfaces are discussed in the context of different types of instabilities observed in emulsions.

9.2.1 Morphology

Emulsions/dispersions are frequently classified according to their morphology. Water (aqueous phase) dispersed in oil forms the W/O emulsion, whereas oil phase dispersed in water (aqueous phase) forms the *oil-in-water* (O/W) emulsion. Under certain conditions, complex, multiple emulsions/dispersions containing heterogeneous drops can be formed. Aqueous drops containing smaller oil droplets suspended in continuous oil phase form oil-in-water-in-oil (O/W/O) emulsions and oil drops containing smaller aqueous drops suspended in continuous aqueous phase form water-in-oil-in-water (W/O/W) emulsions. Multiple emulsions are produced by re-dispersing simple emulsion in presence of appropriate surfactants. For example, dispersing a stable W/O emulsion in water leads to a complex W/O/W emulsion or they can form spontaneously during phase inversion, even in surfactant free systems (Pacek *et al.*, 1994a). Multiple emulsions are frequently used to deliver active components in food and drugs (McClements *et al.*, 2007, Okochi and Nakano, 2000) but their structures, as well as other properties, are strongly system specific and are not discussed here.

9.2.2 Volumetric Composition

Volumetric composition is determined by the required properties and application of emulsion based products and it is not affected by chemical composition or by processing conditions. The volume of dispersed phase affects drop size distribution, average drop size, stability and rheology as well as the appearance and physical properties of emulsions (apparent density, thermal conductivity etc.). Typically it is expressed as a volume fraction:

$$\phi = \frac{V_d}{V} \tag{9.1}$$

or less frequently as a mass fraction:

$$\phi_{mass} = \frac{m_d}{m} \tag{9.2}$$

Volume fraction can be calculated if the mass fraction is known:

$$\phi = \frac{\phi_{mass}\,\rho_c}{\phi_{mass}\,\rho_c + (1-\phi_{mass})\rho_d} \tag{9.3}$$

and mass fraction can be calculated if the volume fraction is known:

$$\phi_{mass} = \frac{\phi\rho_d}{\phi\rho_d + (1-\phi)\rho_c} \tag{9.4}$$

When densities of both phases are the same the mass fraction is equal to the volume fraction.

9.2.3 Drop Size Distributions and Average Drop Sizes

The main aim of all emulsification processes is to break a certain amount of one phase into droplets of the required size and to disperse these droplets uniformly into the whole volume of the second phase. In practice, all types of emulsification equipment produce drops within certain size range (poly-dispersed emulsions) and emulsions in which all drops have the same size (mono-dispersed emulsions) practically do not exist. Therefore, an accurate description of the size of the dispersed phase requires knowledge of the drop size distribution. In many practical applications, rather than using drop size distribution (function) to describe the population of drops, certain average/mean size (number) is frequently used. Differently defined average drop sizes are discussed in detail later in this section.

Different techniques used for measurements of drop size distributions are discussed by McClements (2005). The selection of the technique depends on required accuracy of measurements, concentration of dispersed phase and the range of drop size as well as physicochemical properties of both phases. Drops in the range of 0.5–2000 μm are frequently measured using laser light diffraction techniques and the size of drops in nano-range (0.6–6000 nm) is determined using Dynamic Light Scattering (www.malvern.com/LabEng). The main advantage of these techniques is that the instruments are user friendly and are supplied with software, enabling full statistical analysis. The main disadvantage is that only very diluted samples can be analysed. For drops larger than 5 μm photographic techniques might be attractive as they can cope with more concentrated emulsions. In all these techniques the size of hundreds/thousands of drops are measured and differently defined size distributions are calculated, using the following (or a very similar) algorithm (Beddow, 1980):

1. The full size range (difference between the size of the largest and the smallest drop) is divided into classes (bins) limited by d_i and d_{i+1} and the total number of drops N_T is binned into i classes. It is assumed that all drops in a bin have the same size calculated as an average of the bin limits:

$$d_{iav} = 0.5 * (d_i + d_{i+1}) \quad (9.5)$$

2. Volume and number frequency distributions are calculated from:

$$f_{iv} = \frac{n_i * d_{iav}^3}{\sum_{j=1}^{i} n_i * d_{iav}^3} * 100 \quad (9.6a)$$

$$f_{in} = \frac{n_i}{\sum_{j=1}^{i} n_i} * 100 \quad (9.6b)$$

3. Volume and number cumulative distributions are calculated from:

$$F_{iv} = \sum_{j=1}^{i} f_{iv} \quad (9.7a)$$

$$F_{in} = \sum_{j=1}^{i} f_{in} \quad (9.7b)$$

4. Probability density functions with the following property: $\int_0^\infty \Phi(x)\,dx = 1$ are defined as:

$$\Phi_{iv} = \frac{f_{iv}}{d_{i+1} - d_i} \quad (9.8a)$$

$$\Phi_{in} = \frac{f_{in}}{d_{i+1} - d_i} \quad (9.8b)$$

The last two functions are used to calculate the number of drops or the volume of dispersed phase, contained between drops of different sizes. For example, the number of drops between drop of size d_1 and larger drop of size d_2 can be calculated from:

$$n(d_1, d_2) = N_T \int_{d1}^{d2} \Phi_n(d)dd \quad (9.9a)$$

and the volume of those drops:

$$V(d_1, d_2) = V_T \int_{d1}^{d2} \Phi_n(d)dd \quad (9.9b)$$

Table 9.1 *Volumetric drop size distributions calculated according to the algorithm in equations 9.5–9.8*

d_i /μm/	d_{i+1}/μm/	d_{iav}/μm/	n_i	f_{iv} /%/	F_{iv}/%/	Φ_{iv}/μm^{-1}/
0.20	0.28	0.24	0	0.00	0.00	0.00
0.28	0.39	0.34	52	0.74	5.6e-4	5.08e-5
0.39	0.55	0.47	209	2.99	0.01	4.00e-4
0.55	0.77	0.66	432	6.17	0.04	1.62e-3
0.77	1.08	0.92	611	8.73	0.18	4.49e-3
1.08	1.51	1.29	1063	15.19	0.84	0.02
1.51	2.11	1.81	1226	17.52	2.93	0.03
2.11	2.95	2.53	1350	19.29	9.23	0.07
2.95	4.13	3.54	1101	15.73	23.33	0.12
4.13	5.79	4.96	552	7.89	42.73	0.12
5.79	8.10	6.94	340	4.86	75.52	0.14
8.10	11.34	9.72	50	0.71	88.75	0.04
11.34	15.87	13.61	10	0.14	96.01	0.02
15.87	22.22	19.05	2	0.03	100.00	0.01
22.22	31.11	26.67	0	0.00	100.00	0.00

This algorithm is illustrated in Table 9.1. The first three columns contain bin sizes, the numbers of drops in each bin are given in column 4 and volume distribution functions are given in columns 5 to 7 and compared in Figure 9.1.

It is not always necessary to describe the population of drops in terms of size distributions and in many practical applications description in terms of a mean/average drop size is sufficient. The mean drop size is defined in terms of moments of size distribution function (Beddow, 1980):

$$M^k = \int_0^\infty d^k f(d)dd \qquad (9.10)$$

where k is an integer. The first four moments of drop size distribution have the following meaning: *0th* moment ($k = 0$) is equal to the total number of drops, *first* moment ($k = 1$) is equal to sum of diameters of all drops, *second* moment ($k = 2$) is equal to the total surface area of all drops (interfacial area between dispersed and continuous phase) and the *third* moment ($k = 3$) is equal to the total volume of all drops (volume of dispersed phase).

The mean drop size is defined as a ratio of two moments:

$$d_{p-q} = \left[\frac{\int_0^\infty d^p f(d)\partial d}{\int_0^\infty d^q f(d)\partial d}\right]^{\frac{1}{p-q}} \qquad (9.11)$$

where p and q are integers and $p > q$.

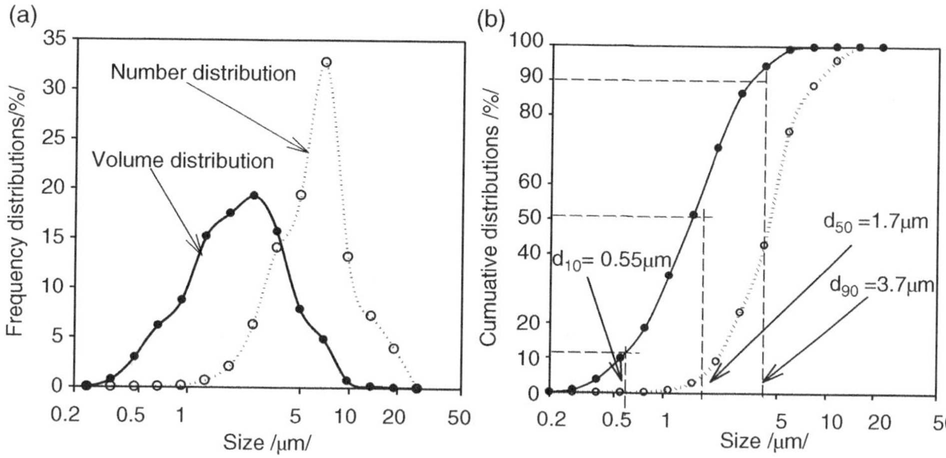

Figure 9.1 *Frequency and cumulative size distributions corresponding to the data in Table 9.1*

Equation 9.11 implies that it is possible to define several mean/average sizes for the same population of drops and Table 9.2 summarizes the most common mean diameters used for characterization of emulsion.

The Sauter mean diameter is frequently used to describe efficiency of emulsification processes and it relates specific interfacial area to the volume fraction of dispersed phase:

$$a = \frac{6\phi}{d_{32}} \tag{9.12}$$

It is important to realize that using mean drop size to describe a polydisperse emulsion has certain consequences. A polydisperse emulsion has four basic properties: number of drops, total linear dimension (sum of diameters of all drops), total interfacial area (sum of surface of all drops) and total volume of dispersed phase (sum of volumes of all drops) and each of those parameters can be accurately calculated from drop size distribution functions. By introducing an average drop size, e.g., replacing/modelling the polydisperse emulsion with a monodisperse one, only two out of four of these properties are preserved. For example, d_{10} preserves the number of drops and total linear dimension but the volume of dispersed phase and the surface area are not preserved. On the other hand, d_{32} preserves volume and surface area but the total number of drops and their total length are not preserved. This problem can be illustrated by considering the number of drops calculated by dividing the volume of dispersed phase by the volume of drop of certain mean diameter. The mean diameters in Table 9.2 are different; therefore, such a calculation would produce different numbers of drops whereas only the number of drops calculated by dividing total volume of dispersed phase by the volume of drop with diameter equal to d_{30} is the same as the total number of drops in polydisperse emulsion.

The last column in Table 9.2 indicates that, in order to avoid misunderstanding, it is necessary to precisely define the mean diameter used to describe the population of drops.

Table 9.2 *Different definitions of mean drop size*

p	Q	Name	Definition		Value [μm] (based on Table 9.1)
1	0	Number–length d_{10}	$\frac{\int_0^\infty d^1 f(d)\partial d}{\int_0^\infty f(d)\partial d}$	$\frac{\sum_{i=1}^n d_{iav} n_i}{N_T}$	2.51
2	0	Number–surface x_{20}	$\left[\frac{\int_0^\infty d^2 f(d)\partial d}{\int_0^\infty f(d)\partial d}\right]^{\frac{1}{2}}$	$\left[\frac{\sum_{i=1}^n d_{iav}^2 n_i}{N_T}\right]^{\frac{1}{2}}$	3.07
3	0	Number–volume d_{30}	$\left[\frac{\int_0^\infty d^3 f(d)\partial d}{\int_0^\infty f(d)\partial d}\right]^{\frac{1}{3}}$	$\left[\frac{\sum_{i=1}^n d_{iav}^3 n_i}{N_T}\right]^{\frac{1}{3}}$	3.67
3	2	Area–volume (Sauter) d_{32}	$\frac{\int_0^\infty d^3 f(d)\partial d}{\int_0^\infty d^2 f(d)\partial d}$	$\frac{\sum_{i=1}^n d_{iav}^3 n_i}{\sum_{i=1}^n d_{iav}^2 n_i}$	5.24

It is worth noticing that mean diameters calculated from high order moments are larger than those calculated from lower moments, for example, $d_{32} > d_{10}$. Also, the high moment's diameters are strongly biased towards large drops and small increases in the number of large drops leads to a substantial increase of d_{32} or d_{43}. Therefore, such diameters might frequently be misleading.

There are also certain characteristic diameters associated with cumulative drop size distributions (see Figure 9.1b), such as:

$\bar{d}_{10}$ – 10% of drops are smaller than this diameter
$\bar{d}_{50}$ – 50% median size separating top and bottom half of a population
$\bar{d}_{90}$ – 90% of drops are smaller than this diameter.

There are also analytical expressions describing drop size distributions such as the normal, also known as Gaussian, distribution used to describe a bell-shaped, symmetrical frequency distribution:

$$f(d) = \frac{1}{\sigma\sqrt{2\pi}} exp\left[\frac{-(d-d_{10})^2}{2\sigma^2}\right] \tag{9.13a}$$

$$\sigma = \sqrt{\frac{\sum N_i (d_{iav} - d_{10})^2}{N_T}} \tag{9.13b}$$

and a log-normal frequency distribution for distributions skewed towards large drops (Beddow, 1980):

$$f(lnx) = \frac{1}{ln\sigma\sqrt{2\pi}} exp\left[\frac{-(lnd - lnd_{10})^2}{2ln^2\sigma}\right] \quad (9.14a)$$

$$ln\sigma = \sqrt{\frac{\sum N_i(lnd_{iav} - lnd_{10})^2}{N_T}} \quad (9.14b)$$

$$lnd_{10} = \frac{\sum N_i lnd_i}{N_T} \quad (9.14c)$$

From what has been said already, it is clear that drop size distributions (detailed description of population of drops) as well as drop mean sizes (simplified description of population of drops) can be defined several ways. Therefore, it is always necessary to precisely define the mean/average size, otherwise the frequently used term *mean/average drop diameter* is meaningless.

9.2.4 Rheology

The word rheology is used to describe the behaviour of both single phase liquids, as well as multiphase emulsions, subjected to shear force. The way fluids respond to applied shear is commonly used to classify them into two groups: Newtonian and non-Newtonian fluids. The latter one can be further subdivided into; plastic, shear thickening and shear thinning fluids as shown in Figure 9.2. In this section, only the basic concepts of rheology are discussed and for more detailed information on each type of fluid the reader is referred to Barnes *et al.* (1998).

In Newtonian fluids, shear stress (τ) is directly proportional to the shear rate ($\dot{\gamma}$):

$$\tau = -\eta\dot{\gamma} \quad (9.15)$$

and the proportionality coefficient, called *shear viscosity* (η), is independent of shear rate. Viscosity is a physical property of a Newtonian fluid, practically independent of pressure and it decreases with temperature according to the Arrhenius equation (Barnes, 1998):

$$\eta = Aexp(-B/T) \quad (9.16)$$

where A and B are liquid specific constants. Viscosity is measured using different type of rheometers and for simple liquids viscosity can be estimated from the molecular theory of liquids (Sibley and Alberty, 2001).

In non-Newtonian fluids, dependency between the shear stress and the shear rate can take a different form as shown in Figure 9.2. There are several models relating shear stress (or viscosity) to shear rate and the Carreau model is frequently used (Barnes *et al.*, 1998):

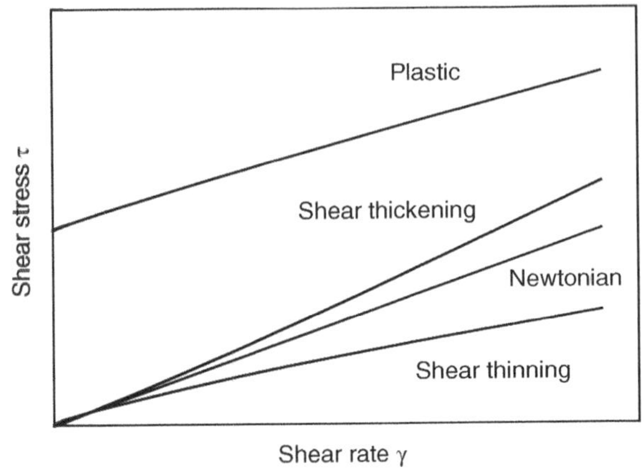

Figure 9.2 *Flow curves for various types of fluids*

$$\frac{\eta - \eta_\infty}{\eta_0 - \eta_\infty} = \frac{1}{\left[1 + (C\dot{\gamma})^2\right]^{m_1}} \tag{9.17}$$

For moderate viscosities, this model reduces to the very well-known power-law model:

$$\eta = K\dot{\gamma}^{n-1} \tag{9.18}$$

In this model, the power law index n indicates the fluid's behaviour with respect to shear rate and for Newtonian fluids $n = 1$, for shear thinning fluids $n < 1$ and for shear-thickening (dilatant) fluids $n < 1$. Whilst shear thinning fluids/emulsion are rather quite common, shear thickening behaviour has been observed only in concentrated solid/liquid suspensions (Barnes *et al.*, 1998).

The common feature of the fluids discussed here is that they flow even at infinitely small shear stress. There is also a class of fluids, the so called Bingham plastic fluids, which do not flow if applied shear stress is smaller than a certain critical value called *yield stress*. In such fluids, the total shear stress is a sum of yield stress (static) and the product of 'viscosity' and the shear rate (dynamic):

$$\tau = \tau_0 + \eta_B \dot{\gamma} \tag{9.19}$$

The rheological properties of certain non-Newtonian fluids dependent on shear stress and time. In thixotropic fluids at constant temperature viscosity decreases with time, whereas in rheopetic fluids at constant shear and temperature, viscosity increases with time (Schramm, 1992).

In principle, the concept of viscosity has been developed for homogeneous liquids. Emulsions are heterogeneous, two phase liquid/liquid systems and their flow can be analysed using different models such as the mixture model or separated flow model (Kleinstreuer, 2003). Separated flow models are used to describe the movement of drops in the continuous phase and might be used to analyse stability of emulsions. The mixture models assume that an emulsion can be treated as a single phase fluid with certain apparent viscosity (η_{ap}) and density (ρ_{ap}). Within this approach, shear stress can be calculated using apparent viscosity of emulsion in Newton's law and all rheological models discussed earlier are frequently used to describe the behaviour of emulsions. The apparent viscosity of emulsions depends on:

1. Volume fraction of dispersed phase (ϕ) and drop size distribution
2. Viscosity of continuous phase (η_c)
3. Temperature
4. Type and concentration of surfactant
5. For the non-Newtonian continuous phase or at the high volume fraction of dispersed phase, apparent viscosity also depends on shear rate.

There are several models that can be used to calculate (estimate) viscosity of emulsion if the viscosities of both the dispersed and continuous phases, as well as the volume fraction of the dispersed phase, are known. Assuming that interaction between particles can be neglected, Einstein developed a theoretical expression for viscosity of the very diluted ($\phi < 0.05$) suspension of spherical, solid particles that also can be used for diluted emulsions (Barnes *et al.*, 1998):

$$\eta_r = \frac{\eta_c}{\eta_{ap}} = 1 + 2.5\phi \tag{9.20}$$

To account for the effect of the viscosity of the dispersed phase and circulation inside drops on the apparent viscosity of emulsion, the Einstein model has been modified (Derkach, 2009):

$$\eta_r = 1 + \phi \frac{\eta_c + 2.5\eta_d}{\eta_c + \eta_d} \tag{9.21}$$

The effect of drop size on relative viscosity of diluted emulsions can be estimated from the Peclet number (*Pe*) describing the ratio of the hydrodynamic and Brownian contributions to the movement of drops in the emulsion:

$$Pe = \frac{\dot{\gamma}\eta_c R^3}{\kappa_B T} \tag{9.22}$$

If $Pe \ll 1$, the movement of drops is controlled by Brownian motion and the apparent viscosity is independent of drop size, and if $Pe \gg 1$, hydrodynamic forces control drop movement and again viscosity is independent of drop size. At *Pe* values between those two extremes, the apparent viscosity of emulsion increases with decreasing drop size (Briceno, 2000).

In the range of an intermediate volume fraction of dispersed phase and Newtonian continuous phase, the Krieger–Dougherty equation is frequently used to relate viscosity of emulsion to volume fraction of dispersed phase (Schramm, 1992):

$$\eta_r = \left[1 - \frac{\phi}{\phi_m}\right]^{-[\eta]\phi_m} \tag{9.23}$$

This equation, originally developed for solid/liquid suspensions, contains three adjustable constants: volume fraction of dispersed phase at maximum packing (ϕm) and intrinsic viscosity $[\eta]$. For suspensions of solid particles $\phi_m \in 0.6 - 0.75$ and $[\eta] \in (2.7 - 9.87)$ (Barnes *et al.*, 1998). The major difficulty with the Krieger–Dougherty equation, when applied to liquid/liquid emulsions, is the estimation of these two constants. They are system specific and might also depend on processing conditions, especially on the width of drop size distributions; therefore, they should be calculated from experimental flow curves using regression methods.

The combined effect of volume fraction and viscosity of dispersed phase on apparent viscosity of Newtonian emulsions has been accounted for in semi-theoretical models developed by Choi and Schowlater (1975):

$$\eta_r = 1 + \frac{2\left[5\lambda - (\lambda - 1)\phi^{7/3}\right]}{4(\lambda + 1) - 5(5\lambda + 2)\phi + 42\lambda\phi^{5/3} - 5(5\lambda - 2)\phi^{7/3} + 4(\lambda - 1)\phi^{10/3}}\phi \tag{9.24}$$

and by Pal (2001):

$$\eta_r \left[\frac{2\eta_r + 5\lambda}{2 + 5\lambda}\right]^{1.5} = \left(1 - \frac{\phi}{\phi_m}\right)^{-2.5\phi_m} \tag{9.25}$$

The last equation fits experimental data rather well for different systems up to $\phi \approx 0.6$, with the volume fraction at maximum packing being practically the same as volume fraction at maximum packing for solid particles.

Viscosity of highly concentrated emulsions, where volume fraction of dispersed phase exceeds maximum packing ($\phi > 0.7$), can be related to the drop's Reynolds number $Re_d = \frac{\rho_c r^2 \dot{\gamma}}{\eta_c}$ and maximum packing (Krynke and Sek, 2004):

$$\phi_m^{0.5}\left(1 - \eta_r^{-1/\varsigma[\eta]}\right) = A_0 + A_1 \log Re_d + A_2 (\log Re_d)^2 \tag{9.26}$$

Under certain conditions, drops might form large flocs that strongly affect viscosity of emulsions. In such cases drops are held together by the surface forces and it is possible to relate viscosity of flocculated emulsions to the energy barrier (Quemada and Berli, 2002):

$$\eta_r = \left[1 - \frac{\phi}{\phi_m}\right]^{-2.5\phi_m} + C_1 \phi exp\left(\frac{\Delta U}{\kappa_B T} - \frac{C_2}{\phi} \frac{\tau d^3 \tau}{\kappa_B T}\right) \tag{9.27}$$

where C and C_1 are experimental constants and ΔU is energy barrier between two drops discussed in Section 9.3.

This discussion of rheological properties is limited to relatively simple pharmaceutical emulsions used as drug delivery systems (up to 10% of dispersed phase), artificial blood (up to 20% of dispersed phase) or parenteral fat emulsions (10–20% of dispersed phase) (Nielloud and Marti-Mestres, 2000). There are also very complex, semi–solid emulsions (creams) used for topical drug delivery in dermatology, exhibiting viscoelastic or viscoplastic properties, and the rheology of such systems has been discussed by Peramal *et al.* (1997) and Derkach (2009).

9.3 Emulsion Stability and Surface Forces

In general terms, emulsion stability can be understood to be the ability of emulsion to resist changes in morphology and functional properties with time. The functional properties of emulsions are determined by the chemical composition and morphology. An emulsion is chemically unstable if the chemical composition of the dispersed/continuous phase or interface changes as a result of an undesirable chemical reaction, for example oxidation. These types of instabilities are system specific and they are not discussed here. McClements (2005) briefly discussed chemical/biochemical instabilities of food emulsions and certain problems typical for food systems might be also relevant in pharmaceutical emulsions.

The other type of instability results in changes of morphology of emulsion that might occur both during processing and during storage. During storage the morphology can change because of: (1) change of drop size caused by coalescence or Ostwald ripening, (2) change of spatial distribution of dispersed phase caused by flocculation and by gravitational separation of dispersed phase and (3) some of these phenomena occurring simultaneously. These changes of morphology can be related to surface and hydrodynamic forces, therefore relatively universal models, discussed next, can be used to predict developments of such instabilities. Morphology also changes during processing and typically drop size is reduced in a controlled manner until it meets product specification. However, under certain processing conditions an emulsion becomes unstable and a catastrophic change of morphology occurs, with the dispersed phase becoming continuous and the continuous phase becoming dispersed e.g., phase inversion occurs (Pacek *et al.*, 1994a). This type of instability is highly undesirable, except in a few cases where it is used to produce an emulsion (Fernandez *et al.*, 2004) and it is also briefly discussed in this section.

9.3.1 Surface Forces

Surface forces strongly affect flocculation and coalescence, and determine size, shape, porosity and strength of flocs as well as the stability of dispersed systems in general. They are discussed in depth by Israelachvili (1994), therefore only basic concepts within engineering approximations are briefly summarized next.

9.3.1.1 van der Waals Forces

van der Waals interactions between two dispersed entities are practically always attractive and depend on the material of dispersed and continuous phases, distance between dispersed entities and their shape. For two identical drops of radius r, interaction energy can be calculated from:

$$W^{vdW}(h) = -\frac{r\,Ha}{12h} \tag{9.28}$$

The Hamaker constant (Ha) for many systems, as well as the methods allowing its calculation, can be found in the literature, and for organic drops suspended in water it is of the order of $10^{-20}[J]$ (Israelachvili, 1994).

9.3.1.2 Electrostatic Interactions

The surface of drops suspended in liquid of high dielectric constant is practically always charged because of the dissociation of surface groups or adsorption of ions from the bulk of the continuous phase (Israelachvili, 1994). The presence of identical charge on the surface of drops leads to electrostatic repulsive forces that are one of the main forces stabilizing emulsions. In simple terms, the charge on drops surface in the presence of a surfactant can be seen as a result of 'directional adsorption' of the surfactant molecules. For the O/W type of emulsions, a hydrophobic group of surfactant molecule will orientate towards oil whereas the hydrophilic group will 'stick out' into the water. The charge of the interface leads to a formation of the layer of counter-ions surrounding the drops surface known as the diffuse electric double layer (Israelachvili, 1994). When two drops of the same charge approach each other, the diffuse electric double layers overlap, resulting in a strong repulsive force between drops that prevents coalescence and flocculation. Electrostatic repulsive force increases with the surface coverage by surfactant molecules and with the size of the drops (the larger the drops the stronger the repulsive interactions). It also strongly depends on the electrical properties of drop surface and ionic strength of continuous phase. At high ionic strength the range of electrostatic interactions is short and it increases as the ionic strength decreases. The extent of electrostatic interaction is determined by the Debye length (Israelachvili, 1994):

$$\kappa^{-1} = \left[\frac{e^2 \sum \rho_i z_i^2}{\varepsilon \varepsilon_0 \kappa_B T}\right]^{-0.5} \tag{9.29}$$

Distribution of repulsive energy in the space between two drops can be calculated by integrating the Poisson–Boltzmann equation with appropriate boundary conditions (Israelachvili, 1994). At a constant surface potential ψ, and for separation between drops much smaller than the drop size, the distribution of repulsive energy in the gap between drops (Quemada and Berli, 2002) can be simplified to:

$$W^{elec}(h) = 2\pi\varepsilon\psi^2 R ln\{1+\exp[-\kappa_B h]\} \quad \text{for} \quad \kappa_B h > 5 \tag{9.30a}$$

$$W^{elec}(h) = 2\pi\varepsilon\psi^2 R exp[-\kappa_B h] \quad \text{for} \quad \kappa_B h < 5 \tag{9.30b}$$

In practical situations, the Stern layer potential ψ can be replaced by measured values of the ξ potential which enables simple calculations of repulsive energy at any point between approaching drops.

9.3.1.3 Steric Interactions

Repulsive steric interactions occur in emulsions containing large molecules adsorbed at drop surfaces. With some simplification, steric interaction can be seen as a 'mechanical' barrier separating two drops by a distance corresponding to the dimensions of those molecules sticking out of drop surfaces. Steric interactions are strongly repulsive and their range increases with the thickness of the adsorbed layer of large molecules and with the drop size. The quantitative theoretical description of steric repulsive energy is still not possible but several semi-empirical expressions have been developed for certain food emulsions (McClements, 2005).

9.3.1.4 Hydrophobic Interactions

Hydrophobic interactions are strongly attractive and they occur between non-polar surfaces separated by a film of water. Their exact nature is not very well understood and the majority of the literature information is based on system specific experimental data, but in general the strength of hydrophobic interactions increases with temperature and with interfacial tension (Israelachvili, 1994). The hydrophobic forces act both at long, as well as at short, separation:

$$W^{hyd}(h) = A_1 exp\left(-h/\lambda_1\right) + A_2 exp\left(-h/\lambda_2\right) \tag{9.31}$$

where decay lengths $\lambda_1 \cong 1-3nm$ dominates at short separation and $\lambda_2 \cong 5-15nm$ dominates at large separation (Christenson and Claesson, 2001).

For separations up to 10 nm, simpler, one term exponential decay has been proposed (McClements, 2005):

$$W^{hyd}(h) = -2\pi r\sigma\varphi_H exp\left(-h/\lambda_0\right) \tag{9.32}$$

where $\sigma[mJ/m^2]$ is interfacial tension between non-polar groups and water, ϕ_H is the measure of hydrophobicity of drop surface, and $\lambda_0 \cong 1-2nm$ is the decay length. Strong hydrophobic attraction can destabilize emulsions as it leads to flocculation or even coalescence. This can be prevented by ensuring full (or multilayer) coverage of drop surface by surfactant molecules.

9.3.1.5 DLVO Model

The simultaneous effect of van der Waals attractions and electrostatic (double layer) repulsion on total interaction energy is accounted for in the DLVO model developed independently in 1942 by Derjaguin and Landau in Russia and Verwey and Overbeek in Holland (Vincent, 2005):

$$W^T(h) = W^{vdW}(h) + W^{elec}(h) = -\frac{r\,Ha}{12h} + 2\pi\varepsilon\varepsilon_0 R\psi^2 ln[1+\exp(-\kappa h)] \tag{9.33}$$

Typical distributions of all components of DLVO model as a function of distance between two surfaces are summarized in Figure 9.3.

In the emulsions where steric and hydrophobic interactions can be neglected, the DLVO model can be used to estimate the total interaction between drops as they approach each other. In the absence of surfactants the electrostatic charge on oil drops in water is weak and drops are strongly attracted by van der Waals forces that increase as the separation decreases. This strong attraction takes drops to the primary minimum where they coalesce. In practice, van der Waals attraction cannot be controlled (the Hamaker constant is a property of the system). Therefore to prevent coalescence and to stabilize emulsion drops have to be charged. The strength of electrostatic repulsion can be controlled by the type and concentration of surfactant and concentration of ions in the continuous phase. At a very high charge when the absolute value of zeta potential is larger than 40 mV (www.malvern.com) the total interaction is repulsive and emulsions are stable. The reduction of charge either by reduction of concentration of surfactant or by addition of salt leads to a reduction in repulsive energy and the total interaction energy develops two minima (primary and secondary) and one maximum (the so called energy barrier). If the total energy of two approaching drops is higher than the energy barrier, drops can reach a primary minimum where they coalesce. If the total energy

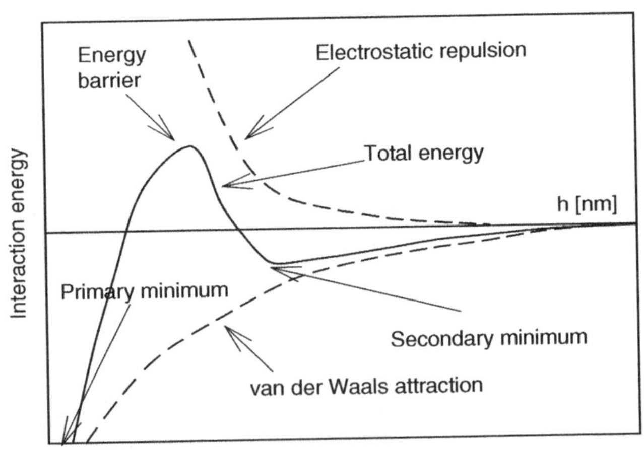

Figure 9.3 *Schematic distributions of all components of DLVO model as a function of separation distance. Reprinted with permission from* Intermolecular and Surface Forces, *Jacob N. Israelachvili, p. 253–289. Copyright (2011) Elsevier*

of approaching drops is lower than the energy barrier they stay in the secondary minimum where they form weak flocs. Those flocs can be easily broken by gentle mixing.

In principle, the classical DLVO model can be extended by including hydrophobic and/or steric interactions (Pacek *et al.*, 2007). However, understanding and quantitative description of other types of interactions is system specific; therefore the extended DLVO model has limited applicability.

9.3.2 Emulsion Stability

The detailed analysis of stability of pharmaceutical emulsions, even under quiescent conditions during storage, is difficult, because the interactions between drops in concentrated emulsions in the presence of a surfactant is rather complex. Simplified descriptions of most common instabilities such as: gravitational separation (creaming or sedimentation), flocculation, coalescence, Ostwald ripening and phase inversion are briefly discussed next.

9.3.2.1 Gravitational Separation

Gravitational separation results from the density difference between the continuous and the dispersed phase. If the density of the dispersed phase is lower than the density of the continuous phase, drops tend to move upwards and form a concentrated, closely packed layer at the top part of a container with the bottom part occupied by the continuous phase. This type of gravitational instability (Figure 9.4b) is typical for O/W emulsions and is frequently called creaming because it has been used to produce cream from fresh milk. If the density of dispersed phase is higher than density of the continuous phase (typically W/O emulsions), drops move towards the bottom of the container where they form a concentrated, closely packed layer of water drops with the top of container occupied by oil.

If, during separation, drops do not coalesce, the separation rate can be approximated by terminal velocity of a single drop calculated from the Stokes equation:

$$v_{St} = \frac{2gr^2\left|\rho_d - \rho_c\right|}{9\eta_c} \tag{9.34}$$

In principle, this equation is valid for a single solid particle moving through a large volume of fluid but it can also be used for drops smaller than approximately 50 μm in diluted emulsions with a non-viscous continuous phase. For larger drops moving through the viscous

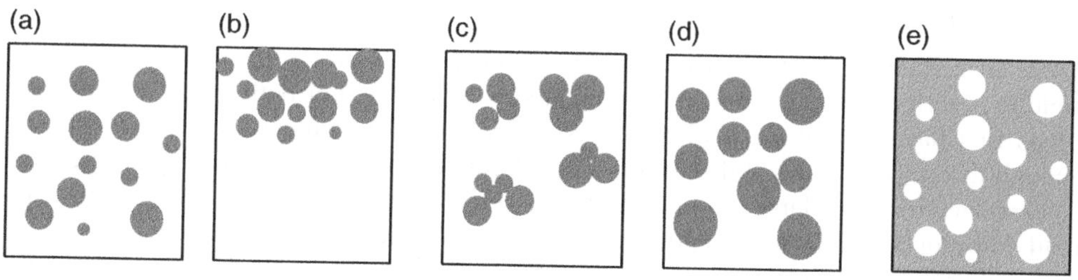

Figure 9.4 *Typical instability in emulsions: (a) stable emulsion, (b) gravitational separation/creaming, (c) flocculation, (d) Ostwald ripening or coalescence, (e) phase inversion*

continuous phase, the circulation within the drop leads to a slip on the interface and the increase of terminal velocity (Dickinson, 1992):

$$v_{St}^{l} = v_{st}\frac{3(\eta_d + \eta_c)}{3\eta_d + 2\eta_c} \tag{9.34a}$$

Description of the movement of a single drop in concentrated emulsions is more complex and semi-empirical correlations for terminal velocity are common (McClements, 2005):

$$v_{St}^{c} = v_{St}\left(1 - \frac{\phi}{\phi_m}\right)^{k\phi_m} \tag{9.35}$$

where k and ϕ_m are experimental constants with ϕ_m being close to maximum packing. The sedimentation velocity in flocculated emulsions can be estimated from the modified Stokes equation replacing radius and density of drop by radius and density of flocs (McClements, 2005). However, it is not always possible to estimate those two parameters, as well as the shape of flocs.

In pharmaceutical emulsions where drops are typically smaller than 5 μm, Brownian motion can affect separation rate and in such cases the volume fraction of dispersed phase at a certain distance y from the top of emulsion can be related to drop size, density difference and temperature (Walstra, 1996):

$$\phi(y) = \phi exp\frac{-4\pi r^3 gy\Delta\rho}{3\kappa_B T} \tag{9.36}$$

Gravitational separation can be prevented/reduced by: (1) increasing viscosity of the continuous phase, (2) reducing drop size, (3) increasing the volume fraction of dispersed phase or by a combinations of all those parameters. However, in pharmaceutical emulsions the volume fraction of the dispersed phase, viscosity of continuous phases and drop size strongly affect functional properties of emulsion based drugs, therefore it is frequently impossible to adjust them to ensure stability of emulsion. If the flocculated drops do not coalesce after forming concentrated layers the morphology of emulsion can be easily reinstated by gentle shaking or stirring.

9.3.2.2 *Flocculation/Coalescence*

There are certain similarities between those two processes (Figure 9.4c and d) and it is possible to describe flocculation as non-completed coalescence. For both processes to occur drops first have to collide. If after successful collision the attractive forces are strong enough to completely destabilize a thin film of continuous phases separating drops, they coalesce and form one large drop. If the attractive forces cannot break the film but they can hold drops together as separate entities, drops flocculate. Because coalescence is one of the two main processes occurring during formation of emulsions, collision frequency and factors affecting stability of film separating drops after collision are discussed in detail in Section 9.4.

9.3.2.3 Ostwald Ripening

Ostwald ripening occurs in the systems where drops (or at least one of their components) are partially soluble in the continuous phase. The dissolution rate of dispersed phase is proportional to Laplace pressure and solubility. Both solubility and Laplace pressure:

$$c(r) = c_{\infty} exp\left(\frac{2\sigma V_m}{RTr}\right) \tag{9.37}$$

$$\Delta P = \frac{2\sigma}{r} \tag{9.38}$$

depend on the curvature of the interface and the smaller the drops the higher the solubility and the higher the Laplace pressure (Tadros and Vincent, 1983). Therefore, the concentration of dispersed phase (or one of its components) dissolved in continuous phases surrounding small drops is higher than concentration in the continuous phase around large drops; e.g., the concentration gradient of the dispersed phase dissolved in continuous phase develops. Concentration gradient causes molecular diffusion of dispersed phases from the small drops to the large ones and a reduction of mass (size) of the small drops and an increase in mass (size) of large drops. The reduction of the volume of small drops can be estimated from simple mass balance of the component of the dispersed phase soluble in the continuous phase (Kabalnov and Shchukin, 1992):

$$v_d(t) - v(0) = \frac{\sigma V_m C_{\infty} D_{d-c}}{RT} t \tag{9.39}$$

Ostwald ripening can be reduced by reducing interfacial tension and by ensuring that phases forming emulsions are either completely insoluble in each other or that the solubility is minimal.

9.3.2.4 Phase Inversion

In manufacturing of emulsion based drugs, the first question that has to be answered is whether oil dispersed in water (O/W emulsion) or water dispersed in oil (W/O emulsion) should be used with a given formulation. The type (morphology) of emulsion mainly depends on the application and it has very strong effect on the functional properties of the final product. For instance, in the majority of parenteral fat emulsions, the oil phase is practically always dispersed (O/W emulsions) whereas emulsions for ophthalmic use can be either W/O or W/O (Nielloud and Marti-Mestres, 2000). Morphology of emulsions depends on the volumetric composition, properties of surfactant and processing conditions. Oil soluble surfactants with an HLB <9 are used to produce and stabilize W/O emulsions whereas water soluble surfactants with an HLB >10 are used for O/W emulsions (Schramm, 1992).

The morphology of surfactant free liquid/liquid systems, important during the preparation of coarse emulsion, strongly depends on the volumetric composition, physical/surface properties of liquids and hydrodynamic conditions. For such systems processed in stirred vessels there are two rules of thumb: (1) if volume fraction of either liquid is below 30% v/v, this liquid will be dispersed, and (2) if an agitator is started in a liquid it tends to be continuous. For liquid/liquid mixtures in pipe flow maps, relating morphology to Re number, volumetric composition and physical/interfacial properties of both liquids are available (Brauner and Ullmann, 2002).

In all emulsion based products, and in a great majority of manufacturing processes, it is essential that morphology does not change unexpectedly, that is phase inversion does not occur. The term phase inversion is used to describe rapid change of morphology of a liquid/liquid system when the dispersed phase becomes continuous and the continuous phase becomes dispersed. It occurs in emulsions stabilized by surfactants (Brooks *et al.*, 1998; Song *et al.*, 2009) and in surfactant free systems both during processing of liquid/liquid systems in a stirred vessels (Pacek and Nienow, 1995) and two phase flows in pipes or in static mixers (Piela *et al.*, 2008).

In surfactant free liquid/liquid systems phase inversion occurs when the volume fraction of the dispersed phase is higher than a certain critical value that depends on type of liquid, type of processing equipment and intensity of hydrodynamic conditions (Pacek *et al.*, 1994a,b). This critical volume fraction varies between 0.5 and 0.9, however, O/W systems invert at a much higher volume fraction of the dispersed phase than W/O systems formed from the same liquids. In other words, in the absence of a surfactant, O/W emulsions are more stable than W/O ones (Pacek and Nienow, 1995). Phase inversion in surfactant free systems has a catastrophic nature, the transition from O/W to W/O is completed within a few seconds but it might be proceeded by a time delay during which a gradual change of morphology occurs, including formation of droplets-in-drop structures (Pacek *et al.*, 1994a,b).

In emulsions stabilized by surfactants, phase inversion might occur when the volume fraction of dispersed phases exceeds a certain critical value or when the temperature of emulsion is changed in such a way that it passes through the so called phase inversion temperature, PIT (Shinoda and Kunidea, 1983). In the first case, phase inversion is catastrophic (Jahanzad *et al.*, 2009) whereas, in the second case it is transitional (Sajjadi, 2006). The temperature induced phase inversion can be explained by the change in solubility of the non-ionic surfactant from oil soluble at temperatures below PIT to the aqueous phase soluble at temperatures above PIT. Therefore, at temperatures lower than PIT O/A emulsions are formed and at temperatures higher than PIT A/O emulsions are formed. At PIT, interfacial tension reaches a minimum that leads to very small, unstable drops that have to be stabilized by fast cooling (Tadros and Vincent, 1983).

Despite extensive research, the exact mechanism of catastrophic phase inversion is still not understood. It has been postulated that, as the volume fraction of the dispersed phase increases, droplets of the continuous phase appear inside the drops of the dispersed phase (droplets-in-drops phenomena) that leads to a reduction of volume fraction of the continuous phase, reduction in the thickness of the film separating closely packed drops and catastrophic coalescence (Pacek *et al.*, 1994a,b, Pacek and Nienow, 1995, Jahanzad *at al.*, 2009). Attempts have been made to develop quantitative models enabling prediction of phase inversion both within the framework of the population balance model (Hua *et al.*, 2006) and by minimizing free energy of dispersion (Brauner and Ullmann, 2002). However, because of the complexity of the interactions between drops in concentrated dispersions/emulsions and a lack of understanding of all factors governing stability of the continuous phase, those theoretical models have limited accuracy and applicability.

Whilst most of the investigations of phase inversion are system specific, there are two findings that the majority of researchers agree on; (1) catastrophic phase inversion is associated with large pressure fluctuations in pipe flows or fluctuations of torque in stirred vessels and (2) drops after phase inversion are smaller and have a narrower size distribution than before phase inversions. The first phenomenon has an adverse effect on processing of emulsions and should be avoided either by careful control of the temperature of the emulsion and/or volume fraction of dispersed phase. The second phenomenon has been exploited in several manufacturing processes. In food processing, phase inversion has been used in margarine manufacturing for many years (Dickinson, 1992) and recently, PIT based methods are frequently used to manufacture micro- and nano-emulsions (Fernandez *et al.*, 2004, Sajjadi, 2006; Jahanzad *et al.*, 2009). Temperature induced phase inversion seems to be particularly attractive in manufacturing pharmaceutical emulsions (Anton and Vandamme, 2009) where the maximum drops size should not exceed 5 μm. However, as phase inversion changes morphology of the systems, it might also affect the kinetics of the drug released (Ma and McHugh, 2007); therefore, more work aimed at tailoring the PIT method to manufacturing pharmaceutical emulsions is needed.

9.4 Principles of Emulsion Formation

One of the most important properties of the majority of pharmaceutical emulsions, especially those administered intravenously, is a drop size that should not exceed a few microns (Nielloud and Marti-Mestres, 2000). Drops larger than 5–7 μm are mechanically trapped in the capillary of the lung, drops in the range 0.1–0.3 μm are taken up by reticuloendothelial system and only drops below 0.1 μm will circulate in the blood through the body (Okochi and Nakano, 2000). Preparation of emulsions with such small drops and relatively narrow drop size distribution is a multistage process involving: (1) preparation of an aqueous and oil phase by dissolving surfactants, glycerol, vitamins, drugs and so on, (2) preparation of a coarse dispersion with drops in the order of tens of microns by mixing and sterilizing both phases in a stirred vessel at elevated temperature, (3) final emulsification to produce emulsion with drops between 1–5 μm and (4) filtration to remove all drops larger than 5 μm, adjustment of pH, pasteurization and packing (Cuéllar *et al.*, 2005).

In the first stage, distribution of active components (chemical/biochemical) between aqueous and organic phases and the limits of processing conditions such as temperature and pH have to be determined. Also the type and concentration of surfactant that can be used with the given chemistry to form the required morphology, and that complies with regulations (Nielloud and Marti-Mestres, 2000) can be selected. This stage is drug and application specific and requires an interdisciplinary approach; therefore, it is not discussed in this chapter.

Both coarse and fine emulsions are non-equilibrium systems and an energy input is necessary to form emulsions. The formation of drops increases the interfacial area between the liquids by ΔA, therefore, the interfacial energy increases by $\Delta A \cdot \sigma$. It is well known that the amount of energy necessary to form emulsion is an order of magnitude higher than the increase of surface energy and that there is no correlation between the increase of surface energy and the energy input necessary for emulsification. On the other hand, it is also well known that the smaller the drops, the higher the energy input required to produce an emulsion. According to energy demand, one can distinguish between low and high energy emulsification.

9.4.1 Low Energy Emulsification

Recently, low energy emulsification methods have been proposed for the manufacturing of nano-emulsions (Gutierrez *et al.*, 2008, Anton and Vandamme, 2009, Solans *et al.*, 2005), however, considering that in many pharmaceutical emulsions drops are smaller than 1 μm, similar methods can be employed in manufacturing of pharmaceutical emulsions (Sadurni *et al.*, 2005). In those methods based on phase transitions, physicochemical properties of liquid-liquid-surfactant systems are exploited to produce emulsions with sub-micron drops from coarse emulsions at a very low input of mechanical energy. The phase transition in the liquid-liquid-surfactant system is frequently induced by change in temperature, the so called PIT method (Shinoda and Kunidea, 1983). In the PIT method, the aqueous phase, organic phase and non-ionic surfactant are mixed at the room temperature forming an O/W emulsion with the surfactant dissolved in the aqueous phase. When this emulsion is heated the solubility of surfactant in the organic phase increases. At the PIT the surfactant becomes fully soluble in organic phase and the system inverts from the O/W type to a W/O emulsion. Also interfacial tension is very low, 10^{-2} to 10^{-5} mN/m (Solans *et al.*, 2005) that, on the one hand leads to very small drops and makes emulsification easier, but, on the other hand increases coalescence rate leading to the separation of the emulsion into two layers of liquids. This can be prevented by rapid reduction of the temperature of emulsion just after phase inversion.

An alternative method of low energy emulsification involves inducing phase inversion by increasing the volume fraction of the aqueous phase. In this method the aqueous phase is added to the oil/surfactant whilst stirring at constant temperature. At a volume fraction of the aqueous phases of the order of 90% the system inverts from oil continuous to aqueous continuous with oil drops in the range of 10–40 nm depending on the oil/surfactant ratio (Sadurni *et al.*, 2005).

Spontaneous emulsification is an extremely low energy process. A good example of spontaneous emulsification is the well-known *ouzo effect*. After addition of water, the traditional Greek spirit (ouzo) turns from a completely transparent, colourless liquid into a milky, two phase emulsion with drops of aniseed oil suspended in the mixture of alcohol and water. In this case, addition of water to the transparent solution of alcohol water and anise oil leads to supersaturation and homogeneous nucleation (Vitale and Katz, 2003). Presence of bi-layer structures in close proximity to the water-oil interface is the prerequisite to spontaneous emulsification and there is a connection between equilibrium interfacial tension and dynamics of spontaneous emulsification (Shahidzadeh *et al.*, 2000). During spontaneous emulsification, fluctuation of interfacial tension leads to development of dispersed structure at oil/aqueous interface that, with time, spreads into a whole volume of fluid (Wojciechowski and Kucharek, 2009). Lab scale experimental results indicate that low energy methods can produce stable emulsions with narrow drop size distributions and, depending on the method, drops are in the range of tens of nanometres (phase inversion methods) to a few microns (spontaneous emulsification). The major problems with low energy emulsification methods are: the great majority of the published results were obtained on the laboratory scale, results are system/equipment specific and it is difficult to predict mean drop size. All these factors make the implementation of a low energy method on an industrial scale rather difficult. Therefore, considering that the cost of energy necessary for emulsification in developing/manufacturing emulsion based products is typically not a major factor, whereas reproducibility and robustness of the process are the key factors, high energy, mechanical/ultrasound emulsification methods are still common in industry.

9.4.2 High Energy Emulsification

Course dispersions are typically formed in stirred vessels and in general their formation is a two-step process. First, at the commencement of agitation, flat interface separating layers of aqueous and organic phase becomes unstable because of velocity/density differences across the interface, and jets or very large drops are formed. Next, those large drops/jets are broken down into smaller drops of a certain size distribution that depends on the type and intensity of flow and on the physical/interfacial properties of both phases. In engineering applications the first step is ignored and only the mean size of drops formed in the second step is considered. Currently, there are no models allowing theoretical prediction of drop size distributions, instead simple mechanistic models relating maximum stable drop size to the hydrodynamic conditions and physical/interfacial properties of both phases are used.

Mean drop size can be estimated considering the cohesive (τ_c) and disruptive (τ_d) stress acting on the drop in a highly diluted suspension where the collisions with other drops (and stresses resulting from them) are negligible. In general, cohesive stress depends on interfacial tension (σ), viscosity of dispersed phase (η_d) and radius of the drop (r) and for non-viscous dispersed phase it is frequently approximated by:

$$\tau_c \approx \frac{\sigma}{r} \tag{9.40}$$

Disruptive stress depends on the viscosity of the continuous phase (η_c), radius of drop (r), type of flow (laminar or turbulent) and its intensity described by shear rate ($\dot{\gamma}$), in laminar flow and specific energy dissipation rate ($\dot{\gamma}$) in turbulent flow. The drop is stable if $\tau_d < \tau_c$ but becomes unstable and breaks if:

$$\tau_d \geq \tau_c. \tag{9.41}$$

The ratio of disruptive to cohesive stress τ_d/τ_c is frequently called the capillary number (Ca) if the flow is laminar, and the Weber number (We) if the flow is turbulent, and it is commonly used to relate drop size to hydrodynamic conditions and physical properties of the dispersed and continuous phases. At low capillary numbers cohesive stress dominates therefore, the drop might deform but does not break. When disruptive stress dominates at certain critical values of the capillary number (Ca_{cr}), the drop becomes unstable and breaks. From definition, the critical capillary number should be in the order of 1 and in fact, for laminar elongational flow (see Figure 9.5) as well as for fully developed turbulent flow,

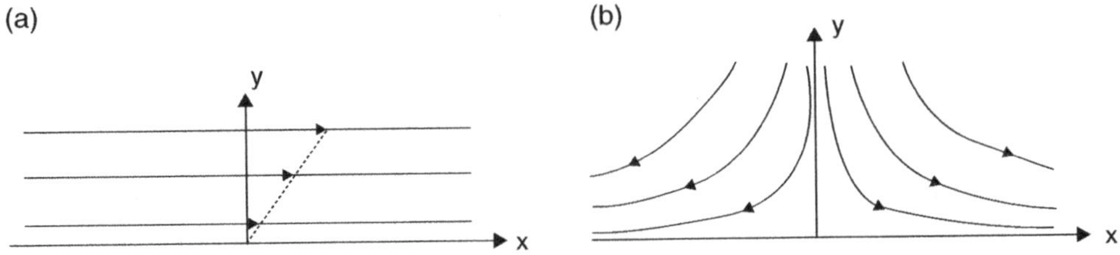

Figure 9.5 *Types of laminar flow: (a) simple shear flow, (b) hyperbolic flow*

it is close to 1. However, for simple shear flow as well as for extensional flow, this is not the case. This discrepancy can be explained by the complexity of deformation processes of the drops and different mechanisms of breakage (Stone, 1994).

9.4.2.1 Maximum Stable Drop Size in Laminar Flow

In the first approximation, laminar flow can be defined as a flow where fluid flows in separated layers and where there is no flow in the direction perpendicular to those layers. Two model flows are relevant in processing equipment: simple shear flow (streamlines are straight) and hyperbolic flow (streamlines are hyperbolas), which are shown in Figure 9.5.

Simple shear flow occurs in the fluid contained between two concentric cylinders separated by a narrow gap and either rotating in opposite directions or one rotating and one stationary. This type of flow might approximate flow in colloidal mills. Hyperbolic flow occurs when a jet of liquid hits the surface and it is an approximation of the flow in certain types of high pressure homogenizers. In both types of flows, drops are deformed and eventually broken by shear stress resulting from velocity gradient across the drop.

$$\tau_d = \mu_c \frac{dv_z}{dy} = \mu_c \dot{\gamma} \tag{9.42}$$

The capillary number at which breakage occurs defines the maximum stable drop size and is called the critical capillary number:

$$Ca_{cr} = \frac{\dot{\gamma}\, \mu_c d_{max}}{\sigma} \tag{9.43}$$

The critical capillary number in laminar flow depends on the type of flow and the viscosity ratio $\lambda = \frac{\mu_d}{\mu_c}$ and it can be determined from stability curves (frequently called Grace's curves) shown in Figure 9.6. The two top curves were first reported by Grace (1971) and since then they have been commonly used to calculate maximum stable drop size in laminar flows.

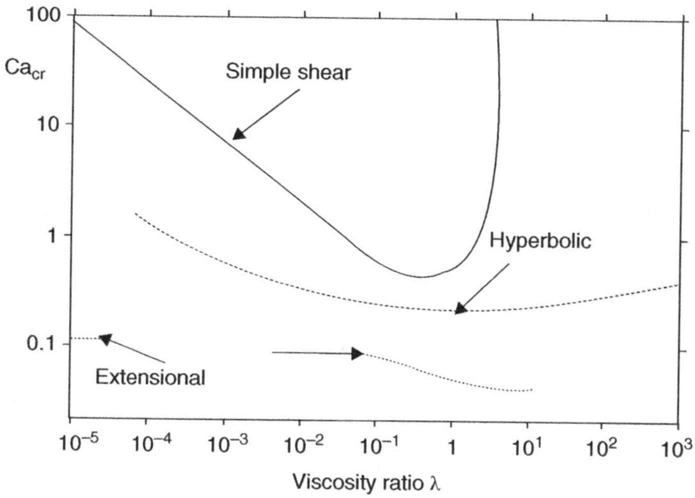

Figure 9.6 *Critical capillary number for different types of laminar flows*

If the viscosity ratio and interfacial tension are known the above curves can be used to find the maximum stable drop size at a given shear rate or to determine whether at a given shear rate existing are stable. If the value of the capillary number is larger than the critical capillary number for a given type of flow (a point with coordinates $\lambda = \frac{\mu_d}{\mu_c}$, Ca is above an appropriate curve), the drop will break and if it is lower, the drop is stable.

Elongational and hyperbolic flows are more efficient in terms of breakage than the simple shear flow. In hyperbolic flows, Ca_{cr} is very weakly dependent on the viscosity ratio and is of the order of 1 throughout a very wide range of viscosity ratios. In the simple shear flow the critical capillary number strongly depends on the viscosity ratio. At a high viscosity ratio (above 4), even at a very high shear rate the drop will not be broken but it will rotate; for example, such type of flow is unsuitable for processing emulsions with a very viscous dispersed phase.

An alternative way of assessing whether the drop in a laminar flow is stable or not is to calculate the deformation parameter at a given capillary number:

$$D = \frac{5(19\lambda + 16)}{4(1+\lambda)\left[(19\lambda)^2 + \left(\frac{20}{Ca}\right)^2\right]^2} \tag{9.44}$$

If the deformation parameter is in the order of 0.5, the drop becomes unstable and breaks.

9.4.2.2 *Maximum Stable Drop Size in Turbulent Flow*

Turbulent flows can be characterized by chaotic, random changes of fluid velocity both in space and time. Analysis of velocity distribution in turbulent flows is very complex and discussion of different methods used to describe turbulent flows can be found elsewhere

(Baldyga and Bourne, 1999). Turbulent flows in emulsification devices are commonly described in terms of energy dissipation (scalar) rather in terms of local velocity (vector) by the well-known Kolmogorov's model. In brief, this model assumes that homogeneous turbulence can be described as an energy cascade and that it can be modelled as a population of differently 'sized' eddies ('size' of eddy is a measure of the energy it contains) undergoing continuous breakage associated with energy transfer from the largest (energy containing) eddies that break into smaller ones without losing energy. The smallest eddies corresponding to Kolmogorov's length scale cannot be broken down any further and at that scale mechanical energy is dissipated into heat. As during the emulsification the amount of energy transferred from dispersed to continuous phase determines the maximum stable drop size, this model is well suited to describe dispersion processes and has been commonly used since 1955 (Hinze, 1955). It is sufficient to quantify the disruptive stress exerted by continuous phase on the drops of dispersed phase (Hinze, 1955); however, the underlying assumptions of this model, such as homogeneous and isotropic turbulent flow, are often far from flow conditions existing in the majority of emulsifying devices.

Within this model, stress acting on drops depends on the size of the drop relative to the 'size' of eddies and to Kolmogorov's length scale:

- drops larger than Kolmogorov's length are 'bombarded by the eddies' of sizes similar to the drop size that results in a normal disruptive stress acting on the drop,
- drops smaller than Kolmogorov's length scale are immersed in the smallest eddies and they are exposed to disruptive shear stresses resulting from the flow existing within the eddies.

Based on this description of turbulence, Hinze (1955) developed an expression relating maximum stable drop size to local energy dissipation. Drops larger than Kolmogorov's scale are exposed to a disruptive normal stress:

$$\tau_d \approx \rho_c (\varepsilon d)^{2/3} \tag{9.45}$$

Inserting this equation and equation 9.40 into the general definition of maximum stable drop size (equation 9.41):

$$\frac{\sigma}{d_{max}} = C_1 \rho_c \left(\varepsilon d_{max}\right)^{2/3} \tag{9.46}$$

the expression for a maximum stable drop size in a turbulent flow takes the form:

$$d_{max} = C_2 \sigma^{0.6} \varepsilon^{-0.4} \rho_c^{-0.6} \tag{9.47}$$

where the experimental constant $C_2 \approx 0.725$ (Hinze, 1955).

Drops smaller than Kolmogorov's scale are exposed to shear flow inside the smallest eddies. The shear stress inside those eddies can also be related to the energy dissipation rate (Baldyga and Bourne 1999):

$$\dot{\gamma} = C_3 \left(\frac{\varepsilon}{\nu_c} \right)^{0.5} \tag{9.48}$$

and the maximum stable drop size can be calculated from:

$$Ca_{cr} = \frac{d_{max} \mu_c \dot{\gamma}}{\sigma} = f(\lambda) \tag{9.49}$$

The last expression is similar to the expression for the maximum stable drop size in a laminar flow, but instead of Grace's curves the analytical expression for Ca_{cr} as a function of viscosity ratio has been suggested (Shinnar, 1961):

$$f(\lambda) = 16 \frac{(\lambda + 1)}{19\lambda + 16} \tag{9.50}$$

In summary, the maximum stable drop size in a laminar flow is related to the shear stress that can be estimated if the local shear rate (velocity gradient $\dot{\gamma}$) and geometry of the flow are known, whereas maximum stable drop size in turbulent flow can be estimated if the local energy dissipation rate (ϵ) is known. In processing equipment, the spatial distributions of both shear rate in a laminar flow and energy dissipation in a turbulent flow are not known, therefore an average shear rate or energy dissipation rate calculated from semi-empirical correlations developed for different types of equipment are used to calculate the maximum stable drop size. In a laminar flow in stirred vessel the average shear rate is proportional to impeller speed with the proportionality constant depending on the type of impeller from (Nienow, 1997):

$$\dot{\gamma} = KN \tag{9.51}$$

The average energy dissipation rate in a turbulent flow in a stirred vessel is calculated from

$$\varepsilon = \frac{P}{\rho V} \tag{9.52}$$

where the total power input P depends on impeller type, diameter and speed:

$$P = Po \rho N^3 D^5 \tag{9.53}$$

and Po, the so-called power number, is a proportionality coefficient that depends on the type of impeller and Re number (Nienow, 1997). In flow-through emulsification devices such as static mixers and valve homogenizers, average energy dissipation rate ε can be calculated from the pressure drop (Pacek *et al.*, 1999b):

$$\varepsilon = 2f \frac{v_0^3}{D_0} = \frac{u_c \Delta P}{l_m \rho_c} \tag{9.54}$$

Correlations for mean drop size in different emulsifying devices are discussed in Section 9.4.

9.4.2.3 Kinetics of Breakage

The above considerations allowed an estimation of the maximum stable drop size but did not reveal the mechanisms of drop breakage. Whilst under steady state conditions mean drop size is frequently sufficient to describe the emulsion the analysis of transients requires a more detailed description of the breakage process. There has been extensive research into breakage in liquid/liquid systems and different models available in the literature have been compared recently (Liao and Lucas, 2009). Most of the models postulate that breakage occurs when the turbulent energy transferred from continuous phase to drops exceeds a certain critical value. It is frequently assumed that a drop breaks when the kinetic energy it acquires from the continuous phase is larger than its surface energy and breakup frequency is related to energy dissipation rate, surface tension and drop size (Tavlarides and Stamatoudis 1981):

$$\theta(d_i) \approx d_i^{-2/3}\,\varepsilon^{1/3}\exp\left[-\frac{\sigma}{\rho_d \varepsilon^{2/3} d_i^{5/3}}\right] \tag{9.55}$$

To close the description of breakage kinetics it is necessary to define the number of fragments the drop is broken into (so called daughter drops) and their size distributions. It is frequently assumed that a drop breaks into two daughter drops and their sizes are described by Gaussian distribution. Models of the kinetics of breakage are used within the population balance equation discussed later in this section.

9.4.2.4 Kinetics of Coalescence

Coalescence in dispersions/emulsions might occur both during formulation/processing and during storage. During processing coalescence and breakage occur simultaneously and drops size distributions, as well as average drop size, result from the dynamic equilibrium between those two processes. During storage of emulsion based products coalescence is one of the major mechanisms destabilizing emulsion (McClements, 2005). Understanding the effect of hydrodynamics conditions and physical/interfacial properties of both phases on coalescence rate enables better design of processing equipment as well as the selection of the optimal methods preventing coalescence. The complexity of coalescence phenomena does not allow fully theoretical prediction of coalescence rate but there are several mechanistic models relating collision frequency and coalescence efficiency to physical/interfacial properties of both phases and the type/intensity of the flow (Tavlarides and Stamatoudis, 1981, Chesters, 1991, Man, 1998, McClements, 2005,). Those models can be used to predict the evolution of drop size distribution due to coalescence but, practically all models are semi-theoretical and they require experimental data to close them.

The majority of the models assume that coalescence is a second order process (e.g. only coalescence between two drops is possible) and that coalescence rate $\omega(d_1, d_2)$ is proportional to the product of the number of coalescing drops $n_1 n_2$ and two proportionality coefficients: one describing coalescence efficiency $\vartheta(d_1, d_2)$ and the second describing collision frequency $\beta(d_1, d_2)$:

$$\omega(d_1,d_2) = \vartheta(d_1,d_2)\beta(d_1,d_2)n_1n_2 \tag{9.56}$$

In stagnant emulsions, collisions between drops can be induced by Brownian motion or by gravity forces. Drops smaller then 1–3 μm move randomly due to the Brownian motion and gravity forces are frequently negligible and the coefficient describing collision efficiency is independent of the drop size (McClements, 2005):

$$\beta_{Br} = \frac{8}{3}\frac{\kappa T}{\eta_c} \tag{9.57}$$

Collision due to gravity forces results from the difference of terminal velocities of drops of different sizes and in such cases the coefficient describing collision frequency depends on the density difference, viscosity of the continuous phase and drop size (Lyklema, 2005, Dukhin *et al.*, 2007):

$$\beta(d_1,d_2) = \frac{2g\pi\Delta\rho}{9\eta_c}\left(\frac{d_1}{2}+\frac{d_2}{2}\right)^3 \tag{9.58}$$

In laminar shear flow, the coefficient describing collision frequency depends on the shear rate and drop size (Chesters, 1991):

$$\beta(d_1,d_2) = \frac{1}{6}\dot{\gamma}(d_1+d_2)^3 \tag{9.59}$$

In turbulent flows the collision mechanism strongly depends on the size of the drops relative to Kolmogorov's length scale ranging from tens microns in stirred vessels down to a few microns in a more energy intensive processing equipment. Drops smaller than Kolmogorov's length scale are exposed to a shear flow and the collision efficiency can be estimated from equation 9.61 with the shear rate expressed in terms of the energy dissipation rate (Tavlarides and Stamatoudis, 1981):

$$\beta(d_1,d_2) = \left(\frac{\pi}{15}\right)^{0.5}\left(\frac{\varepsilon}{\nu}\right)^{0.5}(d_1+d_2)^3 \tag{9.60}$$

Collisions between very small drops can be also affected by Brownian motion and turbulent shear (Saffman and Turner, 1956):

$$\beta(d_1,d_2) = \frac{1}{3}\frac{\kappa T}{\mu_c r}(d_1+d_2) + \left(\frac{\pi}{15}\right)^{0.5}\left(\frac{\varepsilon}{\nu}\right)^{0.5}(d_1+d_2)^3 \tag{9.61}$$

Drops larger than Kolmogorov's scale are interacting with randomly moving eddies; therefore it is commonly assumed that they also move randomly. By analogy to the kinetic theory of gases, collision frequency between drops in a turbulent flow depends on relative velocities and can be related to the energy dissipation rate (Tavlarides and Stamatoudis, 1981):

$$\beta(d_1,d_2)=\frac{\pi}{2}(d_1^2+d_2^2)\left(d_1^{2/3}+d_2^{2/3}\right)^{1/2}\varepsilon^{1/3} \tag{9.62}$$

After drops collide they stay in close proximity for a certain period of time, the so called contact time (t_c). For drops to coalescence this time must be longer than the time necessary for two drops to merge into one, so called coalescence time (t_{col}) and coalescence efficiency can be defined as (Tavlarides and Stamatoudis, 1981):

$$\vartheta(d_1,d_2)=exp\left(-\frac{t_col}{t_c}\right) \tag{9.63}$$

Contact time depends on the drop size and the intensity of the flow of continuous phase. It can be related to an average shear rate in a laminar flow (Chesters, 1991) or the energy dissipation rate in turbulent flow (Tavlarides and Stamatoudis, 1981):

$$t_c \approx \frac{(d_1+d_2)^{2/3}}{\varepsilon^{1/3}} \tag{9.64}$$

Coalescence time in surfactant free systems is equal to the time necessary for the film separating two drops to drain to a critical thickness at which drops coalesces instantaneously. It depends on the force squeezing the drops together, conditions on the film/drop interface and on whether drops deform on impact. Typically, in surfactant free oil/water systems drops smaller than approximately 50 μm can be treated as rigid drops (non-deformable), whereas in the presence of surfactant even drops of 10 μm diameter can be considerably deformed (McClements, 2005).

Film drainage time for deformable drops is proportional to the force compressing the drops and to the drop size (Tavlarides and Stamatoudis, 1981)

$$t_{dr}(d_1,d_2)\approx\frac{\mu F}{\sigma^2}\left[\frac{d_1d_2}{(d_1+d_2)}\right]^2 f(h,h_{cr}) \tag{9.65}$$

The force in equation 9.65 is typically of a hydrodynamic nature and it can be related to energy dissipation rate in a turbulent flow and shear rate in laminar flow. The function $f(h,h_{cr})$ depends on properties of the interface (or in other words on the boundary conditions for film drainage) and it has different form for mobile, semi-mobile and immobile interface as shown in Figure 9.7 (Man, 1998).

For each of these cases, different expression for coalescence efficiency can be obtained (Man, 1998) and, for example, for fully mobile interface the coalescence efficiency can be calculated from:

$$\vartheta(d_1,d_2)=exp\left(-\frac{C\rho_c d^{5/3}\varepsilon^{2/3}}{\sigma}\right) \tag{9.66}$$

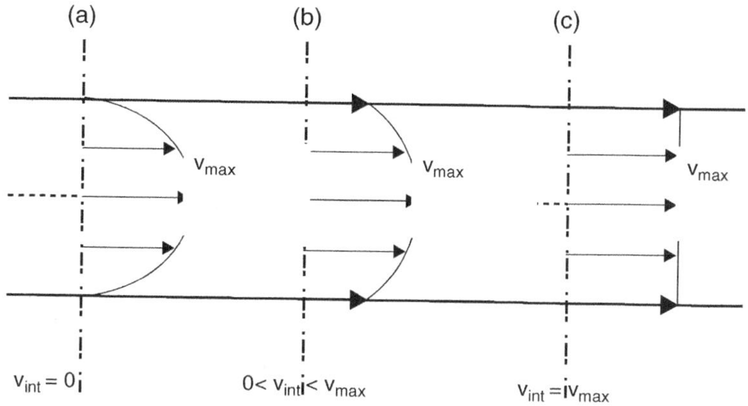

Figure 9.7 *Different types of interfaces between two deformed drops and thin film separating them: (a) immobile interface, non-slip boundary condition; (b) semi mobile interface, partial slip boundary condition; (c) fully mobile interface, full slip boundary condition*

The film drainage is also affected by the viscosity of both phases and as the viscosity of the dispersed phase increases, the interfacial mobility is reduced and coalescence time increases (Jeelani and Windhab, 2009). It is commonly assumed that, in surfactant free systems, when the thickness of the film reaches a certain critical value, h_c, the film ruptures instantaneously and the drops coalesce. This critical thickness depends on the Hamaker constant, interfacial tension and for two drops of the same size can be calculated from (Chesters, 1991):

$$h_c \approx \left(\frac{Had}{24\pi\sigma}\right)^{1/3} \tag{9.67}$$

The last equation implies that for the same oil/aqueous system the critical thickness of the oil film separated aqueous drops is the same as the critical thickness of the aqueous film separating oil drops, which implies that at the same hydrodynamic conditions stability and coalescence rate in aqueous/oil dispersions are the same as in oil/aqueous dispersions. Experimental evidence, however, clearly indicates that, without surfactants, oil in water dispersions are much more stable than water in oil dispersions and that the coalescence rate in the former is typically much lower (Pacek and Nienow, 1995). Those differences can be explained by enhanced stability of oil drops arising from the presence of electrostatic charge on the surface of oil drops suspended in water and affecting the critical thickness of the film (Pacek *et al.*, 1997):

$$h_c \approx \left(\frac{Hd}{24\pi\sigma}\right)^{1/3}\left(1-\frac{6\pi\Phi_0 h_c^3 exp(-\kappa h_c)}{H}\right)^{1/3} \tag{9.68}$$

In the absence of the electrostatic charge, the second term in the bracket becomes zero and the last equation simplifies to the form suggested by Chesters (1991).

Analysis of the stability of a thin film separating two drops suggests that, in the presence of a surfactant, film rupture does not occur instantaneously but results from the instability of the film surface developing over a certain period of time. The amplitude of capillary waves on the film surface caused by thermal fluctuations grows with time, and when amplitude is of the order of half of film thickness, holes in the film are formed and drops merge (Kabalnov, 1998).

The coalescence models discussed here were developed for two phase liquid-liquid systems exposed to intensive hydrodynamic conditions; therefore, they stress the effect of hydrodynamic on interactions between two drops and between drops and continuous phase. They have been used to predict the evolution of drop size distribution during processing within the concept of the population balance model, discussed in the next section. An alternative approach to coalescence in the emulsions where the movement of the drops is not very intensive, for example, movement of drops in a stagnant emulsion, has been discussed by McClements (2005). In such cases the coalescence efficiency can be related to the total interaction energy between drops as described by DLVO (see Section 9.3.1.5). If the energy barrier is low and short range repulsive forces are negligible, drops tend to coalesce immediately after collision and coalescence rate is controlled by the collision frequency. For drops staying together in the secondary minimum, coalescence is controlled by the time necessary for the transfer to the primary minimum and, once in the primary minimum, drops will coalesce after a certain period of time. In the latter case the film rupture discussed previously is a rate limiting step (McClements, 2005).

9.4.2.5 Population Balance Model

The population balance model (also known as the drops number continuity equation) has been frequently used to predict evolution of drop/particles size distributions in processes where breakage and coalescence occur simultaneously. The continuous form of population balance is a rather complex integro-differential equation discussed in depth by Ramakrishna (2000) and, in general, it can only be solved numerically. Different methods used to solve the population balance equation in batch systems were discussed by Rigopoulos and Jones (2003). In continuous flow systems, solution of the population balance model is even more complex because it has to be solved simultaneously with momentum balances for continuous and dispersed phases. Recently, transient drop size distribution in liquid-liquid dispersion during the flow through the static mixers has been predicted and found to be in good agreement with experimental results (Pianko-Oprych and Jaworski, 2009).

In perfectly mixed batch systems, where all spatial gradients are equal to zero, drops can only break or coalesce and population balance can be simplified to the set of ordinary differential equations:

$$\frac{dn_i}{dt} = c_i - b_i \tag{9.69}$$

Number of drops in class '*i*' (n_i) can increase as a result of coalescence of smaller drops and/or breakage of larger drops (often describe as a 'birth' in the literature) and it can also be reduced because drops from that class are broken into a smaller drops or they also coalesce forming larger drops (often described as 'death' in the literature). Coalescence between two drops is modelled as the product of the number of coalescing drops and coalescence efficiency (second order process):

$$c_i = \frac{1}{2}\sum_{j=1}^{i=1} k^c(i, j-1)n_i n_{j-1} - \sum_{j=1}^{N} k^c(i,j)n_i n_j \tag{9.70}$$

and breakage is modelled as the first order process that depends on the number of drops undergoing breakage and breakage efficiency:

$$b_i = -k^b(i)n_i + \sum_{j=i+1}^{N} k^b(j)n_j \tag{9.71}$$

Coefficients k^b *and* k^c are frequently called breakage and coalescence kernels, respectively, and they can be related to the coalescence and breakage models:

$$k^c = \beta(i,j)\vartheta(i,j) \tag{9.72}$$

$$k^b = \theta(i)\nu(i)g(i,j) \tag{9.73}$$

where $\nu(i,j)$ is the number of daughter drops formed during breakage of drop i and $g(i,j)$ is the daughter drop size distribution.

Equations 9.69–9.71 can be integrated directly starting from drop size distributions at the beginning of the process (initial condition) and drop size as a function of time, processing conditions and physical/interfacial properties of both phases can be predicted. In this case it is necessary to know how to relate (in a closed form) breakage and coalescence kernels (Equations 9.72 and 9.73) to processing conditions and physical/interfacial properties of emulsion.

Alternatively, population balance can also be used to calculate coalescence and breakage kernels by solving the so called inverted population balance with the help of experimental transient drop size distributions. In this case two approaches are possible: (1) black box approach and (2) application of phenomenological models of breakage and coalescence (see equations 9.55–9.65). In a black box approach the mechanisms of breakage and coalescence are not considered. Initial values of coalescence and breakage kernels are assumed which enables solution of equation 9.69–9.71 (Laso and Steiner, 1987) and calculation of approximated number of drops in each bin n_i^{theory}. The solution of the inverted problem giving correct values of initially assumed kernels is obtained from:

$$\left| n_i^{exp} - n_i^{theory} \right| = min \tag{9.74}$$

In phenomenological modelling, equations 9.72 and 9.73 can be used to relate both breakage and coalescence kernels to the processing conditions and physical/interfacial properties of the system (see equations 9.57 and 9.69). Introduction of the theoretical description of both kernels makes them more general but again leads to the introduction of empirical constants. Those constants can also be calculated from the experimental data by solving the inverted problem defined by equation 9.74 (Tsouris and Tavlarides, 1994).

Obviously, application of the population balance equation in the analysis of emulsification processes is much more demanding than predicting maximum stable drop size but, if the knowledge of full drop size distribution during processing is important, there is no other option.

9.5 Emulsification Equipment

Manufacturing of pharmaceutical emulsions is a multistep process, the number of steps is frequently formulation specific and in formulation of emulsion for intravenous nutrition seven steps are necessary (Arii, 1999) whereas formulation of parenteral emulsions requires only four steps (Cuéllar *et al.*, 2005). However, in practically all pharmaceutical formulations the following steps are essential:

1. Preparation of aqueous and organic phases
2. Sterilization and reparation of coarse dispersion frequently carried out at an elevated temperature
3. Fine emulsification, reduction of drop size to below 5 μm
4. Filtering out of drops larger than 5 μm.

Preparation of aqueous and organic phases involves addition and dissolution of drugs, emulsifiers, vitamins and son on, in water and/or oil depending on the solubility of ingredients and application of emulsion. The selection of oils and emulsifiers for application in pharmaceutical emulsions is rather restricted to products approved by different regulatory bodies (Nielloud and Marti-Mestres, 2000) and discussion of this topic is well outside the scope of this chapter. This process is hardly discussed in the literature on preparation of pharmaceutical emulsions and is typically brushed off by the statement 'phases were prepared in water bath using magnetic stirrer'. However, in industrial, or even on large laboratory scales, dissolution of certain components in viscous oil or in viscous aqueous phase with simultaneous, uniform heating of resulting solution to 70–80°C is not always a simple task. Dissolutions and sterilizations are frequently carried out in a jacketed stirred vessel fitted with four baffles and an appropriate impeller. Baffles typically have a width equal 1/10 of vessel diameter and they are essential to ensure good mixing. The selection of impeller depends mainly on the viscosity of the fluid, and low viscosity fluids can be mixed with a propeller type impeller rotating at high speed and very viscous fluids require a ribbon or helical impeller rotating at low speed. There is a variety of impeller designs and in depth discussion of all factors affecting the selection of impeller/vessel configuration has been recently published (Paul *et al.*, 2004). Depending on the scale and configuration of the emulsification process, a coarse emulsion can be prepared in a stirred vessel (typically batch process) or in a static mixer (continuous process). The batch stirred vessels are recommended for small scale productions whereas static mixers are more efficient in large scale continuous processes. The final emulsification can be carried out in high shear mixers, high pressure homogenizers or ultrasonic homogenizers briefly discussed below.

9.5.1 Stirred Vessels

The diagrams of a stirred vessel and impellers frequently used for preparation of liquid/liquid dispersions are shown in Figure 9.8.

Impellers are characterized by power numbers, *Po*, a coefficient that relates energy dissipation rate to the liquid density, impeller diameter and speed (equation 9.53). Radial flow Rushton turbines, often called 'high shear impellers', have been traditionally considered especially efficient for processing gas/liquid and liquid/liquid dispersions (Nienow, 1997). Low *Po* impellers, such as axial flow hydrofoils (Chemineer HE3) and special 'ultra high shear' impellers (Chemineer CS2 and CS4) shown in Figure 9.8, with *Po* of the order of 0.3, run at very high speeds (around 1000 rpm) have been recently developed for producing fine liquid-liquid emulsions. They produce smaller drops with narrower size distributions than high power number, 'high shear' agitators at the same mean energy dissipation rates; they also do so more rapidly (Pacek *et al.*, 1999a). These clearly indicate that there are processing advantages to be gained from choosing a low *Po* impeller when small drops of narrow size distributions are required.

As discussed in Section 9.3.2, drop size in a liquid/liquid system is determined by the balance between cohesive and disruptive forces. In stirred vessels, the ratio of these forces is called the tank Weber number, $\left(We = \frac{N^2 D^3 \rho_c}{\sigma}\right)$, and this number is commonly used to calculate the Sauter mean diameter. For the non-viscous dispersed phase the following general correlation is frequently used:

$$\frac{d_{32}}{D} = C_1(1 + C_2\phi)We^{-0.6} \tag{9.75}$$

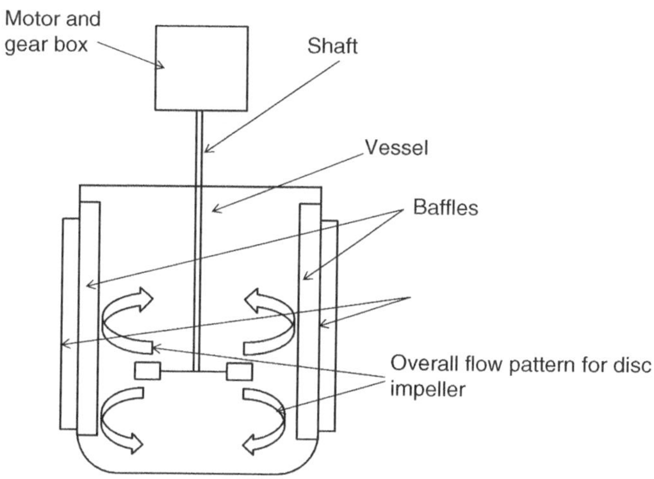

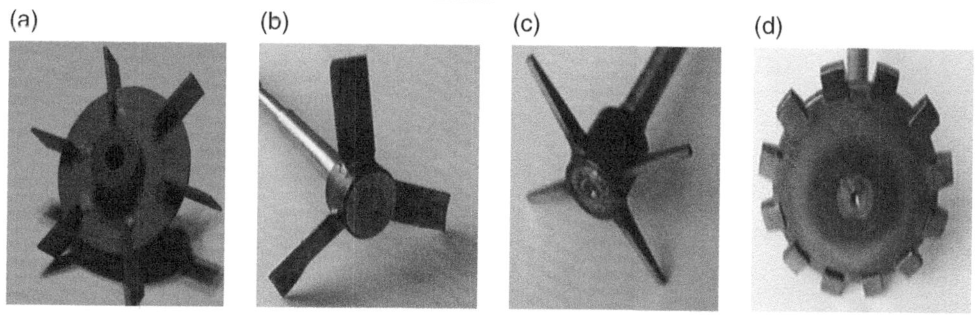

Figure 9.8 *Stirred vessel and impellers used for preparation of liquid/liquid dispersions: (a) Rushton turbine; (b) Chemineer HE3, (c) Chemineer CS2 and (d) Chemineer CS4. Reprinted with permission from High-pressure homogenization as a process for emulsion formation, by S. Schulz, G. Wagner, K. Urban and G. Ulrich,* Chemical Engineering and Technology, *361–368. Copyright (2004) John Wiley & Sons*

The proportionality constant, C_1, depends on the impeller type, especially the power number, whereas C_2 is a measure of the tendency to coalescence and it has higher values for the systems where coalescence is fast. Typically constants are in the range of $0.04 < C_1 < 0.06$ and $3 < C_2 < 20$ (Pacek *et al.*, 1999a).

In the case of the viscous dispersed phase, the Sauter mean diameter can be calculated from (Calabrese *et al.*, 1986):

$$\frac{d_{32}}{D} = 0.054(1+3\phi)We^{-0.6}\left[1+4.42Vi(1-2.5\phi)\left(\frac{d_{32}}{D}\right)^{0.33}\right]^{0.6} \tag{9.76a}$$

$$Vi = \left(\frac{\rho_c}{\rho_d}\right)^{0.5} ND\left(\frac{\mu_d}{\sigma}\right) \tag{9.76b}$$

The great majority of correlations for mean drop size in agitated stirred vessels available in the literature are valid for the Rushton turbine (Figure 9.8a) but there are also correlations developed for other impellers (Leng and Calabrese, 2004).

9.5.2 Static Mixers

Static mixers are formed from differently shaped elements inserted directly into the pipe and the energy necessary for dispersion comes from pressure drop across these elements. There are many different designs and manufacturers of static mixers but the two best known are Kenics, manufactured by Chemineer (Figure 9.9), and Sulzer, manufactured by SulzerChemTech.

In continuous emulsification, static mixers might offer an attractive alternative to the stirred vessels for preparation of coarse emulsions. They have several advantages over stirred vessels such as a narrow drop size distribution, a compact design and a lack of moving

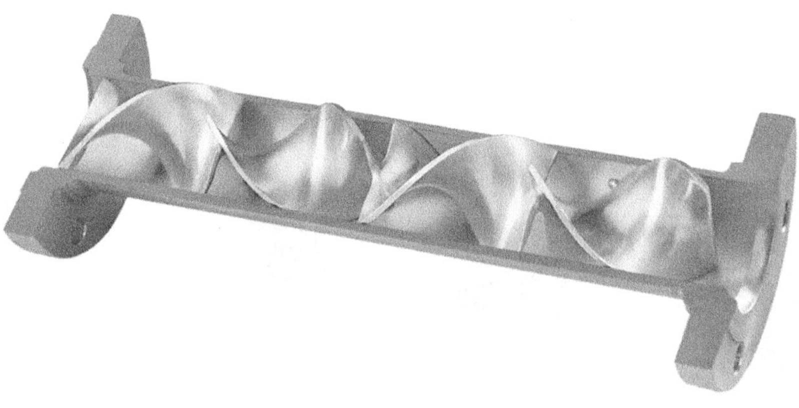

Figure 9.9 *Static mixers: (a) Kenics adapted from www.chemineer.com/kenics_products.php, Reprinted with permission from* Chem. Eng. Res. Des., *Static mixers: Mechanisms, applications, and characterization methods – A review by Akram Ghanem, Thierry Lemenand, Dominique Della Valle, Hassan Peerhossaini, 92, 2, 205–228. Copyright (2014) Elsevier*

parts, which makes them very reliable. Also heat exchangers might be installed inside mixing elements offering larger specific heat fluxes than heating jackets in stirred vessels that might be advantageous during sterilization. The main disadvantages of static mixers are: high pressure drop and rather limited information on their performance in the open literature.

Selection of a static mixer is rather difficult because of very limited information on their performance in the open literature. Manufacturers often offer to select the best mixer for a given process but in order to do that they need to know details of the process, which might not be acceptable for manufacturers. The Sauter mean diameter in liquid-liquid dispersion in static mixers is typically correlated with the Weber number (We_c) and Reynolds number (Re_c) defined in terms of superficial velocity of continuous phase with pipe diameter as a characteristic dimension. In Kenics mixers, the Sauter mean diameter also depends on the viscosity group (Pacek *et al.*, 1999a):

$$\frac{d_{32}}{D} = 0.247 We_c^{-0.47}(1 + 0.11 Vi^{0.05}) \tag{9.77}$$

whereas, in the SMX Sulzer it is also affected by number of mixing elements (Theron *et al.*, 2010):

$$\frac{d_{32}}{D} = 0.15 We_c^{-0.6} Re_c^{0.1} n_e^{-0.2} \tag{9.78}$$

The pressure drop in a fully developed flow in static mixers is calculated from the experimentally determined friction factor related to Re_c (Joshi, 1995):

$$f = 0.316 Re_c^{-0.25} \tag{9.79}$$

In the SMX Sulzer, the volume of mixing elements in Sulzer mixers is typically much greater than the volume of mixing elements in the Kenics mixer. Therefore, pressure drop and the friction factor in Sulzer mixers is much higher than in Kenics mixers (Theron *et al.*, 2010):

$$f = 24 Re_c^{-0.25} \tag{9.80}$$

The higher pressure drop in Sulzer mixers gives a higher energy dissipation rate (see equation 9.55) and a smaller average drop size than in the Kenics mixer, however, in both types of static mixers, as well as in stirred vessels, typically drops are of the order of tens of microns in size.

9.5.3 High Shear Mixers

High shear mixers are commonly used in pharmaceutical, food and cosmetic industries for the most demanding applications such as blending liquids of very different viscosities and for forming fine, stable emulsions and suspensions (Myers *et al.*, 1999; Atiemo-Obeng and Calabrese, 2004). There are various designs of rotor-stator mixers from different vendors Silverson (www.silverson.com), Ross (www.highshearmixers.com), Ystral (www.ystral.de), Chemineer (www.chemineer.com) and IKA Works (www.ikausa.com) but the common feature of practically all designs is a high speed rotor closely surrounded by a stator. The rotor speed is of the order of thousands of rpm giving typical tip speeds in the range of 10–50 m/s (Atiemo-Obeng and Calabrese, 2004). With the gaps between rotors and stators between 100 and 3000 μm (Karbstein and Schubert, 1995) the shear rate in the gap is in the range of 20 000–100 000 s^{-1} (Atiemo-Obeng and Calabrese, 2004). The kinetic energy supplied by the rotor dissipates mainly in a very small volume around stator, therefore, local energy dissipation rate is in the range of 10^4 to 10^6 W/kg (Utomo *et al.*, 2009). The combination of a very high shear rate with a very high energy dissipation rate enables manufacturing of emulsions with drops between hundreds of nanometres and a few microns.

High shear mixers can be broadly classified into colloid mills and axial/radial discharge rotor-stator mixers (Atiemo-Obeng and Calabrese, 2004). Colloid mills have limited pumping capacity and usually operate as in-line mixers with emulsions pumped through the mixer by an external pump. Axial and radial discharge rotor-stator mixers have considerable pumping capacity; therefore, they can operate both as batch and as in-line mixers. When viscous emulsion/liquids are processed in batch systems an additional impeller such as an anchor or a helical ribbon impeller should be used to enhance bulk mixing (Myers *et al.*, 1999).

9.5.3.1 Rotor-Stator Mixers

Although rotor-stator mixers have several advantages over stirred vessels or static mixers and have been used extensively in many industrial applications, there is very limited information on their performance available in the public domain. Figure 9.10 illustrates the general principle of emulsification in rotor stator mixers:

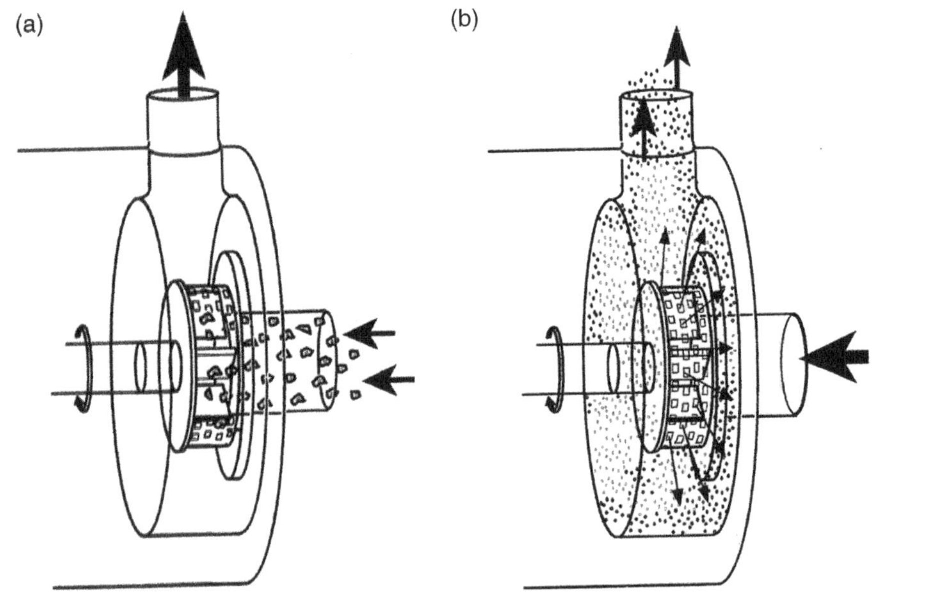

Figure 9.10 *Emulsification in rotor stator mixers. Reprinted with permission from Silverson Machines. Copyright (2014) Silverson Machines*

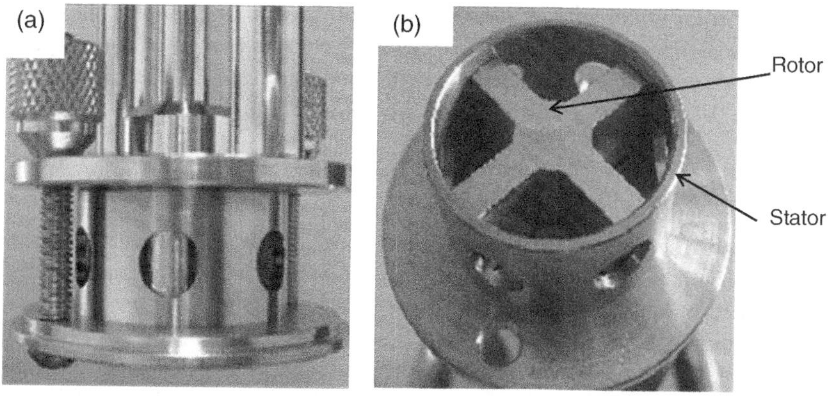

Figure 9.11 Radial discharge rotor-stator mixer Silverson L4RT; (a) mixing head fitted with disintegrating stator, (b) bottom view of the mixing head (rotor diameter approx. 26 mm). Reprinted with permission from Silverson Machines, Copyright (2014) Silverson Machines and from Chem. Eng. Res. Des., Dispersion of water into oil in a rotor–stator mixer. Part 1: Drop breakup in dilute systems by Paul E. Rueger, Richard V. Calabrese, 91, 11, 2122–2133. Copyright (2013) Elsevier

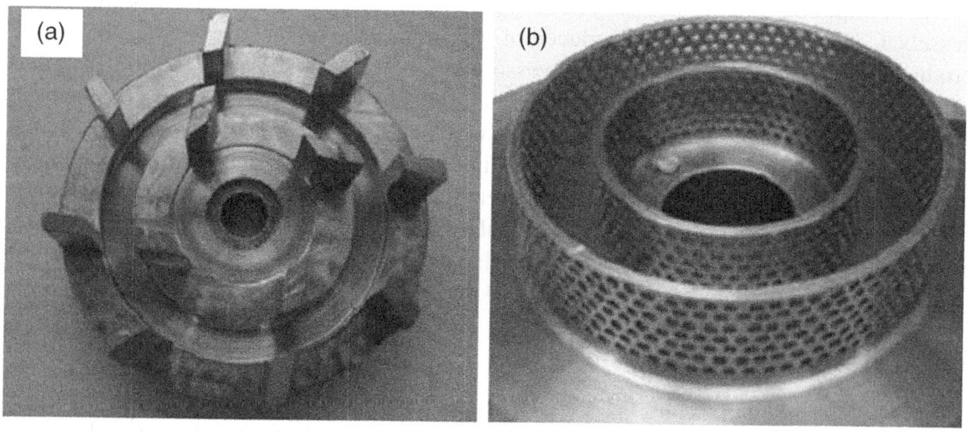

Figure 9.12 150/250 Silverson in-line rotor-stator (a) rotor, (b) stator – diameter of inner screen approx. 38 mm, diameter of outer screen approx. 63 mm. Reprinted with permission from Silverson Machines. Copyright (2014) Silverson Machines and from Chem. Eng. and Proc., Dispersion of oil droplets in rotor–stator mixers: Experimental investigations and modeling by Magdalena Jasińska, Jerzy Bałdyga, Steven Hall, Andrzej W. Pacek. Copyright (2014) Elsevier

High speed rotation draws the coarse dispersion into rotor/stator head (Figure 9.10a) from where it is forced through a narrow gap between the rotor and through perforation of the stator (Figure 9.10b) where large drops are broken into fine droplets. The details of rotor and stator of batch high shear mixer are shown in Figure 9.11 and rotor and stator of in-line rotor/stator double gap mixer is shown in Figure 9.12.

In high shear rotor-stator mixers, drops can be broken by the laminar shear, turbulent eddies, mechanical impact with solid surfaces or a combination of these (Myers *et al.*, 1999). Mean drop size (Sauter mean diameter) in batch rotor stator mixer, similar to the one shown in Figure 9.11, can be correlated with We number (Calabrese *et al.*, 2000):

$$\frac{d_{32}}{D} = 0.040We^{-0.58} \tag{9.81}$$

The same researchers suggested that in rotor stator mixers shear in the gap is not the predominant droplet breakage mechanism but drops are broken by impingement on the stator surfaces and by turbulent eddies in the jets emerging from stator slots.

Sauter mean diameter in liquid/liquid emulsions produced in a range of different types of emulsifying devices can be correlated with volumetric energy dissipation rate ε_v and mean residence time. Mean drop size in rotor-stator mixers can be calculated from following 'practical approximation' (Schubert *et al.*, 2004):

$$d_{32} \approx (\varepsilon_v t_r)^{-b} \approx E_v^{-b} \tag{9.82}$$

Exponent b depends on the mechanism of breakage and for inertial breakage by turbulent eddies and for breakage by turbulent shear, $b \approx 0.4$ (Schubert and Engel, 2004), whereas for breakage by laminar simple and elongational shear, $b \approx 1$ (Schubert *et al.*, 2004). The energy dissipation rate in rotor-stator mixers is higher than in the static mixers and stirred vessels. Consequently, droplets produced in the rotor-stator mixers are smaller than those produced in the static mixers or stirred vessels and they range from 0.5–100 μm (Atiemo-Obeng and Calabrese, 2004). This implies that high-shear rotor stator mixers can be used for manufacturing of emulsion for pharmaceutical applications both in a small scale (batch processing) as well as in a larger scale (continuous processing). Indeed, the Ultra-Turrax high shear mixer has been used to produce emulsion based lipid carriers (Formiga *et al.*, 2007) and to produce coarse intravenous emulation containing vitamin E (Lu *et al.*, 2008). A high shear rotor stator homogenizer was also used to prepare a complex W/O/W emulsion containing vancomycin (Okochi and Nakano, 2000).

9.5.3.2 Colloid Mills

Colloid mills, shown in Figure 9.13, are typically used as in-line mixers where emulsion is forced by an external pump through a narrow gap between a high speed rotor and a stator where large, even very viscous drops are broken into submicron droplets.

The stators are frequently fitted with cooling jackets to keep the temperature of emulsion approximately constant and to avoid hot spots that could damage the products. As these devices are frequently used in food processing to ensure cleanliness the wetted parts are designed in such a way that they can be easily dismantled and cleaned (Myers *et al.*, 1999).

The mechanism of breakage in colloid mills depends on the size of the gap (frequently adjustable www.ikausa.com) and the finish of the surfaces of rotor and stator. When the gap is very narrow and the surfaces of rotor and stator are smooth the flow is predominantly laminar (Schubert, 1997) and drops are broken both by a simple and an elongational shear. A simple shear results from the tangential velocity of the rotor and elongational shear results from velocity gradient in the direction of the flow caused by the reduction of width of the gap in this direction. Presence of both type of shear makes those devices very efficient

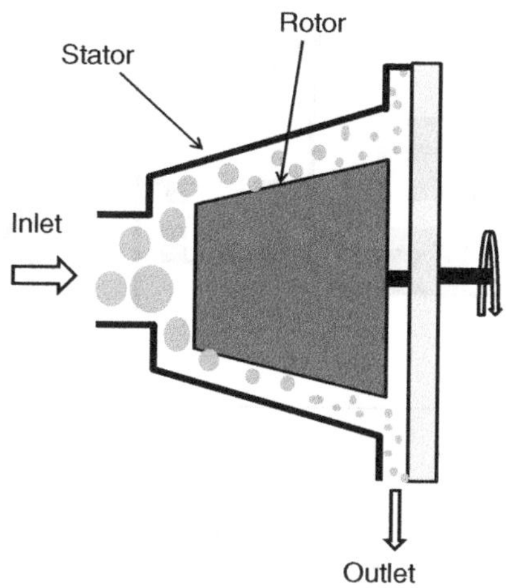

Figure 9.13 *Operating principle of a colloid mill*

in laminar breakage of very viscous drops and in this case the drop size can be estimated using Grace's curves shown in Figure 9.6.

Frequently, the surfaces of rotor and stator are roughened or toothed and in such cases turbulence breakage predominates (Schubert, 1997) and the maximum stable drop size can be related directly to the volumetric energy dissipation rate in a similar way as in the homogeneous turbulent flow and for low viscosity drops (Schuchmann and Schubert, 2003):

$$d_{max} \approx \rho_c^{-0.2} \sigma^{0.6} \varepsilon_v^{-0.4} \tag{9.83}$$

whereas for very viscous drops

$$d_{max} \approx \rho_c^{-0.5} \mu_d^{0.75} \varepsilon_v^{-0.25} \tag{9.84}$$

There are several features of modern designs that make colloid mills attractive for pharmaceutical applications. The cooling jacket enables simultaneous sterilization and emulsification that can be carried out both in batch and continuous operations. The drop size can be adjusted according to the product specification by adjusting the width of the *s* (shear rate) between the conical rotor and stator and hygienic design enables easy cleaning of all moving parts.

9.5.4 High-Pressure Homogenizers

High pressure homogenizers are commonly used to break large (tens of microns) drops in coarse emulsion into sub-micron droplets in fine emulsion in food (McClements, 2005) and in pharmaceutical industries (Lu *et al.*, 2007), but cannot be used for direct emulsification from completely separated phases. They consist of two major parts: a high pressure pump (up to 300 MPa) feeding the coarse emulsion into high pressure-drop dispersing unit. There are many different types of high pressure homogenizers developed by different

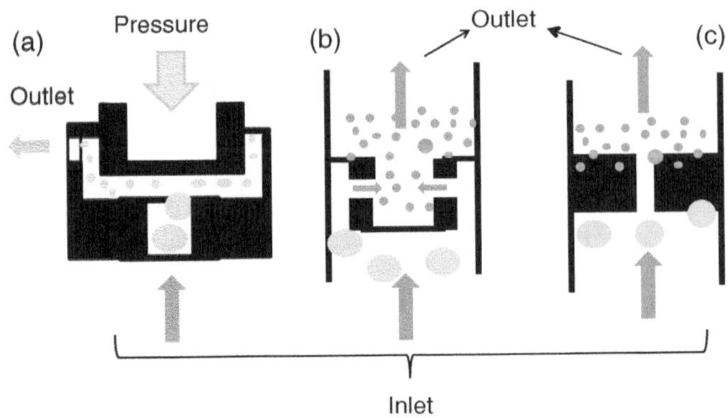

Figure 9.14 Flow patterns in different types of high pressure homogenizers; (a) radial flow homogenizer, (b) counter jet homogenizer, (c) axial flow nozzle homogenizer. Reprinted with permission from Chem. Eng. Technol., *27, 4, 361–368. Copyright (2004) WILEY-VCH Verlag GmbH & Co. KGaA, Weinheim*

vendors that can be classified into three groups according to the flow pattern into: radial flow devices (Figure 9.14 a), counter jet devices (Figure 9.14b) and axial flow nozzle devices (Figure 9.14c) (Schultz *et al.*, 2004).

Within each group there are devices with differently shaped and sized valves, channels or nozzles. The exact mechanism of drop breakage in high pressure homogenizers is still not well understood and it depends on the flow arrangement. In the radial flow devices (Figure 9.14a), also known as valve homogenizers, a variety of mechanisms controlling drop size was postulated ranging from laminar extensional shear through inertial turbulent forces with certain influence of cavitations It has been established experimentally that in this type of homogenizers the viscosity of the dispersed phase have strong effect on the mean drop size whereas the drop size is only weakly dependent on the volume fraction of dispersed phases (Schultz *et al.*, 2004).

Breakage in the counter jets (also known as the micro-fluidizer) and nozzle devices is even less understood than breakage in the valve homogenizers. It appears that drops are broken by extensional shear in the orifices and turbulent forces (both shear and inertial) in mixing chambers with geometry of nozzles and chambers having a very strong effect on drop size (Schultz *et al.*, 2004). Similar mechanisms were postulated for nozzle devices. In all those types of homogenizers, viscosity and the volume fraction of the dispersed phase have a relatively small effect on the drop size.

Correlations for average drop size and average volumetric energy dissipation rate developed for high shear homogenizers (Equation 9.82) can also be used for estimation of average drop size in high pressure homogenizers by substituting $\varepsilon_v = \Delta p$ with $0.35 < b < 1$ (Schubert *et al.*, 2003).

The common perception is that in the large scale continuous emulsification with submicron drops can be produced either in a high-shear or in high pressure homogenizers. However, in many formulations with viscous dispersed phase is frequently necessary to use two-stage high pressure homogenizer or high shear mixer in recirculation loop.

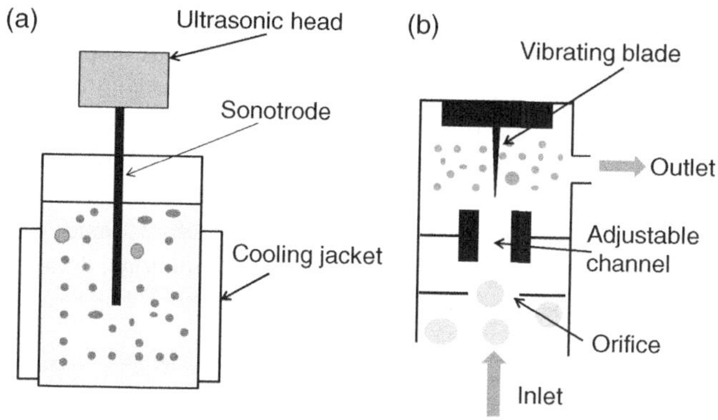

Figure 9.15 *Ultrasonic homogenizers: (a) batch, (b) continuous (also called the liquid whistle)*

9.5.5 Ultrasonic Homogenizers

High intensity acoustic energy has been used to produce emulsions from separated liquids, reduce drop size in already existing emulsions (Gaikwad and Pandit, 2008) and also to break solid aggregates suspended in liquids (Ding and Pacek, 2008). This energy is generated by a piezoelectric transducer in batch homogenizers (Figure 9.15a) or by the oscillations of the blade induced by the liquid flow (Figure 9.15b) in continuous flow homogenizers (frequently called liquid whistles). The batch homogenizers can easily be converted into continuous systems by pumping the suspension through the flow cell.

In both types of homogenizers, low frequency (in the range of KHz) and high power ultrasound waves are employed giving very high energy density (of the order of 10^9 Jm^{-3}) dissipated in a small volume around the tip of the sonotrode or around the vibrating blade. Practically all this energy is dissipated into heat as only a very small part is used to reduce drop/aggregates size. Whilst in continuous systems the temperature increase is limited because of a very short residence time in the flow cell, in batch systems flow cells are practically always fitted with cooling jackets.

The exact mechanism of breakage in ultrasound field is still not well understood. It has been postulated that drops exposed to ultrasound energy are broken because of instability of their interface resulting from oscillation of whole volume of the drop caused by ultrasonic waves (Behrend *et al.*, 2000). Cavitations of bubbles generating local, high velocity liquid jets (up to 100 m/s) and pressure gradients up to 20 GPa/cm appear to control drop size in many practical applications (Aoki, 1987). It has been experimentally established that the increase in irradiation time leads to an increase of volume fraction of dispersed phase and reduction of average drop size (Gaikwad and Pandit, 2008) and that the drop size is also affected by the design of ultrasound homogenizers (Leong *et al.*, 2008). Typically, average drop size depends on the physical properties of both, but mainly the continuous phase and in the presence of surfactants, drops between 0.1–3 μm are produced but optimization of composition of emulsion and energy input can lead to further reduction of drop size down to 40 nm (Leong *et al.*, 2008).

Whilst ultrasound is a very effective way of producing fine emulsions as well as nano-emulsions, it might affect biochemical properties of both dispersed and continuous phases (Chemat *et al.*, 2004) as well as the surfaces of processing equipment. The latter problem can be overcome by appropriate design of the flow cells (Freitas *et al.*, 2006). Ultrasound proved to be particularly useful in sterilization, however, after prolonged periods of processing the erosion of fine metal particles from the sonotrode leading to contamination of the emulsion was observed (Freitas *et al.*, 2006). Considering all this, before ultrasound is employed in processing of pharmaceutical emulsions, detailed analysis of the sonochemistry of all components should be carried out.

9.6 Concluding Remarks

The quality of emulsions and the efficiency of emulsification processes depends on the composition and physical/interphasial properties of both phases, in other words on formulation, and the processing/hydrodynamic conditions. In surfactant free systems, physical properties are practically independent of hydrodynamic conditions and the coalescence/breakage models discussed in this chapter are sufficient for many applications. In the presence of surface active agents the interfacial properties become dynamic and they frequently vary with the intensity of processing conditions and with the processing time. These variations are the result of adsorption/desorption of a surfactant and they affect interfacial rheology and stability of the interface. Current understanding of the interactions between hydrodynamic conditions in the bulk of both continuous and dispersed phase and the conditions on the interface separating them is very limited and further research in this area is necessary. Improved models of the dynamic behaviour of the interface can be incorporated into existing CFD codes that would enable a more detailed analysis of both the emulsification process and the stability of the resulting emulsions.

Nomenclature

A – experimental constant in equation Eq 9.16	[Pas]
A_0, A_1, A_2 – experimental constants	[–]
b_i – change of number of drops in class i due to breakage	[$s^{-1}m^{-3}$]
B – experimental constant in equation Eq 9.16	[K]
c_i – change of number of drops in class i due to coalescence	[$s^{-1}m^{-3}$]
$c(r)$ – solubility of the solute when it is contained in a drop of radius r	[kmol m^{-3}]
c_∞ – solubility of the solute in the phase of infinite curvature	[kmol m^{-3}]
C, C_1, C_2, C_3 – experimental constants	
d – drop diameter	[m]
D – rotor diameter	[m]
D_0 – static mixer diameter	[m]
$D_{d\text{-}c}$ – diffusion coefficient of dispersed phases in continuous phase	[m^2s^{-1}]
e – electron charge	[C]
E – energy density	[kJ kg^{-1}]
f – friction factor	[–]
f_{iv} – volume frequency	[%]

f_{in} – number frequency [%]
F_{iv} – cumulative volume distribution [%]
F_{iN} – cumulative number distribution [%]
h – distance between drops [m]
Ha – Hamaker constant [J]
k^c – coalescence kernel [m^3s^{-1}]
k^b – breakage kernel [m^3s^{-1}]
K – consistency constant in Eq 9.18 [Pa s^n]
l_m – length of static mixer [m]
m_d – mass of dispersed phase [kg]
m_I – constant in Eq 9.17 [–]
m – total mass of emulsion [kg]
n – power law index in Eq 9.18 [–]
n_i – number of drops in the bin i [–]
N – rotor speed [s^{-1}]
P – pressure [Pa]
Po – power number [–]
r – drop radius [m]
R – universal gas constant [J K^{-1} mol^{-1}]
$Pe = \frac{\dot{\gamma}\eta_c R^3}{\kappa_B T}$ – Peclet number [–]

$Re_c = \frac{\rho_c v_0 D}{\mu_c}$ – continuous phase Reynolds number [–]

$Re_d = \frac{\rho_c \dot{\gamma} R^2}{\eta_c}$ – drop Reynolds number [–]

t – time [s]
t_c – contact time [s]
t_{col} – coalescence time [s]
t_{dr} – film drainage time [s]
T – absolute temperature [K]
u_c – superficial velocity [ms^{-1}]
v_0 – volumetric flow rate [m^3s^{-1}]
v_{St} – terminal velocity [ms^{-1}]
v_d – volume of drop [m^3]
V_d – volume of dispersed phase [m^3]
V – total volume of emulsion [m^3]
V_m – molecular volume of solute [m^3kmol]
W^{elec} – electrostatic interaction energy [J]
W^{hyd} – hydrophobic interaction energy [J]
W^{vdW} – van der Waals interaction energy [J]
$We_c = \frac{\rho_c v_0^2 D}{\sigma}$ – Weber number [–]

z – valency [–]

Greek symbols

β – collision frequency [s^{-1}]
$\dot{\gamma}$ – shear rate [s^{-1}]
ε – energy dissipation rate [$W\ kg^{-1}$]
η_c – viscosity of continuous phase [Pas]
η_d – viscosity of dispersed phase [Pas]
η_{ap} – viscosity of emulsion [Pas]
$\eta_r = \eta_c / \eta_{ap}$ – reduced viscosity of emulsion [–]
η_B – constant (measure of viscosity in Equation 9.19) [Pas]
η_0 – asymptotic value of viscosity at very low shear rate [Pas]
η_∞ – asymptotic values of viscosity at very high shear rate [Pas]
θ – breakup frequency [s^{-1}]
$\kappa_B = 1.81 * 10^{-23}$ – Boltzman constant [JK^{-1}]
κ^{-1} – Debye length [nm]
$\lambda = \eta_d / \eta_c$ – viscosity ratio [–]
ν – kinematic viscosity [m^2s^{-1}]
ρ_c – density of continuous phase [$kg\ m^{-3}$]
ρ_d – density of dispersed phase [$kg\ m^{-3}$]
σ – interfacial tension [Nm^{-1}]
τ – shear stress [Pa]
τ_0 – yield stress [Pa]
ψ – electrostatic potential [V]
ω – coalescence rate [$m^{-3}s^{-1}$]
ϵ – permittivity of continuous phase [$C^2J^{-1}\ m^{-1}$]
ϕ – volume fraction of dispersed phase [–]
ϕ_{mass} – mass fraction of dispersed phase [–]
ϕ_m – volume fraction at maximum packing [–]
Φ_{in} – number probability density function [m^{-1}]
Φ_{iv} – volume probability density function [m^{-1}]

References

N. Anton and T.F. Vandamme, The universality of low energy nano-emulsification, *International Journal of Pharmaceutics*, **377**, 142–147 (2009)

M. Aoki, T.A. Ring, and J.S. Haggerty, Analysis and modelling of the ultrasonic dispersion technique, *Advanced Ceramic Materials*, **2**, 209–212 (1987)

K. Arii, Y. Fukuta, T. Kai and Y. Kokuba, Preparation of fine emulsified particles for intravenous nutrition, *European Journal of Pharmaceutical Sciences*, **9**, 67–73 (1999)

V.A. Atiemo-Obeng and R.V. Calabrese, High shear mixers, in E.L. Paul, V.A. Atiemo-Obeng, S.M. Kresta, (eds) *Handbook of Industrial Mixing*, John Wiley & Sons, Inc., New Jersey, 2004

J. Baldyga and J.R. Bourne, *Turbulent Mixing and Chemical Reactions*, John Wiley & Sons, Chichester, 1999

H.A. Barnes, J.F. Hutton, K. Walters, *Introduction to Rheology*, Elsevier, Amsterdam, 1998

P. Becker (ed.), *Encyclopedia of Emulsion Technology, Volume 2: Applications*, Marcel Dekker, New York, 1985

J.K. Beddow, *Particulate Science and Technology*, Chemical Publishing Co., Inc, New York, 1980

O. Behrend, K. Ax and H. Schubert, Influence of continuous phase viscosity on emulsification by ultrasound, *Ultrasonics Sonochemistry*, **7**, 77–85 (2000)

S. Bjerregaard, I. Soderberg and C. Vermehren, Formulation and evaluation of release and swelling mechanism of a water-in-oil emulsion using factorial design, *International Journal of Pharmaceutics*, **193**, 1–11 (1999)

N. Brauner and A. Ullmann, Modeling of phase inversion phenomenon in two-phase pipe flows, *International Journal of Multiphase Flow*, **28**, 1177–1204 (2002)

M.I. Briceno, Rheology of suspensions and emulsions, In *Pharmaceutical Emulsions and Suspensions*, F. Nielloud and G. Marti-Mestres (eds), Marcel Dekker, Inc, New York, 2000

B.W. Brooks, H.N. Richmond and M. Zerfa, Phase inversion and drop formation in agitated liquid-liquid dispersions in the presence, of non-ionic surfactants, in *Modern Aspects of Emulsion Science*, B.P. Binks (ed.), The Royal Society of Chemistry, Cambridge, UK, 1998

R.V. Calabrese, M.K. Francis, V.P. Mishra and S. Phongikaroon, Measurements and analysis of drop size in a batch rotor-stator mixer, *Proceedings of 10th European Conference on Mixing Delft*, The Netherlands, Elsevier, H.E.A van den Akker, J.J. Derkse (eds), Elsevier, July 2–5, 2000

R.V. Calabrese, C.Y. Wang and N.P. Bryner, Drop breakup in turbulent stirred-tank contactors. Part III: Correlations for mean size and drop size distribution, *AIChE Journal*, **32**, 677–680 (1986)

A.K. Chesters, The modelling of coalescence processes in liquid-liquid dispersions: a review of current understanding, *Trans. Inst. Chem. Eng.*, **69**, 259–270 (1991)

S.J. Choi and W.R. Schowalter, Rheological properties of non-diluted suspensions of deformable particles, *Physics of Fluids*, **18**, 420–427, (1975)

F. Chemat, I. Grondin, A. Shum Cheong Sing and J. Smadja, Deterioration of edible oils during food processing by ultrasound, *Ultrasonics Sonochemistry*, **11**, 13–15 (2004)

H.K. Christenson and P.M. Claesson Direct measurements of the force between hydrophobic surfaces in water, *Advances in Colloid and Interface Science*, **91**, 391–436 (2001)

I. Cuéllar, J. Bullón, A.M. Forgarini, A. Cárdenas and M.I. Briceño, More efficient preparation of parenteral emulsions or how to improve a pharmaceutical recipe by formulation engineering, *Chemical Eng. Science*, **60**, 2127–2134 (2005)

S.S. Davies, J. Hadgraft and K.J. Palin, Medical and pharmaceutical applications of emulsions, in *Encyclopedia of Emulsion Technology*, vol 2, P. Becher (ed.), Marcel Dekker, Inc. New York 1985

S.W. Derkach, Rheology of Emulsions, *Advances in Colloid and Interface Science*, **151**, 1–23 (2009)

P. Ding and A.W. Pacek, Effect of pH on de-agglomeration and rheology/morphology of aqueous suspensions of goethite nano-powder, *Journal of Colloid and Interface Science*, **325**, 165–172 (2008)

E. Dickinson, *Introduction to Food Colloids*, Oxford University Press, Oxford, 1992

A.S Dukhin, S.S. Dukhin and P.J. Goetz, Gravity as a factor of aggregative stability and coagulation, *Advances in Colloid and Interface Science*, **134**, 35–71 (2007)

P. Fernandez, V. André, J. Rieger and A. Kühnle, Nano-emulsion formation by emulsion phase inversion, *Colloids and Surfaces A: Physicochem. Eng. Aspects*, **251**, 53–58 (2004)

F.R. Formiga, I.A.A. Fonseca, K.B. Souza, A.K.A. Silva, J.P.F. Macedo, I.B. Araujo, et al., Influence of a lipophilic drug on the stability of emulsions: An important approach on the development of lipidic carriers, *International Journal of Pharmaceutics*, **344**, 158–160 (2007)

S. Freitas, G. Hielscher, H.P. Merkle and B. Gander, Continuous contact and contamination free ultrasonic emulsification – a useful tool for pharmaceutical development and production, *Ultrasonics Sonochemistry*, **13**, 76–85 (2006)

S.G. Gaikwad and A.B. Pandit, Ultrasound emulsification: Effect of ultrasonic and physiochemical properties on dispersed phase volume and droplet size, *Ultrasonic Sonochemistry*, **15**, 554–563 (2008)

J.C. Godfrey and M.J. Slater, Liquid-liquid extraction equipment, John Wiley & Sons, Inc., New York, 1994

H.P. Grace, Dispersion phenomena in high viscosity immiscible fluid systems and application of static mixers as dispersion devices in such systems, *Chem. Eng Communications*, **14**, 225–237 (1971)

J.M. Gutierrez, C. Gonzalez, A. Maestro, I. Sole, C.M. Pey and J. Nolla, Nanoemulsions: new applications and optimization of their preparations. *Current Opinion in Colloid and Interface Science*, **13**, 245–251 (2008)

J.O. Hinze, Fundamentals of hydrodynamic mechanism of splitting in dispersion processes, *AIChE Journal*, **1**, 289–295 (1955)

B. Hua, O.K. Matarb, G.F. Hewitt and P. Angelia, Population balance modelling of phase inversion in liquid–liquid in pipeline flows, *Chemical Engineering Science*, **61**, 4994–4997 (2006)

J. Israelachvili, *Intermolecular and Surface Forces*, Academic Press, 1994

F. Jahanzad, G. Crombie, R. Innes and S. Sajjadic, Catastrophic phase inversion via formation of multiple emulsions: A prerequisite for formation of fine emulsions, *Chemical Engineering Research and Design*, **87**, 492–498 (2009)

T. Jansen, M.P.M. Hofmans, M.J.G. Theelen and V.E.J.C. Schijns, Structure–activity relations of water-in-oil vaccine formulations and induced antigen-specific antibody responses, *Vaccine*, **23**, 1053–1060 (2005)

S.A.K Jeelani and E.J. Windhab, Drop coalescence in planar extensional flow and gravity, *Chem. Eng Sci.*, **64**, 2718–2722 (2009)

N. Joshi and N. Nauman, The Kenics static mixer: new data and proposed correlations, *Chem. Eng. J.*, **59**, 265–271 (1995)

A.S. Kabalnov, Coalescence in emulsions, in *Modern Aspects of Emulsion Science*, B.P. Binks (ed.), The Royal Society of Chemistry, Cambridge, 1998

A.S. Kabalnov and E.D. Shchukin, Ostwald ripening theory: applications to fluorocarbon emulsion stability, *Advances in Colloid and Interface Science*, **38**, 69–97 (1992)

H. Karbstein and H. Schubert, Developments in the continuous mechanical production of oil-in-water macro-emulsions,' *Chem. Eng. Process.*, **34**, 205–211 (1995)

C. Kleinstreuer, *Two-Phase Flow: Theory and Application*, Taylor & Francis, New York, 2003

K.K Krynke, and J.P. Sek, Predicting viscosity of emulsions in the broad range of inner phase concentrations, *Colloids and Surfaces A-Physicochemical and Engineering Aspects*, **245**, 81–92 (2004)

M. Laso, L. Steiner and S. Hartland, Dynamic simulation of agitated liquid-liquid dispersions, *Chem. Eng. Science*, **42**, 2429–2436 (1987)

D.E Leng and R.V. Calabrese, Immiscible Liquid-liquid systems, in *Handbook of Industrial Mixing*, E.L. Paul, V.A. Atiemo-Obeng, S.M. Kresta, (eds), John Wiley & Sons, Inc., New Jersey, 2004

T.S.H. Leong, T.J. Wooster, S.E. Kentish and M Ashokkumar, Minimising oil droplet size using ultrasonic emulsification, *Ultrasonic Sonochemistry*, **16**, 721–727 (2009)

Y. Liao and D. Lucas, A literature review of theoretical models for drop and bubble breakup in turbulent flow, *Chem. Eng. Science*, **64**, 3389–3406 (2009)

Y. Lu, Y.J. Wang and X. Tang, Formulation and thermal sterile stability of a less painful intravenous clarithromycin emulsion containing vitamin E, *International Journal of Pharmaceutics*, **346**, 47–56 (2008)

J. Lyklema, Pair interactions, in *Fundamentals of Interface and Colloid Science*, J. Lyklema (ed.), London, 2005

D.J. Ma and T. McHugh, The interplay of phase inversion and membrane formation in the drug release characteristics of a membrane-based delivery system *Journal of Membrane Science*, **298**, 156–168 (2007)

C.C Man, *Drop Size and Coalescence Rates in Oil-in-Aqueous and Aqueos-in-Oil Dispersion in Stirred Tank*, PhD Thesis, University of Birmingham, Birmingham, 1998

D.J. McClements, *Food Emulsions, Principles, Practise and Techniques*, CRC Press, London, 2005

B. Mishra and J.K. Pandit, Prolonged release of pentazocine, from multiple O/W/O emulsions, *Drug Dev Ind. Pharm.*, **15**, 1217–1230 (1989)

K.J. Myers, M.F. Reeder, D. Ryan and G. Daly, Get a fix on high shear mixing, *Chem. Eng Progress*, **95**, 33–42 (1999)

F. Nielloud and G. Marti-Mestres, *Pharmaceutical Emulsions and Suspensions*, Marcel Dekker, New York, 2000

A.W. Nienow (1997), *Mixing in the Process Industries, 2nd Edition*, Butterworth Heinemann, London,

H. Okochi and M. Nakano, Preparation and evaluation of w/o/w type emulsions containing vancomycin, *Advanced Drug Delivery Reviews*, **45**, 5–26 (2000)
A.W. Pacek, I.P.T. Moore, A.W. Nienow and R.V. Calabrese, Video technique for measuring dynamics of liquid-liquid dispersion during phase inversion, *AIChE Journal*, **40**, 1940–1949 (1994a)
A.W. Pacek, A.W. Nienow and I.P.T. Moore, On the structure of turbulent liquid–liquid dispersed flows in an agitated vessel. *Chem. Eng. Sci.*, **49**, 3485–3498 (1994b)
A.W. Pacek and A.W. Nienow, A problem for the description of turbulent dispersed liquid–liquid systems, *Int. J. Multiphase Flow*, **21**, 323–328 (1995)
A.W. Pacek, C.C. Man and A.W. Nienow, Coalescence Rates in Water (Aqueous)-In-Oil and Oil-In-Water (Aqueous) Dispersions, 9th European Conference on Mixing, Paris, 18–21 March, *Groupe Francouis de Genie des Procedes,* Nancy, France, vol. I, pp. 263–270 1997
A.W. Pacek, A. Aylianawati and A.W. Nienow, Breakage of oil drops in Chemineer static mixer. Part 1 Experiments and correlations, *Proceedings of 3rd International Symposium on Mixing in Industrial Processes,* Osaka, Japan, 115–122 1999a
A.W. Pacek, S. Chamsart, A.W. Nienow and A. Bakker, The influence of impeller type on mean drop size and size distribution in an agitated vessel, *Chem. Eng. Sci.*, **54**, 4211–4222 (1999b)
A.W. Pacek, P. Ding and A.T. Utomo, Effect of energy density, pH and temperature on de-aggregation in nano-particles/water suspensions in high shear mixer, *Journal of Powder Technology*, **173**, 203–210 (2007)
R. Pal, Novel viscosity equations for emulsions of two immiscible liquids, *J. Rheology*, **45**, 509–520 (2001)
E.L. Paul, V.A. Atiemo-Obeng and S.M. Kresta (eds) *Handbook of Industrial Mixing*, John Wiley & Sons, Inc., New Jersey, 2004
V.L. Peramal, S. Tamburic and D.Q.M. Craig, Characterization of variation in the physical properties of commercial creams using thermogravimetric analysis and rheology, *Int. Journal Pharm.*, **155**, 91–98 (1997)
P. Pianko-Oprych and Z. Jaworski, CFD modelling of two-phase liquid-liquid flow in a SMX static mixer, *Polish Journal of Chemical Technology*, **11**, 41–49 (2009)
K.R. Piela, R. Delfos, G. Ooms, J. Westerwee and R.V.A. Oliemans, On the phase inversion process in an oil–water pipe flow, *International Journal of Multiphase Flow*, **34**, 665–677 (2008)
D. Quemada and C. Berli, Energy of interaction in colloids and its implications on rheological modelling, *Advances In Colloid and Interface Science*, **98**, 51–85 (2002)
D. Ramakrishna, *Population Balances, Theory and Applications to Particulate Systems in Engineering*, Academic Press, New York, 2000
S. Rigopoulos and A.G. Jones, Finite-element scheme for solution of dynamic population balance equation, *AIChE Journal*, **49**, 1127–1139 (2003)
N. Sadurni, C. Solans, N. Azemar and M. Garcia-Celma, Studies on the formation of O/W nano-emulsions, by low-energy emulsification methods, suitable for pharmaceutical applications, *European Journal of Pharmaceutical Sciences*, **26**, 438–445 (2005)
P.G. Saffman and J.S. Turner, On the collision of drops in turbulent clouds, *J. Fluid Mech.*, **1**, 16–30 (1956)
S. Sajjadi, Nanoemulsion formation by phase inversion emulsification: On the nature of inversion, *Langmuir*, **22**, 5597–5603 (2006)
L.L. Schramm, *Emulsions, Fundamentals and Applications in the Petroleum Industry*, American Chemical Society, Washington, D.C., 1992
H. Schubert, Advances in the mechanical production of food emulsions, in: *Proceedings of the 7th International Congress on Engineering and Food.* Part 1, S. pp. 82–87 (1997)
H. Schubert and R. Engel, Product and formulation engineering of emulsions, *Chemical Engineering Research and Design*, **82**, 1137–1143 (2004)
H.P. Schuchmann and H. Schubert, Product design in food industry using the example of emulsification, *Eng. Life Science*, **3**, 67–76 (2003)
S. Schultz, G. Wagner, K. Urban and J. Ulrich, High-pressure homogenization as a process for emulsion formation, *Chem. Eng. Technol.*, **27**, 361–368 (2004)
N. Shahidzadeh, D. Boon, J. Menunier, M. Nabavi, M. Airau and M. Morvan, Dynamics of spontaneous emulsification for fabrication of oil in water emulsions, *Langmuir*, **16**, 9703–9708 (2000)

R. Shinnar, On the behaviour of liquid-liquid dispersions in mixing vessels, *Proc Royal Soc*, **10**, 259–275 (1961)
K. Shinoda and H. Kunidea, Phase properties of emulsions: PIT and HLB, in *Encyclopaedia of Emulsion Technology Vol. 1*, Paul Becher (ed.), Marcel Dekker, New York, 1983
R.J. Sibley and R.A. Alberty, *Physical Chemistry*, John Wiley & Sons, Inc., 2001
A. Silva-Cunha, M. Chéron, J.L. Grossiord, F. Puisieux and M. Seiller W/O/W multiple emulsions of insulin containing a protease inhibitor and an absorption enhancer: biological activity after oral administration to normal and diabetic rats, *International Journal of Pharmaceutics*, **169**, 33–44 (1998)
C. Solans, P. Izquierdo, J. Nolla, N. Azemar and M.J. Garcia-Celma, Nano-emulsions, *Current Opinion in Colloid & Interface Science*, **10**, 102–110 (2005)
D. Song, W. Zhang, R.K. Gupta and E. Melby, Droplet size and viscosity of tackifier emulsions formed via phase inversion, *Canadian Journal of Chemical Engineering*, **87**, 862–868 (2009)
H.A. Stone, Dynamics of drop deformation and breakup in viscous fluids, *Annu. Rev. Fluid Mech.*, **26** 65–102 (1994)
T.F. Tadros and B. Vincent, Emulsion stability, in *Encyclopaedia of Emulsion Technology, Vol. 1*, P. Becher (ed.), Marcel Dekker, New York, 1983
L.L. Tavlarides and M. Stamatoudis, The analysis of interphase reactions and mass transfer in liquid-liquid dispersions, *Advances in Chemical Engineering*, **11**, 199–273 (1981)
F. Theron, N. Le Sauze and A. Ricard, Turbulent liquid-liquid dispersion in Sulzer SMX Mixer, *Ind. Eng. Chem. Res.*, **49**, 623–632 (2010)
C. Tsouris and L.L. Tavlarides, Breakage and coalescence models for drops in turbulent dispersions, *AIChE Journal*, **40**, 395–406 (1994)
A. Utomo, M. Baker and A.W. Pacek, ‚Effect of stator geometry on flow pattern and energy dissipation rate in a rotor-stator mixer, *Chem. Eng. Res. Des.*, **87**, 533–542 (2009)
B. Vincent, Introduction to colloidal dispersions, in *Colloid Science, Principles, Methods and Applications*, T. Cosgrove (ed.), Blackwell Publishing, 2005
S.A. Vitale and J.L. Katz, Liquid droplet dispersions formed by homogeneous liquid–liquid nucleation:'The ouzo effect,' *Langmuir*, **19**, 4105–4110 (2003)
P. Walstra, Disperse systems: Basic Consideration; In *Food Chemistry*, O.R. Fenneman (ed.), Marcel Dekker, New York, 1996
K. Wojciechowski and M. Kucharek, Interfacial Tension Oscillations without Surfactant Transfer, *J. Phys. Chem. B*, **113**, 13457–13461 (2009)

10

Mixing of Pharmaceutical Solid-Liquid Suspensions

Mostafa Barigou[1] *and Frans L. Muller*[2]
[1] *School of Chemical Engineering, University of Birmingham, UK*
[2] *AstraZeneca, Hursfield Industrial Estate, UK*

10.1 Introduction

10.1.1 Linking Solid-Liquid Processing to Critical Quality Attributes

As outlined in Figure 10.1, as the project progresses, the quantities of both drug substance and product required for toxicology, formulation development and clinical trials increase. So, although process development is typically done in 20 mL to 3 L equipment, the scale of manufacturing of DS material increases to 20 L to 100 L in a large scale (or kilogram) laboratory. For phase 2 and phase 3 trials, material is typically manufactured at 500 to 2000 L scale in a pilot facility or 1000–10000 L for an agile manufacturing unit. As processes are scaled up many things can change compared to the scale at which the process was developed. In order to identify where scale-up can impact on a critical quality attribute (CQA) one needs to have an understanding of the nature of equipment, operations and mixing required at the various scales. Table 10.1 provides an overview of equipment characteristics at a range of scales used in development. It lists a number of physical attributes of the equipment as well as equipment capabilities like isolation methods, containment, heat and mass transfer and so on.

To understand the impact of scale-up on a CQA requires a general understanding of the interaction between a process and the equipment, and which processing duties are important

Pharmaceutical Blending and Mixing, First Edition. Edited by P.J. Cullen, Rodolfo J. Romañach, Nicolas Abatzoglou and Chris D. Rielly.

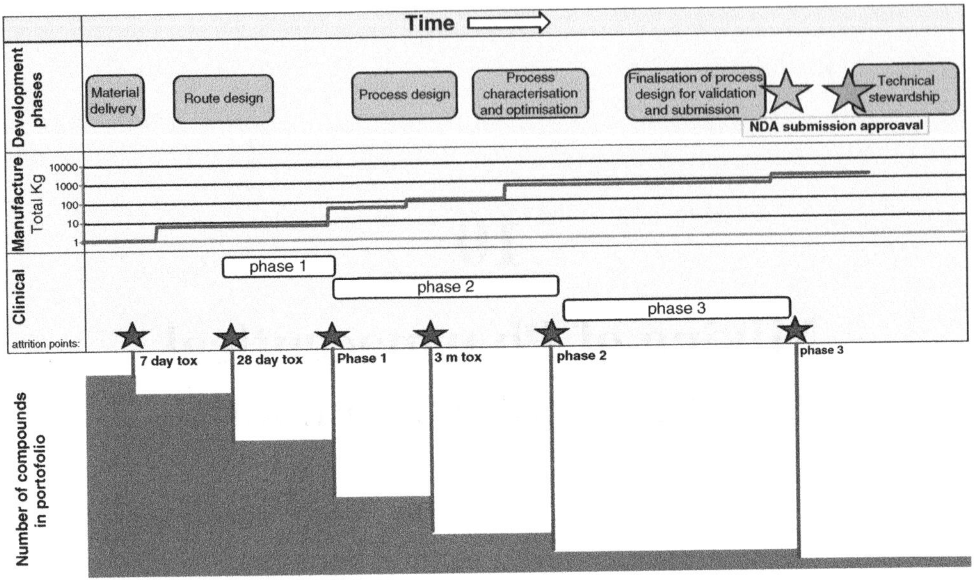

Figure 10.1 Lining up clinical trials, attrition points and process development

to the final drug product quality. A list of possible changes and their impact on CQAs is discussed next.

10.1.2 Material Properties and Composition

As scale increases, so do the required quantities of raw materials, the time it takes to order the materials as well as the time it takes to process them. Material purchased in large quantities can be different from material bought in small quantities for lab work. In our experience, particle size, polymorphic form, impurity profile and solvent content can all change. Some of these may be picked up by the specification of the material (e.g. solvent, impurity levels). However, polymorph, particle size and new unknown impurities are often not specified for raw materials, but can be important to solid-liquid (S-L) processes (e.g. crystallization, suspension mass transfer), and thus impact on the CQA for impurities, assay and/or chirality.

10.1.3 Impact of Blending and Homogenization

If the solids are well suspended, then just as for single phase systems, the mixing time in S-L systems is also inherently worse at a larger scale. The bulk mixing time scales for instance with the reciprocal of the agitator speed $1/N$. From Table 10.1, it follows that on scale-up the mixing time increases from seconds on the small scale to minutes or even tens of minutes at the larger scale.

The distribution of solids over the vessel contents is strongly dependent on the agitation rate. At low agitation rates a significant fraction of the solids may remain in a solid bed on the bottom of the vessel. This results in very long blend times as there is little exchange

Table 10.1 *An overview of equipment used in drug substance processing across a range of scales*

Scale	Screening equipment	synthetic laboratory	development laboratory	Large (kg) scale laboratory	Pilot scale plant
Volume	10 mL	20–250 mL	100–5000 mL	20–100 L	200–2000 L
Description	Hydrogenation, stemblock, well plates; typically all in reactions	Round bottom flasks; surface addition	Glass jacketed vessels with quickfit lids; surface addition	Glass jacketed reactors; surface addition	Glass lined mild steel jacketed reactors, surface addition. Occasional reactors may be Hasteloy
starting Materials	<5 gr	1–10 gr	10–100 gr	1 to 10 kg	20–50 kg
Ordering time	day	day	day	day – weeks	weeks – months
Processing time/ campaign time	hours	hours-days	hours-days	days – week	weeks
PAT	temperature, pressue	temperature, pressure	temperature, Pressure, in situ IR, UV, viscosity, particle size	temperature, Pressure, in situ particle size	Temperature, Pressure, Volume
Auxillaries	few, manufacturer specific	quickfit glass overheads heating mantles, dricold	over head stirring and heater chiller external baths, vaccuum ovens	fixed vapour uplift, condensers and receivers. Open Nutch filters, tray drier ovens, some batch centrifuges	fixed vapour uplift, condensers and receivers. Closed pressure filters or batch centrifuges + dryer.
Agitation	flee, shaking, sometimes overhead agitated	flee, some overhead stirring, minimal baffling	Glass and metal agitators, mininimal baffling. Typical retreat curve or pitch blade. Occasional anchor	Glass retreat curve and general metal impellers (RTD, PBT). Occasional finger baffle	Glass retreat curve and general metal impellers (RTD, PBT). Occasional finger baffle
tip speed					
power per unit volume					
Attrition, grinding	severe attrition when stirred with flee	severe attrition when stirred with flee			
minimum Addition time	seconds	seconds	10s of seconds	minutes	10's of minutes

(continued)

Table 10.1 (continued)

Scale	Screening equipment	synthetic laboratory	development laboratory	Large (kg) scale laboratory	Pilot scale plant
Heat transfer	High, set point reached in minutes	High, set point reached in minutes. Significant heat losses through top half of vessel	Medium, set point reached in 10s of minutes (limited by jacket). Significant heat losses through lid	low - medium, eq. set point reached in 30 min. Limited by internal heat transfer. Significant heat losses through lid and vapour up lift	low eq. Temperature reached in 30–60 min. Limited by internal heat transfer, low heat loses
Mass transfer	typically low, but OK for some specialised equipment	low	low to high	low - medium, but typical for hydrogenators	low - medium, but typical for hydrogenators
Solid suspension	in homogeneous	in homogeneous	well distributed providing agitation is sufficient	well distributed providing agitation is sufficient	well distributed providing agitation is sufficient
Isolation	syringe filter	buchi filter, open to air, dried by passing air through the cake, and vacuum oven	buchi filter, open to air, dried by passing air through the cake then vacuum oven	nutch filter open to air, dried by passing air through the cake then vacuum oven. Some times possebility to use an inline filter to screen out solids	Pressure filter or centrifuge combined with a drier. Dried by applying vaccum or (hot) nitrogen through the cake. Some times possible to use in line filters (gaff bags, micron sized filters)
Inertion	none	by nitrogen or argon if required	by nitrogen or argon if required	by nitrogen if required	by nitrogen
Distillation	none	high refractionation through heat losses in overheads	high refractionation through heat losses through lid and overheads	high refractionation through heat losses through lid and overheads	low refractionation, minimum heat losses
Containment	fumehood	fumehood	fumehood	fumehood	plant
Risk processes	paper assessment + DSC	paper assessment + DSC & , adiabatic stability test as required	paper assessment + DSC & , adiabatic stability test as required	Full hazard assesment based on calorimetry, adiabatic and isothermal stability tests	Full hazard assesment based on calorimetry, adiabatic and isothermal stability tests. Plant compatibility check

between the liquid in the bed at the bottom and the bulk. If the 'just suspended speed', N_{js}, is exceeded particles no longer remain on the base, but the solid concentration will still be significantly higher near the bottom compared to the top. In concentrated slurries (>10 wt%) a clear interface can form between a dense solid suspension phase and a lighter clear liquid above it. In such systems mixing between the two layers can be very slow (Bujalski *et al.*, 1999).

So the presence of solids can result in severe inhomogeneity. In drug product manufacturing this leads to concentration variations of the formulated product (Dose CQA), whilst in drug substance manufacturing processes this can have a large impact on the reaction profile (impurity CQA).

10.1.4 Impact of Turbulence

Many S-L duties are dependent on the degree of turbulence, for example, mass transfer, deagglomeration and particle size reduction. For these it is often sufficient to keep either the tip speed (πND) or the power per unit volume (P/V) constant. This can be achieved over a wide range of processing scales. Clearly, changes in these duties, and scale-up using the wrong criteria can lead to significant changes in processing times (possibly impacting on the impurity CQA) and/or changes in particle size distribution (affecting the product dissolution CQA).

10.1.5 Impact of Heat Transfer

Heat transfer and heat loss are another classical example of an equipment capability that reduces on scale-up; this is no different for S-L systems: systems have less heat transfer area per unit volume at larger scales. There are two major consequences: (1) exothermic reactions need to be controlled, which is typically done by slowing addition rates on scale-up and (2) the maximum operating temperature is reduced to prevent thermal runaway reactions[1]. A consequence of the reduction in heat transfer with scale-up is that process times increase, which could lead to additional impurities through degradation or overreaction. Alternatively, some species may be supersaturated and given more time at large scale may nucleate, whereas this would not have occurred on a smaller scale. In both cases the impurity CQA may be affected.

Cooling crystallizations are often used as a final processing stage to control the polymorphic form of the drug substance. This is very important as both the drug stability and its successful delivery are strongly dependent on the polymorphic form.

On scale-up, the wall and batch temperature fluctuations may become larger, and as a result unstable polymorphic forms may nucleate, with a disastrous impact on the Form CQA.

10.2 Scale-Up of Operations Involving Solid Suspensions

10.2.1 The Nature of Suspensions

The manufacture of pharmaceutical intermediates, drug substances and drug products relies on mechanically agitated batch vessels. Often, solid-liquid systems will occur at some point in these manufacturing processes. Typical solid-liquid unit operations in the

[1] Large exothermic systems are close to adiabatic operation because thermal losses are low. If cooling fails, even an initially slow rate reaction could heat up the reactor; thus leading to reaction acceleration and eventually to "runaway", which can cause an unplanned disassembly event.

pharmaceutical industry are: charging solids to a liquid (for fine, hydroscopic, coarse, light, dense solids), homogenizing, dissolution, reaction and fermentation, crystallization, deagglomeration, particle size reduction and filtration.

The purpose of the solid in a process ranges from reagent, catalyst, to product or excipient. The key reason for processing suspensions is that it allows more concentrated processing; volumetric efficiency is much increased if solids can be used. Product concentrations during drug substance manufacture are typically 5–20 L solvent per kg starting material, or 50 to 200 gL^{-1}. In drug product processes this can be significantly higher, up to 500 gL^{-1}. In both cases the loading is well above the solubility limit (typically less than 20 gL^{-1}, but of course there are many examples where complete dissolution is obtained).

There are many words used to describe a solid-liquid dispersion, and the literature does not provide clear definitions as descriptions are used interchangeably. Here, we will use suspension as a general word to describe a solid-liquid dispersion. Alternatives in order of increasing concentration are dilute suspension, slurry and then paste. Suspensions can generally be categorized into two broad classes on the basis of their particle size:

- Type I represents a suspension of fine particles that are fairly uniformly distributed in the liquid with little separation occurring.
- Type II suspensions consist of coarse particles that tend to separate out. Though such a classification is evidently not very clear cut, as it is influenced by a number of other factors including solids loading, density difference and the nature of the flow field, it serves as a useful practical basis for classifying the general behaviour of solid-liquid suspensions.

Pharmaceutical particles are usually small; in drug substance processes fine (<30 μm) to coarse (<1 mm) particles are used. Drug product is typically micronized (<10 μm) and excipients range again between fine and coarse. The continuous phase (suspending fluid) tends to be a low viscosity Newtonian fluid in drug substance processes. In drug product processing, fluids with a non-Newtonian rheology are frequently encountered and the corresponding apparent viscosities can be high.

The solid particles discussed here may also be classified in two categories, (1) those with little particle-particle interaction, which are assumed to be stable in suspension and have little influence on the system rheology other than through the concentration effect; and (2) particles that have some form of interaction allowing them to form structures like flocs, weak agglomerates or strongly entangled systems that align under shear. Suspensions of this second category can often resist a certain amount of shear, but once disrupted require some time to rebuild. As a result, the rheology of type II slurries tend to exhibit a yield stress combined with a strongly time-dependent behaviour.

Pharmaceutical systems are thus in general of type I, although in some cases high density differences can lead to type II suspensions (e.g. caesium carbonate base in an organic solvent). Interaction between particles is uncommon; charged solids typically have little interaction, although static electricity may sometimes cause string agglomeration. If solids form during processing, then again, particles with little particle-particle interactions are desired, as these are easier to process. If during processing the solids generated do have strong interactions, rheology may become complex and processing issues often result. For instance, if uncontrolled crystallization occurs, particles with a high aspect ratio can 'spot weld' resulting a 3-D network of connected particles that can have a significant yield strength (Muller, 2009).

10.2.2 Scale-Up and Scale-Down Rules

As outlined in Table 10.1, during development a range of scales is covered. Most scale-up issues are addressed in order to manufacture drug substance and drug product for clinical trials. Equipment tends to be fixed; large scale laboratory and pilot plants are expensive and not easily reconfigured. Lab scale often geometrically mirrors the larger development scales. This does not hold true for the smallest of scales, typically <250 mL.

As a consequence, experimental information is usually obtainable in a geometrically relevant system. Experiments are carried out for many reasons and data for scale-up of mixing processes can usually be obtained from experiments that are also required for other reasons (e.g. chemistry development, stability trials, formulation tests).

Scale-up is based on the assumption that the *principle of similitude* is respected, that is, geometric, kinematic and dynamic similarity are satisfied (note that dynamic similarity implies geometric and kinematic similarity). In stirred vessels, however, the principle of similitude is usually violated due to a number of practical limitations. For instance, the size of the particles remains the same while the equipment is scaled up. When scale-up is done in the manufacturing facilities of outsource partners, it is not likely to have exact (or even approximate) geometrical similarity. There have certainly been examples of outsource companies using anchor agitators when implementing processes designed using pitch-blade, hydrofoil or retreat curve impellers. Even when the same agitator is used, it is not a given that exact geometric similarity is maintained. The blade thickness, impeller hub dimensions and even the actual surface roughness are usually not identical at plant, large scale laboratory and bench scales.

Scale-up of mixing in non-Newtonian fluids has its own added difficulties as the apparent viscosity is shear-dependent and may also be time-dependent. Thus, for example, changes in the apparent viscosity may shift the Reynolds number into the transitional or laminar flow regimes, which affects other dimensionless groups such as power number and flow number. For suspensions, the objective of scale-up is to determine the design and operating conditions necessary to ensure that the relevant CQAs are met at all scales, notwithstanding differences in geometry.

Assuming a reasonable degree of geometrical similarity, general scaling rules exist for most mixing problems, but quantitative correlations exist only for a subset of suspension mixing operations. A general scaling rule has been suggested (Zlokarnik, 1991; Tatterson, 1994):

$$ND^a = constant \tag{10.1}$$

When scaling up, the value of the parameter a changes depending on the nature of the *critical agitator duty*. This is the aspect of agitation that is most likely to impact a CQA. Figure 10.2 demonstrates this for a number of agitator duties. Starting with a 'large' pilot scale vessel, the agitator speed at smaller scales is calculated using scale-up rules with different values of a:

- Constant tip speed (ND)
- Constant power per unit volume ($ND^{2/3}$)
- Solids are just suspended, Zwietering criterion ($ND^{0.85}$)
- Constant circulation time (also constant mixing time) (ND^0 i.e. N).

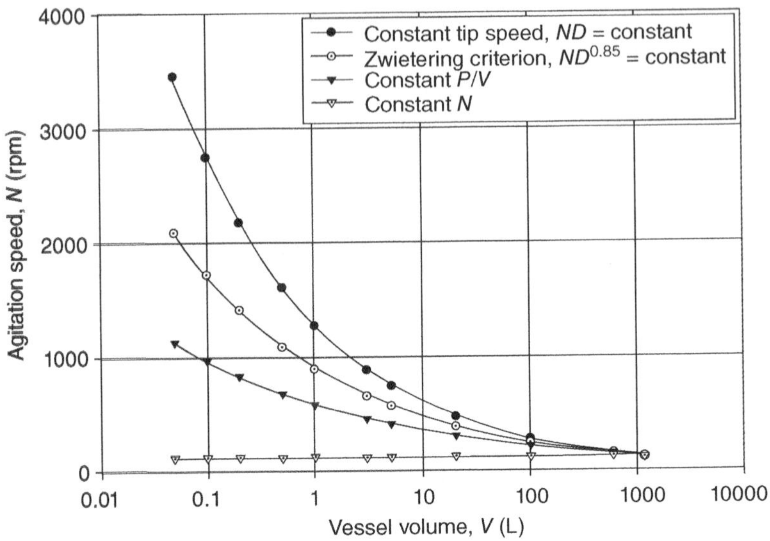

Figure 10.2 *Scale-down using different scale-up rules*

This last criterion should *never* be used for scale-down; turbulence will be so uncharacteristically low that basic mixing and heat transfer will not be sufficient at small scale.

It is clear that depending on the critical duty and relative scale, the agitation speed in the lab must be chosen with some care. In general, one should at least scale down using constant *P/V*. Using lower agitation rates leads to uncharacteristic turbulence behaviour on the small scale.

10.2.3 Identification of Agitator Duties

When discussing agitation problems with development teams it is often instructive to check '*why does the agitator need to be on?*'. The minimum speed at which the agitator is required to run is determined by the *duty* of the agitator. The duty of the agitator refers to the objective a particular process requires from the agitator. When developing processes there are many reasons to 'have the agitator on'. Typical agitator duties for solid-liquid systems are: (1) charging and homogenization, suspension and dispersion of particles; (2) heating and cooling of the system; (3) dissolution and mass transfer; (4) chemical reaction between the solid and liquid phases; (5) crystallization; (6) deagglomeration, particle size reduction or avoidance of this and (7) homogeneous discharge.

Note that within a single processing step the agitator can have a range of duties; for example, during a reaction mass transfer may be important, whilst near the end of the reaction the product may crystallize, and preventing the system from setting solid may be the key objective. For a formulation process, initially solid draw-down may be important, but when discharging homogeneity may be the key duty. All these duties do not necessarily scale up according to the same rule. A range of duties frequently encountered in development are described in Table 10.2 and their basic scale-up rules provided. These duties are described in more detail in later sections.

Table 10.2 *Common solid-liquid mixing duties and their scale-up rules (the scale-up rules are explained in more detail in subsequent sections)*

Duty	Scale-up rule	Experimental verification	Likely to be an issue when
Solid suspension	$N > N_{js}$, then $ND^{0.85}$ constant	Increase agitation speed until no solids remain at the bottom of the vessel	Vessel shape conical Large dense solids
Solid distribution homogenization	P/V constant	Increase agitation speed and note speed at which solids are distributed across the vessel	Clear layer is observed at the top of vessel
Blending in solid-liquid systems	No clear liquid on the surface, $N > N_{js}$, then P/V constant	Mixing time correlations hold only if solids are well distributed.Reduce H (suspension height) or add a second agitator to improve mixing	Fast reactions Solids do not reach the surface; clear liquid layer on top Solids not well suspended
Mass transfer	$N > N_{js}$, then P/V constant	Monitor time to equilibrium	Solubility of solid in the liquid is low Reaction could be mass transfer limited Mass transfer usually not limited in crystallizations as crystal growth is generally slow
Solid draw-down	P/V constant	Add solids fast, and observe draw-down from the surface is complete	When $\rho_p < \rho_L$, high surface tension, agglomeration, or solids that form gels at high concentration
Nucleation	Constant difference between the wall and bulk temperature	Use jacket temperature control to avoid large wall temperature fluctuations; accept slightly larger temperature difference on plant	Nucleation is very unpredictable Seeded crystallizations are preferred
Crystal growth	Constant cooling profile Constant addition time and at least P/V constant, but ideally N constant on scale-up (not on scale-down!!)	Apply ramp, start very slow and optimize from there	In all cases
Break up of structure Formation of structure/ solid networks	ND constant Rate of crystal formation and spot welding	Identify agitation rate at which slurry remains mobile Reduce cooling rate or hold times, seed or dilute	When slurry becomes immobile Uncontrolled crystallization, aspect ratio of crystals > 10
Attrition and size reduction	ND constant	Observe changes in particle size at high lab speed (900 rpm) and check with microscope; scale down plant speeds on constant ND	Particles at high agitation speeds High aspect ratio, thin plates and complex 3-D shapes are generally more fragile than cubes and rods
Vortex formation	Fully turbulent: N^2D constant Transitional: ND constant	Note speed at which vortex reaches the agitator	High P/V requirements in unbaffled systems

In order to establish what duty is most important and needs to be controlled by scale-up, a risk assessment of the process can help to identify what operations are most likely to impact on certain CQAs (Muller and Latimer, 2009). Pharmaceutical equipment tends to be multi-purpose as many potential products require manufacturing. Pharmaceutical process development is therefore focussed on two key mixing questions:

1. *Can I avoid a problem with respect to mixing sensitivity?*
   Often equipment at a range of scales is similar. So, if problems are identified in the laboratory before scale-up, then it is often easier to modify the process so as to make it more robust with respect to agitation. For instance, in the case of a solid suspension of Caesium Carbonate in DMF, suspension is likely to be an issue as $CsCO_3$ is very dense. By selecting a fine grade material and using a vessel with a pitched-blade or hydrofoil type impeller, a reasonable agitation speed will provide satisfactory solid suspension.
2. *Is the equipment right for the process?*
   If the process is in the later stages of development, process modifications are less desirable. In this case, it is important to check that the equipment selected for manufacture is suitable for the process. If, for example, an outsource company comes back and indicates that it wants to run this process in a vessel with an anchor agitator, whereas the lab work was all done with a retreat curve impeller, the outsource team may then ask this question. A simple calculation should suffice to indicate that this is not suitable, and a vessel with a more appropriate agitator should be selected.

Note that this is different from conventional engineering which tends to be focused on agitator selection and design. It is noteworthy that virtually all of the knowledge and correlations for the various S-L duties stem from chemical engineering research. Pharmaceutical materials have not been used in the vast majority of published works. In particular, suspensions of solids in a non-Newtonian continuous phase have received little attention. However, usually most of the established correlations and rules of thumb can be applied as a first approximation for the design of pharmaceutical mixing operations.

It is often advisable to use experimentation and pilot scale tests and then apply established scale-up rules. The usual assumption in pharmaceutical development teams is that experimental work in the lab on the 'real' system is easy to do, and that the agitators, vessels, baffling are similar at laboratory and manufacturing scales. In such circumstances, one can scale down the plant operation using scaling rules, and then experimentally verify in the laboratory whether a particular duty is critical or not. If the duty is critical, either the process or the agitation can be changed. As stated previously, early in development, it is often judged best to change the process (i.e. avoid the problem), but in later development, it may become necessary to optimize the mixing (i.e. minimize the impact).

10.2.4 Solid-Liquid Unit Operations

It is usually easier to identify a critical operation first, and then evaluate the duties to determine the likelihood they are critical. Typical solid-liquid mixing operations in pharmaceutical processing include charging and homogenization, solid dissolution, and cooling or antisolvent crystallization. The key solid-liquid mixing duties for these operations are identified in Table 10.3.

Table 10.3 Typical solid liquid operations and their relevant duties

Operation	Duty
Solid charging, homogenization, particle size reduction	Addition rate Vortex formation Solid draw-down Solid suspension Solid distribution Break up of structure (see also yield stress) Attrition and deagglomeration
Solid dissolution, reaction, fermentation	Solid suspension Solid distribution Mass transfer Solid draw-down
Cooling or antisolvent crystallization	Heat transfer Solid suspension Solid distribution Mass transfer Nucleation Crystal growth Attrition Formation and break up of structure (see also yield stress)

10.3 General Principles of Solid-Liquid Suspensions

10.3.1 Rheological Behaviour of the Continuous Phase

In pharmaceutical processing, the continuous phase can often be approximated by the Newtonian model:

$$\tau = \mu\dot{\gamma} \tag{10.2}$$

where τ is shear stress, $\dot{\gamma}$ is shear rate and the proportionality constant μ is the Newtonian viscosity, which is independent of both shear rate and (theoretically) time. Many real fluids including gases and low viscosity liquids exhibit Newtonian behaviour over a wide and important range of shear stress, for example, water, solvents and solutions of low-molecular-weight liquids. However, for drug product processes the continuous phase may consist of polymer solutions or concentrated surfactant solutions that display non-Newtonian behaviour. The internal structure of the continuous phase is then such that the viscosity depends on the rate at which the fluid is sheared and may also depend on the duration of shearing. An apparent viscosity, η, which may vary with time and shear rate is defined for these fluids as:

$$\eta = \tau/\dot{\gamma} \tag{10.3}$$

Non-Newtonian fluids may be classed as time-independent or time-dependent.

10.3.1.1 Time-Independent Rheology

In this case, the viscosity is only a function of shear rate. There are three sub-categories:

1. *Shear-thinning or pseudoplastic:* this is the most common type of time-independent non-Newtonian behaviour. The flow curve of this type of fluid typically shows two end-regions of Newtonian behaviour in which the viscosity is almost constant and a middle region of decreasing, shear-thinning viscosity. Commonly, the shear-thinning region spans several decades of shear rate and is often described by the power-law model because of its simplicity:

$$\tau = k\dot{\gamma}^n \tag{10.4}$$

   where k is the consistency index and n is the power-law or flow behaviour index. The model is used to describe the widely familiar shear-thinning fluids with $n < 1$, such as polymer solutions, concentrated surfactant solutions and creams. Other rheological models can be used that are more accurate but at the expense of more complexity.
2. *Shear-thickening or dilatant:* typically, the flow curve of a shear-thickening suspension of particles exhibits some shear-thinning at low shear rates. At higher shear rates, the deformation of this type of fluid causes rearrangement of its microstructure leading to an increase in viscosity as the shear rate is increased. These are much less common than shear-thinning fluids, but most concentrated suspensions of non-aggregating solid particles show some shear-thickening behaviour given the correct conditions, for example, concentrated suspensions of drug substance. Over the shear-thickening region, the behaviour can be represented by equation (10.4) but with $n > 1$.
3. *Viscoplastic*: this type of fluid appears to require an apparent yield shear stress, τ_y, which has to be exceeded before flow takes place; that is, it has a sufficiently rigid solid-like structure that can resist any stress less than the yield stress and no motion appears to occur. At stresses above τ_y, the structure of the material disintegrates and the fluid flows. Examples frequently encountered in the pharmaceutical industry are gels, polymer solutions/mixtures, concentrated slurries and slurries of particles that have weak or strong particle-particle interactions like in some crystallizing systems.

Yield stress is postulated as the result of the formation of a structure or network formed by particles or molecules that have strong inter-particular interactions (e.g. entangled polymers, crystallising solids that spot weld together, surfactants that form 3-D lamellae). The yield stress of a fluid is associated with the stress required to be able to break (some of) the networks bonds. Note that after a bond is broken, it may take time to build back up (a diffusional process); as a result, most yield stress fluids also tend to have time-dependent behaviour. In some cases, the bond formation is very rapid (e.g. polymers) and the time scale is much smaller than the time scale of disruption, which is typically the circulation time in a stirred vessel. In such cases, the fluid behaves as a 'true' reversible time-independent yield stress fluid.

Though the concept of apparent yield stress is useful in engineering applications, its existence is regarded by some as dubious (Barnes *et al.*, 1989). Viscometric measurements often cannot be made at sufficiently low shear rates to determine whether a yield stress exists, or whether there is extreme shear-thinning behaviour and a very large zero-shear viscosity in the limit as $\dot{\gamma} \to 0$.

For this type of fluid, the Bingham plastic and the Herschel–Bulkley models are the most popular:

1. *Bingham plastic model* – the constitutive equation for a Bingham plastic fluid is:

$$\begin{aligned} \tau &= \tau_y + \eta_B \dot{\gamma} \quad & \tau > \tau_y \\ \dot{\gamma} &= 0 & \tau < \tau_y \end{aligned} \tag{11.5}$$

   where the constant η_B is known as the plastic viscosity. The Bingham fluid, mathematically, appears to flow as a Newtonian fluid under an applied stress τ - τ_y.
2. *Herschel–Bulkley model* – this is also called the generalized power-law model as it represents power-law behaviour with an apparent yield stress, that is,

$$\begin{aligned} \tau &= \tau_y + k\dot{\gamma}^n \quad & \tau > \tau_y \\ \dot{\gamma} &= 0 & \tau < \tau_y \end{aligned} \tag{10.6}$$

The model can also be regarded as a generalization of the Bingham model to include the non-linear flow curve. It is interesting to note that a viscoplastic fluid exhibits an apparent viscosity that decreases with increasing shear rate. One could therefore regard these materials as possessing a particular type of shear-thinning behaviour.

10.3.1.2 Time-Dependent Rheology

In these systems, the viscosity depends not only on the magnitude of the applied shear rate but also on the time the shearing has been applied. These fluids may be subdivided into two classes according to whether the apparent viscosity (or corresponding shear stress) decreases or increases with time when the fluid is sheared at a constant rate. Both phenomena may be reversible, partially reversible, or irreversible.

1. *Thixotropic behaviour:* this is reversible time-dependent thinning. Examples include Gelucire mixtures (Ratsimbazafy *et al.*, 1999) and crystallising systems (Muller, 2009). The viscosity decreases with time of shearing as a result of breakdown of structures within the fluid, but the product regains its structural characteristics after shearing has ceased as the structure reforms (sometimes structural recovery is obtained only after the material has rested for a sufficient time free from stress). However, with a number of fluids the structure is irreversibly broken down, and this phenomenon is called rheomalaxis or rheodestruction; crystallizing systems are an example of such a system.
   As described in the previous Section 10.3.1.1, many viscoplastic or yield stress fluids also display time-dependent behaviour. For some systems, however, the timescale of reforming the structure bonds is so short that for the purpose of agitation and mixing the rheology may be considered time-independent (e.g. some polymer solutions such as Carbopol).
2. *Rheopectic behaviour:* this is reversible time-dependent thickening. Rheopexy (or negative thixotropy) can be obtained with shear-thickening fluids where the apparent viscosity (or corresponding shear stress) increases with the duration of deformation, that is, there is a gradual development of structure by shear with time. This is a rare phenomenon, but it has been observed in highly-concentrated starch pastes, protein solutions, coal-water slurries as well as in some Gelucire-drug mixtures (Ratsimbazafy *et al.*, 1999).

There are no simple mathematical models of general validity to predict time-dependent rheological behaviour. It is usually necessary to make measurements over the required range of conditions. Flow curves are of limited utility unless they correspond to the particular history of interest in the application.

10.3.1.3 Viscoelastic Fluids

Complex, structured fluids, behave neither as pure viscous liquids nor as pure elastic solids, that is, they simultaneously show viscous and elastic behaviour and, hence, in the absence of the time-dependent behaviour discussed earlier, are known as viscoelastic fluids. Many polymeric liquids deform in this way; their long chain molecules interact, forming chemical or physical cross-links, so that a deformation of one part of the fluid is transmitted to all other entangled chains, that is, the fluid shows some elastic properties. These interactions can give rise to elasticity within the polymer network, large elongational viscosities and normal stress differences, as well as shear-thinning behaviour. Some substances are predominantly liquid, for example polymer melts, gels, hydrocolloid dispersions; and some are predominantly solid, for example glassy crystalline polymers.

10.3.2 Rheology of Suspensions

10.3.2.1 Suspensions with Low Concentration of Non-Interacting Inert Particles

Fine particles tend to form reasonably homogeneous suspensions and are usually treated as such. The apparent slurry viscosity of inert particles may be empirically described as a function of solid content (Gay *et al.*, 1969; Borghesani, 1985; Heymann *et al.*, 2002):

$$\eta_{slurry} = \frac{\eta(\theta)_{solvent}}{\left(1-\left(\frac{\varphi}{\varphi_{crit}}\right)^{a}\right)^{b}} \tag{10.7}$$

Here, $\eta(\theta)_{solvent}$ represents the apparent solvent viscosity (a function of temperature θ), φ the volume fraction of the solid phase and φ_{crit} the critical or maximum solid volume fraction the liquid can contain. For instance, the values $a = 2$ and $b = 1$ were used to successfully describe concentrated slurries of glass ballotini, as displayed in Figure 10.3 (Muller, unpublished industrial work). The data show that for (non-interacting) suspensions of ballotini no significant increase in viscosity is expected at solid concentrations below 20 vol%. Most pharmaceutical drug substance processes and many formulation processes fall into this category. Clearly, when a system displays a complex rheology at low solid concentrations, the particles must interact in a way different to that described by equation (10.7).

10.3.2.2 Suspensions with High Concentration of Non-Interacting Inert Particles

At high solid concentrations, particles under normal agitation conditions have low settling velocities compared to the liquid flow velocities. Under conditions of turbulent flow, particles are maintained in suspension by the eddies in the liquid. Such conditions tend to prevail in

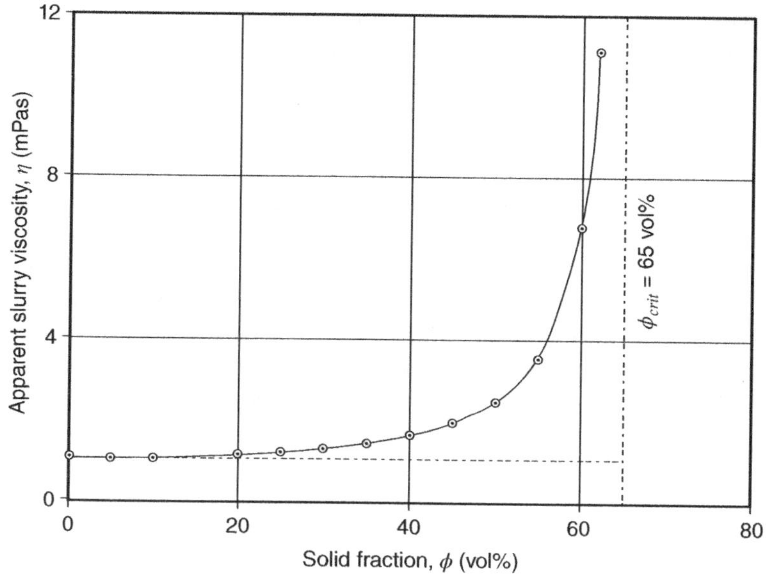

Figure 10.3 *Typical effect of solid concentration on viscosity in a slurry of non-interacting particles (glass ballotini)*

practice unless the suspension becomes viscous at solid concentrations significantly larger than 20 vol%.

Concentrated suspensions often tend to exhibit a non-Newtonian behaviour, and they behave essentially like single-phase pseudoplastic fluids. Existing models for describing these pseudo-homogeneous systems apply the concept of effective or average density and viscosity. Amongst the situations where non-Newtonian behaviour is most important is the suspension of polydisperse slurries. As the concentration of solids increases, the suspension more and more takes on the character of a shear-thinning (pseudoplastic) fluid caused by the presence of a large amount of fine particles. Such a behaviour can often be described by the power-law model (equation 10.4). Typically, the suspension first becomes moderately shear-thinning and as the concentration increases, this behaviour is enhanced, that is, the consistency index k steadily increases reflecting an increase in viscosity and the power-law index n is reduced showing further departure from Newtonian behaviour.

Above a certain concentration, the suspension becomes viscoplastic, that is, n becomes so small (typically at $n < 0.2$) that it appears the fluid exhibits an apparent yield stress like a Bingham plastic (equation 10.5) or Herschel–Bulkley fluid (equation 10.6). Then both k and τ_y increase further with increasing solids concentration. In certain cases, highly concentrated pastes may exhibit dilatant behaviour. Such systems are not common in drug substance manufacture, but could occur during formulation.

10.3.2.3 Suspensions with Particle–Particle Interactions

Where particles can interact with each other, a major impact on the suspension rheology can result. Interactions can be through entanglement (fibres), spotwelding (in crystallizing systems), charge (clay) or van der- Waals interactions (flocs). These systems exhibit non-Newtonian behaviour, which is time-dependent. Depending on the nature of the interaction, the rheology is either reversible as particle-particle interactions reform in areas of low turbulence (e.g. interactions based on electrostatic and van der Waals forces), or irreversible if the interactions cannot be reinstated (e.g. deagglomeration, breakage of solid contact points between particles).

These systems can exhibit an apparent yield stress or display other forms of non-Newtonian behaviour at solid concentrations much below 20 vol%. Møller *et al.* (2006) described systems of reversibly interacting particulates (avalanches), and Muller (2009) applied a similar analysis to model the rheology of irreversible interactions.

In these highly non-Newtonian and time-dependent systems, the average centre point distance between two particles must be less than the length of the particles, so that particles can overlap and form a structure that can bridge the whole of the system volume. Muller (2009) derived a simple rule for needle shaped particles:

$$\frac{\ell_p}{d_p} \geq \sqrt{1/\varphi} \tag{10.8}$$

where d_p is the average of the width and depth of the needle and ℓ_p is its length. If the aspect ratio of the needles is more than 10, a 1 vol% dispersion could potentially form a structure that could significantly affect suspension rheology.

To form a significant structure, the particles need to interact. Figure 10.4 illustrates two possible forms of interaction. If the particles form dense agglomerates or flocs, the aspect ratio of the new super particle will typically be smaller, and thus a larger volume of solid is required before rheology is dramatically affected. If, however, the particles remain randomly dispersed through the continuous phase, structures can be formed that potentially change the fluid into a soft solid (yield stress behaviour). Note if the agglomerates are one or two-dimensional structures (e.g. strings or sheets) their aspect ratio is still high and significant changes in rheology may still be expected.

The strength of the structure formed is dependent on the concentration of connection points between the particles. Concentrated systems and particles with high aspect ratios have more contact points per volume, and thus in any given plane. In order to shear a given plane, these junctions need to be broken. Therefore, if the number concentration of junctions in the fluid is C_j (number/m^3), the shear stress that structure can withstand is proportional

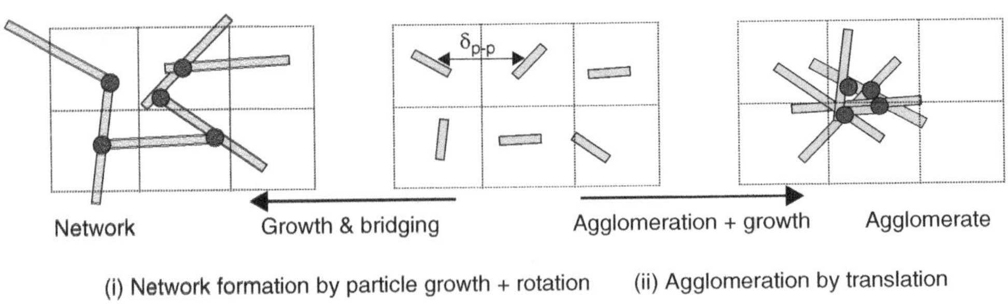

Figure 10.4 *Structure formation from seed crystals*

to the number of junctions in a plane (number/m^2) that equals $C_j^{2/3}$. The force per unit area required to break these junctions is the structure yield stress τ_y, which can be expressed as:

$$\tau_y = C_j^{2/3} \tau_j \tag{10.9}$$

in terms of τ_j, the average force required to break a single junction. The time-dependent aspects of these systems were reviewed by Møller *et al.* (2006) who modelled the dependence of the parameters in a rheological model $\left(\tau = f(\dot{\gamma})\right)$ on a structure parameter like the concentration of junctions C_j:

$$\tau = \tau_y(C_j) - \dot{\gamma}\eta(C_j, \dot{\gamma}) \tag{10.10}$$

$$\frac{\partial C_j}{\partial t} = f(C_j, \dot{\gamma}) - g(C_j, \dot{\gamma}) \tag{10.11}$$

where t is time and η is apparent viscosity. This model was successfully used to describe avalanches, but has not found widespread application in the description of complex rheologies in agitated vessels.

10.3.3 Terminal Velocity of Particles

A particle with a density different from that of the fluid will travel at a velocity u relative to the fluid, known as slip velocity. A number of quantities are defined on the basis of the slip velocity such as particle Reynolds number and drag coefficient, as discussed next. Such a velocity, therefore, is needed for hydrodynamics as well as mass/heat transport calculations. In a mechanically agitated suspension, the definition of slip velocity can be further complicated by the possible superimposition of other components of motion, namely rotation of the particle about its centre and turbulent fluctuations of the particle in complex situations of turbulence. In a stirred suspension, u will be a function of particle size and will vary from point to point. Attempts to measure it or estimate it on the basis of Kolmogorov's theory have predominantly been unsuccessful. Recently, however, using positron emission particle tracking (PEPT), estimations of local time-averaged particle slip velocities have been obtained by tracking the solid and liquid phases separately, one at a time, and determining their local velocities (Barigou, 2004; Barigou *et al.*, 2009; Guida *et al.*, 2009).

In practice, however, it has been customary in stirred vessels to take the free terminal settling velocity of the particle, u_∞, as a representative of its mean slip velocity. This assumption, albeit crude, seems for example to give reasonable mass transfer predictions at N_{js}, but not above it (Nienow, 2000).

The settling tendency of the particles has a dominating influence on the behaviour of the suspension in processing equipment, and u_∞ has been used to classify suspension problems as illustrated in Table 10.4. The particle settling velocity is, thus, an important parameter and as such deserves some attention.

When a solid particle settles under gravity in a stationary fluid, it undergoes an initial acceleration after which it attains its constant terminal settling velocity, u_∞.. The terminal velocity is approached very rapidly in Newtonian and power-law fluids. For example, a particle settling in creeping flow will reach u_∞ after a distance equivalent to only a few

Table 10.4 *Illustration of power requirement for different suspension criteria and settling velocities (adapted from Oldshue, 1983)*

	Power ratio		
	$u_\infty = 0.51–3.05$ mms^{-1}	$u_\infty = 20.3–40.6$ mms^{-1}	$u_\infty = 81.3–305$ mms^{-1}
State of suspension	Easy problem	Moderate problem	Difficult problem
Complete particle motion	1	1	1
Complete off-bottom suspension	2	3	5
Homogeneous suspension	4	9	25

particle diameters. When a particle in a fluid is in relative motion to it, the *drag* is defined as that component of the resultant force acting on the particle in the direction of the relative motion. The total (or profile) drag force acting on a particle in a fluid is made up of two contributions: the *form* (or *pressure*) drag, arising from the non-uniform pressure distribution on the particle, and the *skin friction* (or *viscous*) drag, the force on the particle due to the fluid shear stress at the surface. The total drag force F on a particle is made dimensionless by use of the drag coefficient C_D defined as:

$$C_D = \frac{F}{\frac{1}{2}\rho_L u^2 A} \tag{10.12}$$

where A is the area of the particle's projection on a plane normal to the direction of relative motion, and ρ_L is the fluid density. For a spherical particle, A is the area of the circle having the sphere diameter d_p and hence the following equation results:

$$F = C_D\left(\frac{1}{2}\rho_L u^2\right)\left(\frac{\pi d_p^2}{4}\right) \tag{10.13}$$

The velocity of a particle settling in a gravitational field will increase until the drag force becomes equal to the apparent weight of the particle (particle weight – buoyancy force), that is for a sphere:

$$F = \left(\frac{\pi d_p^3}{6}\right)(\rho_p - \rho_L)g = C_D\left(\frac{1}{2}\rho_L u^2\right)\left(\frac{\pi d_p^2}{4}\right) \tag{10.14}$$

where ρ_p is the particle density. For a sphere settling in creeping flow in a Newtonian liquid (i.e. $Re_p \leq 0.2$), Stokes law using equation (10.17) below leads to the following equation:

$$u_\infty = \frac{g d_p^2(\rho_p - \rho_L)}{18\mu} \tag{10.15}$$

For systems at higher Reynolds numbers where C_D is a strong function of Re_p, as well as non-Newtonian fluids, an iterative procedure is usually required to solve equation (10.14). The sections that follow review the drag coefficient for different liquid phase rheologies.

10.3.3.1 Drag on a Sphere in a Newtonian Fluid

Both contributions to the profile drag can be calculated if the pressure and shear stress distributions around the particle are known. The shear stress and pressure distributions can, in principle, be derived by solving the continuity and momentum equations. General solutions do not exist, however, and numerical solutions are often sought even at low Reynolds numbers. A detailed treatment of this subject for Newtonian fluids can be found in Clift *et al.* (1978), and for non-Newtonian fluids in Lareo *et al.* (1997) and Chhabra (2006). The following sections, however, give a summary of the main results.

In general, both skin friction and form drag depend on the particle Reynolds number defined as:

$$Re_p = \frac{\rho_L u d_p}{\mu} \tag{10.16}$$

Therefore, C_D is a function of Re_p, but also depends on factors such as particle shape and surface roughness, the turbulence in the fluid, and the acceleration of the fluid relative to the particle.

For a sphere moving in creeping flow, that is, $Re_p \leq 0.2$, the well-known Stokes law $(F = 3\pi\mu d_p u)$ and equation (10.13) lead to the following relationship, a different form of Stokes law:

$$C_D = \frac{24}{Re_p} \tag{10.17}$$

More generalized theoretical treatments are in general difficult, and it is usually necessary to rely on experimental data. Such data for drag are most conveniently represented in graphical form by plotting C_D versus Re_p. The drag curve for a rigid sphere is called the *standard drag curve*. It should be noted that in stirred vessels, C_D for large particles ($d_p >$ ~1.5 mm) is higher than shown by the standard drag curve due to the high level of turbulence, so a value of 1.0 instead of 0.44 should be used in the Newton's flow region (i.e. ~ $1000 < Re_p < 2 \times 10^5$), (Nienow, 2000).

Many other empirical expressions, often highly complex, have been suggested for C_D throughout the standard drag curve. These have been reviewed and critically evaluated by Clift *et al.* (1978).

10.3.3.2 Drag on a Sphere in Power-Law Fluids

These fluids are described by equation (10.4) and a simple dimensional analysis would show that for such fluids:

$$C_D = f(Re_p, n) \tag{10.18}$$

Thus, C_D is a function of the power-law index n and the corresponding particle Reynolds number is now defined as follows:

$$Re_p = \frac{\rho_L u^{2-n} d_p^n}{k} \tag{10.19}$$

For a power-law fluid in creeping flow, the drag coefficient can be expressed in terms of Stokes law (equation 10.17) using a correction factor $Z(n)$:

$$C_D = \frac{24}{Re_p} Z(n) \tag{10.20}$$

The numerical values of $Z(n)$ have been reported by Chhabra and Richardson (1999) for both shear-thinning and shear-thickening behaviour. The data show that shear-thinning increases drag whereas shear-thickening reduces it. Experimental results and numerical simulations indicate that creeping flow in shear-thinning liquids occurs up to $Re_p \sim 1.0$. For shear-thickening liquids creeping flow occurs up to $Re_p \sim 0.2–0.5$.

Experimental results are available in the literature for Re_p values up to 1000 and $0.38 \leq n \leq 1$ (Chhabra, 1990). It is found that the standard drag curve for Newtonian liquids adequately correlates the results in power-law liquids in the region $1 \leq Re_p \leq 1000$ within ±30%. The impact of Non-Newtonian behaviour also diminishes with increasing Re_p and predictions using the standard drag curve improve accordingly.

Numerical predictions of the drag coefficient of a sphere in a power-law liquid are available up to $Re_p = 130$, with a maximum error of 10% using the following expressions for shear-thinning liquids developed by Graham and Jones (1994):

$$C_D = \frac{35.2(2)^n}{Re_p^{1.03}} + n\left(1 - \frac{20.9(2)^n}{Re^{1.11}}\right) \quad 0.2(2)^n \leq Re_p \leq 24(2)^n \tag{10.21}$$

$$C_D = \frac{37(2)^n}{Re_p^{1.1}} + 0.25 + 0.36n \quad 24(2)^n \leq Re_p \leq 100(2)^n \tag{10.22}$$

10.3.3.3 Drag on a Sphere in Viscoplastic Fluids

Bingham Plastic Fluid. Numerical finite-element simulations of a sphere in creeping flow in a Bingham plastic liquid (equation 10.5) have suggested the use of a correction factor such that (Lareo *et al.*, 1997):

$$C_D = \frac{24}{Re_B} Z \tag{10.23}$$

in which Re_B is the Bingham–Reynolds number $\left(Re_B = \frac{\rho_L u d_p}{\eta_B}\right)$, and Z is a function of the Bingham number $Bi = \frac{\tau_y d_p}{\eta_B u}$, thus:

$$Z = 1 + a(Bi)^b \tag{10.24}$$

where $a = 2.93, b = 0.83$ for *Bi* values up to 1000. Note that as *Bi* decreases, *Z* tends to 1 (i.e. Newtonian flow). The higher drag ($Z > 1$) in a viscoplastic medium is due to the combined effects of viscosity and yield stress. The criterion for creeping flow in viscoplastic liquids is found to be the Bingham Reynolds number, the upper limit for which is as follows:

$$Re_{Bmax} \approx 100Bi^{0.4} \tag{10.25}$$

Thus, the greater *Bi* (i.e. the greater τ_y) the higher the upper Bingham Reynolds number for creeping flow.

Herschel–Bulkley Fluid. For these fluids (equation 10.6), the following semi-empirical correlation has been proposed for C_D (Atapattu *et al.*, 1995):

$$C_D = \frac{24}{Re_p}(1 + Bi^*) \tag{10.26}$$

where Bi^* is the modified Bingham number $Bi^* = \tau_y / k\left(\frac{u}{d_p}\right)^n$. This correlation covers the ranges of values $10^{-5} \leq Re_p \leq 0.36$, $0.25 \leq Bi^* \leq 280$, and $0.43 \leq n \leq 0.84$.

Beyond creeping flow, drag data are reasonably well represented by the standard drag curve for Newtonian liquids. Thus, the non-Newtonian effects seem to be much more important at low Re_p values and they gradually diminish as inertial effects become more and more significant.

10.3.3.4 Effects of Particle Shape on Terminal Settling Velocity and Drag

Drag on particles is strongly influenced by their shape and orientation to the flow, which must be specified before the drag force can be estimated. In consequence, the drag force on non-spherical particles is much more difficult to determine than for spheres, and often the effect of shape on particle settling must be determined experimentally. Experimental data for non-spherical particles are presented in the same way as for a sphere, that is, in the form of a drag curve representing $\log(C_D)$ *versus* $\log(Re_p)$. The particle Reynolds number for a non-spherical particle is based on the diameter of an equivalent sphere having the same volume. A different curve is obtained for each particle shape and for each orientation. For Newtonian liquids, data exist in the literature for a number of different shapes, for example cylinders, plates, discs and so on (Clift *et al.*, 1978).

Spheroidal particles (oblates and prolates) have been studied in pseudoplastic and dilatant liquids for Reynolds numbers up to 100 over the range ($0.4 \leq n \leq 1.8$). For a given Reynolds number and aspect ratio (minor/major axis), the drag on an oblate particle is less than on a sphere of equal volume, whereas it is higher for a prolate particle. A summary of the relevant literature is given by Lareo *et al.* (1997) and Chhabra and Richardson (1999).

As observed for a sphere, in the creeping flow regime, the drag on a non-spherical particle in shear-thinning liquids is higher than in Newtonian liquids under otherwise identical conditions. As Re_p increases, the shear thinning effect (i.e. the n effect) diminishes. In dilatant liquids, the drag is lower than in Newtonian liquids. Results concerning other particle shapes (cylinders, rectangular prisms, discs and cones) settling at their terminal velocity in power-law media have been published, but no general correlation has emerged. There is at present rather a paucity of data concerning the drag on non-spherical particles in viscoplastic and viscoelastic liquids.

The problem discussed here relates to the motion of a single isolated particle in an effectively infinite medium. The boundaries of the fluid container in which the particle is settling will also affect its terminal velocity. Moreover, to characterize a multiple particle system, single particle behaviour must be understood, but most solid-liquid suspensions are of such a high solid fraction that single particle data are not usually sufficient. Such details are beyond the scope of this chapter and the reader is referred to more specialized publications such as Lareo *et al.* (1997) and Chhabra (2006).

10.3.4 Turbulence

Power dissipation per unit volume in a turbulent system is one or two orders of magnitude larger than for laminar flow. Energy dissipation, however, still occurs by viscous forces, so in turbulent systems the volume-averaged shear rate is significantly higher than the shear rate in a laminar system. How does turbulence manage that?

In turbulent systems, fluid flow does not follow well-defined streamlines. On a micro-scale, a turbulent system can be viewed as an ensemble of eddies or vortices (with a finite length and diameter) dispersed through a 'continuous' liquid phase. The vortices move in a manner similar to gas molecules (random, but with an average direction and speed). Unlike gas molecules, however, the eddies can have a range of sizes so that small eddies may reside in (much) larger eddies, as well as in the 'continuous phase' of these larger eddies. The 'continuous phase' of an eddy refers to the volume of liquid in which eddies of similar size do not occur. This vision of turbulence was captured in a poem by L.F. Richardson (1922, a famous meteorologist) in 'The supply of energy from and to atmospheric eddies'[2]:

'Big whorls have little whorls
that feed on their velocity,
and little whorls have lesser whorls
and so on to viscosity.'

10.3.4.1 Generation and Dissipation of Turbulence

The three-dimensional flow field inside a mechanically agitated vessel displays complex features depending on the mixer configuration used and the physical properties of the phases involved. The regime of flow is determined by the impeller Reynolds number $\left(Re = \dfrac{\rho_L N D^2}{\mu}\right)$. Even when the flow field is fully turbulent (i.e. $Re > 2 \times 10^4$) the spatial

[2]The rhyme is a play on a famous Jonathan Swift poem on fleas and the parody of Swift by Augustus De Morgan: 'A Budget of Paradoxes.'

distribution of the local energy dissipation and turbulent shear rates is highly non-uniform. Energy dissipation is highest in the impeller flow region, being an order of magnitude greater than the mean value in the tank and consequently much lower in the bulk circulation region.

Turbulence is generated by the agitator and behind the impeller blades there are trailing vortices. These are generally not random and they do introduce the circular fluid motion from which other eddies result. The bulk fluid motion generated by the agitator also interacts with the wall baffles resulting in turbulent motion. It is worth noting that baffles increase power dissipation by a factor of 2–10.

Once formed, an eddy starts to lose energy, a little through viscous dissipation, but the majority due to the generation of new smaller eddies, which themselves dissipate energy due to the formation of even smaller eddies and so on. However, the smaller the eddy, the larger the area exposed to the continuous phase in which it moves, and the greater the viscous forces on it. So finally, the eddies reach a size so small that viscous dissipation becomes large compared to the energy contained in the spinning liquid. Such an eddy is called a Kolmogorov eddy, which stops spinning a short while after it is formed and becomes part of the continuous phase. This smallest scale of turbulence, or smallest eddy size, is characterized by the Kolmogorov length (Kolmogorov, 1941a,b). Associated with this smallest length scale are also the timescale over which this eddy decays, and the small scale velocity fluctuations that result from this kind of eddies. Table 10.5 provides the definition of the Kolmogorov scales as well as an example of typical values in water.

10.3.4.2 Turbulent Velocities

The turbulent eddy structure described causes the local fluid velocity in the vessel to fluctuate strongly in both magnitude and direction. An estimate of the root-mean-square (rms) velocity fluctuations near a drop in a turbulent field was first derived by Kolmogorov (1941a,b) and Hinze (1955). The velocity fluctuations relevant to a particle of size d_p were assumed to be dependent only on eddies of equal size or smaller than the particle. The rms velocity fluctuations near the particle may be approximated by:

$$u' = (\varepsilon d_p)^{1/3} \propto Po^{1/3} \frac{D}{T} d_p^{1/3} N D^{2/3} \tag{10.27}$$

in which $\varepsilon = P/\rho V$ is the local rate of energy dissipation or power dissipation per unit mass. For geometrically similar systems, the velocity fluctuations can be shown, by using the power number *Po*, to scale with tip speed (i.e. *ND*). Typically, the particle size d_p remains constant on scale-up, in which case a constant power per unit volume is required to keep the velocity fluctuations near the particle the same. As the local velocities near the surface

Table 10.5 *Definition of Kolmogorov scales and typical values in turbulent water*

Local rate of energy dissipation ε (Wkg^{-1})	0.01	0.1	0.5	1	20
Kolmogorov length scale $\lambda = (\nu^3/\varepsilon)^{1/4}$ (μm)	100	56	38	32	15
Kolmogorov time scale $\tau_\lambda = (\nu^3/\varepsilon)^{1/4}$ (ms)	10	3.2	1.4	1.0	0.224
Kolmogorov velocity scale $u = (\nu\varepsilon)^{1/4}$ (ms^{-1})	0.01	0.02	0.03	0.03	0.07

of a particle enhance heat and mass transfer, but also cause attrition and deagglomeration, it follows that to ensure these parameters remain constant on scale-up, constant P/V is the correct scale-up rule.

10.3.4.3 Turbulent Rate Processes

Many processes depend on either the formation of eddies (e.g. blending) or the interaction of eddies with an object (e.g. vessel wall, disperse phase). We have already seen that the rate of eddy formation is proportional to power input, and thus power dissipation in the system. The rate of a process in which two objects interact is normally proportional to the concentration of the two objects. It is thus important to understand the 'concentration' of eddies, and how that changes with power input.

As the smallest eddies all have the same rate of decay determined by viscosity, to dissipate more energy requires proportionally more eddies. Although it does not necessarily follow that this is also the case for larger eddies, in general, rate processes can be assumed to depend on power dissipation. Note that for a process requiring very high power dissipation (i.e. more than the average ε in the vessel) the effective volume in which that process occurs will only be a small fraction of the total vessel volume. Typically the impeller region, or even specific locations within that region like the trailing vortices, is the only place where the power dissipation is high enough for some processes. Consequently, in order to process the bulk of the fluid, it may need to pass many times through the impeller region before steady state is achieved.

10.3.4.4 Turbulent Forces on Particles

In general, the impact of fluid motion on a particle is studied by evaluating the forces acting on the particle. These forces can be either 'disruptive', trying to pull the particle apart, or cohesive, trying to keep the particle together and are generally expressed as a pressure or shear force.

The shear force is a disruptive force exerted by the continuous phase on the dispersed phase and is proportional to μN; e.g. the force exerted by the continuous phase as it moves. This force will act on the whole particle. The maximum shear rate in a system is near the edge of the impeller blades and may be assumed proportional to N (Metzner and Otto, 1957).

In turbulent systems, velocity fluctuations generate pressure fluctuations in the continuous phase (Bernoulli's law) that can interact with surfaces and particles that are in close proximity to the eddy. The local velocity fluctuations result in disruptive forces on the particle and may lead to breakage of fluid drops, and deagglomeration and even attrition of solid particles. The pressure fluctuations, ΔP_p, near the particles are given by:

$$\Delta P_p \propto \rho_L u'^2 = \rho_L (\varepsilon d_p)^{2/3} \tag{10.28}$$

The maximum value of ε is found in the impeller region and near the baffles, and can be as much as 30–60 times higher than the average power dissipation. In Table 10.6 estimations are presented of the disruptive force on particles in water for a range of power inputs and particle sizes. The gravity force is also provided for comparison. The results suggest that for typical pharmaceutical particle sizes the pressure fluctuations dominate. Of course, there are some reagents with high density as well as some vessels with low power inputs for which gravity can be dominant, resulting in lack of suspension, dispersion and homogeneity.

Table 10.6 *Turbulent forces on particles in water* ($\Delta\rho = 400$ kgm^{-3})

ε (Wkg^{-1})	0.01	0.1	0.5	1	20	$gd_p\Delta\rho$ (Pa)
d_p (μm)	$\Delta P_p \propto \rho_L u'^2 = \rho_L(\varepsilon d_p)^{2/3}$ (Pa)					
30			0.6	1.0	7.1	0.1
50		0.3	0.9	1.4	10.0	0.2
100	0.1	0.5	1.4	2.2	15.9	0.4
300	0.2	1.0	2.8	4.5	33.0	1.2
500	0.3	1.4	4.0	6.3	46.4	2.0
1000	0.5	2.2	6.3	10.0	73.7	3.9

10.4 Solids Charging

10.4.1 Charging to Batch Vessels

In the pharmaceutical industry, charging to batch vessels occurs in a whole range of manners, but typically the operation is either (1) batchwise, which typically involves a manual element; or (2) for some formulation processes inline equipment is used to mix solids and a continuous flow of fluid. Both methods will be briefly described in this section.

The draw-down of solids in stirred vessels has been little investigated. So, in general, avoiding problems by changing the way in which solids are added to the process is often much more effective than trying to find a solution to the draw-down problem. In practice, the following strategies can be adopted:

The rate at which solids are fed could be reduced by changing from manual charging to controlled charging using a rotary valve or a screw feeder, and ensuring the powder is well spread over the surface. Reducing the feed rate and/or making it more steady will aid the process, but it will also prolong processing times. In order to keep the flux of particles (kgm^{-2}s^{-1}) constant on scale-up, the addition time increases proportionally with the vessel diameter T as the mass to be charged increases proportionally to T^3 and the area with T^2: 6 min in the lab (1 L), would be 1 hr on the plant (1 m^3).

The rate at which particles agglomerate on the surface could be minimized by changing the physico-chemical properties of the system, for example improving the wettability of particles by adding surfactants enhances the rate at which they can be incorporated. For hydrating solids, a reduction in temperature will alter the rate at which the solid absorbs water. If the swelling rate is reduced, more time is available to incorporate the particles and the agglomeration rate will be reduced.

10.4.1.1 Vortex Formation

For dense solids that are easily wetted by the solvent they are charged to, the charging operation need not be an issue. These can be charged in slugs that will break easily through the surface. Dispersion problems may result, however, if particles build up at the surface, which may occur for solids that:

- have a lower density than the solvent;
- form agglomerates that contain significant amounts of gas allowing them to float (boats);

- are difficult to wet, liquid may not be able to enter the pores making a lump difficult to dissolve/disperse;
- are made from substances that hydrate to give viscous fluids at high concentration; gel-like particles with a virtually dry centre may be formed "(fish eyes)". Once drawn into the liquid these can be very difficult to break up, requiring very high shear.

Finally, if much material builds up at the surface a skin can form, which stops powder incorporation altogether as surface movement now is very low.

In such systems, turbulence at the surface is required to transfer the material from the surface to the bulk. The preferred vessel configuration for these systems would be to have submerged baffles, and an axial or mixed flow impeller. In pharmaceutical multipurpose vessels, many systems are glass-lined to cope with the aggressive and varied nature of the reagents used. As a result, baffling can be minimal and is often non-existent.

In unbaffled, or minimally baffled vessels, the liquid will start to swirl around. Due to the action of centrifugal forces, the flow will be primarily rotational with little or no axial mixing and a vortex forms. For most impellers, the flow near the centre of the vessel is towards the impeller. It is therefore advantageous to feed solids into the vortex, so that as and when they are drawn in through the surface they quickly experience high shear in the impeller region. This enhances deagglomeration and dispersion of the solid phase.

Nagata (1975) modelled vortex formation assuming there are two different regions in the vessel: (1) a zone in the centre of radius r_o, the 'forced vortex', which rotates as a solid body at the same speed as the agitator; and (2) near the wall is a concentric cylinder where no torque is applied to the fluid and the tangential velocity profile is hyperbolic. The model demonstrates the importance of the Froude number ($Fr = N^2D/g$). Most existing correlations, however, are based on dimensional analysis. Markopoulos and Kontogeorgaki (1995) reviewed the literature data for a range of agitators and compiled the relevant correlations. In these correlations, the Galileo Number also appears influential ($Ga = Re^2/Fr$). They defined a 'vortex factor' C_v:

$$C_v = \frac{h_v}{DFr} = \frac{gh_v}{N^2D^2} \tag{10.29}$$

where h_v is the vortex depth below the initial surface level, and C_v increases with *Re* tending towards a constant value, typically 3–6, at high *Re*. So, for systems operating in the turbulent regime ($Re > 5000$) the absolute vortex depth scales with tip speed. More relevant is the ratio of vortex depth to agitator diameter, that is, the relative vortex depth (h_v/D), which is unchanged if on scale-up the Froude number is kept constant (i.e. $ND^{1/2}$ = constant). Data for a range of agitators are plotted in Figure 10.5. In general, under the same conditions, the vortex depth created by a flat six-blade paddle and a six-blade disc turbine is greater than that of downward pumping turbines, and is about twice that of three pitched-blade turbines. In addition, the relative vortex depth decreases with increasing D/T and with an increase in liquid viscosity.

10.4.1.2 Draw-Down

Solid incorporation from the surface can be a very energy intensive process compared to solid suspension. The key to surface draw-down is surface movement to prevent particle

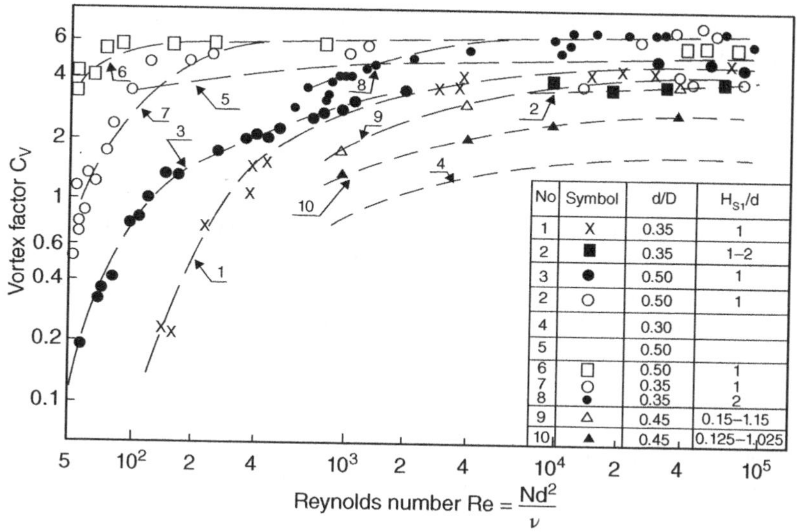

Figure 10.5 The Vortex Factor $C_v = h_v g/(ND)^2$ as á function of Re for various impeller types: 1–3 and 9: Rushton disk turbine; 4: propeller; 5: grid agitator; 6–8: 4 blade flat paddle, 10: pitched-blade turbine. Reprinted with permission from Chem. Eng. and Tech., Vortex depth in unbaffled single and multiple impeller agitated vessels by Joannis Markopoulos, Eleni Kontogeorgaki, 68–74. Copyright (2004) John Wiley & Sons, Ltd

build-up. Thus, solids draw-down in baffled vessels is effected by the intensity of turbulence and mean circulation velocity of the liquid at the surface, and the distribution of solids in the tank is strongly affected by the vertical circulation patterns. Khazam and Kresta (2009) identified three main modes of incorporation:

1. The central vortex in an unbaffled vessel draws in solid and can (if the vortex extends far enough) transport solid directly into the agitator zone. Note that particle distribution in this mode of operation will be very poor.
2. Turbulent eddies near the surface draw liquid and solid from the surface into the bulk. This mode can dominate in systems with an agitator at low distances below the surface.
3. Mean drag: through strong circulation fresh liquid wells up thus returning some surface fluid and particles into the bulk. The axial component of the mean velocity near the surface must be larger than the particle (or agglomerate) slip velocity at some point close to the liquid surface for this mechanism to be effective.

If systems are well baffled (two or more baffles) then sufficient surface turbulence may be generated by the agitator. The usual configuration for vessels where the main duty is surface draw-down is to ensure that the baffles are submerged, thus, generating a vortex that helps prevent build-up of material. A second impeller mounted just below the surface will help promote surface turbulence.

Initial work on draw-down focussed on the speed at which gas just started to be entrained from the surface into the fluid: the critical speed for surface aeration (N_{CSA}). Patwardhan and Joshi (1998) reviewed the correlations for N_{CSA} for a range of agitators. For fully-baffled vessels with a *single radial impeller* (Rushton turbine), the correlation proposed by Greaves and Kobbacy (1981) may be used:

$$N_{CSA} = K\left(\frac{TH}{D^3}\right)^{2/3}\left(\frac{S}{H}\right)^{1/3} \tag{10.30}$$

where S is the submergence of the agitator, that is, the distance below the liquid surface, and the constant $K = 0.4$–0.5 for different aqueous systems. Analysis of a limited data set in Zeneca (Muller, not published) indicated that the speed at which particles are just drawn down, N_{jd}, is typically ~ 60–80% of the speed at which gas is ingested; so, for example:

$$N_{jd} = 0.6 \times N_{CSA} \tag{10.31}$$

The speed for critical surface aeration equation (10.30) may be used to calculate the critical power per unit volume corresponding to N_{jd} for the solid:

$$\left(\frac{P}{V}\right)_{jd} \propto \frac{\rho_L N_{NCA}^3 D^5}{T^2 H} = \frac{\rho_L (TH)^2}{D^6} \times \frac{S}{H} \times \frac{D^5}{T^2 H} = \rho_L \frac{S}{D} \tag{10.32}$$

This shows that the critical P/V is proportional to S/D, so that larger diameter turbines positioned lower under the surface reduce the power required to draw solids in (for radial flow impellers!). This demonstrates that in geometrically similar systems (i.e. S/D constant) the onset of draw-down scales with P/V.

Özcan-Taskin (2006) also found that for up-pumping axial flow impellers constant P/V gives reasonable scale-up. However, for down-pumping impellers equivalent correlation with conventional parameters was not attained. This can also be observed from earlier work on 45° pitched-blade turbines by Joosten *et al.* (1977) who proposed the following correlation for N_{jd}:

$$Fr_{jd} = \frac{N_{jd}^2 D}{g} = 0.036\left(\frac{D}{T}\right)^{-3.65}\left(\frac{\Delta\rho}{\rho_L}\right)^{0.42} \tag{10.33}$$

in which small deviations in D/T are strongly amplified. In a recent study, however, it was found that whilst half baffles are very similar to full baffles in performance, surface baffles offer several advantages: a significant reduction in N_{jd} and more robust performance at large submergences for both up-pumping and down-pumping axial flow impellers; a better distribution of solids, a longer circulation time below the surface, and finally allowing impeller placement deep in the tank to avoid air entrainment (Khazam and Kresta, 2008; 2009). The N_{jd} observed for an up-pumping pitched-blade turbine is more sensitive to both submergence and baffle configuration than a down-pumping one.

The number of baffles, their dimensions and location, however, are still the subject of much controversy in the literature, which underlines the complexity of the problem and that experimental studies are ultimately required for reliable design and scale-up.

10.4.2 Charging Difficult Powders

For systems with a very low density, or a strong tendency to form "fish eyes" or "boats", introducing the solids to a flowing stream is more effective than feeding to a batch vessel. Two classes of systems exist:

1. Eductor system: a vacuum caused by the fluid flowing past an eductor draws powder into the fluid. Process upsets often make this equipment useful for only the easiest to disperse solids.
2. Rotating mixing chambers: the fluid phase is pumped into a rotating mixing chamber, which is essentially a high shear rotor rotating in the horizontal plane inside a screen that retains large clumps until they are broken down. The fluid discharged from the mixing chamber creates a vacuum, drawing powder into the chamber. A valve should deliver a steady shower of particles, not a slug of powder, into the mixing chamber. The two common set-ups are the Tri-Blender® and the Silverson.

10.5 Solid Suspension

10.5.1 States of Solid Suspension

The state of suspension in a stirred vessel can be defined in a number of ways. In a design or scale-up problem, it is important to use the appropriate definition and correlation as different processes require different degrees of suspension. The basic common suspension regimes are described next in order of increasing homogeneity, as schematically illustrated in Figure 10.6.

State of nearly complete suspension with filleting. Most of the solid particles are suspended while a small fraction is allowed to loosely aggregate and form fillets on the base of the vessel in relatively stagnant regions behind baffles, in corners or below the agitator. This state of suspension may sometimes be acceptable provided the fillets do not grow and the solids do not cake. This, however, would be undesirable in operations such as crystallization or where mass/heat transfer is involved.

State of complete particle motion. No fillets exist, and solids that are not suspended are in a state of motion on the bottom. These particles will have considerably reduced mass/heat transfer coefficients than the suspended ones because of their non-uniform exposure to

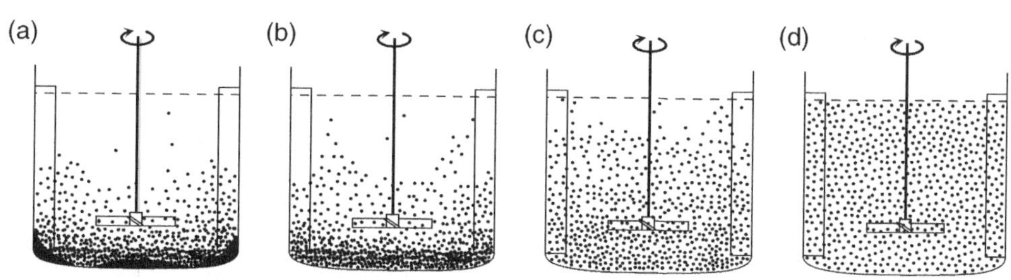

Figure 10.6 *States of solid suspension: (a) nearly complete suspension with filleting; (b) complete particle motion; (c) complete off-bottom suspension; (d) uniform or homogeneous suspension*

the liquid. Such a condition, however, is sufficient in some cases such as the dissolution of highly soluble solids even if only a relatively small fraction of solids are suspended.

State of complete off-bottom suspension. In this state, all solids are suspended and no particle remains on the bottom of the vessel for more than 1 or 2 s approximately, a condition known as Zwietering's criterion (Zwietering, 1958). Under this 'just suspended' condition, the maximum solid area is exposed to the fluid but there are usually concentration gradients in the vessel and there may be a significant region of clear liquid near the top. Much of the mixing research in this area has been devoted to the determination of the minimum agitation speed, N_{js}, necessary to achieve this state of suspension. As such, N_{js} is one of the most important design requirements. This is usually measured in a well-illuminated transparent vessel by gradually increasing the impeller speed until the condition is visually satisfied. It should be noted, however, that whilst the concept of N_{js} is simple, its accurate measurement is not, especially under conditions of high solids concentration, as generally found in real industrial processes, or where a third gas phase is also present. Determination of N_{js} tends to be somewhat subjective and measurements by different workers can differ by a significant margin. However, in a given experiment a single experimentalist can achieve results with a good precision.

Complete suspension is often an energy intensive operation with power requirements of the order of 1 kWm^{-3} being rather common, depending on impeller and vessel geometry. A more relaxed definition of N_{js} would include where appropriate the state of nearly complete suspension with filleting, as described previously. Since power dissipation is proportional to N^3, this state of suspension offers substantial savings in power requirement compared to Zwietering's criterion, which may more than outweigh the deficiency in suspended solids.

State of homogeneous or uniform suspension. Homogeneous suspension exists when the solids are practically uniformly distributed throughout the vessel volume, that is, there are no solids concentration gradients, and for a polydisperse system the particle size distribution should also be approximately the same everywhere. This regime is discussed further in Section 10.6.

10.5.2 Prediction of Minimum Speed for Complete Suspension

The mechanisms of particle lift-off and suspension are governed by the flow field adjacent to the base of the vessel, whereas the general flow pattern in the bulk dictates the way particles are held in suspension and distributed in 3-D space. Attempts have been made to develop physical and theoretical models capable of explaining particle suspension. Such models, however, have in the main considered particles that are already in suspension or just about to be lifted at the base of the vessel. These two situations are distinctly different and it is important to treat them as such, because the fluid mechanics that facilitate particle lift-off are undoubtedly different from those needed to maintain the particles in suspension and distribute them.

Particle lift-off from a stationary bed of particles on the bottom of the vessel occurs as a result of the drag and lift exerted by the moving fluid. The flow near the base has been described as boundary layer flow, which causes particles to be swept across the base of the vessel (Bourne and Zabelka, 1980). Once small fillets of particles have been formed, particle lift-off is usually seen to be caused by sudden turbulent bursts originating in the turbulent bulk flow above. Kolmogorov's theory of isotropic turbulence has been exploited to some advantage in analysing fluid-particle interactions in this type of flow (Kolmogorov, 1941a,b).

As discussed earlier, eddies relatively large compared to a particle will tend to entrain it and it is, therefore, the large eddies (near the base) generated by the impeller motion that are responsible for the suspension of particles. Consequently, different agitator designs and configurations yield different flow signatures, that is, generate different convective flows and, thus, achieve different levels of solids suspension at the same power input. Once suspended, neutrally-buoyant or nearly-neutrally buoyant particles will follow the motion of the fluid. It is then relatively easy to keep them in suspension and distribute them throughout the vessel. Heavier particles, however, will have significant slip velocities and will tend to settle out, so the fluid flow field must be such that the combined fluid drag and lift generated are sufficient to keep them suspended. At high concentrations, once particles are suspended, they may significantly damp fluid turbulence and, consequently, greater energy inputs are necessary to achieve and maintain suspension.

The minimum impeller speed to produce complete off-bottom suspension has been an issue receiving attention in the literature for decades. For example, Brujes *et al.* (1998) compiled most of the correlations for estimating N_{js} published over a 40 year span, and tested them against experimental measurements obtained in baffled and unbaffled tanks of microcapsule suspensions. Since then many more papers have been published on the topic. Many workers have measured N_{js} using different instruments and approaches, but Zwietering's approach remains the most popular (Zwietering, 1958).

Zwietering's classical correlation, which stands as a reference in the field, was developed from dimensional analysis and was based on experiments covering by far the widest range of fluid and particle properties, particle size and concentration, impeller type and size, and vessel geometry, thus:

$$N_{js} = S\nu^{0.1} d_p^{0.2} \left(\frac{g\Delta\rho}{\rho_L} \right)^{0.45} D^{-0.85} X^{0.13} \tag{10.34}$$

where S is a shape factor called Zwietering constant, a dimensionless parameter, which accounts for geometrical effects including impeller type, impeller off-bottom clearance, and impeller-to-tank diameter ratio; X is solids concentration by weight × 100, and ν is liquid kinematic viscosity. Subsequent independent studies (e.g. Nienow, 1968; Baldi *et al.*, 1978; Rao *et al.*, 1988) generally corroborated Zwietering's correlation for process conditions similar to those covered by Zwietering. For conditions very different from Zwietering's, equation (10.34) may be much less reliable and where a state of complete off-bottom suspension is deemed essential, it is advisable to measure N_{js} experimentally if at all possible.

10.5.2.1 Influence of Physical Properties

Zwietering's correlation, which is based on turbulent flow, indicates a low dependence on fluid viscosity ($\nu^{0.1}$) which is expected in a turbulent flow field. Results on suspensions where the liquid is viscous are scarce, however. Shamlou (1993) reported on the basis of some limited experimental data obtained in high-viscosity liquids, that N_{js} values estimated by correlations such as Zwietering's are too high by as much as a factor of 2.5. Using Newtonian liquids, Ibrahim and Nienow (1994) found that at viscosities of about 1 Pas the Zwietering correlation fails to predict N_{js} with as much as 90% error. The influence of the suspending fluid rheology on solids suspension has generally received scant attention in the literature. When the suspending medium is non-Newtonian, the hydrodynamics inside a stirred vessel become even more complex with a non-uniform viscosity field. Some recent experiments and Computational Fluid Dynamics (CFD) simulations seemed to indicate that large glass particles ($d_p = 4.5$ mm) tend to suspend and distribute better in a shear-thinning fluid compared to pure water in a vessel agitated by a pitched-blade turbine (Pianko-Oprych *et al.*, 2006). This could be due to increased drag on the particles in such a shear-thinning fluid (Section 10.3.3). Despite their industrial importance, these rheologically complex suspensions have been inadequately researched and are not well understood.

The low dependence on particle size $\left(d_p^{0.2}\right)$ has been confirmed for particles in the range 0.2–1 mm. For solids smaller than 0.2 mm higher exponents have been reported, but since N_{js} seems to fall off more rapidly than equation (10.34) suggests, the latter expression is still considered to give conservative predictions (Baldi *et al.*, 1978). For d_p greater than about 1 mm, however, there are indications in the literature that N_{js} may be insensitive to particle size but these have not been widely confirmed. On the other hand, it has been reported that Zwietering's correlation is not as reliable at high d_p/D values (Choudhury *et al.*, 1995). Little information exists on the suspension of such coarse particles, and especially so in viscous and non-Newtonian media.

The solid-fluid density difference, $\Delta\rho$, is the property with the largest influence on N_{js}. Its exponent reflects the effect of the settling velocity of the solids. The exponent on D represents the influence of scale.

10.5.2.2 Influence of Solid Concentration

The dependence on X seems fairly small, but it has been reported that Zwietering's correlation is not as reliable at low solids concentrations below 2 vol% and high concentrations above 15 vol% (Choudhury *et al.*, 1995). As discussed previously, though a lot of work has been done on measuring N_{js}, there is still a need for considerably more high quality experimental data in which both N_{js} and local energy dissipation rates are measured. This is needed to improve the prediction of N_{js} through better understanding of particle lift-off from a stationary bed of particles and particle settling, especially in rheologically complex media where information is scarce.

10.5.2.3 Influence of Geometric Parameters

The influence of impeller design, impeller size D/T, impeller off-bottom clearance C/T, and vessel configuration are represented by the dimensionless parameter S in equation (10.34). Graphs of S as a function of T/D and T/C have been presented by Zwietering (1958) and Nienow (1968) for three different impellers (propeller, disc turbine, flat paddle) in flat-base cylindrical vessels equipped with four baffles of $0.1T$ width, where $H = T$. These data can be represented by a correlation of the form:

$$S = p\left(\frac{T}{D}\right)^q \qquad (10.35)$$

where the constants p and q are a function of impeller design and T/C. Other forms of correlation have been proposed by different workers (Armenante *et al.*, 1998). Values of S for different types of impellers and mixer configurations are listed in Table 10.7. Such

Table 10.7 *Values of the Zwietering constant S for different impellers and mixer configurations*

Impeller	Number of blades	Blade width w/D	Pitch	Pumping direction	Vessel	Impeller diameter D/T	Impeller clearance C/T	Zwietering constant S	Reference
Flat paddle	2	1/2	–	radial	flat base	1/5.5–2	1/7–1/2	$S \propto (T/D)^{1.3}$	Zwietering (1958)
	2	1/4	–			1/5.5–2	1/20–1/2	$S \propto (T/D)^{1.3}$	
Disc turbine	6	1/5	–	radial	flat base	1/6–2	1/7–1	$S \propto (T/D)^{1.3}$	Zwietering (1958)
	6	1/5	–	radial	flat base	1/4	1/4	12.2	Chapman *et al.* (1983)
	6	1/5	–			1/3	1/4	7.1	
	6	1/5	–			1/2	1/4	4.25	
Pitched-blade turbine	4	1/5	45°	down	flat base	1/3	1/5	5.7	Wong *et al.* (1987)
	4	1/5	45°			1/3	1/4	6.2	
	4	1/5	45°			1/3	1/3	6.8	
	4	1/5	45°			1/3	1/2	11.5	
	4	1/5	45°	down	flat base	1/2	1/4	5.8	Chapman *et al.* (1983)
	4	1/5	45°			1/4	1/4	7.1	
	6	1/5	45°	down	flat base	1/3	1/4	3.94	Ibrahim *et al.* (1996)
	6	1/5	45°			1/2	1/6	5.4	
	6	1/5	45°	up		1/2	1/6	5.1	
	6	1/5	45°	down	flat base	1/2	1/4	6.4	Bujalski *et al.* (1988)
	6	1/5	45°	up		1/2	1/4	6.9	
	4	1/2.5	30°	down	torispherical base	1/3	1/4	6.4	Mak (1992)
	4	1/2.5	30°			1/3	1/6	7.1	
	4	1/2.5	30°			1/3	1/8	7.2	
	4	1/2.1	45°			1/3.3	1/4	4.5	
	4	1/2.1	45°			1/3.3	1/8	4.3	

(continued)

Table 10.7 *(continued)*

Impeller	Number of blades	Blade width w/D	Pitch	Pumping direction	Vessel	Impeller diameter D/T	Impeller clearance C/T	Zwietering constant S	Reference
	4	1/3.5	45°			1/3	1/4	4.8	
	4	1/3.5	45°			1/3	1/6	4.6	
	4	1/3.5	45°			1/3	1/8	4.2	
	4	1/2.8	45°			0.4	1/4	4.7	
	4	1/2.8	45°			0.4	1/8	3.4	
	4	1/3.5	45°			1/2	1/4	5.2	
	4	1/3.5	45°			1/2	1/6	4.2	
	4	1/3.5	45°			1/2	1/8	3.7	
	4	1/6	45°			1/2	1/4	5.5	
	4	1/6	45°			1/2	1/8	5.5	
	4	1/3.5	45°			1/1.7	1/4	6.7	
	4	1/3.5	45°			1/1.7	1/6	5.1	
	4	1/3.5	45°			1/1.7	1/8	4.4	
	4	1/4.3	45°			1/1.7	1/4	6.8	
	4	1/4.3	45°			1/1.7	1/8	3.8	
	4	1/5	45°			1/1.4	1/4	5.4	
	4	1/5	45°			1/1.4	1/8	4.5	
	4	1/4	60°			1/3	1/4	4.4	
	4	1/4	60°			1/3	1/6	4.1	
	4	1/4	60°			1/3	1/8	3.7	
	4	1/5	90°	radial		1/3	1/4	4.4	
	4	1/5	90°			1/3	1/6	4.1	
	4	1/5	90°			1/3	1/8	4.1	
Vaned disc	12 vanes	0.1*D*	–	radial	flat base	1/5.5–2	1/6–1/2	$S \propto (T/D)^{1.3}$	Zwietering (1958)
Marine propeller	3	–	–	axial	flat base	1/6.5–1/2	1/4–1/2.5	$S \propto (T/D)^{0.82}$	Zwietering (1958)

Lightnin A310 hydrofoil	3	–	–	axial	flat base	1/3	1/5	7.6	Wong *et al.* (1987)
	3	–	–			1/3	1/4	7.9	
	3	–	–			1/3	1/3	8.4	
	3	–	–			1/3	1/2	9.6	
	3	–	–	axial	flat base	1/3	1/4	7.8	Guerci *et al.* (1986)
	3	–	–	axial	flat base	1/2	1/4	6.0	Ibrahim *et al.* (1996)
	3	–	–	axial	torispherical base	1/2.4	1/4	6.9	Mak (1992)
	3	–	–			1/2	1/4	7.1	
Chemineer HE3 hydrofoil	3	–	–	axial	flat base	1/2	1/4	6.2	Ibrahim *et al.* (1996)
	3	–	–			1/3	1/4	7.2	

data show that S is generally smaller for smaller C/T values; that is, at low off-bottom clearances, and at larger D/T values, that is, when using wider impellers, but only up to a practical limit beyond which performance declines. Literature data also show that axial flow agitators, that is, propellers and hydrofoil impellers such as Lightnin A310 and Chemineer HE3 are the best performers as they have the lowest power dissipation rates at N_{js}. They have a low power number (Po ~ 0.25) compared to a pitched-blade turbine (Po ~ 1.6) or a Rushton turbine (Po ~ 4.2), and tend to run at higher speeds, which allows the use of lighter shafts and motors. These high efficiency impellers develop a stronger axial flow field near the base of the vessel where particles deposit, than radial (disc turbine, flat paddle) or mixed flow (pitched-blade turbine) impellers. Such an axial flow is effective in lifting off particles and suspending them, and enables these impellers to cope better when positioned at relatively high clearances. Their low power demand is relatively independent of D/T, which means that larger impeller diameters with lower rotational and tip speeds can be used to minimize damage to shear sensitive particles. Large D/T ratios combined with low clearances, however, lead to a weak axial flow causing particle accumulation in the centre directly beneath the agitator, and should be avoided.

When solid suspension is the main duty of a vessel, it is advised to use fully baffled vessels with a mixed flow or axial flow agitator with a large diameter; D/T ~ 0.5, mounted closer to the bottom than for liquid blending duties ($C = T/6$ to $T/4$ vs $T/3$ for blending duties). Note, centreline jets aimed at the bottom are also very efficient in suspending solids but not as good at dispersing them due to the low overall power input.

Both axial and mixed-flow impellers are more efficient at suspending solids when used in the down-pumping mode. Some more recent studies, however, have shown that up-pumping axial hydrofoil impellers provide considerable advantages over down-pumping ones in single phase mixing (Aubin *et al.*, 2001) and in three-phase gas-solid-liquid mixing (Nienow, 1999). This is also true for mixed-flow impellers. In the down-pumping mode, one circulation loop is produced and velocities in the upper part of the vessel are very weak, resulting in poor mixing in that region. In the up-pumping mode, fluid circulation in the upper part of the tank is considerably improved as two distinct circulation loops are established, which is beneficial to gas retention and dispersion.

Data reported by Guerci *et al.* (1986) suggest that N_{js} is more easily achieved in dished bottom vessels (~20% lower) and vessels equipped with a draught tube, as they have smaller S values than flat based vessels, but deep dishes are usually less energy efficient because of the proximity of the impeller tip to the base. In this respect, however, there is no significant difference between different dish shapes, for example, hemispherical or elliptical.

It should also be pointed out that, whilst the use of more than one impeller improves solids distribution, this should not have any significant effect on N_{js} as the settled solids would only feel the effect of the action of the bottom agitator. Power draw, however, would increase proportionally to the number of agitators used. Varying the liquid height also has no effect on N_{js} as the hydrodynamics associated with particle lift-off from the sediment on the bottom of the vessel remain unaffected.

10.6 Solid Distribution

To understand solid-liquid mixing, it is necessary to know the states of solid distribution occurring in the stirred vessel. In accordance with operational demands, it is possible to conduct solid-liquid mixing either in the just suspended mode or in the homogeneous suspension mode. Homogeneity is required, for example, when it is necessary to obtain uniform treatment of all the particles, when a suspension must be discharged at a constant concentration to ensure for instance the CQA covering the dose for patients is met. Another example would be in a crystallizer where a non-uniform solids distribution may cause high local supersaturation levels and, hence, a non-uniform crystal growth or worse secondary nucleation. The following sections describe the different regimes encountered and the effects of the various important parameters.

10.6.1 Agitator Speed

As the agitation speed is increased from rest, the following states of solid suspension and distribution can be identified. Initially, the solids form a thick layer at the bottom of the vessel from which, at low speeds, a small quantity of particles are lifted up and distributed in the vessel. With increasing N, a clear interface appears separating the solid-rich suspension and a virtually solid-free liquid layer in the upper part of the vessel; the height of the suspension from the bottom to the interface is usually referred to as *cloud height*. As N is increased further, Bujalski *et al.* (1999) reported that the cloud height first drops significantly before increasing again as N_{js} is approached and the solids are fully suspended. However, the data from Hicks *et al.* (1997) do not show this fall, and cloud height increases monotonically with N. Increasing N above N_{js}, gradually increases the cloud height and eventually the solid-liquid mixture reaches the surface. The formation of the liquid layer is attributed to the upward liquid axial velocity falling below the particle settling velocity. This phenomenon is usually observed in concentrated mixtures (>10 wt%).

It is important to note that when a clear liquid layer is present, the mixing time in the system will be very much increased as there is very little exchange of liquid between the fluidized zone and the clear layer. Mixing is very slow in the liquid layer, as much as 20 times slower than in the cloud region, as very little energy dissipation occurs there (Bujalski *et al.*, 1999). This effect is much more serious when solids are small and light and, therefore, require low energy dissipation rates for suspension, leading to mixing times more than two orders of magnitude longer compared to mixing liquid alone. The use of multiple impellers increases power consumption in proportion to the number of impellers used, but reduces the likelihood of an interface forming and the mixing time is then only slightly longer than for liquid alone. The best separation between impellers is $3D$. At this separation, dual impellers generate a single large flow loop. Higher separations reduce the cloud height, and at ~ $3.7D$ two separate flow loops are formed and the cloud height drops to the same value as for a single impeller.

The following correlation for axial hydrofoil impellers is valid for $0.154 < D/T < 0.52$ for solids with a terminal settling velocity less than 143 mms^{-1} (Bittorf and Kresta, 2002):

$$\frac{Cloud\,height}{T} = \frac{N}{N_{js}}\left[0.84 - 1.05\frac{C}{T} + 0.7\frac{(D/T)^2}{1-(D/T)^2}\right] \qquad (10.36)$$

So, cloud height increases linearly with agitation speed, and a larger D/T and smaller C/T result in a higher cloud height. It is generally accepted that at $1.5N_{js}$ to $2N_{js}$ the solid is well distributed. Depending on the size and density of the particles, a significant concentration difference may still exist between the bottom and the top of the vessel. Further increases in agitator speed cause the solids to redistribute to the outside of the circulation loops. Cloud height reduces with larger particles and higher solids loading.

10.6.2 Homogeneity

In general, a considerably higher power input is required to achieve a state of homogeneous suspension than just complete suspension. Such an increase in power demand is higher for faster settling particles, as shown in Table 10.4. For nearly-neutrally buoyant particles homogeneity is easier to achieve than in many other industrial processing applications where it is not usually economically feasible. In many such cases, however, the minimum condition of suspending all particles in the fluid is sufficient to satisfy the process requirements and, thus, suspensions in the process industries are often designed to operate under a heterogeneous regime, that is, at N_{js} or slightly above it.

At the much higher impeller speeds generally required to achieve homogeneity, however, there is the additional possible problem of surface aeration. Considerable amounts of air can be drawn into the vessel, which can have negative effects on the process, especially when mixing very viscous or viscoplastic fluids. Under such conditions, surface aeration must be guarded against to avoid a severe entrapment of unwanted air in the suspension that can cause great difficulties, including the mass/heat transport limitations that may ensue due to a blanketing of the particle surfaces.

Whilst solids tend to suspend fairly uniformly across the radius of the vessel at agitation speeds above N_{js}, vertical homogeneity is much harder to achieve. The vertical distribution is usually non-uniform and is generally characterized by a local maximum occurring above the impeller plane giving rise to what is sometimes called a 'belly plot' for different impellers whether radial or axial (Barresi and Baldi, 1987; Guida *et al.*, 2009, 2010). Above this maximum, the solid concentration decays exponentially with height, but as N increases, the distribution tends towards the mean value. Visual observation is most commonly used to measure N_{js}, as discussed previously, but is also used in practice to qualitatively gauge the degree of homogeneity. This is a crude but rapid procedure that enables a quick basic comparison to be made between different geometries or processing conditions, and can enable salient features and problems to be identified such as stagnant areas and solids accumulation. Whilst visual observation becomes increasingly more difficult at high solids loadings due to the increased opacity of the system, the method is still useful in acquiring a rough picture of the general flow patterns.

A quantitative description of homogeneity is harder to formulate, however. The degree of homogeneity can be quantified in terms of the coefficient of variation, a statistical parameter defined as:

$$C_v = \frac{\sigma}{\bar{C}} = \frac{\sqrt{\frac{1}{n-1}\sum_{i=1}^{n}(C_i - \bar{C})^2}}{\bar{C}} \tag{10.37}$$

where σ is the standard deviation, $\bar{C}$ is the mean solids concentration in the vessel, C_i is the local solids concentration of location i, and n is the number of samples (Rieger *et al.*, 1988). Whereas σ gives a measure of how different the values are from each other and from the mean, C_v is a measure of the spread of the distribution relative to its mean; the larger the C_v, the more significant the σ relative to the mean.

The state of homogeneous suspension is difficult to achieve and to measure in practice. When a liquid layer exists above the suspension, it has been proposed that a suspension should be assumed homogeneous when the cloud height reaches 90% of the liquid height (Zlokarnik, 2001). A 100% uniform suspension would imply $C_v = 0$ which would be impractical if a particle free layer is present near the surface, so in practice, homogeneity is usually deemed adequate if $C_v \leq 0.05$.

Whilst the definition of the coefficient C_v is simple, its measurement is far from trivial. The method requires a large number of local measurements of solids concentration, something not readily achievable in practice. Withdrawal of samples has been attempted in the past, but it is fraught with problems as it is difficult to achieve representative isokinetic sampling in most regions of the vessel (Nasr-El-Din *et al.*, 1996). So far, other attempts at local measurements have been mainly confined to the investigation of axial solid concentration profiles at relatively low concentrations using intrusive conductivity or capacitance probes (Yamazaki *et al.*, 1986; Barresi and Baldi, 1987; Mak *et al.*, 1997; Montante *et al.*, 2001, 2002; Brunazzi *et al.*, 2004; Spidla *et al.*, 2005). There are, however, no instruments that can be used to reliably probe concentrated suspensions and provide detailed pointwise measurements of solids concentration. A better more reliable criterion for uniformity of suspension may, thus, also be needed. The novel PEPT technique, however, is able to measure the 3-D local particle concentration distribution and local phase velocities in a stirred vessel provided one of the particles can be radioactively labelled and used as a representative tracer for the solid phase. PEPT has recently been used to accurately determine the 3-D velocity field as well as solids distribution developed during the mixing of monodisperse and polydisperse slurries of glass ballotini, at mass concentrations up to 40 wt% (Barigou *et al.*, 2009; Guida *et al.*, 2009, 2010).

10.6.3 Geometry

It is known that cloud height is lower for a pitched-blade turbine than a Rushton turbine. In our recent PEPT work, a down-pumping pitched-blade turbine achieved a significantly better 3-D homogeneity than an up-pumping turbine in suspending glass particles (1–3.3 mm) in water (Guida *et al.*, 2009, 2010). It is not entirely clear, however, what the pumping direction of axial-flow impellers does to the 3-D distribution of particles and, hence, to the homogeneity of a suspension. In addition, when the suspending liquid is viscous leading to transitional flow, such impellers are known to exhibit almost radial flow, and in this case again it is not entirely clear *à priori* which pumping configuration would be more advantageous both in suspending the solids and achieving a good spatial distribution. For $N > N_{js}$, increases in particle settling velocity and solids loading both reduce homogeneity for identical mixing conditions, and for constant power input large *D/T* ratios enhance homogeneity.

10.6.4 Practical Guidelines

In practice, several indicators can be used to evaluate if a solid distribution problem is likely:

- *Compare N_{js} to the mixing time*: if the agitator speed required for mixing is significantly larger than N_{js}, the distribution of solids is more likely to be tending towards homogeneous.
- *Check the particle Reynolds number*: if it is laminar, particles will tend to follow the fluid streamlines and be well distributed.
- *Compare the particle terminal velocity to the impeller tip speed*: if the terminal velocity is several orders of magnitude smaller than the impeller tip speed, particles are likely to be well suspended and distributed. Alternatively, compare turbulent forces to gravity (see Table 10.6).
- *Compare particle size to the Kolmogorov length scale*: if particles are of a similar size to the smallest turbulent eddies, they are very likely to be well distributed (see Table 10.5).
- *Experiment*: if a strong concentration gradient is suspected and a homogeneous slurry is required, it is best to conduct an experiment. Experiments have shown that solid distribution is similar scales with constant P/V.

10.7 Blending in Solid-Liquid Systems

10.7.1 Mixing Time

When a vessel has a solid suspension duty, there is typically also a blending duty associated with the vessel (e.g. a slurry feed vessel). When calculating the power input and mixing time, the fluid properties (density, viscosity) should be those for the slurry. At high solid loadings, these properties can be significantly different from the properties of the continuous phase and there is likely to be some rheological complexity too.

The applicability of the available mixing time correlations depends on the degree of solid mixing in the system:

- $N < N_{js}$ – solid bed on the bottom: mixing time correlations may not hold, as the bed provides a dead zone;
- $N > N_{js}$ – but solids have still not reached the surface: mixing time correlations will not hold as there is little circulation between the clear liquid layer on top and the fluidized zone. A second agitator should be added to improve blending. Note that mixing times can be extremely long for a system with a clear liquid layer on top.
- $N >> N_{js}$ – solids well dispersed: mixing time correlations hold; volume-averaged fluid properties should be used, and the effect of solids on rheology should be taken into account. Note that unbaffled vessels may suffer from maldistribution of solids. (Tamburini *et al.*, 2009).

10.7.2 Viscoplastic Slurries Yield Stress and Cavern Formation

In the mixing of viscoplastic slurries, the impeller creates a 'cavern' within which liquid is in flow, but in the bulk where shear stresses are below the yield stress the fluid is stagnant, a phenomenon that around the cavern can be disastrous for many mixing operations. With increasing agitator speed, the cavern of mobilized fluid will grow until eventually it reaches the wall and the surface when the system should be well mixed. Some work has been done on measuring the size of caverns in transparent yield stress fluids using 2-D visualization methods (Elson, 1990). Nienow and Elson (1988) used X-rays in a shear-thickening slurry; this method only gave rough estimates of flow patterns, however. Recently, a Planar Laser Induced Fluorescence (PLIF) technique and CFD were used to visualize and study caverns in transparent non-Newtonian fluids (Adams and Barigou, 2007). The PLIF technique also gave a measure of the rate of fluid mixing within such caverns, a problem not studied before.

Similarly, 'pseudo-caverns' are formed when other fluids are agitated such as shear-thinning fluids or even highly-viscous Newtonian fluids, especially in the laminar and transitional flow regimes. Outside a pseudo-cavern the fluid is in motion but the velocities are small. The presence of stagnant zones is detrimental to mixing, heat and mass transfer and should be avoided. For a proper understanding and design of these processes, it is essential to establish the size of the cavern region as a function of fluid rheology and agitation conditions. This is a real industrial problem, but progress in this area has been hampered by the lack of techniques suitable for flow visualization and measurement in these complex fluids that are usually opaque. Recently, however, using PEPT the 3-D flow field within such caverns has been investigated for the first time, as shown in Figure 10.7, giving accurate measurements of all velocity components. The flow inside the cavern is mainly tangential, which suggests poor mixing (Barigou *et al.*, 2009).

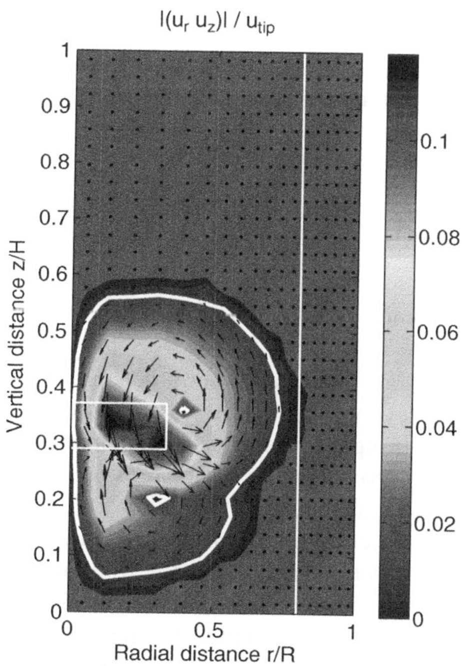

Figure 10.7 *Mixing of an opaque shear-thinning viscoplastic slurry: visualization of cavern around the impeller and determination of flow field using PEPT*

The size of the cavern can be estimated from a force balance where the torque on the agitator shaft is balanced against the moment generated by the yield stress on the cavern surface, thus:

$$\frac{P}{2\pi N} \propto D_{cav} \times Area_{cav} \times \tau_y \propto D_{cav}^3 \tau_y \tag{10.38}$$

where $P/2\pi N$ is the torque on the agitator shaft and D_{cav} is the diameter of the cavern. If the cavern is treated as a cylinder with a height proportional to the diameter, the area of the cavern on which the yield stress acts is then proportional to $D_{cav}^{\ 2}$. The ratio of cavern diameter to agitator diameter is therefore:

$$\left(\frac{D_{cav}}{D}\right)^3 \propto \frac{P}{\tau_y ND^3} \propto \frac{Po\rho_S N^2 D^2}{\tau_y} \propto PoRe_y \tag{10.39}$$

where, ρ_S is the slurry density and

$$Re_y = \frac{\rho_S N^2 D^2}{\tau_y} \tag{10.40}$$

is the yield-stress Reynolds number, which is the ratio of the turbulent stresses to the yield stress. From equation (10.39) it follows that when scaling up or down, if *D/T* and *Po* are kept constant, the cavern will remain at constant size subject to *ND* being kept constant. Thus, it appears that for problems with cavern formation, the correct scale-up rule should be constant tip speed, not constant *P/V*.

For a system with a cavern, the apparent slurry viscosity inside the cavern may be calculated using the well-known postulate of Metzner and Otto (1957):

$$\tau_{cav\ wall} = \tau_y = \eta k_s N$$

So, the apparent viscosity is

$$\eta = \frac{\tau_y}{k_s N} \tag{10.41}$$

where k_s is the mixer shear-rate constant, slightly dependent on impeller type and size (Metzner *et al.*, 1961). The Reynolds number based on η is Re_y as defined above. In reality, yield stress fluids display a strong time-dependent behaviour (similar to avalanches!), and in many cases the time it takes to reform the structure is not achieved in the agitator zone, which thus remains free flowing (Muller, 2009).

It may be helpful to view a yield stress fluid as a two-phase system: (1) a low viscosity continuous phase, with (2) a 'sticky' dispersed phase. If left unstirred, the sticky dispersed phase will cross-link and form a network that spans the whole of the vessel. To agitate the slurry, the network needs to be broken up and that requires a certain minimum force, that is, a yield stress force. However, the network does not break up into tiny particles. Initially, it will be large blobs that then reduce in size over a period of time due to interaction with turbulent eddies (see Section 10.9 on size reduction). Using a force balance, it can be shown that Re_y is associated with the maximum size of a structure that can still resist the turbulent forces:

$$d_{structure} < \frac{D}{Re_y^{3/2}} \qquad (10.42)$$

Here, $d_{structure}$ is the diameter of the largest blob that cannot be broken up by the turbulent eddies. For systems not to have a cavern, Re_y must be greater than 30 (if $T/D = 3$), which means that the largest blob is <1% of the impeller diameter.

A number of theoretical cavern/pseudo-cavern models have been proposed assuming a cylindrical, spherical or toroidal shape. These have been recently reviewed and compared to CFD predictions and experimental PLIF measurements, with the toroidal shape model giving the better agreement in terms of shape and size for both caverns and pseudo-caverns (Adams and Barigou, 2007). When using a Carbopol solution, fluorescent dye injected near an impeller blade is seen to mix relatively fast near the centre but mixing progresses very slowly outwards towards the cavern boundary. Small localized regions of low energy dissipation below the impeller are observed that may ultimately only mix by molecular diffusion. As pointed out earlier, recent PEPT measurements within opaque slurry caverns also revealed low radial and axial flow velocities, and poor momentum transfer between different regions of the cavern (Barigou *et al.*, 2009).

The cylindrical cavern model, although simplistic in terms of cavern shape representation, it gave a good approximation to cavern size, but only at low Reynolds numbers. The spherical cavern model of Amanullah *et al.* (1998) for a yield stress fluid, did not fit the cavern shape well and over-estimated the cavern size. This model was extended by Adams and Barigou (2007) to a toroidal cavern shape, giving a better agreement with experimental measurements. The toroidal cavern model of Amanullah *et al.* (1998), agreed reasonably well with CFD simulations of pseudo-caverns formed in a power-law fluid at low Reynolds numbers, where the pseudo-cavern is confined to a small region around the impeller.

10.8 Mass Transfer

A survey of the vast literature shows that a number of approaches have been used to model mass transfer from suspended solids including slip velocity theory, penetration theory, Kolmogorov's theory, and dimensional analysis. Whilst all these approaches have received partial support from experimental studies, none of them has proved able to successfully predict the effects of all the relevant parameters affecting solid-liquid mass transfer. It is not the aim here to discuss these theories in detail but to present the key points upon which there is consensus.

The rate of diffusional mass transfer, M, from a solid to a liquid can be described by the following equation:

$$M = k_{SL} a_p (C^* - C) \qquad (10.43)$$

The mass transfer rate across the interface is, therefore, a function of the volumetric mass transfer coefficient $k_{SL}a_p$ (where k_{SL} is the bulk diffusion mass transfer coefficient and a_p the interfacial area for mass transfer), and a driving force that is given by the distance to equilibrium, and it is represented by the difference between the concentration of the solute at the solid surface (for crystallization, this is the solubility of the solute in the liquid), C^*, and the concentration of the solute in the liquid phase, C. As the dissolution process progresses and the concentration of solute in the liquid phase increases, the driving force decreases, and therefore the mass transfer rate decreases. Therefore, generating concentrated solutions might require long times. In addition to this, the driving force will be low when the thermodynamic solubility of the solute in the solvent is low (e.g. K_2CO_3 in DMF). If the driving force is sufficiently low, mass transfer from the solid phase to the liquid phase might become a rate limiting process. Efficient mixing that ensures homogeneity of the dissolved solute across the vessel will be critical to avoid zones with high concentrations and a small driving force. This is particularly important in the case of high-concentration slurries that are pseudoplastic or viscoplastic to avoid stagnant regions.

The volumetric mass transfer coefficient depends strongly on the interfacial area available for mass transfer. Research has shown that an increase in the agitation rate below N_{js} results in a large increase in this coefficient, but above N_{js}, $k_{SL}a_p$ increases only slightly. The reason for this lies behind the increase in the area of the particle exposed to the liquid when the agitation rate is increased in the region below N_{js}, as well as an increase in k_{SL} as the hydrodynamics near the surface of the particles are enhanced by the agitation. The influential hydrodynamic parameters are the slip velocity and the thickness of the diffusional boundary layer at the solid surface and its rate of renewal, which are a function of the local convective velocity and turbulence intensity.

Above N_{js}, the particles are fully suspended and no increase in the surface area of the particles exposed to the liquid results from increasing the agitation rate, but k_{SL} continues to increase albeit at a much lower rate. At N_{js}, the value of k_{SL} has been found to be independent of the geometry of the vessel, impeller design or specific power consumption. Thus, in terms of power consumption, a mixer configuration that is efficient for solid suspension is also efficient for mass transfer. This can be achieved in most cases by using a low-speed hydrofoil impeller of large diameter, or a pitched-blade turbine of $D/T \sim 0.4$.

Several correlations are available in the literature to estimate k_{SL} as a function of the pertinent variables. In general, decreasing particle size ($a_p \propto d_p^{-1}$), increasing phase density difference, increasing molecular diffusivity, decreasing viscosity, and increasing power dissipation increase k_{SL}. However, these correlations have been found to be subject to considerable errors. Furthermore, because the diffusivity of a solute in a liquid medium is strongly influenced by the presence of other solutes, it is usually recommended that the mass transfer coefficient is measured experimentally in the given mixture for systems where mass transfer is important. The available correlations, however, remain a useful guide and provide insight into the expected effects of the various parameters on mass transfer in agitated systems (Doraiswamy and Sharma, 1984).

Mass transfer coefficients for well suspended systems may be estimated from the Frössling (1938) equation that correlates the Sherwood number, Sh, to a diffusion and a convective term:

$$Sh = \frac{k_{SL} d_p}{\mathcal{D}} = 2 + C_1 \mathrm{Re}_p^{1/2} Sc^{1/3} \tag{10.44}$$

Here, $\mathcal{D}$ is the diffusion coefficient of the solute in solution, d_p is a characteristic length scale of the particle, Re_p the particle Reynolds number based on this length scale, and $Sc = \mu/\rho_L\mathcal{D}$ is the Schmidt number.

The constant C_1 as well as the exponents of Re_p and Sc do vary in the literature. C_1 ranges from 0.4 to 0.72 for solid particles, whilst the exponent of Sc in empirical correlations varies from 1/3 to 0.38. Note that using the value 0.38 results in a ~ 40% increase in predicted mass transfer over the value 1/3.

Nienow (1975) and Nienow and Miles (1978) demonstrate that k_{SL} is independent of power per unit volume at $N = N_{js}$ (note that k_{SL} does increase with N!). This implies that for particles with a significant settling velocity, the velocity term in Re_p is the terminal velocity (u_∞) of the particles:

$$Sh = \frac{k_{SL}d_p}{\mathcal{D}} = 2 + C_1\left(\frac{\rho_L d_p u_\infty}{\mu}\right)^{1/2} Sc^{1/3} \tag{10.45}$$

For small particles, or for particles with a low $\Delta\rho$, the terminal velocity tends to zero. In such cases, the relevant velocity is that of the turbulent fluctuations $u' = (\varepsilon d_p)^{1/3}$ (equation 10.27). With $\varepsilon \propto N^3D^2$, then $u' \propto ND(d_p/D)^{1/3}$ and, in consequence, if the turbulent fluctuations are larger than the terminal velocity, then:

$$Sh = 2 + C_1\left(\frac{\rho_L d_p (\varepsilon d_p)^{1/3}}{\mu}\right)^{1/2} Sc^{1/3} = 2 + C_2\left(\frac{\rho_L d_p ND}{\mu}\right)^{1/2}\left(\frac{d_p}{D}\right)^{1/6} Sc^{1/3} \tag{10.46}$$

This equation suggests that the scale-up rule for maintaining mass transfer constant is constant energy dissipation rate (P/V). Note that this assumes all particles are suspended and that geometrical similarity and the particle size distribution are maintained between scales.

10.9 Size Reduction, Deagglomeration and Attrition

In the pharmaceutical industry, size reduction may be a blessing or a curse . . . When charging reagents, drug product or excipients, the objective is typically to achieve good dispersion, and the disruption of loose agglomerates and lumps is desirable. In drug product processes this can be very important and often high shear agitators are used to ensure particles are size reduced to the appropriate level associated that is likely to be a drug product CQA. Typical high shear systems are a saw tooth agitator, or proprietary rotor stator devices that operate at high speed.

10.9.1 Breaking Particles through Turbulent Forces

Hydrodynamic stresses on particles in stirred vessels can be important. Damage due to hydrodynamic forces, often loosely referred to as 'shear effect', can be particularly significant where solids are delicate, but little has been reported on this aspect in the literature. In laminar flow, soft particles may be deformed and even damaged by large shear stresses, in the same way that liquid droplets are deformed and broken. In turbulent flow, however, fluid-particle interactions, as pointed out previously, are governed by the relative size of eddies and particles.

This is, for instance, important in fermentations and similar operations, in which biological cells may be destroyed if the local shear rates in the vessel are too high. A lot of work has been reported on the damage caused to cells in fermenters. Ultimately, it was shown that the dominant cell rupture mechanism is caused by the disengagement of bubbles at the surface of the fermenter, rather than turbulence or fluid shear (Nienow, 2006).

Similarly, the impact of agitation by standard impellers on attrition and deagglomeration is also often exaggerated. Turbulent pressure fluctuations resulting from common agitators on their own are unlikely to break droplets with a size of less than 100 μm, let alone solid needles and rods with a length of less than 100 μm. Ordinary agitation cannot be relied upon to achieve controlled particle size reduction. In the formulation of agrochemical products, for instance, an agitator is often used in combination with a high shear device to reduce particle size. Typically, agglomerates are reduced down to 250 μm.

If based on particle imaging it is felt that the particles may be sensitive to fracture, scale-up should be done on the same principles used for liquid-liquid systems. A particle will break if it is exposed to a stress larger than its tensile strength. Roberts *et al.* (1995) reported the tensile stress of some typical pharmaceutical materials in the range of 5–14 MPa. Recently, Macleod and Muller (2011) derived the tensile strength from particle breakage during pressure filtration and found values of 3–17 MPa.

The particles are subjected to turbulent forces, so by analogy with disruptive forces on a liquid drop, one could imagine that an eddy causes a pressure fluctuation resulting in a force on the centre of a needle shaped or plate-like crystal of length ℓ_p, width b and thickness h, where $b \geq h$, thus:

$$F_C \propto \rho_L(\varepsilon \ell_p)^{2/3} \times b\ell_p \tag{10.47}$$

The force required to break the crystal 'beam' is given by:

$$\sigma_T < \frac{6\ell_p F_C}{bh^2} \tag{10.48}$$

where σ_T is the tensile strength of the material. So, a particle will break if:

$$\left(\frac{\rho_L \varepsilon^{2/3} \ell^{2/3}}{\sigma_T}\right)\left(\frac{\ell_p}{h}\right)^2 > \text{constant} \tag{10.49}$$

Even though the constant in equation (10.49) may not be known, it follows that scale-down or scale-up using constant *P/V* will result in a similar breakage rate. So, if no excessive breakage is seen in the lab, it is unlikely to happen on the plant providing *P/V* is kept constant.

10.9.2 Breaking Particles through Impact

In a stirred suspension, particles can incur mechanical damage through comminution or attrition to the extent that the overall quality of the product is affected. Attrition is the unwanted breakdown of particles occurring within a process mainly as a consequence of collisions with other particles or parts of the equipment, i.e. impeller blades or vessel walls.

In a rare contribution about the mechanical damage of soft particles, which is of some relevance to this area of work, Wang *et al.* (2002) measured the damage caused to cooked potato during processing in a continuous scraped surface heat exchanger, which is similar in principle to a mechanically agitated vessel. The material was cut into 7 mm cubes and suspended in a carboxymethylcellulose solution whose rheology was described by the power-law model (equation 10.4). The particle concentration used was rather low at 3.6 particle per kg of liquid, however. Even then, it was shown that a severe reduction in particle size can occur when the particle tissue is soft (i.e. when the cooking time is high in the case of potatoes). The evidence obtained suggested that particle damage was due primarily to particle-blade collisions. A higher liquid viscosity did not offer any protective effect to the particles. The degree of particle attrition was directly affected by the rotor speed that determined the collision frequency, and particle residence time that determined the total number of collisions experienced by each particle.

Much of the relevant work reported to date, however, has been in relation to crystallization processes. The relevant mechanisms involved are abrasion, which is the removal of material much smaller than the particle, and fragmentation/breakage of a particle into smaller parts. Abrasion requires a lower impact energy and tends to prevail in crystal suspensions (see for example, Mazzarotta, 1992).

Crystallization is a key aspect in nearly all small molecule pharmaceutical manufacturing and development including purification of intermediates, formation of the product, or prevention of crystallization in amorphous products. Pharmaceutical intermediates and drug substance crystals tend to be needle shaped, but other regular shapes are of course encountered, for example cubic, tetragonal. Crystal shape is important because it affects other properties such as the angle of repose of stacked crystals and rate of dissolution. Crystal size uniformity is also important because a non-uniform crystal mixture is visually unattractive, the different sizes tend to segregate, and separating the mother liquor from the solids is more difficult. Attrition is the only source of new crystals that is independent of supersaturation. This hydrodynamic phenomenon has a significant effect on nucleation kinetics and hence on the crystal size distribution.

A good treatise on crystal attrition can be found in various works such as Fasoli and Conti (1973), Chianese *et al.* (1986), Shamlou *et al.* (1990), Synowiec *et al.* (1993), and Gahn and Mersmann (1995). Though a number of attrition rates have been defined, such as the number of abrasion fragments produced per abrading particle (Fasoli and Conti, 1973; Nienow and Conti, 1978; Synowiec *et al.*, 1993), the mass-abrasion rate of the fragments (Chianese *et al.*, 1986), and the initial rate of fragment generation (Shamlou *et al.*, 1990), no generally accepted method for quantifying attrition has emerged. In addition to generating large amounts of small fragments, crystal attrition also affects their size distribution as well as their shape. The breakage functions commonly adopted to describe the product of comminution events are not applicable to attrition, since fracture leading to a bimodal size distribution predominates (Kelly and Spottiswood, 1982). Encouraging results were obtained by Mazzarotta (1992) using a model combining abrasion and fracture. However, information about the morphology of crystals that have been subjected to attrition has been limited to qualitative observations gleaned from photographs of the abraded crystals and fragments (Fasoli and Conti, 1973; Conti and Nienow, 1980).

Attrition due to particle interactions with the vessel walls is only significant when there are flow constrictions present, for example when the impeller is installed close to a solid boundary such as when large *D/T* ratios are used, or when inserts are used. In the absence of such flow constrictions, at low solids concentrations inter-particle interactions are rare and relatively weak, and most damage that occurs is due to particle collisions with the impeller blades.

The frequency of particle-impeller collisions, ω, is assumed to be proportional to (Nienow, 2000): (1) the frequency f of particle passage through the impeller volume, represented by the impeller volumetric discharge divided by the vessel volume, $f = ND^3/V$; (2) the probability p of collision during a passage, $p = Nu_\infty$; and (3) the mean solids concentration in the vessel, $\bar{C}$, as shown:

$$\omega \propto \frac{ND^3}{V} \times p \times \bar{C} \tag{10.50}$$

The amount of particle damage due to attrition is assumed to be proportional to the energy of impact, E, which in turn is assumed to be proportional to N^2D^2. For a given fluid-solid system, there is a minimum level of energy that is required at impact before any significant particle damage can occur. Beyond that level, the rate of particle attrition J is then given by the following equation (Nienow, 2000):

$$J \propto \omega E \propto \frac{P}{V} N \tag{10.51}$$

The energy threshold for particle damage to occur needs to be assessed in a controlled experiment using appropriate mechanical testing equipment. Therefore, a higher power input and increasing agitation speed by the use of smaller *D/T* ratios for example, will increase the rate of particle damage. Note, however, that N decreases on scale-up and hence particle damage would be expected to be lower in larger vessels. This implies that the use of large *D/T* ratios and minimum power input – for example, by using high efficiency hydrofoil impellers – would help to minimize particle damage. Conversely, in a crystallization process it may be desirable to promote particle-impeller collisions, and in that case the dissipation of higher power inputs using smaller impellers would be recommended.

In concentrated suspensions, inter-particle collisions would be more frequent and their effects on particle integrity would become predominant, again provided the impact energy levels are high enough. In that case, the rate of particle damage has been described as follows (Nienow, 2000):

$$J \propto \bar{C}^2 \left(\frac{P}{V}\right)^{3/2} d_p^6 \tag{10.52}$$

This suggests that the rate of particle attrition is highly sensitive to particle size and solids concentration. Therefore, concentrated systems with larger particles would generate a lot of attrition provided the solids are soft enough or conversely the impact energies are high enough. Specific power input is again a key to controlling particle damage as J is quite sensitive to *P/V* in this case.

Nomenclature

a_p	interfacial area for mass transfer (m^2)
C	impeller off-bottom clearance (m)
C_D	drag coefficient (-)
D	impeller diameter (m)
$\mathcal{D}$	diffusion coefficient (m^2s^{-1})
d_p	particle diameter (m)
F	drag force (N)
Fr	Froude number (-)
g	gravitational acceleration (ms^{-2})
Ga	Galileo number (-)
H	liquid height in vessel (m)
J	rate of particle attrition (number/(volume × time))
k	flow consistency index (Pa s^n)
k_{SL}	bulk diffusion mass transfer coefficient (ms^{-1})
n	flow behaviour index (-)
N	impeller speed (s^{-1})
N_{js}	minimum agitation speed for complete suspension (s^{-1})
N_{jd}	minimum agitation speed for particle draw-down (s^{-1})
P	power dissipation (W)
Po	power number (-)
Re	impeller Reynolds number (-)
Re_B	Bingham Reynolds number (-)
Re_p	particle Reynolds number (-)
S	shape factor or Zwietering constant (-)
Sc	Shmidt number (-)
Sh	Sherwood number (-)
t	time (s)
T	tank diameter (m)
u	particle slip velocity (ms^{-1})
u'	liquid rms velocity fluctuations (ms^{-1})
u_∞	terminal settling velocity (ms^{-1})
V	volume of vessel contents (m^3)
X	solids concentration by weight × 100 (-)
Z, $Z(n)$	drag correction factor (-)

Greek symbols

$\dot{\gamma}$	shear rate (s^{-1})
η	apparent viscosity (Pas)
η_B	plastic viscosity (Pas)
ε	local rate of energy dissipation (Wkg^{-1})
φ_p	volume fraction of particles (-)
λ	Kolmogorov length scale (m)

μ	dynamic viscosity (Pas)
ν	kinematic viscosity (m^2s^{-1})
$\Delta\rho$	solid-liquid density difference (kgm^{-3})
ΔP_p	pressure fluctuations near a particle (Pa)
ρ_L	liquid density (kgm^{-3})
ρ_p	particle density (kgm^{-3})
ρ_S	slurry density (kgm^{-3})
σ	standard deviation (kgm^{-3})
τ	shear stress (Pa)
τ_j	average force required to break a junction between two particles (N)
τ_y	yield stress (Pa)
ω	frequency of particle-impeller collisions (number/time)

Abbreviations

CFD	computational fluid dynamics
CQA	critical quality attribute
PEPT	positron emission particle tracking
PLIF	planar laser induced fluorescence
csa	critical speed of surface aeration
jd	just drawn down
js	just suspended

References

Adams L., Barigou M., 2007, CFD analysis of caverns and pseudo-caverns developed during mixing of non-Newtonian fluids, *Chem. Eng. Res. Des.*, 85, 598–604.

Amanullah A., Hjorth S.A., Nienow A.W., 1998, A new mathematical model to predict cavern diameters in highly shear thinning power-law liquids using axial flow impellers, *Chem. Eng. Sci.*, 53, 455–469.

Armenante, P.M., Nagamine, E.U., Susanto, J., 1998, Dtermination of correlations to predict the minimum agitation speed for complete solid suspension in agitated vessels, *Can. J. Chem. Eng.*, 76, 413–419.

Atapattu, D.D., Chhabra, R.P., Uhlherr, P.H.T., 1995, Creeping sphere motion in Herschel-Bulkley fluids: flow field and drag, *J. Non-Newt. Fluid Mech.*, 59, 245–265.

Aubin, J., Mavros, P., Fletcher, D.F., Bertrand, J., Xuereb, C., 2001, Effect of axial agitator configuration (up-pumping, down-pumping, reverse rotation) on flow patterns generated in stirred vessels, *Chem. Eng. Res. Des.*, 79, 845–856.

Baldi, G., Conti, R., Alaria, E., 1978, Complete suspension of particles in mechanically agitated vessels, *Chem. Eng. Sci.*, 33, 21–25.

Barigou, M., 2004, Particle tracking in opaque mixing systems: An overview of the capabilities of PET and PEPT, *Chem. Eng. Res. Des.*, 82, 1258–1267.

Barigou, M., Chiti, F., Pianko-Oprych, P., Guida, A., Adams, L., Fan, X., Parker, D.J. & Nienow, A.W. (2009). Using positron emission particle tracking (PEPT) to study mixing in stirred vessels: validation and tackling unsolved problems in opaque systems. *J. Chem. Eng. Jpn.*, 42(11), 839–846.

Barnes, H.A., Hutton, J.F., Walters, K., 1989, *An Introduction to Rheology*, Elsevier, Amsterdam.

Barresi, A., Baldi, G., 1987, Solid dispersion in an agitated vessel, *Chem. Eng. Sci.*, 42, 2949–2956.

Bittorf, K.J., Kresta, S.M., 2002, Prediction of cloud height for solid suspension in stirred tanks, *CHISA Conference Proceedings,* Aug. 25–29, Prague, Czech Republic, P5.166.

Borghesani A. F., 1985, Concentration-dependent behaviour of the shear viscosity of coal-fuel oil suspensions. *Rheol. Acta*, 24, 189–197.

Bourne, J.R., Zabelka, M., 1980, The influence of gradual classification on continuous crystallisation, *Chem. Eng. Sci.*, 35, 533–542.

Brujes, L., Legrand, J., Carnelle, G., 1998, Complete suspension of microcapsules in baffled and unbaffled stirred tanks, *Chem. Eng. Technol.*, 21, 735–744.

Brunazzi, E., Gallettii, C., Paglianti, A., Pintus, S., 2004, An impedance probe for the measurements of flow characteristics and mixing properties in stirred slurry reactors, *Chem. Eng. Res. Des.*, 82, 1250–1257.

Bujalski, W., Takenak, K., Paolini, S. *et al.*, 1999, Suspension and liquid homogenisation in high solids concentration stirred chemical reactors, *Chem. Eng. Res. Des.*, 77, 241–247.

Bujalski, W., Konno, M., Nienow, A.W., 1988, Scale-up of 45° pitch blade agitators for gas dispersion and solid suspension, *Proc. 6th Euro. Conf. Mixing, Pavia, Italy, BHRA*: Cranfield, UK, pp 389–398.

Chapman, C.M., Nienow, A.W., Cooke, M., Middleton, J.C., 1983, Particle-gas-liquid mixing in stirred vessels. Part I: Particle liquid mixing. *Chem. Eng. Res. Des.,* 61, 71–81.

Chhabra, R.P., 1990, Motion of spheres in power-law (viscoinelastic) fluids at intermediate Reynolds numbers: a unified approach, *Chem. Eng. & Process.*, 28, 89–94.

Chhabra, R.P., 2006, *Bubbles, Drops and Particles in Non-Newtonian Fluids*, 2nd edn, CRC Press, Boca Raton, FL.

Chhabra, R.P., Richardson, J.F., 1999, *Non-Newtonian Flow in the Process Industries: Fundamentals and Engineering Applications*, Butterworth Heinemann, Oxford.

Chianese, A., Di Cave, S., Mazzarotta, B., 1986, Secondary nucleation by abrasion of potassium sulphate, *Proc. World Cong. of Chem. Eng.*, vol. 11, Tokyo, p. 937, Sept. 21–25.

Choudhury, N.H., Penney, W.R., Meyers, K., Fasano, J.B., 1995, An experimental investigation of solids suspension at high solids loadings in mechanically agitated vessels, *AIChE Symp. Ser.*, 305(91), 131–138.

Clift, R., Grace, J., Weber, M.E., 1978, *Bubbles, Drops and Particles*, Academic Press, New York.

Conti, R., Nienow, A.W., 1980, Particle abrasion at high solids concentration in stirred vessels-II, *Chem. Eng. Sci.*, 35, 543–547.

Doraiswamy, L.K., Sharma, M.M., 1984, *Heterogeneous Reaction: Analysis, Examples and Reactor Design*, vol. 2, Fluid-Fluid-Solid Reactions, Wiley, New York.

Elson, T.P., 1990, The growth of caverns formed around rotating impellers during the mixing of a yield stress fluid, *Chem. Eng. Comm.*, 96, 303–319.

Fasoli, U., Conti, R., 1973, Crystal breakage in a mixed suspension crystallizer, *Kristall Technik*, 8, 931–946.

Frössling N., 1938, The evaporation of falling drops, *Gerlands Beitr. Geophys.*, 52, 170–216.

Gahn, C., Mersmann, A., 1995, The brittleness of substances crystallized in industrial processes, *Powder Tech.*, 85, 71–81.

Gay, E.C., Nelson, P.A., Armstrong, W.P., 1969, Flow properties of suspensions with high solids concentration, *AIChE J.*, 15, 815–822.

Graham, D.I., Jones, T.E.R., 1994, Settling and transport of spherical particles in power-law fluids at finite. Reynolds number, *J. Non-Newtonian Fluid Mech.*, 54, 465–488.

Greaves, M., Kobbacy, K.A.H., 1981, Surface aeration in agitated vessels, In: *IChem. E. Symp. Ser.,* 64, pp. H1–H22.

Guerci, D., Conti, R., Sicardi, S., 1986, Mixed flow stirrer performance in solids suspension in agitated vessels, *Colloque Agitation Mécanique, ENSIGC*, 11–12 June, Toulouse, France, pp 3–18 to 3–24.

Guida, A., Nienow, A.W., Barigou, M., 2010, PEPT measurements of solid-liquid flow field and spatial phase distribution in concentrated monodisperse stirred suspensions, *Chem. Eng. Sci.,* 65(6), 1905–1914.

Guida, A., Fan, X., Parker, D.J., Nienow, A.W., Barigou, M. (2009). Positron Emission Particle Tracking in a mechanically agitated solid-liquid suspension of coarse particles. *Chem. Eng. Res. Des.*, 87, 421–429.

Heymann L., Peukert S., Akse N., 2002, On the solid-liquid transition of concentrated Suspensions in transient shear flow. *Rheol Acta*, 41, 307–315.
Hicks, M. T., Mayers, K. J., Bakker, A., 1997, Cloud height in solid suspension agitation, *Chem. Eng. Commun.* 160, 137–155.
Hinze, J. O., 1955, Fundamentals of the hydrodynamic mechanism of splitting in dispersion processes, *AIChE J.*, 1, 289–295.
Ibrahim, S.B., Nienow, A.W., 1994, The effect of viscosity on mixing pattern and solid suspension in stirred vessels, in *Proc. 8th Euro. Conf. Mixing, IChemE Symposium Series*, 136, 25–32.
Ibrahim S, Nienow AW. Particle suspension in the turbulent régime: the effect of impeller type and impeller/vessel configuration, 1996, *Chem. Eng. Res. Des.*, 74, 679–688.
Joosten, G.E.H., Schilde, J.G.M., Broere, A.M., 1977, The Suspension of floating solids in stirred vessels, *Trans. Inst. Chem. Eng.*, 55, 220–222.
Kelly, E. G., Spottiswood, D.J., 1982, *Introduction to Mineral Processing*, Wiley, New York, pp. 113–123.
Khazam, O., Kresta, S.M., 2009, Drawdown of floating solids in stirred tanks, *13th Euro. Conf. on Mixing*, 14–17 April, London.
Khazam, O., Kresta, S.M., 2008, Mechanisms of solids drawdown in stirred tanks, *Can. J. Chem. Eng.*, 86(4), 622–634.
Kolmogorov, A., 1941a, Dissipation of energy in the locally isotropic turbulence, *Comptes Rendus de l'Académie des Sciences de l'URSS*, 32, 16–18.
Kolmogorov, A., 1941b, The local structure of turbulence in incompressible viscous fluid for very large Reynolds' numbers, *Comptes Rendus de l'Académie des Sciences de l'URSS*, 30, 301–305.
Lareo, C., Fryer, P.J., Barigou, M., 1997, The fluid mechanics of two-phase solid-liquid food flows, *Food Bioprod. Process.*, 75, 73–105.
MacLeod C., Muller F.L. 2011, On the fracture of crystals during pressure filtration: case studies and mechanistic understanding. *Chem. Eng. Sci.*, 470, 77–87.
Mak, A.T.C., Yang, S., Ozcan-Taskin N.G., 1997, The effect of scale on the suspension and distribution of solids in stirred vessels, *9th Euro. Conf. Mixing, Paris, March 1997, Récents Progrès en Génie des Procédés, Lavoisier, Paris*, vol. 11, pp 97–104.
Mak, A.T.C., 1992, *Solid-liquid mixing in mechanically agitated vessels*, PhD, University College London, UK.
Markopoulos and Kontogeorgaki, 1995, Vortex depth in unbaffled single and multiple impeller agitated vessels, *Chem. Eng. Technol.*, 18, 68–74.
Mazzarotta, B., 1992, Abrasion and breakage phenomena in agitated crystal suspensions, *Chem. Eng. Sci.*, 47, 12, 3105–3111.
Metzner, A. B. and Otto, R. E., 1957, Agitation of non-Newtonian fluids, *AIChEJ*, 3 (1), 3–10.
Metzner. A. B., Feehs, R. H., Ramos, H. L., Otto, R. E. and Tuthill, J. D., 1961, Agitation of viscous Newtonian and non-Newtonian fluids, *AIChEJ*, 7(1), 3–9.
Møller P.C.F., Mewis J., Bonn D., 2006, Yield stress and thixotropy: on the difficulty of measuring yield stresses in practice. *Soft Matter*, 2, 274–283.
Montante, G., Micale, G., Magelli, F., Brucato, A., 2001, Experiments and CFD predictions of solid particle distribution in a vessel agitated with four pitched-blade turbines, *Chem. Eng. Res. Des.*, 79, 1005–1010.
Montante, G., Pinelli, D., Magelli, F., 2002, Diagnosis of solids distribution in vessels stirred with multiple PBTs and comparison of two modelling approaches, *Can. J. Chem. Eng.*, 80, 665–673.
Muller F.L., 2009, On the rheological behaviour of Batch crystallisations. *Chem. Eng. Res. Des.*, 87, 627–632.
Muller F.L., Latimer J., 2009, Anticipation of scale-up issues in pharmaceutical development. *Comput. Chem. Eng.*, 33, 1051–1055.
Nagata, S., 1975, *Mixing, Principles and Applications*, Halsted Press, New York.
Nasr-El-Din, H.A., MacTaggart, R.S., Masliyah, J.H., 1996, Local solids concentration measurement in a slurry mixing tank, *Chem. Eng. Sci.*, 51, 1209–1220.
Nienow, A.W., 1968, Suspension of solid particles in turbine-agitated baffled system, *Chem. Eng. Sci.*, 23, 1453–1459.
Nienow, A.W., 1975, Agitated vessel particle–liquid mass transfer: a comparison between theories and data, *Chem. Eng. J.*, 9, 153.

Nienow, A.W., Conti, R., 1978, Particle abrasion at high solids concentration in stirred vessels, *Chem. Eng. Sci.*, 33, 1077–1086.

Nienow, A. W., and D. Miles 1978. The effect of impeller/tank configurations on fluid–particle mass transfer, *Chem. Eng. J.*, 15, 13.

Nienow, A.W., Elson T.P., 1988, Aspects of mixing in rheologically complex fluids, *Chem. Eng. Res. Des.*, 66, 5–15.

Nienow, A.W., 1999, The versatility of up-pumping, wide-blade hydrofoil agitators, *Proc. 3rd Int. Symp. On Mixing in Industrial Processes, Osaka, Japan*, 19–22 Sept., 173–180.

Nienow, A.W., 2000, The suspension of solid particles, in *Mixing in the Process Industries*, 2nd edn, eds N. Harnby, M.F. Edwards, A.W. Nienow, Ch. 16, pp. 364–393, Butterworth-Heinemann, Oxford.

Nienow, A.W., 2006, Reactor engineering in large scale animal cell culture, *Cytotechnology*, 50, 9–33.

Oldshue, J.Y., 1983, Fluid mixing technology and practice, *Chem. Eng.*, 90, 82–108.

Özcan-Taskin, G. 2006, Effect of scale on the drawdown of floating solids, *Chem. Eng. Sci.*, 61, 2871 – 2879

Patwardhan A.W., Joshi J.B., 1998, Design of Stirred Vessels with Gas Entrained from Free Liquid Surface. *Can. J. Chem. Eng.*, 76, 339–364.

Pianko-Oprych, P., Adams, L., Nienow, A.W., Barigou, M., 2006, CFD simulation of solid-liquid suspension in Newtonian and power-law liquids, *Proc. 12th Euro. Conf. Mixing, Bologna, Italy*, 27–30 June, pp. 503–510.

Rao, K.S.M.S., Rewattkar, V.B., Joshi, J.B., 1988, Critical impeller speed for solid suspension in mechanically agitated contactors, *AIChEJ*, 34, 1332–1340.

Ratsimbazafy V, Bourret E, Duclos R, Brossard C., 1999 . Rheological behaviour of drug suspensions in Gelucire mixtures and proxyphylline release from matrix hard gelatin capsules. *Eur J Pharm Biopharm.*, 48(3), 247–252.

Richardson, L.F., 1922, *Weather Prediction by Numerical Process*. Cambridge University Press, Cambridge, p. 66.

Rieger F., Ditl P., Havelkova O., 1988, Suspension of solid particles – Concentration profiles and particle layer on the vessel bottom, *Proc. 6th Euro. Conf. Mixing, Pavia, Italy, BHRA: Cranfield, UK*, pp 251–258.

Roberts, R., Rowe, R., York, P. 1995, The relationship between the fracture properties, tensile strength and critical stress intensity factor of organic solids and their molecular structure. *Int. J. Pharm.*, 125, 157–162.

Shamlou, P.A., 1993, Suspension of particles in liquids in stirred vessels, in *Processing of Solid-Liquid Suspensions*, ed. P.A. Shamlou, pp 273–286, Butterworth-Heinemann, Oxford.

Shamlou, P.A., Jones, A.G., Djamarani, K., 1990, Hydrodynamics of secondary nucleation in suspension crystallization, *Chem. Eng. Sci.*, 45, 1405–1416.

Spidla, M., Sinevic, V., Jahoda, M., Machon, V., 2005, Solid particle distribution of moderately concentrated suspensions in a pilot plant stirred vessel, *Chem. Eng. J.*, 113, 73–82.

Synowiec, P., Jones, A.G., Shamlou, P.A., 1993, Crystal break-up in dilute turbulently agitated suspensions, *Chem. Eng. Sci.*, 48, 3485–3495.

Tamburini A., Cipollina A., Micale G., Brucato A., 2009. Particle distribution in an unbaffled stirred vessel by a novel laser sheet image analysis technique. *AIDIC Conference Series, Vol.* 9, 319–328.

Tatterson, G.B., 1994, *Scale-up and Design of Industrial Mixing Processes*, McGraw-Hill, New York.

Wang, Y.Y., Russell, A.B., Stanley, R.A., 2002, Mechanical damage to food particles during processing in a scraped surface heat exchanger, *Food Bioprod. Process.*, 80, 3–11.

Wong, C.W., Wang, J.P., Huang, S.T., 1987, Investigations of fluid dynamics in mechanically stirred aerated slurry reactors, *Can. J. Chem. Eng.*, 65, 412–419.

Yamazaki, H., Tojo, K., Miyanami, K., 1986, Concentration profiles of solids suspended in a stirred tank, *Powder Technol.*, 48, 205–216.

Zlokarnik, M., 1991, *Dimensional Analysis and Scale-Up in Chemical Engineering*, Springer Verlag, Berlin.

Zlokarnik, M., 2001, *Stirring: Theory and Practice*, Wiley-VCH, Weinheim, Germany.

Zwietering, N.TH., 1958, Suspending of solid particles in liquid by agitators, *Chem. Eng. Sci.*, 8, 244–253.

Part III

Equipment

11

Powder Blending Equipment

David S. Dickey
MixTech, Inc., USA

11.1 Introduction

Powder blending equipment is ubiquitous in the pharmaceutical industry as many drug dosages are delivered in a solid or tablet form. Most of those tablets are made primarily with a powdered excipient (inactive component) such as lactose. The active pharmaceutical ingredient (API) may either be a liquid or powder representing only a small fraction of the total tablet content. The forms of the API and the bulk behavior of the excipient are important factors in considering which type of blender will work best.

Because the API is a small part of the total, extremely uniform blending is essential at the scale of scrutiny of a single tablet. Pre-blending a small concentration (less than 0.5%) of the API at a higher concentration in part of a major component, may be the best approach in achieving a uniform blend. Maintaining a uniform mixture can be more difficult than creating it in the first place. To keep a blend from segregating, an agglomeration process Capes & Fouda (1984), Parkinson (1989) may add a binder to allow the powder blend to be compacted uniformly into a tablet form. Consequently, blending, liquid addition, agglomeration, and even drying may be carried out in the powder blending equipment. The relative importance of the blending and agglomeration may influence the type of equipment that is most suitable for a particular product.

Some blending equipment used for pharmaceutical applications is specifically designed for the industry. However, similar categories of blending equipment are found in many other industries. Polished stainless steel surfaces are commonly used in powder blending equipment for the pharmaceutical industry. Construction details such as non-contaminating

Pharmaceutical Blending and Mixing, First Edition. Edited by P.J. Cullen, Rodolfo J. Romañach, Nicolas Abatzoglou and Chris D. Rielly.

shaft seal materials and CIP cleaning capabilities are also important Kent (2003). The presence of both powders and solvents may require explosion-proof equipment and installation.

11.2 Blending Mechanisms

Three mechanisms contribute to the blending of a powder Muzzio, et al. (2004). Those mechanisms are convection, shear, and diffusion. Convection involves the motion of powder from one location to another within a blender. Shear is the local relative motion between adjacent portions of the powder. Diffusion is the intermingling of individual particles. Each of these three mechanisms is needed to blend powders thoroughly. The mechanisms are present in different proportions for each type of blending equipment.

Additionally, the bulk behaviors of powders are different, from free-flowing, to cohesive, and even to a paste. The flow characteristics of a powder also will influence the selection of blending equipment best able to handle specific powder properties.

11.3 Blend Time

Blend time for powder mixing can be confusing because longer is not always better and most batches blend quickly, Cox (2000). Simple blending of a free-flowing powder can be rapid, as little as 50 revolutions of a tumble blender or 100 revolutions of a rotating element blender may be sufficient. Those numbers are only generalizations, but represent 1 or 2-min blend times, even for large blenders. Fragile particles may be broken with longer blending, leading to dust and size differences that may cause segregation. The objective should be to find the time necessary to assure complete blending and then to stop.

Measuring blend time and checking for uniformity can be difficult, because sampling of a powder batch is difficult (see Chapter 4). Taking a sample from a batch of powder requires stopping the blender, for safety if nothing else. Once the blender is stopped, the powder is no longer as it was while blending and the blender may be difficult or impossible to restart. Because powder blending happens rapidly, measuring a sample to sufficient accuracy to decide if uniformity has been reached can be as difficult as taking a good sample. To assure uniformity as a measure of blend time, taking samples from the least well mixed locations, such as near the side or end, of a blender may be a better approach than trying to measure bulk uniformity.

Batch time may be something quite different from a blend time. Cohesive powders may require additional blending to achieve uniform bulk properties. The addition of multiple components will extend batch time by the nominal blending time following the addition of the last component. The time required for the addition and uniform distribution of a liquid binder for granulation also will extend batch processing time. If a solvent or some liquid must be removed by drying, a further extension to processing time is necessary. Careful evaluation of process conditions and steps may identify other requirements.

Generally blend times greater than 5 min for small, easy batches or 10 min for large, even difficult batches may be longer than necessary. Many continuous processes have residence times of only a minute or two.

Table 11.1 Bulk densities of some powders

Material	Bulk Density [kg/m³]	Bulk Density [lb/ft³]
dibasic calcium phosphate	700	44
granulated sugar	1,600	100
lactose	530	33
magnesium stearate	340	21
manitol	610	38
sorbitol	590	37
sucrose	850	53

11.4 Fill Level

A frequent reason for extended blend times or poor product uniformity is an overfilled blender. Fill level for powder blending equipment is important. Each type of blending equipment has a range of batch volumes for successful blending Cox (2000). In some equipment that range can be very narrow. In other equipment the range can be much wider. One difficulty with fill level is that the operating volume of a powder batch is the dilated or aerated condition of the material, not the settled or compacted volume or the powder. Since most product formulations are described in mass units, the bulk density of a powder is important in determining the fill level. The bulk density of the powder is also a factor in determining the power requirements and mechanical strengths of a blender Kent (2003). Table 11.1 gives unexpanded bulk densities for several materials found in pharmaceutical production.

Bulk density may be a problem for the scale-up of powder blenders. In a small blender, the material at the bottom of the blender will only be slightly compacted. The same powder in a large blender may be more compacted at the bottom of the blender or the bottom of a storage hopper. Different degrees of compacting affect not only bulk density, but also may affect cohesion and adhesion.

11.5 Segregation

Common segregation mechanisms include sifting, fluidization, air entrainment, and angle of repose. Segregation may result in separation or demixing of a power blend. Sifting is the most common segregation mechanism. Sifting occurs as small particles settle between large particles, causing the large particles to move toward the surface of the powder. Effective blending requires that powder motion associated with convection and shear is sufficient to overcome moderate sifting. Large particles and particle size differences may need to be modified by grinding or other means for uniform blending. Fluidization occurs when air passing through a bed of particles lifts the small particles around the large particles, resulting in the small particles being brought to the surface. Fluidization is most likely to occur in fluidized bed blenders and dryers, but may also occur during discharge from enclosed blenders that do not have adequate vending. If incoming air must pass through the discharging powder, fluidization, and demixing may occur. Air entrainment of the fine particles also may result in dust formation. Angle of repose flow may cause segregation because large particles will roll down a slope more quickly than small particles. These powder properties and segregation mechanisms must be considered in the selection of powder blending equipment.

Segregation by particle size sifting can always cause uniformity problems, even if a batch is initially well blended. After leaving the blender, vibration during handling, packaging, and shipment may cause separation, especially with large particles of different sizes. One reason for granulation is to stick large and small particles together to retain the uniformity of a blend. Various other mechanisms and conditions may contribute to blending problems.

11.6 Powder Processing Difficulties

A study done by the Rand Corporation with a report written by Edward W. Merrow (1986) identifies several consistent difficulties with processing of powders, including blending and agglomeration. Operations producing powdered and solid products have poorer performance, more mechanical difficulties, and greater failure rate than plants producing liquids. The report finds that chemistry, impurities, temperature control, equipment design, mechanical design, material handling (loading and unloading), and waste handling are all significant problem areas for solids processing. Some common causes for these problems include a lack of sufficient material characterization, lack of formal training in particle technology, empiricism in equipment design, lack of scale-up methods, and inadequate attention to equipment specification. Information about single particle properties does not translate directly into bulk material and handling properties. Particle and bulk properties do not always predict blend requirements or equipment specification. While pilot testing is always recommended and cost effective, scale-up is not a direct process, which may cause other difficulties. However, greater knowledge, more testing, and some process engineering always reduce start-up and operating problems.

One of the hardest problems to solve in powder blending is inconsistency. Factors such as moisture content, particle size distributions, surface electric properties, and raw material sources can make a difference in blending results. Measurement and identification of these factors can be difficult and usually needs to be monitored carefully to identify the source of problems. Order of addition and operator procedures often contribute to these potentially interacting effects. About the only salvation is that if some batches are good, the blend is possible. Achieving the desired results every time may be a challenge.

11.7 Blender Classification

Blenders can be classified in a few basic categories: tumble blenders, rotating element blenders, and granulators. The tumble blenders accomplish the mixing action by allowing the material to flow within a rotating shell and may or may not have rotating internal elements. The rotating element blenders accomplish mixing by the rotation of spirals or blades inside a stationary shell. Granulators have been categorized separately because of unique features that emphasize the addition of liquids for agglomeration and processing to compact and sometimes dry the agglomerated blend. Many types of blenders have a combination of features, but commonly with one dominant function.

11.7.1 Tumble Blenders

Tumble blenders accomplish mixing by allowing a free-flowing material to move within a partially filled rotating container. The most common tumble blenders are twin-shell blenders, also known as V blenders. Other types of tumble blenders include the double-cone blender, the horizontal rotary blender, and the tote blender, each of which has some variations. Tumble blenders have some strong features for pharmaceutical blending, but also some limitations. Two of the strong features for the tumble blenders are that they can create very uniform blends of powders and they have a minimum of internal parts, so they can be cleaned easily. The primary limitation to tumble blenders is that they are only good for free-flowing powders. Even moderately cohesive powders may form lumps, which may not blend well. Lumps or large agglomerates must be broken by high-speed rotating bars or breakers. However, liquid addition to form small agglomerates may be used to maintain a uniform blend, especially by attaching the API to the excipient powder.

The basic mechanism for tumble blending involves a free-flowing powder sliding down the upper surface of the powder in the blender. The actual blending occurs in a thin layer on this surface. Tumble blenders filled more than half full may have a center core region where little if any blending takes place, Muzzio, et al. (2004). Because the blending is accomplished by angle of repose flow, large differences in particle sizes may result in segregation, especially at the axis of rotation. If the blender is more than half full, the moving layer does not influence the core of the blender contents and the result will be incomplete or uneven blending. If the blender is less than half full, the capacity is underutilized. The stated capacity for most tumble blenders is this half-full volume, not the geometric volume of the blender.

Blending for too long may create a static charge on the particles. Different materials may develop opposite charges, which may cause segregation. Because most pharmaceutical powders are non-conducting, the charge is not readily dissipated, even in grounded equipment.

Tumble blenders come in capacities from 0.03 m^3 (1 ft^3) to 5.5 m^3 (200 ft^3). The capacity usually represents about 50% of the internal volume of the blender. A tumble blender has almost no flexibility in the batch volume, since over or under filling does not blend well. Power consumption is nominally about 5 kW/1000 kg (5 hp/ton), but varies with the bulk density of the material being blended. Blend times are typically from 2 to 10 min for simple blending. Liquid addition, drying, or other processing will take longer.

11.7.1.1 Twin-Shell Blenders

Twin-shell blenders have two cylindrical shells attached at an angle to form a V. The shell is then rotated about a central axis across the legs of the V, so that free-flowing powder is alternately combined and divided. A typical twin-shell or V blender is shown in Figure 11.1.

For a twin-shell blender to work properly, it should be filled only to the axis of rotation. The capacity of powder blenders is based on volume, so weights must be converted to bulk

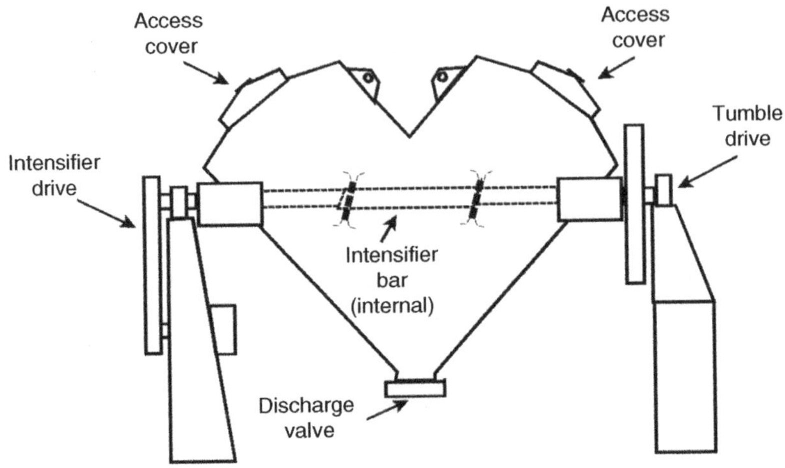

Figure 11.1 Twin-shell tumble blender

volume at the blending condition. The "working capacity" for tumble blenders should be half the open volume inside the blender.

While just tumbling a free-flowing powder will accomplish mixing, some powder applications require additional processing. For example, the addition of a small quantity of API to a large quantity of excipient may be aided by more intense dispersion of the powders for uniform blending. The active ingredient may be a powder, a liquid, or a powder dissolved in a solvent. The form of the active sometimes depends on the method that gives complete and rapid uniformity. A variety of high-speed rotating bars, as shown in Figure 11.2, may be operated along the axis of rotation for the tumble blender.

The liquid disperser bar can add a liquid binder for agglomeration, Pietsch (2003). The active ingredient may be pumped through the rotating slots, past teeth, to disperse both liquid and powder. Liquid addition through a disperser is shown in Figure 11.3.

When a very small quantity (<0.5%) of an ingredient is added to a large quantity, preblending of the small quantity ingredient into all or part of a large quantity ingredient is recommended. The batch for preblending should be done in an appropriately sized blender. If the full-size production blender must be used a quantity of preblend for multiple batches, a master batch, should be made.

Instead of loading the legs of the twin-shell blender from covers at the top of the V, a better initial blend can be loaded with the discharge valve facing upward. Adding and distributing material in both legs of the twin shell will speed initial blending. With multiple materials, the unblended material may have some vertical stratification. If the material is added through the ports on the top of each blender leg, any stratification may be from side to side. Usually, vertical stratification is blended more quickly than side to side stratification. Minor ingredients should be added away from the walls of the blender to avoid surface adhesion. Obviously, the blender must be loaded when it is not running and safety precautions and interlocks are necessary to keep people clear of the blender when it is operating.

Other variations of the basic twin shell design can provide additional process features. A cross-flow design has unequal length legs for the V design. The unequal legs cause the

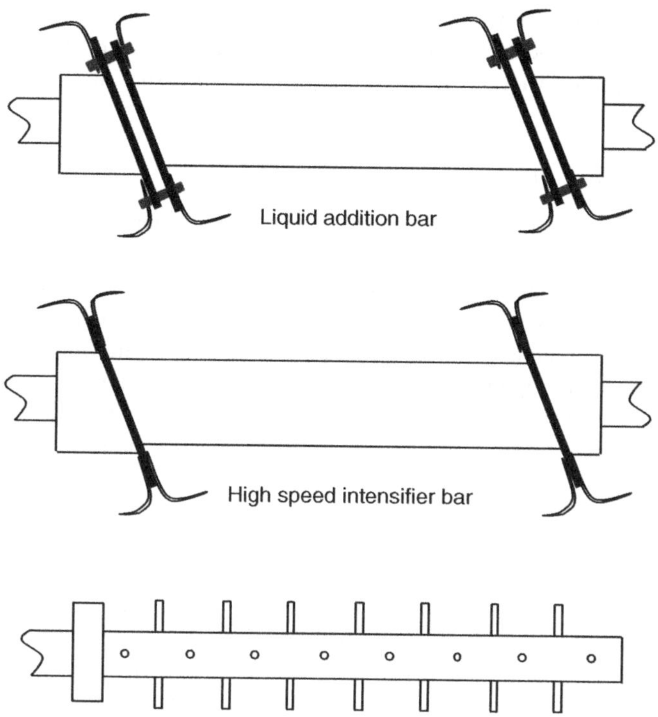

Figure 11.2 High-speed intensifier bars

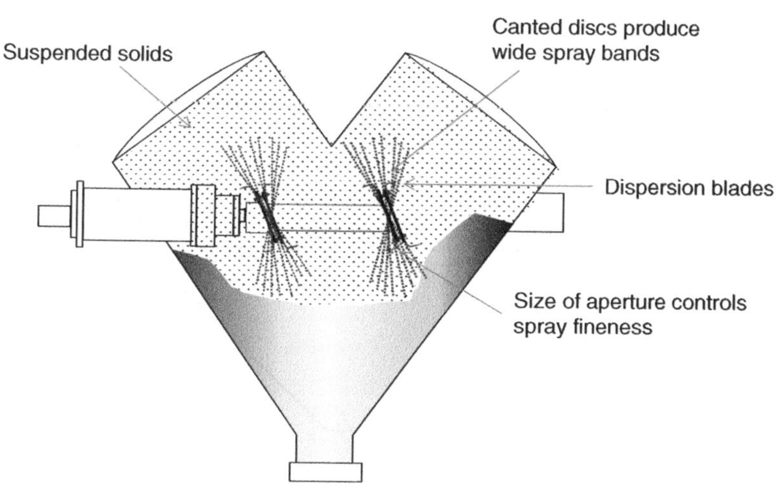

Figure 11.3 Liquid addition by high-speed disperser in a twin-shell blender

blended material to move from side to side and top to bottom for faster blending. A jacket on the shell of a tumble blender may be used to heat the contents of the blender for more rapid drying. An applied vacuum will reduce the vapor pressure and increase the rate of liquid removal.

11.7.1.2 Double-Cone Blenders

Double-cone blenders are similar in function to twin shell blenders. An example of a double-cone blender is shown in Figure 11.4.

As the blender rotates about the central axis, the powder inside the blender alternately flows together when a conical end is down and apart when the ends are horizontal. To achieve good flow, the blender should be filled only half full. Some vendor capacity ratings are closer to 60% of the open volume in the blender, which may leave a poorly mixed region near the center. The double-cone blender generally does not create as uniform blend as the twin-shell blender, because particle size differences are more likely to cause segregation near the central pivot points.

Liquid addition in a double-cone blender is usually done with a spray nozzle aimed at the moving surface of the powder. A series of blades, which look like circular saw blades, may be attached to the high-speed rotating shaft to improve liquid distribution and break lumps. The double-cone design is easier to jacket for heat transfer than the twin-shell design.

Another variation on the double-cone blender is the slant-cone blender, where that central band between the two conical ends is offset (slanted). This offset adds more side to side powder motion, while also helping to blend the potentially poorly mixed locations at the axis of rotation.

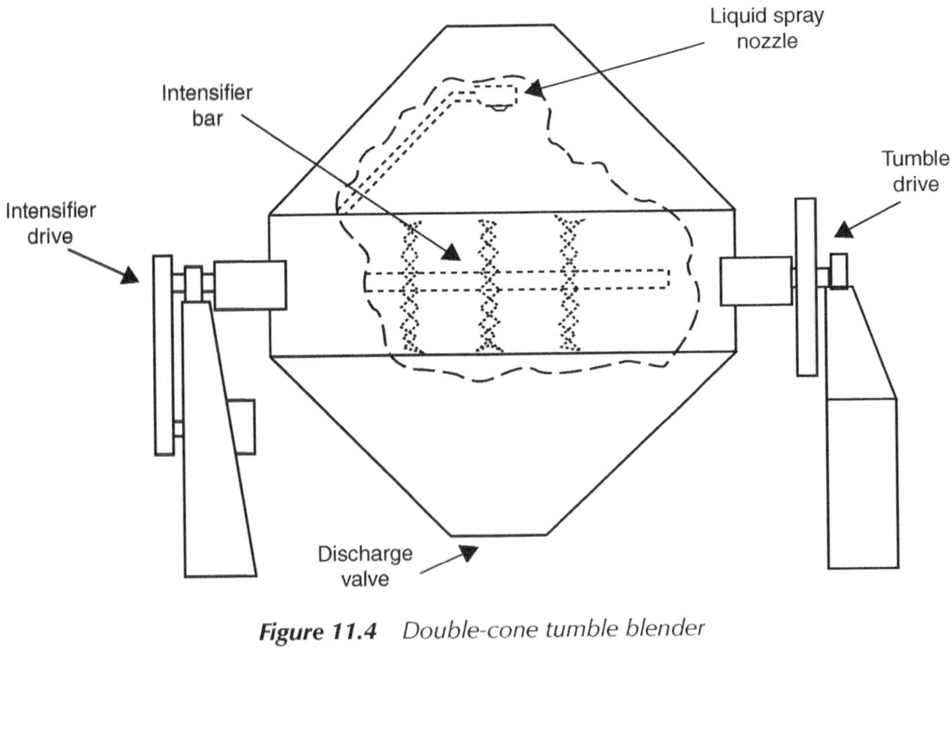

Figure 11.4 *Double-cone tumble blender*

11.7.1.3 Horizontal Rotary Blenders

Horizontal rotary blenders use a combination or a rotating shell and internal baffles to lift and distribute powders. Simply rotating a horizontal cylinder will do some powder blending, but without baffles the process would take a long time for an ingredient added at one end to be distributed along the length of the blender. Placement and angling of the baffles in a horizontal rotary blender not only help end to end mixing, but they also provide a means for discharging material from the blender. The horizontal blender design has the capability of rapidly handling a series of batches or with some modification it can blend continuously. The presence of baffles makes the horizontal rotary blender suitable for blending batches of excipients or a formulation with a large quantity of API. However, the baffles may make it more difficult to clean and inspect the inside of the blender.

11.7.1.4 Tote Blenders

Tote blenders use the tote container to serve both as storage and blender. The tote blender drive simply picks up the tote and rotates it on an angled axis to obtain cross flow in all directions, Figure 11.5.

Tote blenders can only be filled about half full to allow room for powder motion and are not as effective as other tumble blenders because of the corners. However, the ability to avoid transferring blends from storage and back also eliminates some possibilities for contamination and dust release. Several other types of tumble blenders take advantage of other container shapes with some loading or unloading advantages.

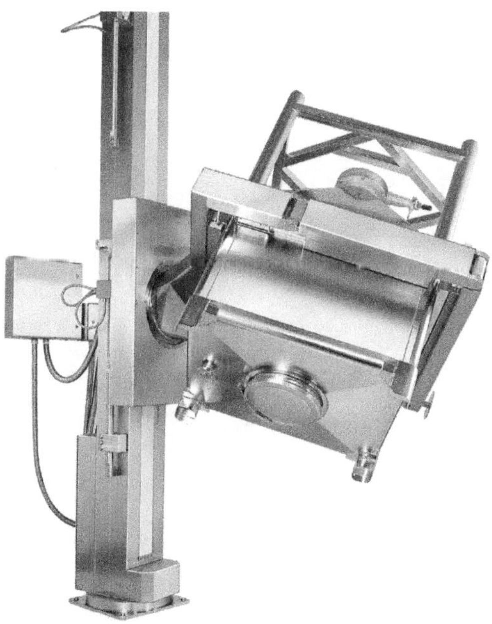

Figure 11.5 *Tote blender mounted to a lifting column. Reprinted with permission from Glatt GmbH Copyright (2014) Glatt GmbH*

11.7.2 Rotating Element Blenders

Rotating element blenders, as the name implies, have some type or rotating device inside a stationary shell or container. Some tumble blenders have an internal rotating element, although the primary mixing is done by the tumbling action inside the rotating shell. Rotating element blenders used for pharmaceutical applications include ribbon blenders, paddle blenders, ploughshare blenders, and vertical-screw blenders. Other special types of rotating element blenders will be discussed in the granulator topic.

For horizontal, rotating element blenders, like ribbon and paddle blenders the optimum fill level is usually just above the horizontal shaft Cox (2000). Below that level, the capacity of the blender is not being used, above that level the trough expands away from the rotating blade, leaving a large gap between the blade and side of the trough. Paddle and ploughshare blenders in a cylindrical container may have a wider range of effective operating levels. Over filling a blender, especially above the height of the rotating blades results in a poor quality blend. Compared with an overfilled blender, two half batches may give both a better quality blend and a shorter blend time.

11.7.2.1 Ribbon Blenders

Ribbon blenders are the most common and widely used of the rotating element blenders. Figure 11.6 shows a typical ribbon blender.

Ribbon blenders are used in a variety of other industries and applications, but with some limitations for pharmaceutical applications. One of the more significant limitations is cleaning the internal surfaces of the blender. The extent and number of surfaces of the ribbon require manual cleaning or several nozzles for CIP.

Ribbon blenders can be used with free-flowing or moderately-cohesive powders. The more cohesive the powders, the more problems for pharmaceutical applications. Cohesive

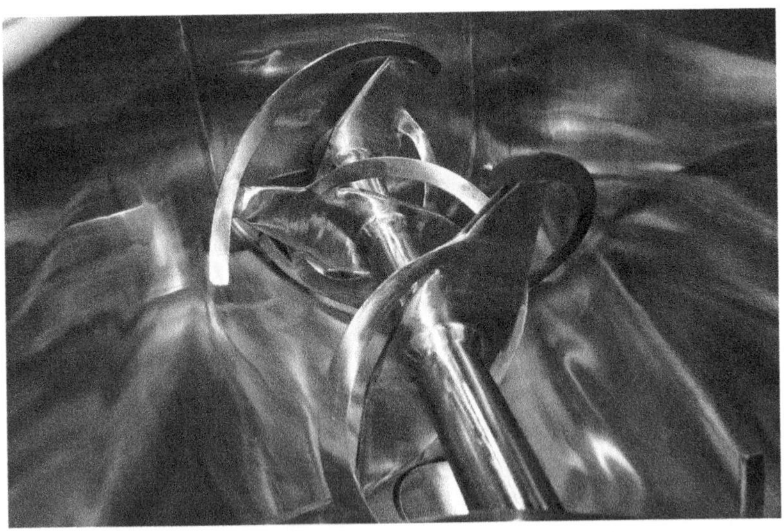

Figure 11.6 *Ribbon blender. Reprinted with permission from American Process Systems Copyright (2014) American Process Systems*

material will stick not only to other powder, but also to the surfaces of the blender. Unless blending is completed in a free-flowing condition, a small quantity of the API may be trapped unevenly between the moving blade and stationary shell. Efforts to form an agglomerating powder only increase the problems of material sticking to blender surfaces.

Ribbons typically have two outside flights mounted on opposite support arms attached to the central shaft. Those outside ribbons push the powder toward the discharge, either at the center or the end of the blender. When pushing toward the center, the flights at one end must have a pitch opposite to those at the other end, so the shaft rotation pushes material in opposite directions with both pushing toward the center discharge. A second set of ribbon blades mounted inside the outer blades push material in the direction opposite to the outside blades. In some blenders, especially larger capacity ones, more than one internal set of blades may be used. The smaller diameter of the inside blades pushes less material in the direction opposite to the outer blades, so multiple inside blades help balance bulk motion in opposite directions

The width of the blades may influence the mechanisms for blending. Wider blades are more effective at creating bulk motion in the blender. The wide blades push material from one place to another. Narrower blades will cut through the powder in the blender, creating more shear. As with all types of powder blenders, a selection procedure or evaluation cannot guarantee an adequate design a blender. Some degree of experience or testing is necessary for selecting the best blender type and design.

Ribbon blenders are available with capacities from 0.06 m^3 (2 ft^3) to 30 m^3 (1000 ft^3). The rated capacity is typically the trough volume measured to the top edge of the outer ribbon. For optimum uniformity, the batch should be limited to the range from 30% to 60% of the rated capacity. Power consumption is from 5 kW/1000 kg (6 hp/ton) to 12 kW/1000 kg (14 hp/ton) depending on the bulk density and cohesiveness of the powder. Blenders are typically loaded and emptied with the blender running. Restarting a full ribbon blender may be difficult to impossible. Typical blend times are from 3 to 12 min, longer with complicated processes.

By far, the most common types of ribbon blenders are horizontal, trough-style blenders. However, ribbon blenders can also be vertical, Figure 11.7.

The vertical ribbon blenders offer some advantages over the horizontal type Cavender & Quick (2000). First, vertical ribbon blenders work well at almost any reasonable fill level, from a small amount as low as 10–100% full at the top of the ribbon impeller. Second, the seal around the rotating shaft is above the powder and therefore less subject to abrasion and contamination. Powders are not compacted against the end of the blender, because a vertical ribbon blender is operated with the blade moving the powder upward. The construction of a vertical ribbon blender is similar to the construction of a helical ribbon blender used for viscous liquids. A vertical ribbon blender can be used with free-flowing dry powders, compacting powders, pastes, viscous fluids, and even low-viscosity liquids. The vessel and seal can even be designed for elevated pressures or vacuum conditions. The surface area of the ribbon may still pose cleaning and inspection problems.

11.7.2.2 Paddle Blenders

Paddle blenders are similar to horizontal ribbon blenders as shown in Figure 11.8.

The paddle arrangement is effectively a variation on the ribbon with more flexibility and options. The paddles can be angled to move powder in a pattern similar to a ribbon or the

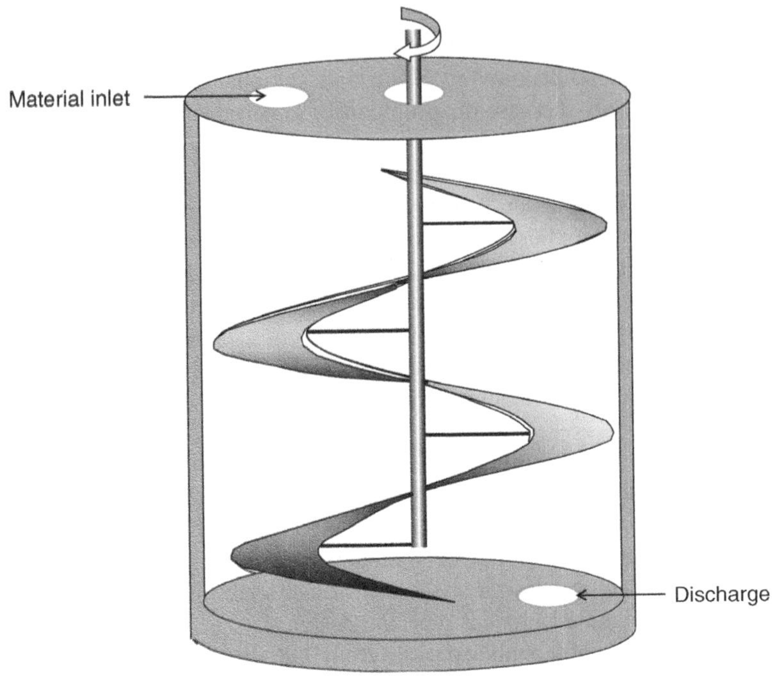

Figure 11.7 Vertical ribbon blender. Reprinted with permission from Glatt GmbH Copyright (2014) Glatt GmbH

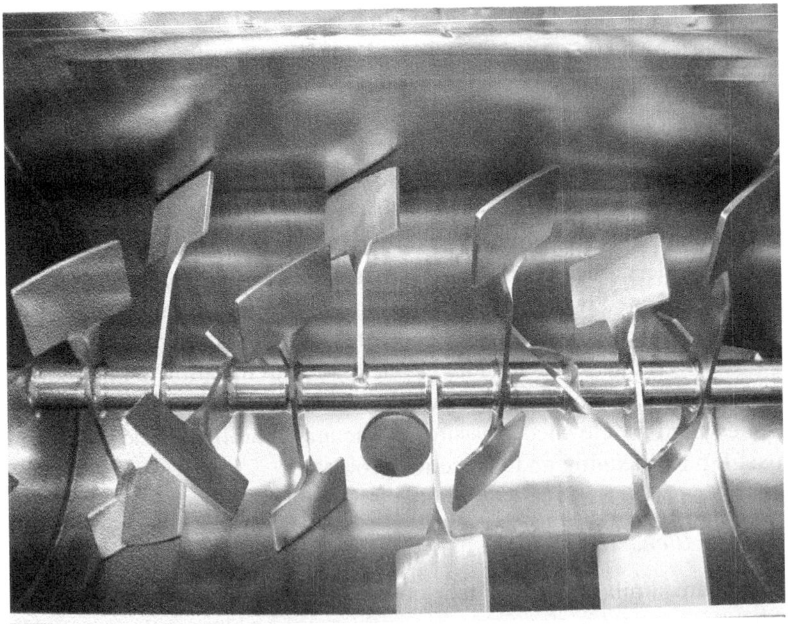

Figure 11.8 Paddle blender. Reprinted with permission from Eirich Machines, Inc. Copyright (2014) Eirich Machines, Inc.

paddles can be oriented in alternating directions to create more cross flow, interaction and shear. The paddle blades that rotate near the curved bottom of the blender are arranged such that they sweep the entire length of the trough, but in discontinuous segments. The opposed area of the paddle blades can be half as much as a ribbon, reducing power and restart difficulties, but with potentially less powder movement. Paddle blenders typically can handle wetter and more cohesive solids than ribbon blenders can.

Paddle blenders are available with capacities from 0.06 m^3 (2 ft^3) to 30 m^3 (1000 ft^3). The rated capacity is typically the trough volume measured to the top of the paddles. For optimum uniformity, the batch should be limited to the range from 25 to 80% of the rated capacity. Power consumption is from 10 kW/1000 kg (12 hp/ton) to 100 kW/1000 kg (120 hp/ton) depending on the bulk density and cohesiveness of the powder. Blenders are typically loaded and emptied with the blender running. Restarting a full blender may be difficult. Typical blend times are from 1 to 6 min or longer with complicated processes.

11.7.2.3 Ploughshare Blenders

Ploughshare blenders provide greater capabilities, but at a higher cost, than other horizontal, rotating element blenders. The blenders are typically enclosed in a complete cylinder, as shown in Figure 11.9, rather than a trough like most horizontal ribbon blenders.

The plough shaped blades are attached to arms on a central shaft. The blade shape lifts material away from the vessel walls and can throw it in both longitudinal directions simultaneously. With a cylindrical shell, the clearance between the ploughs and the wall can be made less than trough blenders. Because the blender can operate over a range of speeds, the intensity can be adjusted to match the particular application. Additional intensity to break large agglomerates and better disperse additives can be provided by choppers. Chopper

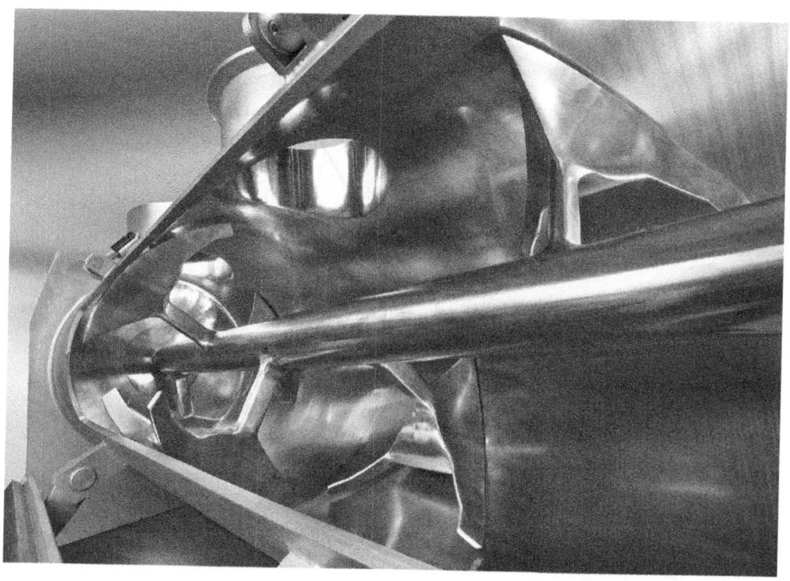

Figure 11.9 *Ploughshare blender. Reprinted with permission from Eirich Machines, Inc. Copyright (2014) Eirich Machines, Inc. and from Gebrüder Lödige Maschinenbau GmbH Copyright (2014) Maschinenbau GmbH*

blades run at motor speed, typically either 3600 (3000) or 1800 (1500) rpm depending on the motor windings and electrical power frequency. The chopper blades can either break agglomerates or intensify the mixing action in the blender.

Ploughshare blenders are available with capacities from 0.6 m^3 (20 ft^3) to 30 m^3 (1000 ft^3). The total volume of the cylinder cannot be used, because some free space is needed for motion and dilation of the powder. For optimum uniformity, the batch should be limited to the range of 30–70% of the cylinder volume. Power consumption is from 10 kW/1000 kg (12 hp/ton) to 100 kW/1000 kg (120 hp/ton) depending on the bulk density and cohesiveness of the powder. Blenders are typically loaded and emptied with the blender running. Restarting a full blender may be difficult. Typical blend times are 0.5–5 min, longer with complicated processes.

11.7.2.4 Orbiting Screw Blenders

Orbiting screw blenders combine the features of a rotating-element blender with the storage capability of a conical bin (Cavender and Quick, 2000), as shown in Figure 11.10.

The orbiting screw has two different actions inside the conical container. When the screw rotates on its own axis, it acts like an auger conveyor. It lifts material from the lower part of the cone, carries it to the powder surface, creates a pile on the surface and allows the material to flow down the angle of the surface away from the screw. The second action of the screw blender rotates the entire auger shaft around the central axis of the cone, allowing the screw to lift material from all parts of the container. The orbiting screw works with free-flowing powders, but also with pastes. However, cohesive powders may cause problems. The orbiting screw blender does not create as high degree of uniformity as other blenders, but it often has greater capacity and can maintain a powder blend in storage.

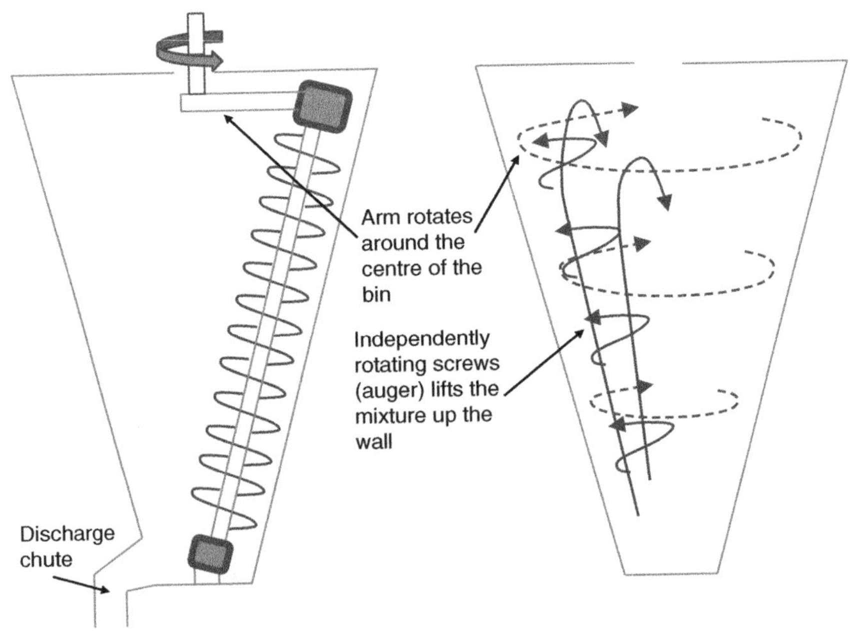

Figure 11.10 *Orbiting screw blender*

Orbiting screw blenders are available with capacities from 0.3 m^3 (10 ft^3) to 60 m^3 (2000 ft^3). The rated capacity of the blenders is usually about 85% of the conical volume. The blenders will work well for volumes from 15 to 85% of the conical volume. Typical blend times are 10 min or more.

11.7.3 Granulators

Granulation is often used to help maintain a powder blend or provide additional cohesion for tableting. Granulation typically involves the addition of a liquid, which will help small particles or different size particles stick together in sufficient uniformity for further handling and processing, as described by Capes and Fouda (1984) and Parkinson (1989). The granules are clusters of particles (see Chapter 8).

11.7.3.1 High Intensity Granulation

High intensity granulation drives small particles together in clusters and breaks large clumps apart. The same high-energy particle-particle and particle-blade collisions that increase granule size and density also reduce the size of large agglomerates to achieve strong and uniform granules. The interior elements of a high-intensity granulator, along with the flow patterns are shown in Figure 11.11.

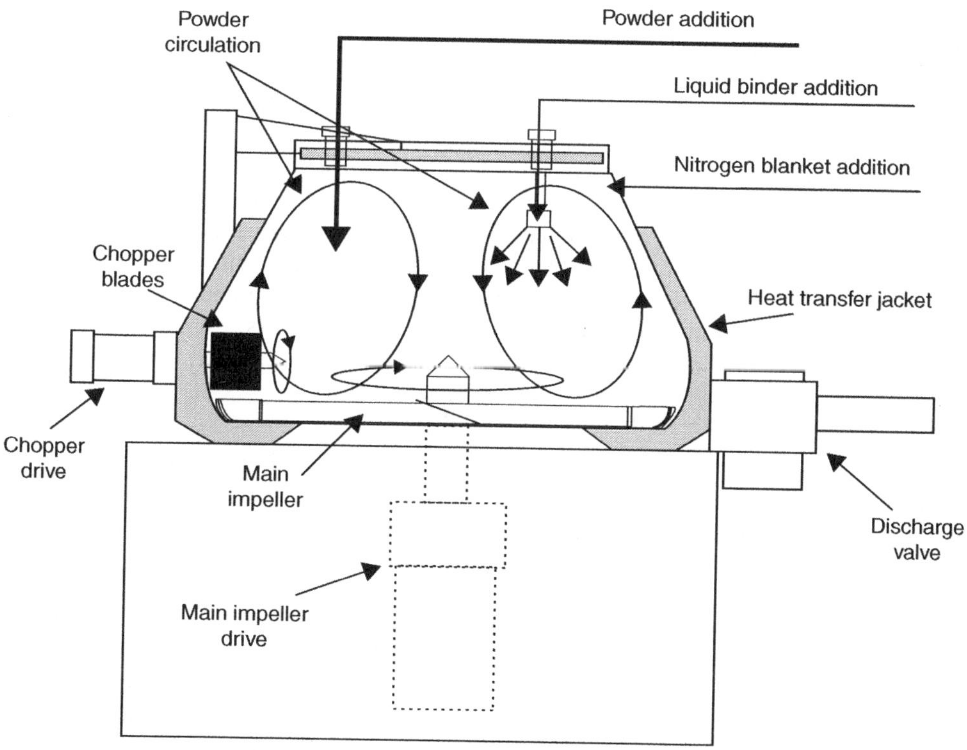

Figure 11.11 *High-intensity bowl granulator*

The bed of powder and resulting granules are circulated within the bowl of the granulator by a large blade contoured to the bottom. As the granules circulate, some pass near or make contact with the chopper blades. The operating volume of a bowl granulator may be from 30 to 65% of the bowl volume. The main blade typically operates on a variable speed drive with a maximum speed in the 200–300 rpm range, resulting in tip speeds from 40 m/s (750 ft/min) to 60 m/s (1000 ft/min). The chopper blades run at 3000 or 3600 rpm, with tip speeds approaching 150 m/s (2700 ft/min). A typical 600 liter (20 ft^3) might have a 37 kW (50 hp) or 56 kW (75 hp) motor on the main blade and a 15 kW (20 hp) motor on the chopper blades. A liquid binder, which can be water, other inert liquid, or a solvent/solute combination, is added to the dry powder blend to promote the granulation.

The granulator is closed during operation to both keep the material in the bowl and to avoid external contamination. The granulator is operated in a batch mode, with the actual granulation process often taking less than a minute, based on experience with the granulator and powder characteristics. Because of the intense agitation of the particles, the power input creates heat, which can raise the temperature of the blend. Cooling is difficult because of the short duration of the blending and the small surface area of the bowl compared with the volume of the batch. Upon completion of a batch, the finished granules can be discharged through a side chute, propelled by the rotation of the main granulator blade.

11.7.3.2 Fluidized-Bed Granulation

Fluidized-bed granulation adds a drying capability to wet granulation. The addition of a liquid to the dry powder in any granulation may leave a sticky particle-particle interaction, which may result in larger lumps forming. With a solvent/solute blend, removal of the solvent may improve the quality and strength of the resulting granules. Granulation may be accomplished in a fluidized-bed granulator or transferred from a high-intensity granulator into a fluidized-bed dryer. A type of fluidized-bed granulation system is shown in Figure 11.12, which uses both a high intensity granulator and fluidized-bed dryer.

A self-contained fluidized bed granulator may have the equivalent of a high intensity granulator in the bottom section of the fluidized bed to form the granules initially. Then without further handling the fluidized bed begins the drying process.

11.7.4 Other Blenders – Mullers and Custom Blenders

Many different types of blending equipment are needed for handling powders because of differences in powder behavior and process requirements. Powders can be free-flowing or cohesive. In the extreme of liquid addition, powders become pastes or slurries. If the powders change properties because of liquid addition, the result may be a dough, gel, or other non-Newtonian material.

One other type of powder blender has its origins in the apothecary. The mortar and pestle were used not necessarily to grind particles, but as a rubbing mechanism to combine different particles into a blend. The modern day version of the mortar and pestle is the muller. The wheels not only roll across the powder, but because of offset axles, skid across the powders to promote blending. Powder can be added into the batch through a funnel in the center as the wheels are powered to rotate about the center of the cylindrical container.

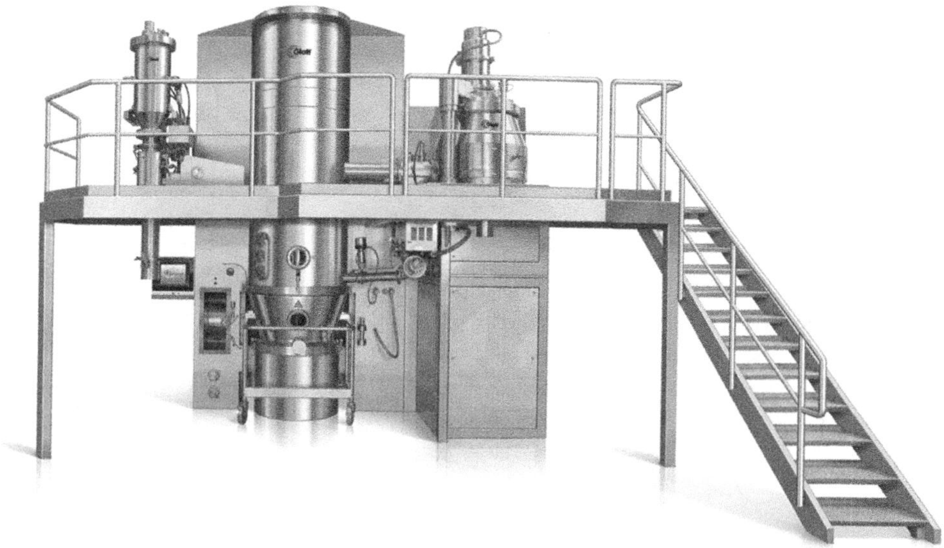

Figure 11.12 *High shear granulation suite. Consisting of high shear granulator (right), fluid bed dryer (middle) and pneumatic conveyer (left). Reprinted with permission from Glatt GmbH Copyright (2014) Glatt GmbH*

Some mullers are fed at the side, with discharge at the center. Scrapers near the center and at the wall push material back under the rollers.

11.8 Continuous Blenders

Although most pharmaceutical products are produced as batches, for identification and control purposes, the economics and volume of continuous production will eventually result in more continuous blending operations. While continuous processing requires the careful control of ingredient addition for proper formulation, separate steps of weighing, loading, blending, and discharging associated with batch processes are all handled in a single continuous operation. The result is larger quantities of a product from smaller blenders, along with the reduced labor requirements and fewer opportunities for individual errors (see Chapter 6).

For many blender types a variation on the equipment is available for continuous processing. For tumble blenders, the rotating body of the blender must have an inlet for material, some length of a tubular section for blending, and an outlet for continuous operation. The tubular section can be of a zigzag arrangement, or more practically contain baffles similar to the horizontal rotary blender. For rotating element blenders, such as ribbon, paddle, and plough share blenders, the body of the continuous blender is longer and narrower than a similar size batch blender, as shown in Figure 11.13. All blenders, batch or continuous have outer ribbon or paddles pushing toward the discharge, to be able to empty the blender completely.

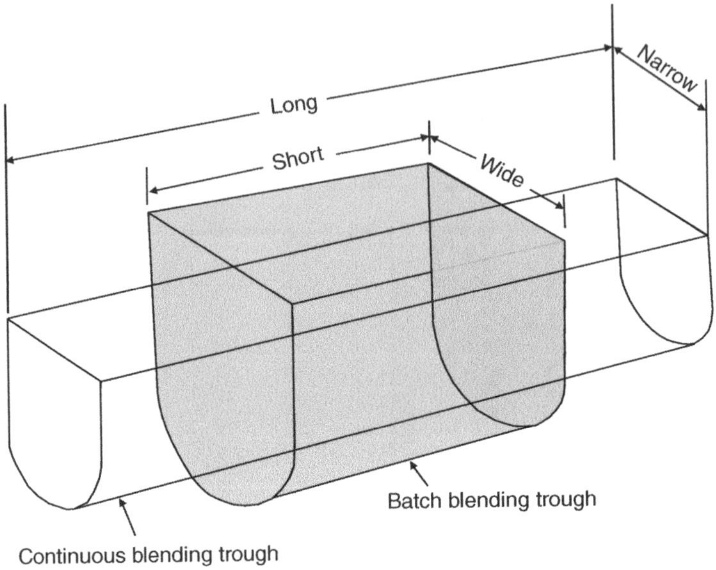

Figure 11.13 *Batch blenders are typically short and wide, while continuous blenders are long and narrow*

Continuous blending in a rotating element blender could easily handle ten times the capacity of the same size blender operating in batch mode. The greater capacity in continuous blending is a result of shorter blend times and reduced loading and unloading times. The capacity of a blender is an inverse function of the residence time in the blender. The residence time for a continuous blender is usually short, a minute or two, and controlled by the feed rate. Level in the blender is most often controlled by an exit weir plate that helps retain the desired level of powder in the blender.

The high-intensity granulators are not usually operated in continuous mode. However, fluidized bed dryers could be adapted for continuous operation. Mullers used for continuous processing typically have two adjacent tubs with rollers and an opening between them. Material enters and is mixed in the first tub before it is pushed into the next tub before leaving. In each tub, the inlet and exit are on the opposite sides of the rotating rollers.

11.9 Blender Selection

Selection of the best blender for a particular application should be a combination systematic evaluation and applied experience. Two factors that influence blender selection are particle strength and flow properties, such as segregating, free flowing, cohesive, or pasty (see Chapter 5). The chart in Figure 11.14 attempts to show general operating ranges for different types of powder blending equipment.

Some blenders like fluidized beds operate over a narrow range of powder flow behavior. Others like the ploughshare blenders operate over a wider range. The orbiting screw

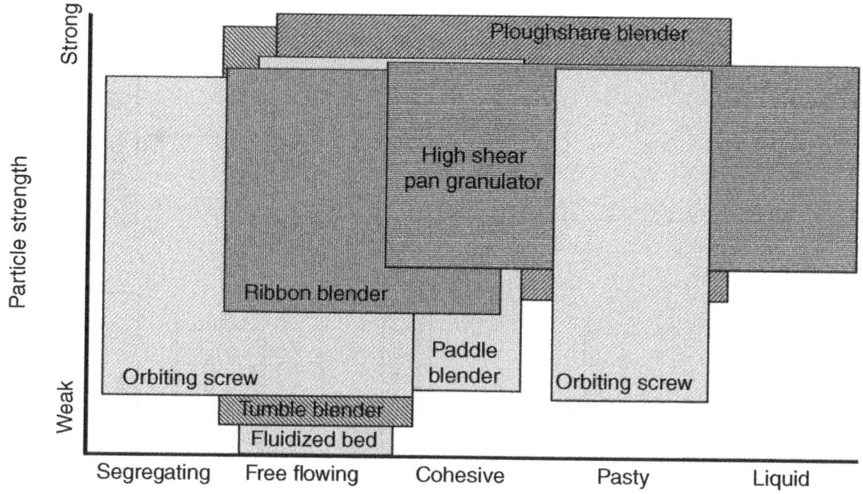

Figure 11.14 *Blender operating ranges. Reprinted with permission from Glatt GmbH Copyright (2014) Glatt GmbH*

blenders work in different ranges, like free flowing powders and pasty materials, but not in cohesive powders.

A more systematic method of blender selection is represented in the flow chart in Figure 11.15.

Several decisions need to be made concerning the process requirements and flow characteristics. Each of those decisions lead to a different set of decisions, process considerations, or equipment selections. The first decision about the percentage of a minor ingredient is a result of the formulation. The next decision concerns the flow characteristics and whether the powder is free-flowing or not. Other decisions concern replacing or grinding the raw materials. The blender selections at the end of each path are just suggestions based on the primary considerations. Those selections are not all of the possibilities and for reasons not tested by the flow chart may not be suitable for a specific application.

11.10 Equipment Specifications

For equipment to be suitable for pharmaceutical applications, some basic characteristics must be met. First, the equipment cannot contaminate the pharmaceutical product. Second, the equipment must be easily cleaned. These two characteristics are linked together by the materials of construction and the finishes on those materials. Chapter 14 on cleaning validation provides more detail about GMP. Beyond the construction of the blender, all blenders have some source of power, usually an electric motor. For safe operation, certain features of electric motors are necessary depending on the product. Other drive components, include gear reducers, belts, chains, and bearings. Seals are also rotating components in contact with the powders (Kent, 2003).

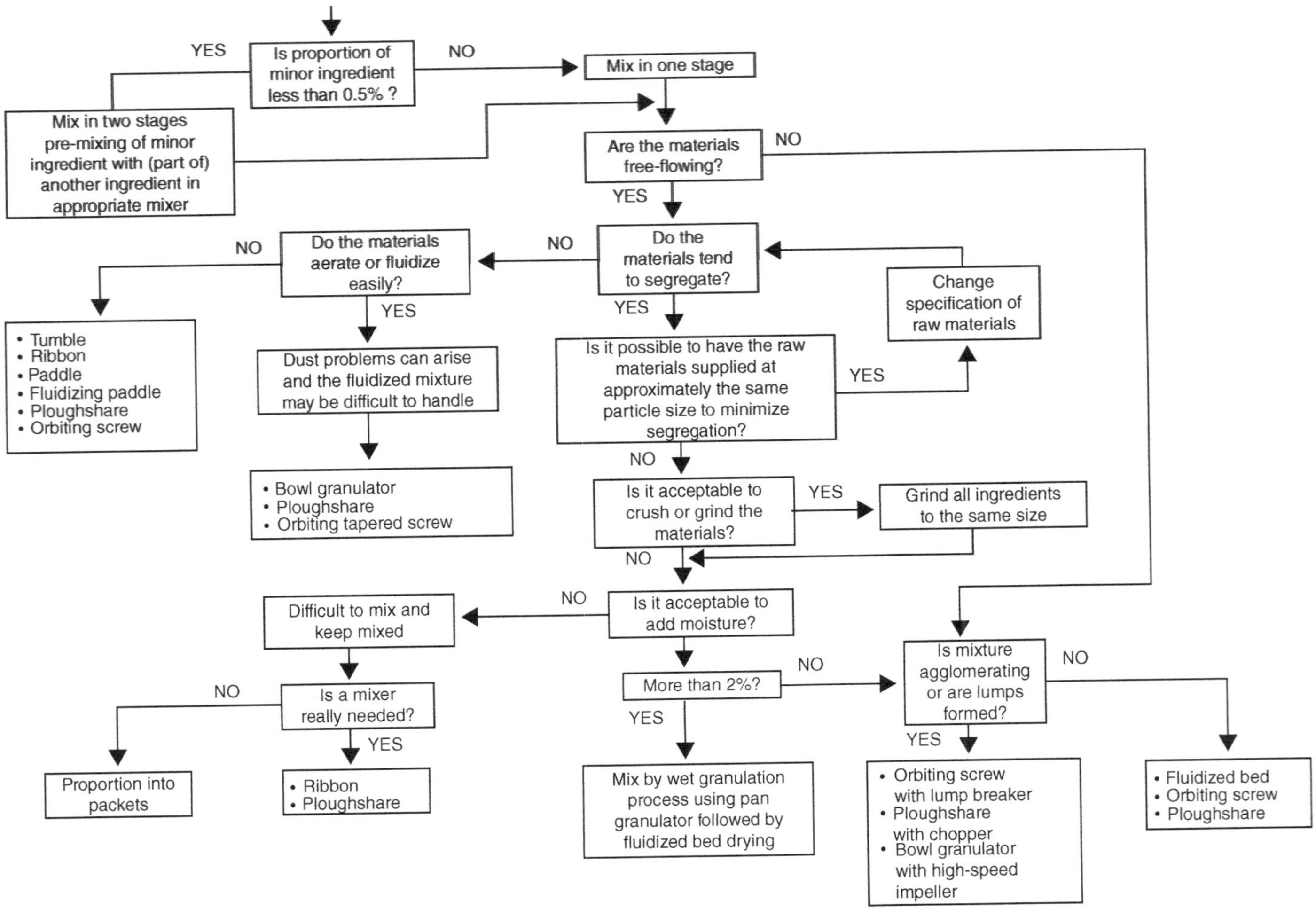

Figure 11.15 *Blender selection flow chart*

11.10.1 Materials of Construction

A stainless steel or other metal alloy metal is usually used as the primary material for powder blending equipment. The finish on the surface of the material may add to either the appearance or ability to clean the surface. Material specification is most often done by a number associated with the alloy composition. The most common stainless steel materials used in pharmaceutical applications are designated as 304, 304L, 316, and 316L. The "L-grade" designation refers to low carbon stainless steel. Low-carbon stainless steel can be welded without creating corrosion problems around welds. However, L-grade stainless is not as strong as the regular stainless, so it is not used for fasteners, like bolts and nuts. A proper specification for equipment construction is "L-grade where welded" not "L-grade only." More detailed information about alloys can be found in Chapter 12, "Fluid Mixing Equipment Design."

11.10.2 Electrical Classification

Electric motor classification includes a combination of factors regarding the safety of a motor for different applications. In most pharmaceutical facilities some degree of ambient control is necessary not only to prevent contamination, but also protect against fires or explosions. Electric motor enclosure classification is usually either "enclosed" or "explosion proof." Enclosed motors simply prevent objects, dust, and sometimes liquid from getting inside the motor. Explosion-proof motors are necessary where solvent vapors or combustible dusts may be present in sufficient quantities to pose an explosion or fire hazard. Motor codes and designations are set by several different groups, including the NEC (National Electrical Code), CEC (Canadian Electrical Code), and the IEC (International Electrochemical Commission). Other designations, such as wash-down duty, may apply to motors for pharmaceutical applications. More detailed information about electric motor classifications can be found in Chapter 12, "Fluid Mixing Equipment Design."

11.10.3 Drives and Seals

Most of the primary rotating components in powder blending and liquid mixing equipment operate at a speed considerably below the output speed of an electric motor. To provide an appropriate speed to drive mechanical components of a blender, various types of speed reduction drives are used. Simple drives, such as belts and chains, can provide small speed reductions (factors of 2 or 3) at modest costs. Gear reducers can accomplish larger speed reductions (factors of 5 to 50) through various types of gears or multiple sets of gears.

Any time a rotating shaft goes through the side of a pharmaceutical mixer, a seal is needed to prevent external contamination or loss of a product to the environment. Seals are difficult to operate and maintain in the presence of powders. Nearly all powders are abrasive to some extent. Most seal materials pose some risk of product contamination. Various types of air purging and dust catchers are used to prevent contact between the seal and product. Careful inspection and maintenance are essential for any mechanical equipment in contact with pharmaceuticals.

References

Capes, C.E. and A.E. Fouda, A.E. (1984). Size enlargement methods and equipment, in *Handbook of Powder Science and Technology*, Fayed, M.E. and Otten, L., (eds), Part 5, Chapter 7, Van Nostrand Reinhold Company, New York.

Cavender, J., Quick, J. (2000). Thorough, and gentle blending with a vertical ribbon mixer, *Powder and Bulk Engineering,* January, p. 46.

Cox, B.D. (2000). Optimize your solids blender, *Chemical Engineering Progress,* October, p. 77.

Kent, M. (2003). How mechanical design and construction affect mixer selection, *Powder and Bulk Engineering,* January, p. 27.

Merrow, E.W. (1986). *A Quantitative Assessment of R&D Requirements for Solids Processing Technology*, Rand Corporation, Santa Monica, CA, R-3216-DOE/PSSP.

Muzzio, J., Alexander, A., Goldridge, C., Shen, E., and Shinbrot, T. (2004). Fundamentals of solids mixing, solids mixing, in *Handbook of Industrial Mixing, Science and Practice*, Part A., Chapter 15, Paul, E.L., Atiemo-Obeng, V.A., and Kresta, S.M. (eds), John Wiley & Sons, Inc., Hoboken, NJ.

Parkinson, G. (1989). Boon for solids handling: Agglomeration, *Chemical Engineering,* August, p. 37.

Pietsch, W., (2003). Mixers for growth-tumble agglomeration, *Powder and Bulk Engineering,* February, p. 19.

12
Fluid Mixing Equipment Design

David S. Dickey
MixTech, Inc., USA

12.1 Introduction

Fluid mixing equipment for the pharmaceutical industry includes conventional and specialized equipment in a range of sizes. Laboratory and development mixing equipment establish the chemistry and basic process requirements for mixing applications. Some applications are easily accomplished with simple portable mixers in cylindrical tanks. Other applications involving larger quantities use various types of top-entering mixers. Top-entering mixers can be used in open or covered tanks. Covered tanks can be designed to prevent ambient contamination or for operation at elevated or vacuum pressures. Bottom-entering, magnetically driven mixers have been developed to handle a range of common applications while providing mixing capability without a rotating shaft seal. Side-entering mixers find applications in storage tanks, where liquid circulation is needed to maintain or improve uniformity. Beyond the conventional tank mixers, other pieces of equipment, such as static mixers, pumps, and special purpose equipment, also accomplish mixing tasks, Couper, et al. (2005), Hemrajani and Tatterson (2004).

Much of the liquid mixing equipment for the pharmaceutical industry requires special features, usually focused on thorough cleaning, no contamination, or sterile conditions. For easy cleaning, surface finish may be especially important. Various degrees of polishing will produce smooth surfaces in stainless steel vessels, Amanullah, et al. (2004). Stainless steel alloys help prevent contamination for most pharmaceutical products. However, glass lining provides advantages for both cleaning and contamination prevention, but at greater expense.

Pharmaceutical Blending and Mixing, First Edition. Edited by P.J. Cullen, Rodolfo J. Romañach, Nicolas Abatzoglou and Chris D. Rielly.

Finally, sterility may involve special closures, like magnetically driven mixers and even single-use disposable mixers. Often overlooked, but important to many aspects of pharmaceutical production, a mixer may be the critical piece of process equipment that brings together the raw materials used to create the product.

12.2 Equipment Description

Mixing equipment can be described by several names: mixer, agitator, stirrer, and blender being the most common. The name "mixer" is generally understood to mean the full range of equipment used to do a variety of applications, although a strict definition of mixing could be the combination of ingredients. Agitator is probably a better general name, since operations such as solids suspension, gas dispersion, liquid-liquid dispersion, and heat or mass transfer may not be mixing in the sense of creating formulation uniformity. Consequently, the terms mixer and agitator are used interchangeably. Stirrer may be another name used for a laboratory mixer and sometimes used in Europe for a general purpose mixer. "Stirrer" implies rotational operation, which includes most mixers. The term blender applies specifically to making a batch more uniform and is commonly applied to dry powder mixers. The difference between a liquid "mixture" and a powder "blend" is that the individual particles in the powder blend retain their chemical identity and may segregate after initial blending because of vibration and or other handling.

Flow patterns in stirred vessels are an important consideration in the effectiveness of mixing. To accomplish mixing, the entire contents of the tank must be in motion. That motion must transport material from one region in the vessel to other regions quickly enough to be effective in providing adequate uniformity for the process.

A deep vortex on the surface and a swirling flow pattern is not a sign of effective mixing. The circular motion only moves the same liquid around in solid-body rotation, without accomplishing any vertical or radial mixing. Even the downward flow in the vortex may require several revolutions before an addition on the surface is gradually drawn down and moved to the center and bottom of the tank. Baffles are used to restrict the rotational motion and contribute to vertical mixing with center-mounted mixers in low viscosity fluids. In each type of mixing equipment, methods to achieve good mixing are different and the desired purpose of the mixer must be considered. Other terms, such as impeller, turbine, disperser, baffle, and so on will be defined more appropriately with respect to individual types of equipment or specific applications.

12.2.1 Laboratory Mixers

Laboratory mixers are usually bench top mixers, used in beakers and flasks, which can be made of glass, plastic, or metal. Probably one of the most common laboratory mixers is the magnetic stirrer with a stir bar, typically used in a glass beaker or flask and sometimes part of a hot plate. Other laboratory mixers or stirrers use a rotating shaft and simple propeller. Also used for mixing are shaker tables for flasks, modified kitchen blenders, and larger bench-top mixers. Common characteristics of laboratory mixers are that blend time is very short and uniformity is obtained rapidly regardless of mixer operation. Most beakers with a stir bar on a magnetic stirrer plate, even without baffles, give rapid mixing to low viscosity liquids. The same mixing equipment may be totally ineffective with a viscous fluid. While laboratory mixing may be difficult to quantify, the effects of mixing are still critical. Without any mixing, almost nothing happens; with some mixing, a reaction occurs; with more mixing the same reaction may go more quickly. The mixing necessary for a successful process must be measured for scale-up to production.

Even with these limitations to laboratory observation of mixing, careful records of the beaker or flask size, the diameter and shape of the stir bar, and the rotational speed can be valuable pieces of information about the mixing requirements. Most small stirrers lack a direct measure of rotational speed and should be calibrated to provide information about mixing intensity. Even the failures of an experiment can be critical for scale-up to production. Sometimes, the best scale-up depends on knowing what conditions to avoid, such as too little mixing or the rapid addition of a reactant. Mixing intensity and flow patterns are different from larger mixers. These characteristics may be unfortunate because some laboratory results can be difficult to use for scale-up.

12.2.2 Development Mixers

Development mixers are the next larger size mixers and are typically associated with process testing. These mixers are designed to more closely represent geometrically and functionally production-size mixers. At this scale, the vessels commonly change from glass or plastic to stainless steel. Development scale mixing is more likely to be a combined function of reaction chemistry, fluid dynamics, and process engineering. Development equipment can be used to study mixing and its effects on process results. Mixing equipment used for developing a new process should be as geometrically similar to the production equipment as practical. Geometric similarity is achieved when all of the length dimensions of the development mixer are in the same proportions as the production scale equipment. Even if not completely similar, basic characteristics, such as impeller type should be as representative as possible. The chapter on scale-up (Chapter 13) provides more detailed guidance.

Properly conducted and documented development scale tests should approximate production results as well as scale-up methods can predict. Also, testing over a range of mixing intensities at the development stage will permit later adjustments in production with minor revalidation of a process for the regulatory authorities.

12.2.3 Portable Mixers

Portable mixers are the simplest and least expensive production-scale mixers. A portable mixer can be attached to the side of or next to a cylindrical tank. Portable mixers are found throughout all types of liquid mixing applications. Although often used in open-top tanks, portable mixers or larger versions may be used on covered tanks in the pharmaceutical industry. Most are fractional horsepower (less than 750W) and operate at speeds greater than 290 rpm (4.8 rps). Impellers are small, between 76 mm (3 inches) and 455 mm (18 inches) in diameter and most often either marine-style propellers or three-blade hydrofoil impellers. The tanks used with portable mixers rarely have baffles, so flow control and effective mixing are achieved by angle mounting the mixers and aiming the direction of flow. The flow patterns resulting from different mounting angles are reflected in the graphics of Figure 12.1.

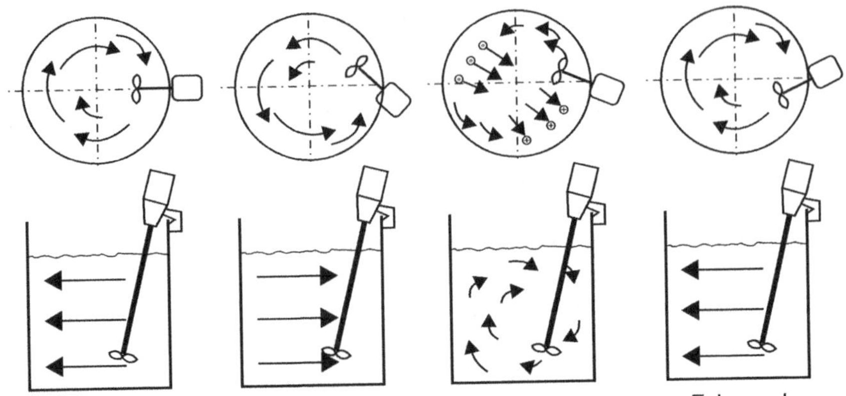

Figure 12.1 *Portable mixer flow patterns depend on mounting angle*

Most portable mixers are mounted at a 10–15° angle from the vertical. This angle keeps the impeller location in the same half of the tank as the mounting. At this angle, the downward flow from the impeller sweeps across most of the bottom of the tank. If the horizontal angle of the mixer is along a radius of the tank, the rotating impeller will create an "inherent" rotational motion to the liquid in the tank. Since nearly all mixers are designed with a clockwise rotation, as viewed from the motor end of the shaft, the liquid rotation will also be clockwise. Because the flow from the impeller is axial, the effect is not unlike that of an outboard motor on a boat, creating some flow in the direction the mixer is aimed. If the mixer is aimed strongly to the right of the radius, an "induced" flow pattern counter acting the inherent flow can be generated. This pattern usually results in the flow being pushed to one corner of the tank with little effective mixing. The "best mixing" is usually achieved when the axial flow from the impeller effectively counteracts the inherent rotational flow. These conditions provide the crucial element of vertical mixing that draws additions on the surface down, through the impeller region and up along the opposite wall of the tank. "Enhanced" rotational flow can be created if the mixer is aimed horizontally in the direction that reinforces the inherent rotational flow.

The "best mixing" flow pattern applies primarily to liquid blending applications. For powder addition on the surface, the surface vortex created with the "inherent" flow pattern may help the process. For mixing moderately viscous fluids, the drag at the tank wall resists rotational flow and the "enhanced flow" positioning of the mixer may be necessary to create motion throughout the tank. The important understanding with any mixing application is not what happens on the surface of the liquid, but how the motion is carried throughout the tank. Often, the strong surface motion with a deep vortex is the least effective mixing because circulation is limited to solid-body rotation with almost no top-to-bottom motion. Each instance of mixing with a portable mixer needs to be considered carefully, and consistency is almost as important as correctness. Special features of portable mixers used in pharmaceutical applications may include stainless steel motor housings, mixer components, and fasteners. Stainless steel is used both to avoid contamination of the products and resist corrosion of the mixer.

12.2.4 Top-Entering Mixers

Top-entering mixers cover an enormous range of mixer types and sizes and can be simple rotating mixers with one or more impeller types or multi-shaft mixers. Top-entering mixers have capabilities for a wide range of applications and are used for mild, to moderate, to intense mixing. Depending on the impeller type used in an application, the flow patterns can be quite different, with corresponding differences in process results. Impellers are the functional element of a rotating mixer. Impellers have different shapes and create different flow patterns for different applications. The impellers are categorized by the type of blades, which includes blade width, blade angle, number of blades, and blade shape. Looking at just three types of impellers, the hydrofoil impeller, pitched-blade turbine, and straight-blade turbine, gives a perspective on mixing characteristics. In low viscosity liquids, these impellers require tank baffles to prevent uncontroller swirling and create either axial or radial flow. Baffles are discussed further in Section 12.2.12, "Baffles."

12.2.4.1 Hydrofoil Impellers

Hydrofoil impellers are a fabricated version of the marine propeller, designed to create axial flow with low drag on the blades. The design concepts follow the characteristics of airfoil design, where an effort is made to have a large lift to drag ratio. The equivalent to lift is axial flow, which should be large for the amount of drag, or power required to rotate the impeller. A couple of typical hydrofoil impellers are shown in Figure 12.2.

While narrow-blades, three-blade hydrofoils are the most common and designed to produce an axial discharge from the impeller. The three-blade, narrow-blade hydrofoils are used in low to moderate viscosity applications for good liquid blending. Wide-blade hydrofoils with three and four blades are also used. The wide-blade hydrofoils are most commonly used for intermediate viscosity or gas dispersion applications. The concave face of the hydrofoil blades is always on the discharge side of the impeller, to create the airfoil effect.

12.2.4.2 Pitched-Blade Turbines

Pitched-blade turbines are versatile and widely used for liquid mixing. They also create an axial discharge, but with a wider spread than hydrofoil impellers. Most pitched-blade

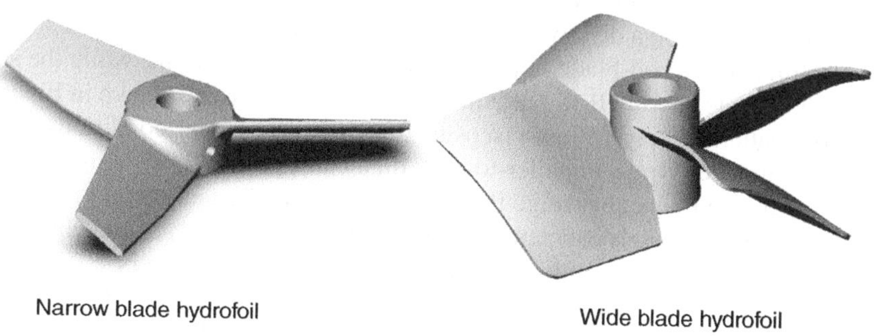

Figure 12.2 *Hydrofoil impellers. Image courtesy of Post Mixing Optimization and Solutions*

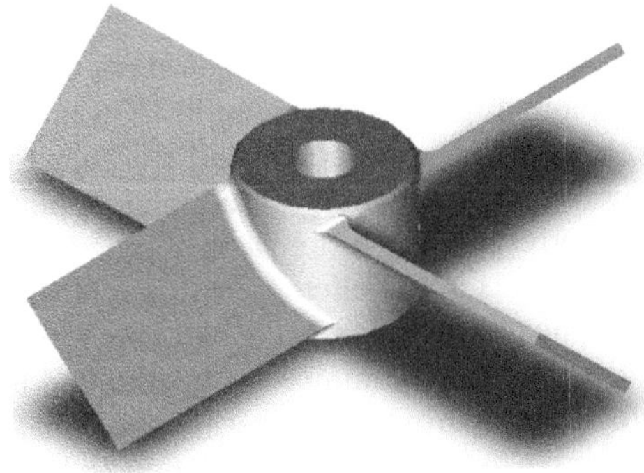

Figure 12.3 *Pitched-blade turbine. Image courtesy of Post Mixing Optimization and Solutions*

turbines have four blades, mounted at a 45° angle, and with an actual blade width one fifth of the impeller diameter, as shown in Figure 12.3.

Other blade angles and widths are practical. Some pitched-blade turbines have blades mounted at either 30 or 60° angles for different amounts of axial flow. Common practice for mixers is for the shaft to rotate in a clockwise direction, when viewed from the mixer drive. To be effective, axial flow impellers should be designed to pump downward toward the bottom of the vessel. Upward pumping impellers do a poor job of lifting flow from the bottom and turning flow at the free surface.

12.2.4.3 Straight-Blade Turbines

Straight-blade turbines have multiple blades mounted to a hub or disk as shown in Figure 12.4.

The use of "turbine" as a designation for an impeller usually means that the blades are made of flat plate material. Impellers need at least two blades for mechanical balance, but usually have 3–8 blades depending on the application and manufacturer. The open style with the hub mount is the lightest and simplest design. The disk mount provides convenient attachment for more blades. In a bolted construction and with additional holes in the disk, the impeller diameter and number of blades can be changed. In a baffled tank, the straight-blade turbines create primarily radial flow. Common proportions for straight-blade turbines have a blade width one-fifth of the impeller diameter and if disk mounted a blade length one-fourth the diameter on a disk two-thirds of the diameter.

The hydrofoil and pitched-blade impellers create axial-flow patterns, while the straight-blade impellers create a radial flow pattern, typical flow patterns are shown in Figure 12.5.

These flow patterns apply to low-viscosity fluids with turbulent conditions in baffled tanks. For the impeller types, impeller-to-tank diameter ratios and off-bottom clearances represented in the figure, local average flow velocities are in the same proportion no matter the absolute size of the vessels or rotational speed of the mixers. The general characteristics of the flow patterns are important to the effective operation of the mixers.

As can be seen from the flow patterns, both the hydrofoil and the pitched-blade impellers create a downward flow near the center of the tank with upward flow near the wall. The downward flow sweeps across the bottom of the tank and recirculates through the upper

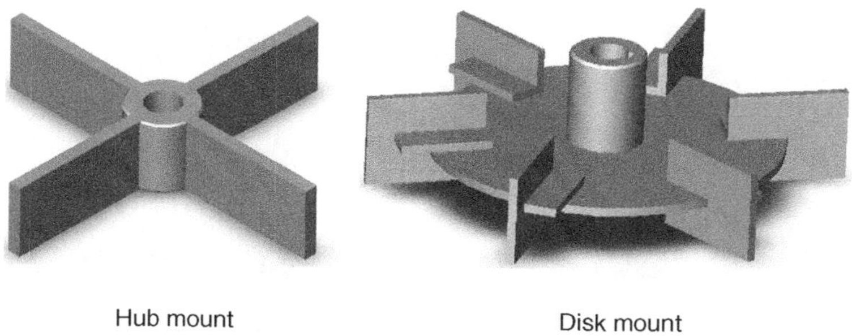

Figure 12.4 *Radial-flow, straight-blade turbine impellers. Image courtesy of Post Mixing Optimization and Solutions*

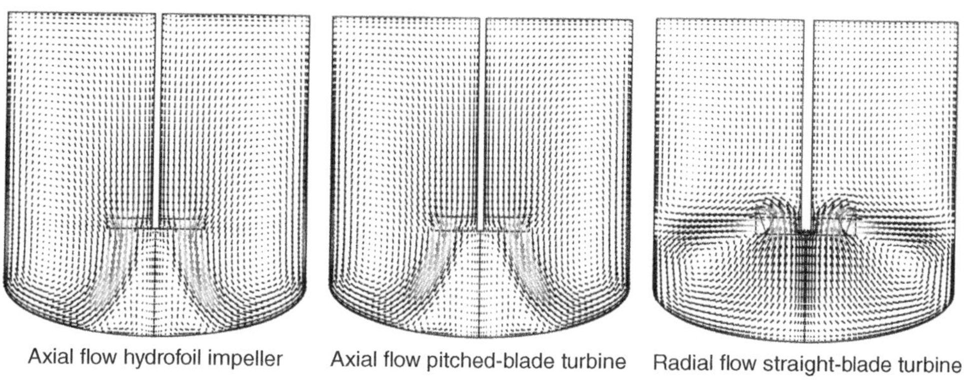

Figure 12.5 *CFD simulated impeller flow patterns for axial flow hydrofoil, axial flow pitched-blade and radial flow straight-blade impellers*

part of the tank, returning to the impeller from above. The rotational flow from the impellers creates additional velocities out of the plane of the two-dimensional representations of the flow profiles. The radial flow with the straight-blade impeller goes out from the blade tips to the tank wall and then both up and down at the wall, recirculating back above and below the impeller. All of the flow patterns in Figure 2.5 are time averages, so fluctuating velocities are not adequately represented. In some locations that appear to have low velocities, such as at the bottom center of the tanks, liquid motion is actually significant, just random in opposite directions, which average to a zero velocity.

The axial-flow impellers are most effective for liquid blending and solids suspension, while the radial flow is most often used for immiscible liquid and gas dispersion. Impeller off-bottom clearance and number of impellers can be changed to handle higher or lower liquid levels. Impeller-to-tank diameter ratios from 0.2 to 0.6 can be used in liquid blending applications, with larger diameter impellers being more effective for moderately viscous fluids. When fluid properties and operating conditions are unique or at the limits of familiar conditions, geometric modeling in development mixers may be needed to be sure that complete and effective liquid motion can be achieved.

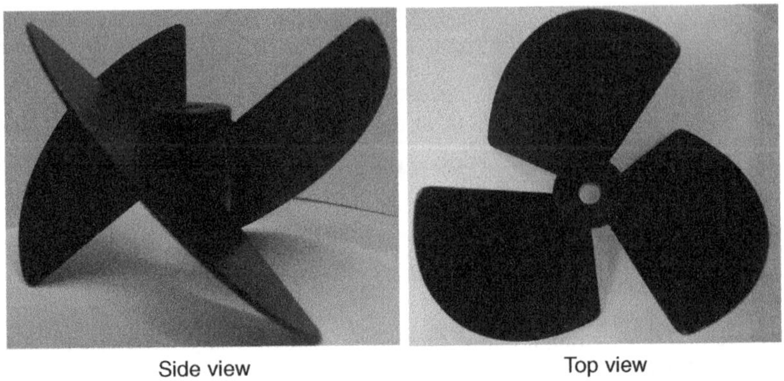

Figure 12.6 *"Elephant Ear" Impeller. Reprinted with permission from* Chem. Eng. Sci., *Axial impeller selection for anchorage dependent animal cell culture in stirred bioreactors: Methodology based on the impeller comparison at just-suspended speed of rotation by Marie-Laure Collignon, Angélique Delafosse, MichelCrine, Dominique Toye, 65, 22, 5929–5941. Copyright (2010) Elsevier*

12.2.4.4 Elephant Ear

"Elephant ear" impellers are almost unique to biotech applications in the pharmaceutical industry, Zhu, et al. (2009). The elephant ear impeller resembles a wide-blade hydrofoil impeller, but has flat plate blades, typically mounted at an angle equal to or greater than 45° from the horizontal. Figure 12.6 shows one type of elephant ear impeller.

Some elephant ear impellers have even wider blades and steeper angles than shown in Figure 12.6. The effective purpose of the wide blades is to have a high power number, which results in high power at a low tip speed. This combination was originally intended to reduce cell damage, although cell damage is rarely caused by mixing impellers.

12.2.5 High-Shear Dispersers

High-shear dispersers are used for immiscible liquid dispersion and breaking powder agglomerates in a liquid suspension. Dispersers use different impellers and systems to create local hydraulic shear capable of breaking agglomerates. Sawtooth impellers operate at high rotationals speeds and have many small blades (teeth) around the perimeter of a disk. The sawtooth impellers have a lower power number than other radial flow impellers to achieve high tip speeds. High tip speeds create velocity gradients that can be used to reduce droplet or agglomerate size. Because the disperser blades are rotated at very high speeds, substantial amounts of power are still input to a batch. Power input creates heat, which can raise the batch temperature. The different size, angle, and number of teeth on the blades adjust the relative amounts of shear and pumping imparted to the fluid.

A different type of high-shear disperser is the rotor-stator style mixer. A rotor-stator impeller has a small impeller (rotator) rotating inside of a stationary housing (stator) with holes or slots. The holes can be large or small or even screen like. Figure 12.7 shows some different types of stator heads.

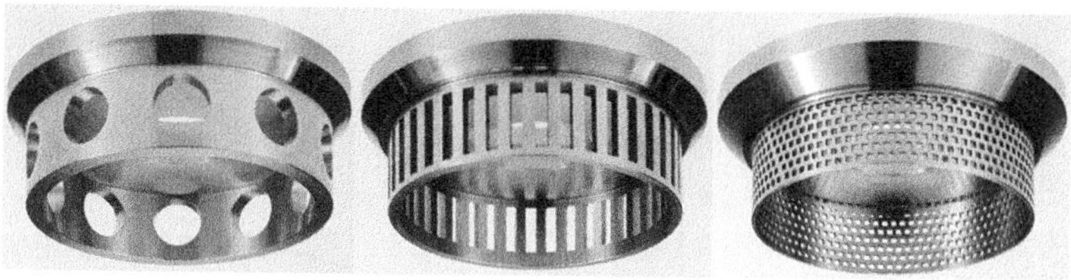

Figure 12.7 *Disperser heads for rotor-stator mixer. Reprinted with permission from Silverson Machines Ltd*

The rotor typically draws fluid from below the head and drives it radially out through the stator. The tip speed of the rotor and size of holes in the stator determine the ultimate drop or particle size produced by the rotor-stator mixer. Hydraulic shear occurs as the fluid flows rapidly through the slots that open and close between the rotor and stator.

12.2.6 High Viscosity Mixers

High viscosity mixers require large diameter impellers, sometimes called sweep impellers. Large impellers are necessary when the viscosity of the fluid is so high that the flow generated by an impeller is damped out before a recirculation pattern can form. A couple of high-viscosity impellers are the anchor and helix shown in Figure 12.8.

The diameters of both the anchor and helix are typically 90 to 95% of the tank diameter. So the gap between the blades and the tank wall is less than half the blade width, which is typically 10% of the impeller diameter. While both impeller types move the fluid near the tank wall by direct application of force. The anchor is only moderately effective for blending uniformity. Because the arms of the anchor are vertical, they provide rotational flow with almost no vertical motion. Anything added on the surface of the liquid may take many impeller revolutions to reach the lower portion of the tank with an anchor impeller. By comparison, the helix can move an additive from the surface to the bottom in only a few revolutions. The problem with the helix is that fabricating one is difficult and therefore more expensive. An alternate to the conventional anchor is one built with angled blades. The angled blades can still be flat if they are cut to an elliptical curve corresponding to the curvature of the tank wall. Tolerances for the tank diameter and the centering of the mixer must be much tighter than for turbine-style mixers to maintain a uniform clearance between a sweep impeller and the tank wall.

12.2.7 Multi-Shaft Mixers

Multi-shaft mixers are used when single-shaft, top-entering mixers do not provide sufficient liquid motion, especially in viscous fluids. When wide ranges of operating conditions are experienced in a batch process, multi-shaft mixers are an effective option. Multi-shaft mixers can provide different types of mixing action in a single tank.

The mixer internals could have both a pitched-blade turbine and a sweep impeller with scrapers at the wall. The pitched-blade turbine, Figure 12.3, would run at a higher rotational speed than the sweep impeller. The pitched-blade turbine could create top-to-bottom motion and more rapid flow with low viscosity conditions, while the sweep would

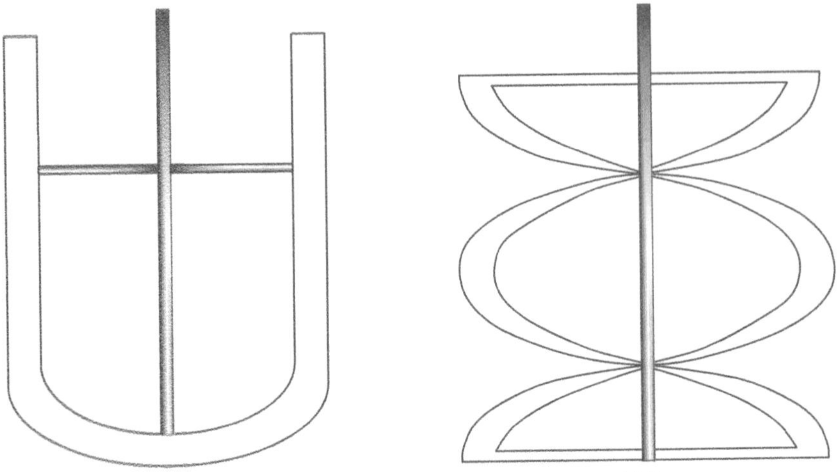

Figure 12.8 High viscosity impellers

prevent stagnation at the tank wall at a higher viscosity. The scrapers attached to the sweep impeller could also help heat transfer, especially for cooling. The turbine impeller in a dual-shaft mixer could also be a hydrofoil impeller, Figure 12.2, or a disk-disperser or a rotor-stator, Figure 12.7, for appropriate applications. The sweep impeller could also be either and anchor or helical impeller, Figure 12.8. For more complicated batch processes more than one high-speed impeller type may operate on another shaft inside a sweep impeller.

Other common types of dual shaft impellers operate in a planetary motion, with individual impellers rotating around their own axis while the both impellers rotate around the central axis of the tank. Some planetary mixers have two open-anchor style impellers, while others have one anchor style and a high-shear disk-style impeller or rotor-stator mixer. Different combinations of impellers can be used depending on the viscosity and shear required for a particular application.

12.2.8 Bottom-Entering Mixers

Bottom-entering mixers for pharmaceutical applications are predominantly magnetic-drive mixers. The magnetic drive eliminates the necessity of a rotating shaft penetration of the vessel and the associated seals in contact with the process fluid. The general arrangement of a bottom-entering, magnetic-drive mixer is shown in Figure 12.9.

The electric motor underneath the tank rotates a high-strength magnet, which is coupled through a stationary housing to magnets on the impeller assembly. The impeller rides on a hard-surface bearing inside the tank. The process liquid provides the necessary lubrication for the impeller bearing. The advantage of the in-tank impeller and bearing is that the vessel can be sterilized and kept closed throughout a process.

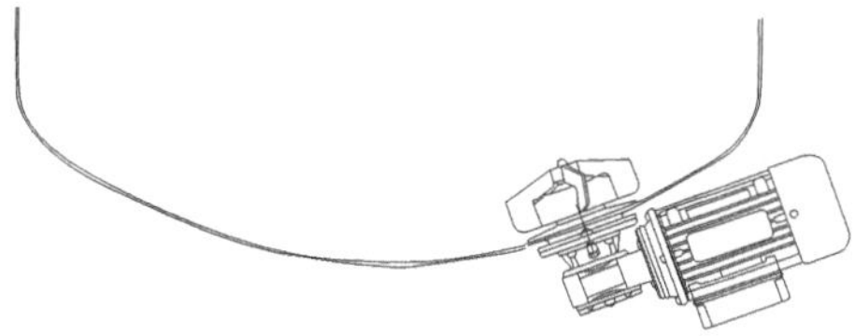

Figure 12.9 Magnetic drive bottom-entering mixer

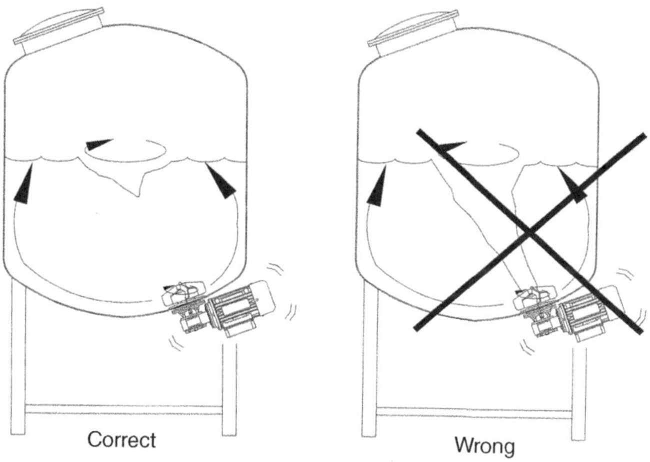

Figure 12.10 Bottom-entering mixer flow patterns

The torque limitations of magnetic drives does mean that most applications are for less than 20,000 l (5000 gal.), but those limits are not a problem for many pharmaceutical applications. Just as for portable mixers, the presence of a strong vortex and swirling motion does not represent effective mixing. Bottom-entering mixers are offset from the center of the tank to limit swirl and provide sufficient vertical motion for good blending. The flow patterns in Figure 12.10 show how a combination of liquid level and rotational speed can be used to obtain a good flow pattern.

Bottom-entering magnetic drive mixers can be combined with a disposable container to be a single-use mixer. The single-use container can decrease external or cross contamination and eliminate cleaning operations between batches. The incremental cost of single-use mixers must be offset by the production of high-value products.

12.2.9 Glass-Lined Mixers and Vessels

Glass-lined mixers and vessels provide both a smooth internal surface for easy cleaning and an inert material in contact with the contents. The glass-lining on the tank and glass-coating on the shaft and impeller are formed by spraying a dispersion of powdered glass on the metal and then heating until the glass melts. The process must be repeated from four to eight times to create a uniform and complete glass coating. Because the glass coating is fragile, especially in tension, the corners of the impellers and baffles are usually rounded. Improvements in glass coating and PTFE lining have reduced some of the coating problems, allowing for more conventional impeller designs.

The advantages of easy cleaning and inert coating are obvious for the pharmaceutical industry. The disadvantages include initial cost and extra care in use. Rapid temperature changes or objects dropped into the tank may break the glass coating. The single, or sometimes dual, baffle arrangement does allow some swirling, especially near the bottom of the vessel. The glass-lined vessels are particularly effective where multiple batch reactions with different chemicals need to be carried out in the same tank.

12.2.10 Side-Entering Mixers

Side-entering mixers are most often used on storage tanks. The advantage of a side-entering mixer on a large or tall storage tank is that a rigid overhead support and long mixer shaft are not needed. Side-entering mixes are located near the bottom of the storage tank, so they remain submerged in the liquid even with a fluctuating liquid level. The recirculation pattern developed by the mixer is sufficient to blend liquids for uniform concentration and temperature, but rarely intense enough for pharmaceutical processing. Side-entering mixers are a cost-effective way of maintaining tank uniformity.

12.2.11 Vessel Geometry

The vessels (tanks) used in the pharmaceutical industry are almost exclusively vertical cylinders. Other geometries, such as horizontal cylinders or rectangular tanks are possible, but rarely used except for storage or special applications. The tank bottoms may be flat, conical, or dished. Flat bottom tanks usually have a slope to one side for complete drainage. Conical bottom tanks also drain well, and usually have a shallow cone just for drainage. Tanks with a deep conical bottom are difficult to mix, especially if solids must be suspended. Dished bottom tanks do not require outside support for large diameters or elevated pressures. The torispherical dish shape can be shallow for a standard head (aka dished bottom), deeper for an ASME or elliptical head, or very deep for a hemispherical head. Very deep heads are difficult to mix, unless the impeller is contoured to the bottom.

For most tanks, the size is specified as an inside diameter, a straight side, and a head type. The tank diameter and standard ratios define the shape of dished or conical heads. The "straight side" is the cylindrical portion of the tank. The length of the straight side is measured from the tangent line of the bottom head to the top of an open tank or the tangent line of the top head for a closed tank. Off-bottom impeller locations and liquid levels are typically measured from the bottom center of a dished or conical head. Other tank dimensions may be important, especially if the tank has a heat-transfer jacket.

Tank wall thickness is determined by pressure load requirements and strength for the material of construction. Those requirements may be set by Section VIII of the ASME Pressure Vessel Code for positive internal pressures above one atmosphere and for vacuum conditions. The ASME Code prescribes not only material thickness, but allowable temperature limits for alloys, welding procedures, and inspection or testing methods. Because the

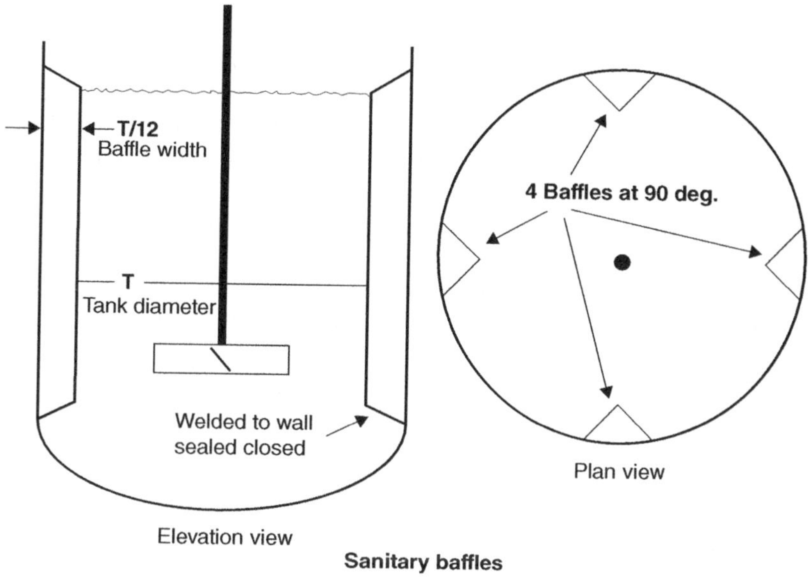

Figure 12.11 Tank baffles for sanitary applications

ASME Code is an integral aspect of safety for pressure vessels, any modification to a Code vessel invalidates the rating and must be reinspected and certified by an ASME Code Shop, with updated calculations and fabrication procedures, even inspection or retesting.

12.2.12 Baffles

To prevent uncontrolled swirling of low viscosity liquids in a stirred, cylindrical tank, baffles are needed. For most industrial vessels, the baffles are four vertical plates mounted at 90° intervals around the tank, or three plates at 120° intervals. The baffles are usually one-twelfth or one-tenth of the tank diameter and set a short distance off the tank wall with two or more supports, depending on tank size. The usual complaint in the pharmaceutical industry is that the flat plates cannot be adequately cleaned by fixed location CIP sprays. The sanitary baffles shown in Figure 12.11 effectively eliminate or greatly reduce cleaning problems.

The baffles are welded continuously to the tank walls and sealed top and bottom, with venting to the tank exterior for the relief of pressure caused by temperature changes.

12.3 Measurements

The measurement and quantification of mixing intensity or success are a difficult aspect of mixing equipment design. The ability to measure the power or torque of a mixer depends on the mixer size and accuracy required. The ability to convert such measurements into mixer performance may or may not be successful depending on the process objective. Some process objectives depend on power input, energy dissipation, or momentum transfer. Other processes depend more on mixer geometry and can be related to other characteristics, such as tip speed.

12.3.1 Power

Being able to estimate, calculate, or measure mixer power has both practical and process implications. At a minimum, impeller power is needed to size a motor and drive correctly. Impeller power is a function of impeller type, diameter, rotational speed, and fluid properties. Sometimes, the ability to relate impeller power to turbulence intensity or length scale may provide guidance for effective process conditions. To size a motor, the actual impeller power is needed. To understand process performance, power per volume or torque per volume are more useful measures.

The easiest and often most effective way of estimating mixer power is by calculation. The dimensionless power number, Eq. 12.1, is a convenient and technically valid way relate mixing power to impeller type.

$$N_P \equiv \frac{P}{\rho N^3 D^5} \tag{12.1}$$

In turbulent conditions the impeller power number is a constant for a given impeller geometry in a baffled tank. Turbulent conditions exist for impeller Reynolds numbers greater than 20,000.The definition of the impeller Reynolds number is shown in Eq. 12.2

$$N_{\mathrm{Re}} \equiv \frac{D^2 N \rho}{\mu} \tag{12.2}$$

Both the power number and Reynolds number are dimensionless, so coherent units or appropriate conversion factors must be used to eliminate dimension dependence. As the Reynolds number becomes smaller with increasing viscosity or smaller impeller diameter, the power number increases. A transition range between turbulent (Chapter 2) and laminar (Chapter 3) conditions typically extends from an impeller Reynolds number of 20,000 down to 10. Laminar conditions exist at Reynolds numbers less than 10. Impeller power numbers as a function of Reynolds number have been published, Grenville and Nienow (2004) for several common impeller geometries, a few of which are shown in Figure 12.12.

Additional power number characteristic curves can be found in other sources, such as Hemrajani and Tatterson (2004) and Couper, et al. (2005).

Using the Reynolds number for specific conditions and the corresponding power number for a geometrically similar impeller, the power number definition can be rearranged to calculate impeller power:

$$P = N_P \rho N^3 D^5 \tag{12.3}$$

Coherent units or appropriate conversion factors are necessary to get proper dimensional results for power. Calculated impeller power values are typically within 10% of measured values and often within 5%. Taking into account the usually minor losses through mixer drives and shaft seals, motor requirements can be calculated. Although motors are rarely loaded to more than 90% of the motor nameplate power because of secondary influences from flow patterns and impeller locations.

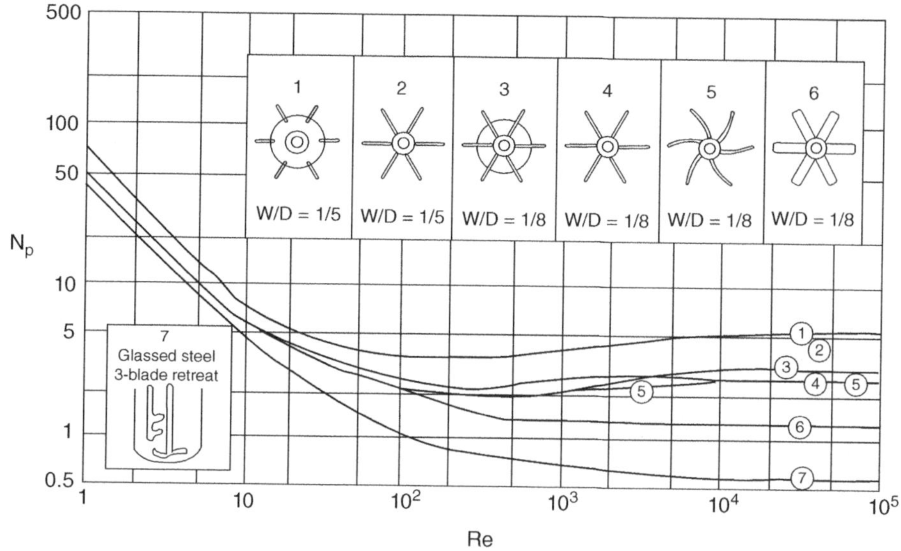

Figure 12.12 *Impeller power number for typical impellers as a function of impeller Reynolds number. Hemrajani & Tatterson (2004) – Figure 6.4*

Other measurements of power can be made in the laboratory or pilot facility using calibrated strain gages on the mixer shaft or a torque arm attached to the mixer drive mounted on a low-friction bearing. Most small-scale power measurements are likely to be research projects requiring care and operating ranges matched to the expected loads. Laboratory mixers with the capability of displaying a power reading usually are not reliable for use with small laboratory impellers, even when the mixer is calibrated at each test speed. An easy check for any power measurement of turbulent mixing conditions should show that power is proportional to the rotational speed cubed, as seen in the power relationship, Eq. 12.3.

Power measurement in production scale equipment can be done using a watt meter, provided no-load conditions have been measured to correct for gear drive or shaft seal losses. Watt meters measure both line voltage and amperage on all three legs of a three-phase power supply to correct for power factor as observed in a phase shift between voltage and current. Provided the electric power is properly connected and the load is within the range of the meter, such readings are reliable within the accuracy of the meter. Measurements with amp probes, even with simultaneous voltage measurements are not reliable, because a lightly loaded motor will draw as much as 50% of the full-load amperage. Motor efficiency is not properly measured by motor current.

Another use for power measurement is as a measure of mixing intensity in terms of power per volume. Actually, the measure should be power per mass, but because the fluid density appears in both the impeller power and fluid mass, the densities cancel and either per volume or per mass works. Power per volume (mass) can be a measure of the micro-scale turbulence in the mixed fluid. In an impeller mixer, the power per mass or energy dissipation is greatest in the region of the impeller. However, for a given stirred tank geometry, the ratio of energy dissipation near the impeller to the average energy dissipation (power per mass) is nearly constant. The local energy dissipation for that geometry, will remain a constant proportion of the average power per mass calculated from the power input and the mass of fluid, density times volume. Extending the idea of energy dissipation to turbulence theory, an estimate can be made for the size of the smallest turbulent eddies, as represented by the Kolmogorov length scale, Eq. 12.4.

$$\eta = \left(\frac{\nu^3}{\varepsilon} \right)^{1/4} \tag{12.4}$$

Turbulent eddy size is important for fast chemical reactions in bringing reactive molecules or ions together. Eddy size has also been used as a guide for the effect fluid shear may have on fragile cells. However, alternative explanations for cell damage, such as gas bubble breakage, may be more correct. For practical purposes, the energy dissipation rate, ε, may be expressed by power per mass, $P/\rho V$, Eq. 12.5

$$\varepsilon = \frac{P}{\rho V} \tag{12.5}$$

Power per volume (mass) may also be used as a conservative scale-up criterion, see Chapter 13 on scale-up for more information.

12.3.2 Torque

Torque is another means of measuring and quantifying mixing intensity. Torque is the related to the angular moment transferred to the fluid by the rotating impeller, and can be represented as power divided by rotational speed (rad/s).

Torque measurement can be done in the laboratory by several means, including the force on a moment arm attached to the mixer drive supported on a low frictionless bearing. Both laboratory and production scale measurements can be made with strain gauges on the mixer shaft and coupled to stationary instruments by slip rings or radio telemetry. Commercially available torque sensors may be mounted in the drive train provided adequate bending support is provided where needed.

The torque required for a mixer application establishes the size of the speed reducer, the shaft diameter, and the impeller-blade thickness. Torque is directly related to component strength requirements and therefore material costs. In practical terms, torque is related to the capital cost of a mixer, while power is related to the operating cost.

Torque per volume (or mass) as a measure of mixing intensity can be generally related to momentum transfer to the fluid. Usually for fluid motion applications, constant torque with different size impellers more nearly matches mixing intensity than equal power. Conceptually, a small impeller operating at a high speed can be expected to produce the same amount of fluid motion as a large impeller operating at a low speed. Those two different impellers and operating speeds are closer to being equal torque for equal fluid velocity, than they are equal power. By the same principles, an application requiring high power input, will require less torque if the impeller is smaller and rotates faster.

12.3.3 Tip Speed

Impeller tip speed, or peripheral velocity, is another measure that can be used to describe the operation of a mixer. The tip speed is closely related to the velocity difference between the blade and the surrounding fluid. Those velocity differences create fluid shear near the blade, often in the trailing vortex system. Those velocity gradients and the related hydraulic shear may determine the ultimate drop size for liquid-liquid dispersion or particle agglomerate size for solid-liquid dispersion. Tip speed is easily calculated, Eq. 12.6.

$$V_{tip} = \pi ND \tag{12.6}$$

12.3.4 Blend Time

Blend time is a practical measure of mixing performance, although only useful to the point that determinations are usually based on additions of small quantities of liquid with similar physical properties. A typical and effective laboratory method for measuring blend time is with a pH color change indicator in a transparent tank. For example, the change from base to acid with phenolphthalein is from pink to clear. Starting with a tank full of water with a pH of about 8.0 and adding a quantity of acid sufficient to change the batch pH to 6.0, the color should disappear at a pH of 7.0 or approximately at the 50% blend point. The advantage of an observed color to clear change, is that the time to when the last point of color disappears does not require any prejudgment for the location of a measurement probe. The location for final color change may move in successive tests, because of random fluid motion. Other methods for observing blend time include pH or ion probes located in the tank, with the addition of an appropriate tracer to observe the time to reach steady or uniform concentration Grenville and Nienow (2004).

Correlations for blend time have been developed for a few impellers using a dimensionless blend time as a function of Reynolds number (Grenville and Nienow, 2004). The dimensionless blend time for a standard pitched-blade turbine involves the rotational speed of the impeller, the impeller-to-tank diameter ratio, and the liquid-level-to-tank diameter ratio, Eq. 12.7.

$$\mathbf{N}_{\Theta_{99\%}} = \Theta_{99\%} N \left(\frac{D}{T}\right)^{2.3} \left(\frac{Z}{T}\right)^{-1.25} n_i^{0.46} \tag{12.7}$$

The dimensionless blend for a pitched-blade turbine in turbulent conditions has a constant value of 6.34. When plotted as a function of Reynolds number, the dimensionless blend time value increases as viscosity increases, Figure 12.13.

Blend time estimates can be made from dimensionless blend time correlations. These times are usually the minimum batch blending or residence times for continuous flow through a stirred tank.

Efforts are sometimes made to estimate blend time from pumping capacity and tank volume, for some number of tank turnovers to achieve uniformity. If a constant dimensionless

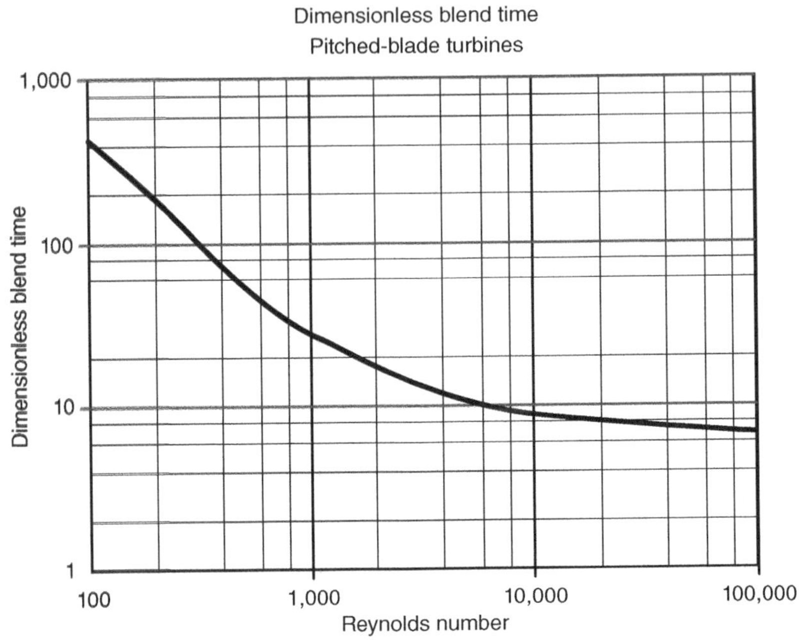

Figure 12.13 *Dimensionless blend time (95%) for pitched-blade turbines*

pumping number is used to estimate impeller pumping capacity, the calculated blend or turnover time will be inversely proportional to the impeller-to-tank diameter ratio (D/T) cubed (3.0 exponent), rather than to the 2.3 exponent as is typical of dimensionless blend time correlations. However, because blend times are rarely treated as precise values, differences may not have a strong influence on mixer designs. Industrial measures of mixer performance based on pumping capacity and tank turnovers are not supported experimentally.

12.4 Mixing Classifications

Because mixing covers such a broad range of applications, even in a single industry like pharmaceuticals, categorization by phases present helps organize the basic elements of equipment design. Whether a process involves only liquid, solids and liquid, gas and liquid, or viscous liquid makes a difference in the types of processes and impellers commonly considered.

12.4.1 Liquid Mixing

Mixing of single-phase liquids is one of the most basic types of mixing, but with many different applications. Immiscible liquid dispersions are less common than miscible liquid processes, but are both important and sometimes complicated.

12.4.1.1 Miscible Liquid Mixing

Miscible liquid mixing can be found in processes for batch formulation, blending to create or maintain concentration uniformity, heat transfer, chemical reactions, and similar continuous processes. Batch formulation may involve the combination of several liquid ingredients, or even quantities of dissolved or soluble solids. The idea of miscible batch formulation and uniformity blending is to combine desired proportions of different ingredients and bring the combination to a uniform composition. Heat transfer also involves creating uniformity, but aimed at temperature uniformity, rather than composition uniformity, although both are involved.

Chemical reactions may involve different rates of liquid blending depending on the rates of reaction and whether side-reactions lead to undesirable products. Simple, but fast reactions, like acid-base neutralization are typically controlled by bulk motion of the liquid, as represented by blend time. Slow chemical reactions, with reaction half-lives longer than blend time, will be controlled by the reaction rate. Chemical reactions with multiple paths and rates will sometimes be strongly influenced by the mixing intensity or the order in which the reactants are added. Which reactant is added to the other may lead to different product distributions. If products of a fast reaction are desired, addition of a reactant in the impeller region will give the most rapid mixing and best product distribution. Chemical reactions and continuous processes never experience the ideal conditions of batch uniformity. Mixing always imposes a time factor on any process.

Most processes involving miscible liquid blending take advantage of impellers with the best pumping or flow characteristics. Hydrofoil impellers are often the best choice for fluid motion. Even with fast reactions, where turbulence is important in bringing species together, the bulk motion from the point of addition to the level of microscale turbulence is the controlling factor in the rate of conversion. Pitched-blade turbines are also effective in creating good bulk blending. Radial-flow impellers, such as straight-blade turbines and dispersion impellers, are more effective at creating local turbulence than bulk flow. Radial flow impellers usually are not used for miscible liquid blending, unless local turbulence or intense mixing is needed to promote a fast reaction.

12.4.1.2 Immiscible Liquid Mixing

Immiscible liquid mixing typically involves either an oil-in-water (O/W) or a water-in-oil (W/O) process, Leng and Calabrese (2004). The most common purposes for such dispersions are to form either a stable emulsion or a dispersion for mass transfer, which can be later separated. A stable emulsion can be formed by some combinations of small dispersed droplets and a stabilizing agent, such as a surfactant. Stable emulsions are used in creams, ointments, and lotions (Chapter 9).

Solvent extraction may be used as a separation process for recovering an ingredient from a chemical process. Solvent extraction involves both droplet dispersion and subsequent coalescence. For optimal results, drop size should be as uniform as possible to use the smallest drops possible that can separated effectively.

Most liquid dispersions are done with disperser disks or rotor stators. Both types of mixers can form small droplets. The ultimate drop size for a given combination of immiscible liquids, stabilizing agent, and mixer is usually closely related to the impeller tip speed. Stable emulsions can be formed by some combination of mixing intensity and stabilizer, typically with a tradeoff between higher tip speed and less stabilizer or more stabilizer and lower tip speed.

12.4.2 Solids Suspension

Solids suspension is used for several categories of applications (Atiemo-Obeng et al., 2004). Solids suspension may be needed while dissolving a soluble solid, reacting or leaching an insoluble solid, making or maintaining a suspension, or in combination with gas dispersion. A three-phase process with solids suspended in a liquid combined and simultaneous gas dispersion may exist in a fermentation process, where the solids are microorganisms. Solids suspension is also a factor in crystallization.

The uniformity to which solids must be suspended for a process usually establishes the design requirement for mixing equipment. Three definitions for solids suspensions are shown in Figure 12.14.

"On-bottom motion" describes the degree of suspension when any solids resting on the bottom are in motion. "Off-bottom suspension" is the intensity when none of the solids rest on the bottom for more than a second, Zwietering (1958). "Uniform suspension" describes a condition when all of the solids are suspended as uniformly as practical (Chapter 10).

Solids suspension is best accomplished with an axial-flow impeller, such as a hydrofoil, Figure 12.2, or a pitched-blade turbine, Figure 12.3. Radial-flow impellers, such as straight-blade turbines, Figure 12.4, are usually only effective when placed near the bottom of a tank. Axial flow is most effective when the flow is down from the impeller, sweeping across the bottom of the tank, and up the sides. Baffles are necessary to control swirl and create effective axial flow. Impeller-to-tank diameter ratio is also an important factor in solids suspension. The optimum impeller-to-tank diameter ratio for solids suspension is between 0.35 and 0.40. Smaller impellers require more power to accomplish the same degree of suspension. Larger impellers begin to block recirculation and require larger amounts of power and torque to accomplish any effective degree of solids suspension.

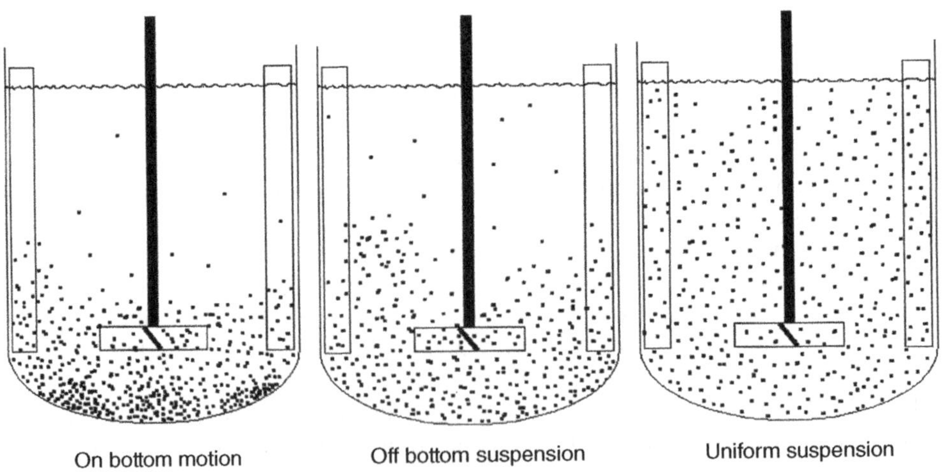

Figure 12.14 *Degrees of solids suspension*

All of the different degrees of solids suspension are a function of the solids being suspended. Small or low density particles may settle slowly enough that only moderate amounts of liquid motion are necessary to suspend them. Large or dense particles may settle more rapidly and require more vigorous motion to keep the solids in suspension. A distribution of particle sizes will require sufficient intensity to keep the most difficult to suspend particles at an appropriate degree of suspension, plus any interaction with other particles in the distribution. Definition of the degree of suspension required for a process can be complicated depending on the particles being suspended. Solids concentration is also a factor in suspension. Higher concentrations of solids are more difficult to suspend than low concentrations. Other factors, such as liquid density and viscosity, will affect solids suspension. Settling velocity alone does not define the conditions necessary for solids suspension in a mixing application.

On-bottom motion is usually the minimum practical degree of solids suspension. Large quantities of permanently settled solids are rarely acceptable, although accumulation of the most difficult to suspend particles may occur in some applications. When all of the particles are in motion on the bottom, some particles will be suspended, sometimes well up into the upper portion of the tank. The degree of uniformity in the tank will depend on how easily particles are to suspend. Easily suspended particles will be more uniformly suspended than rapidly settling particles.

Off-bottom suspension is a characteristic of solids suspension often referenced in literature dealing with mixer evaluation and study. The transition between the on-bottom motion and off-bottom suspension is usually sufficiently observable, especially in a transparent tank, that it can be used as a defined condition. Complete off-bottom suspension is often identified by a rotational speed for the mixer called N_{js}, or the "just suspended" speed. Definitions of other mixer design characteristics are necessary to reduce the off-bottom definition to a rotational speed. Besides the impeller type, impeller-to-tank diameter ratio, the tank bottom shape, impeller off-bottom clearance, solids properties and concentration all need to be defined. The increase in mixing intensity, rotational speed, between on-bottom motion and other degrees of suspension will depend on how difficult the particles are to suspend, Grenville and Nienow (2004), Zwietering (1958).

Uniform suspension is never achieved in an absolute sense. Even with very vigorous mixing intensity the random nature of turbulent motion will always leave some minor variations in the local solids concentration. The greatest variation in local concentration will occur near the free surface of the liquid. Near the surface some regions of lower concentrations will exist, especially with rapidly settling particles. In all cases of solids suspension, rapidly settling particles, will require more mixing intensity for any degree of uniformity and greater differences between the degrees of suspension.

Some processes involve the formation of suspensions or solutions beginning with the addition of dry solids to liquids (Chapter 10). The addition process is different from the suspension process. To successfully add dry powders to liquids requires a sufficient degree of surface motion to draw the solids down and wet them effectively (Ozcan-Taskin and McGrath, 2001, Ozcan-Taskin, 2006, Ozcan-Taskin and Wei, 2003). With impeller mixers, the surface motion may be improved by a second impeller near the surface and baffles cut below the surface. The upper impeller is most often a pitched-blade turbine and may be operated as either down pumping or up pumping. To effectively disperse the powder, it must pass through the hydraulic shear in the impeller region. For the case with particles that are difficult to wet, a rotor-stator mixer may be used instead of impeller mixers. The rotor-stator mixer can disperse clumps of solids to form a dispersion of individual particles. Some inline devices are designed to draw powders into a flowing liquid stream and immediately disperse the powder.

12.4.3 Gas Dispersion

Most mixing applications for gas dispersion involve some reason for mass transfer between the gas and liquid (Middleton and Smith, 2004). Mass transfer of oxygen from the air to water is needed for aerobic biological processes. Microbial fermentation can be used to create some pharmaceutical products (Amanullah, et al., 2004, Paul, et al., 2004). The same dispersed gas that supplies oxygen to the microorganisms may strip away carbon dioxide produced by cellular metabolism. Aerobic treatment also may be used for disposing of process wastes. Dispersed steam may be used for heating or sterilizing.

Similar to solids suspension, gas dispersion is often described in terms of degrees of dispersion, Figure 12.15.

A "flooded" condition for gas dispersion exists when the liquid mixing intensity provided by an impeller is insufficient to disperse the gas. While the flooded condition is rarely acceptable as an operating condition, the transition in mixing intensity to just above flooding, as represented by the "just dispersed" condition in Figure 12.15 is often the condition for maximum efficiency. Gas dispersion efficiency for mass transfer usually is defined as the largest mass transfer rate to power input ratio. This condition is far below the maximum mass transfer rate, but higher rates of mass transfer require more rapidly increasing mixer power than the corresponding increasing transfer rates. In situations where mass transfer

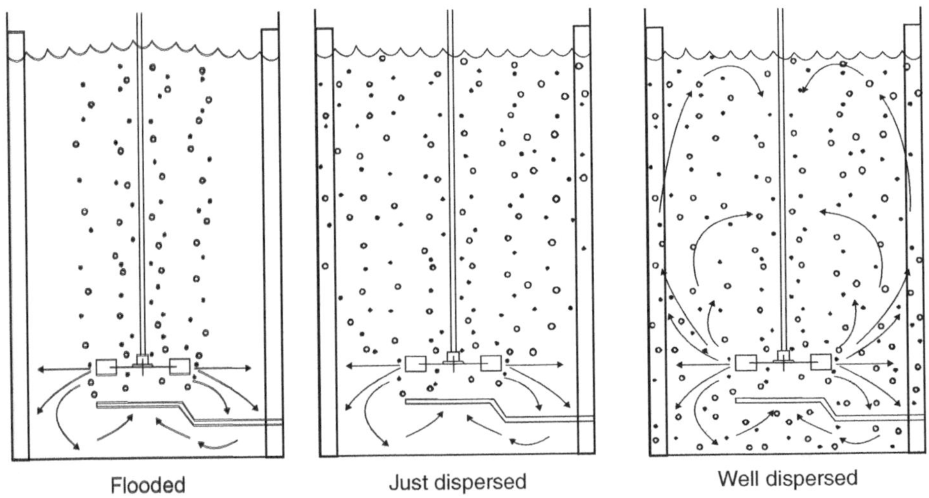

Figure 12.15 *Different degrees of gas dispersion. Reprinted with permission from* Chemical Process Equipment *by James R. Couper, W. Roy Penney, James R. Fair, Stanley M. Walas, 277–327. Copyright (2012) Elsevier*

rates promote productivity, the intense mixing of the "well dispersed" condition will justify the high power input, Nienow, et al. (1977).

The overall mass transfer coefficient for gas dispersion is typically a function involving the superficial gas velocity and the power per volume. Superficial gas velocity is the volumetric flow rate of gas divided by the cross-sectional area of the tank. Superficial gas velocity is related to the hydrodynamic conditions in the tank. If superficial gas velocity is held constant with scale-up for the purposes of mixing control, the gas volume per liquid volume rate decreases. Larger tanks, with greater liquid head and pressure at the bottom, will experience greater depletion of the soluble gas as bubbles rise in the tank. Calculations for overall mass transfer usually require a depth-by-depth, stage-wise calculation because of the changing compressibility and solubility of gas (Benz, 2011).

Mixer design for gas dispersion most often, but not always, begins with a radial-flow impeller. A similar design to a disk-type impeller, Figure 12.4, but with cupped blades, will handle higher gas rates than other radial-flow impellers. Gas is brought into the tank below the impeller through a sparge ring or other gas distribution devices. The sparge ring is typically slightly smaller in diameter than the impeller and located about a blade width below the impeller. The pipe diameter used for the sparge pipe is set appropriately for volumetric flow and pressure of the gas entering the tank. The diameter of the holes in the sparge pipe is selected to avoid plugging, with most of the holes on top of the sparge ring, but with a few on the bottom for drainage. The number of holes in the sparge pipe should be such that the total cross sectional area of all the holes is about half the cross-sectional area of the pipe used for the sparge ring. The reason for the restriction on the size and number of holes is to assure that gas is distributed evenly around the ring.

The classical design for gas dispersion in tall tanks was with multiple radial-flow turbines located about one impeller diameter to two diameters apart on the mixer shaft. While this design provided good gas dispersion at all levels of the tank, better mass transfer has been obtained using axial-flow impellers. Wide-blade hydrofoils, such as the one in Figure 12.2, are used as upper impellers to keep the liquid composition more uniform. A uniform liquid concentration increases the concentration driving force for mass transfer. While hydrofoil impellers work well at low gas rates, high gas rates are best handled by a lower radial-flow impeller and axial-flow upper impellers. The axial-flow upper impellers may pump upward or downward, depending on the gas flow rate.

12.4.4 Viscous Mixing

Viscous mixing involves a range of applications with as many differences as similarities. The definition of "viscous" is a problem with mixing (Chapter 3). Often non-Newtonian viscosity characteristics, such as shear thinning, will cause the apparent viscosity to change with mixer speed. The effect of viscosity is greater in small tanks, just because the Reynolds number is smaller with a smaller length dimension. The effect of size on viscous mixing makes scale-up more difficult. Even just describing viscous mixing can be difficult. Fluid motion dies out before the entire tank contents are in motion. Some applications go from a low viscosity liquid to a high viscosity fluid, such as with the addition of a thickener.

Most viscous mixing ultimately requires some type of close-clearance, large diameter impeller, such as the ones shown in Figure 12.8. However, for the many applications where the viscosity changes, especially by a couple of orders of magnitude or more, a combination of close-clearance and turbine-style impellers may be needed to handle conditions ranging from low to high viscosity. Different combinations of impeller types are used for different applications involving viscous fluids. One of the counter-intuitive understandings about viscous mixing is that lower speed sometimes gives better results, because some amount of time is required for a viscous fluid to flow in response to the rotating impeller.

12.5 Mechanical Design

Beyond the need for effective mixing, the mixer must be designed to be mechanically reliable. Most mechanical design requirements can be satisfied with conventional mechanical design methods for rotating equipment. The unique feature of top-entering mixers is the long overhung shaft required for most applications, Dickey and Fasano (2004).

12.5.1 Shaft Design

Shaft design for mixer applications requires both strength and rigidity. Except for very tall tanks, such as used in large fermenters, most top-entering mixer shafts are supported only by the drive on the top of the tank. For the impeller(s) to be in an appropriate location, the shaft must be long enough to reach more than two-thirds the height of the tank. With such a long shaft, the hydraulic forces associated with mixing can apply substantial torsional and bending moments on the shaft, mixer drive, and tank mounting. The shaft diameter and drive rating will be dictated by the mechanical requirements for the imposed forces.

Calculating the loads imposed on mixer components begins with the rotating torque on the shaft. Shaft torque can be calculated from the power and rotational speed of the mixer shaft, Eq. 12.8:

$$\tau = \frac{P}{2\,\pi\,N} \tag{12.8}$$

Using the motor power and the rotational speed of the mixer shaft will calculate the maximum torque on the shaft. Calculations can also be done to estimate the bending loads imposed by the impellers. Those loads are based on practical experience and measured loads under operating conditions. Equation 12.9 provides a good estimate of the bending load imposed by a mixing impeller.

$$M = \frac{0.048\,Pf_H\,L}{ND} \tag{12.9}$$

This calculation must be repeated for each impeller in a multiple-impeller application, with the appropriate shaft length from the drive to the impeller, the impeller diameter, and the fraction of the motor power at the impeller. The hydraulic service factor, f_H, depends on the type of mixing and whether the mixer operates while the tank is being filled or emptied. Some typical values for f_H are 1.0 for fully submerged operation, 2.0–3.0 for gas dispersion and 3.0 for operation at the liquid level: see Dickey and Fasano (2004) for more complete recommendations

Using basic mechanical engineering calculations for a round bar supported at one end, a minimum shaft diameter for tensile and shear stresses can be determined. The minimum shaft diameter for shear stress is shown in Eq. 12.10.

$$d_s = \left[\frac{16\sqrt{\tau^2 + M^2}}{\pi\sigma_S}\right]^{1/3} \tag{12.10}$$

A similar equation calculates the minimum shaft diameter for tensile stress:

$$d_t = \left[\frac{16\left(M + \sqrt{\tau^2 + M^2}\right)}{\pi\sigma_t}\right]^{1/3} \tag{12.11}$$

Mechanical failures will occur due to fatigue, so the allowable stresses in these equations must be set well below the yield stress of stainless steel. Recommended allowable stresses for stainless steel shafts are 42 MPa (6000 psi) for shear stress, σ_s, and 70 MPa (10,000 psi) for tensile stress, σ_t. Whichever diameter is the larger of the two calculated values will be the minimum shaft diameter. Actual shaft diameters are usually rounded to the next larger size of bar stock.

The same calculations for torque, Eq. 12.8, and bending, Eq. 12.9, can be used to design the mixer drive and the mounting supports. Although additional factors of 2.5 for mounting torque and 3.0 for bending load are recommended for mounting support to assure sufficient rigidity for the dynamic load of the mixer. More information about mixer mounting can be found in Dickey and Fasano (2004).

The other potential problem with mixer shaft design is the natural frequency or critical speed. A cantilevered shaft acts like a long, rigid arm of a tuning fork, so it will vibrate at some frequency associated with the shaft length, shaft and impeller weights. At the critical speed, the vibrations caused by the shaft rotation will match the natural frequency of the overhung shaft, causing undamped vibrations. Operating at the critical speed can result in catastrophic shaft bending or failure. Methods for estimating shaft critical speed can also be found in Dickey and Fasano (2004). Most large mixers operate below the critical speed. Smaller mixers, such as portables, operate above the critical speed. If a mixer is designed to operate above the critical speed, it must accelerate rapidly enough that it passes through the critical speed quickly.

12.5.2 Shaft Seals

Shaft seals are important for pharmaceutical applications, because some products must be confined inside the tank for safety and health reasons. Also, the seal must keep atmospheric and environmental contaminants out. In any case, the seal materials and construction cannot create contamination of their own. One of the simplest seals is called a stuffing-box seal. The stuffing box forms a seal around the rotating shaft by compressing one or more rings of a lubricated, fiber material, called packing, against the housing and shaft. The more rings of packing, the higher the pressure the seal can hold.

Another type of seal found frequently in pharmaceutical applications is a mechanical seal. The seal is formed by a rotating ring of a material such as graphite or ceramic running against a stationary ring of a hard material such as tool-steel or ceramic. Materials of construction depend on the contents of the vessel, temperature, and pressure. Double mechanical seals can make a positive seal, by using a pressurized fluid between the seals, to prevent leakage of the tank contents.

12.5.3 Materials of Construction

Material specification is most often done as a number associated with the metal alloy composition. The most common stainless steel materials used in pharmaceutical applications are designated as 304, 304L, 316, and 316L. Many other types of stainless steels are available for other uses, but are rarely used in pharmaceutical equipment unless a special corrosion or metal contamination issue is involved. For highly corrosive applications a high nickel alloy material such as Hastelloy C276 might be used.

The alloy compositions for these materials are listed as percentages in Table 12.1.

The 304 and 316 stainless steels are primarily composed of iron (Fe) with some added quantities of chromium (Cr) and nickel (Ni). The 316 stainless steels have a molybdenum (Mo) content for greater corrosion resistance. The 304 and 316 stainless steels have some silicone (Si), manganese (Mn), and carbon (C) for strength.

The L-grade stainless steels have a lower carbon content. The low carbon content does two things for the alloys. First, it aids in corrosion resistance where the materials are welded. With the normal carbon content (0.08%) when these metals are heated to sufficient temperature for welding some chromium comes out of the crystal lattice structure, causing rusting to occur along the heat affected part of the weld. Second, the lower carbon content reduces the strength of the steel. The proper designation for specifying materials of construction is "L-grade where welded." "L-grade only" is impractical because all nuts and bolts (fasteners) and other non-welded components can and most likely should be a standard-grade stainless because standard grade stainless is stronger. Many fasteners used in mixers are high-strength variations of the alloys.

Table 12.1 *Metal alloy compositions (percentages)*

Element	304	304L	316	316L	C276
Cr	18–20	18–20	16–18	16–18	14.5–16.5
Ni	8.0–10.5	8–12	10–14	10–14	Balance
Mo			2.0–3.0	2.0–3.0	15–17
C	0.08	0.03	0.08	0.03	0.02
Si	1.0	1.0	1.0	1.0	
Mn	2.0	2.0	2.0	2.0	
W					3.0–4.5
Fe	Balance	Balance	Balance	Balance	4–7

A high alloy, such as Hastelloy C276 is a nickel based alloy with chromium, molybdenum, carbon, and tungsten (W). This material is much more expensive and more difficult to fabricate and weld that 300-series stainless steel. However, it is more corrosion resistant and stronger than stainless.

12.5.4 Surface Finish

Besides the metal alloy used for pharmaceutical mixers, the surface finish is important for appearance and cleaning (Chapter 14). The surface roughness is the primary factor in determining both method and appearance of surface finishing. Surface roughness is typically measured as a Ra (roughness average), Rq (roughness equivalent), or RMS (root mean square roughness). Surface finishing usually involves some sort of grinding or buffing with a grit paper or wheel. The grit describes the number of particles per inch, so a larger number is composed of finer particles and will give a smoother finish. Stainless steel, as it is produced for general purpose applications, has what is known as a "mill finish," as it comes from the steel mill. That finish has a mill No. 3, or a 60-grit finish with maximum surface roughness of Ra 140 microinches, which is equivalent to a Ra of 3.56 micrometers. Any rolling done to shape a cylindrical vessel must be done with stainless steel rolls, otherwise the iron from standard rolls can be forced into the surface, resulting in rust spots.

Besides the basic surface finish resulting from grinding or mechanical polishing, a surface can be electropolished, which removes additional roughness. Electropolishing is similar to plating, except it removes some high points on the metal surface. An electropolished surface has high luster, reflectivity, and brightness, but the final roughness depends on the original surface finish. Electropolishing a No. 3, 60-grit finish, will take if from a Ra of 140 microinches to a Ra between 70 and 90 microinches (Ra 3.56 μm to Ra 1.78–2.25 μm). Table 12.2 shows some typical values for different mill and grit finishes before and after electropolishing.

Although the mill numbers in the table are associated with a grit and roughness, specification of a metal finish should include the grit and Ra value to avoid confusion or misunderstanding.

Table 12.2 *Surface finishes before and after electropolishing*

Mill	Grit	Before electropolishing surface roughness, Ra		After electropolishing surface roughness, Ra	
No.	No.	micrometer	microinches	micrometer	microinches
3	60	3.56 max.	140 max.	1.78–2.25	70–90
4	120	1.14 max.	45 max.	0.58–0.75	23–30
5	150	0.76 max.	32 max.	0.43–0.52	17–21
6	180	0.64 max.	25 max.	0.32–0.40	13–16
7	240	0.20–0.51	8–20	0.10–0.26	4–10
8	320	0.15–0.38	6–15	0.08–0.19	3–8
8	500	0.10–0.25	4–10	0.05–0.13	2–5

A polished No. 4 finish is widely used in restaurant, dairy, kitchen and the exterior of pharmaceutical equipment. It is often available as polished sheet material, eliminating the need for manual polishing after fabrication. Manual polishing may leave some swirls or other visual differences in the surface. The polished sheet may have some directionality to it. A polished No. 5 finish is used for good appearance and pharmaceutical applications, especially with electropolishing. A buffed No. 6 finish has a dull satin finish with low reflectivity. A buffed No. 7 finish is reflective, while a No. 8 finish has the highest reflectivity of the mechanical finishes. Electropolishing will add reflectivity to each of these finishes, with some further reduction in the roughness. Besides polishing, polymer or glass coating may be used to make surfaces more inert or improve cleaning.

Welding will ruin the finish on the area around the weld and will leave some spatter. Welds are usually ground smooth for both appearance and reduction of imperfection. Grinding or filling to remove pits may be done, but requires further finish work. Consideration needs to be given to a balance between the necessary surface finish and the cost.

12.5.5 Motors

Most of the rotational power for all types of pharmaceutical mixers is provided by electric motors. Different types of motors are available from many manufacturers. Some motor types include general purpose, premium efficiency, explosion proof, severe duty, brake, inverter duty, two-speed, and wash-down duty motors. Severe duty and wash-down duty motors have materials and coatings that resist corrosion in contact with chemicals or cleaning solutions. Inverter duty motors are designed to operate with variable frequency controllers to control the mixer speed.

Motors also come in a wide range of standard sizes and are typically specified by power, voltage, although frequency affects the normal operating speed of a motor. Common motor enclosures are either totally enclosed or explosion proof. Explosion proof motors come in different divisions, classes, and groups depending on the environment and possible exposure to different chemicals. Motors come in industrially accepted standard sizes, such as those shown in Table 12.3.

Table 12.3 *Standard motor sizes (metric and horsepower)*

KW	hp	KW	hp	KW	hp
0.18	0.25	5.5	7.5	75	100
0.25	0.33	7.5	10	90	125
0.37	0.5	11	15	110	150
0.55	0.75	15	20	132	175
0.75	1	18.5	25	150	200
1.1	1.5	22	30	155	250
1.5	2	30	40	220	300
2.2	3	37	50	300	400
3	4	45	60	330	450
4	5.5	55	75		

12.5.6 Drives

Mixer drives typically serve two purposes, speed reduction from the motor and support of the mixer shaft. Most electric motors operate nominally at either 1500 rpm (with 50 Hz power) or 1800 rpm (60 Hz). Some small portable mixers operate at the motor speed, but larger portable mixers often operate at either 290 rpm or 350 rpm, with a 5:1 speed reduction. Nearly all large liquid mixers operate at or below 125 rpm, with many viscous mixers operating below 30 rpm. Speed reduction is usually done with an enclosed gear reducer for pharmaceutical applications. The selection of the mixer drive must match the motor input and shaft output requirements.

12.6 Static Mixers

Static or motionless mixers are pipeline mixers that use obstructions and divisions to cause the flowing fluid to mix. Mixing is accomplished by various combinations of flow division, rotation, radial motion, separation, and recombination. The altered flow path for the fluid increases the pressure drop through the mixer. The power required to force the fluid through the mixer causes the mixing to take place. Most static mixers accomplish adequate mixing in a few pipe diameters. Similar mixing might not happen in hundreds of pipe diameters of open pipe.

12.6.1 Twisted Element

One of the most common static mixers is the twisted element design. A sanitary version of a twisted element mixer, with removable elements is shown in Figure 12.16. The mixer can be removed from a pipeline using clamp connections on both ends of the mixer.

Flow entering the mixer is split by the first element so that the flow follows two twisted paths, with the material near the centerline of the pipe being rotated to the outside of the pipe. The second element of the mixer, splits the flow a second time at 90° to the exit of the first element and twists the flow in the opposite direction. With multiple splits and rotations, mixing occurs in turbulent flow in just a few elements. Viscous mixing requires more elements.

12.6.2 Structured Element

Other static mixer designs use various combinations of plates, baffles, and splitters to accomplish mixing. Some designs are simple flow splitters that redirect the flow. Others have multiple splits or corrugated elements to accomplish mixing. Many of these other

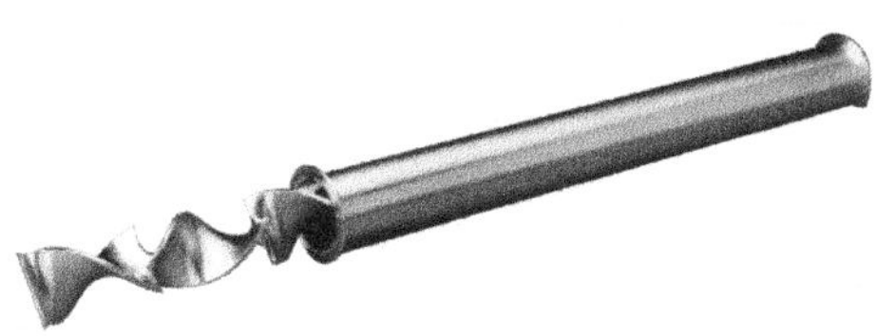

Figure 12.16 *Sanitary twisted-element static mixer. Reprinted with permission from Chemineer*

designs are sufficiently complicated or difficult to inspect and consequently are more likely to be used in chemical applications than in pharmaceutical applications.

12.6.3 Basic Design

The basic design of a static mixer follows pipe design. A typical static mixer is the same diameter as the pipe into which it is installed. Flow velocities of between 1.5 m/s (5 ft/s) and 4.0 m/s (13 ft/s) would be typical for turbulent applications. The importance of these velocities is not only that mixing can be accomplished, but that it occurs rapidly. The length of time that a flowing fluid remains inside the mixer can be as little as a fraction of a second. Mixing continues after the fluid leaves the mixer. Ideally, a static mixer should be preceded by at least 5–10 pipe diameters of straight pipe. Flow exiting the static mixer should go through perhaps 10–20 pipe diameters of straight pipe. Obviously, if the mixer is ahead of or behind a centrifugal pump, those lengths may be meaningless.

Other important aspects of static mixer design are the method of injecting material ahead of the mixer and the physical property differences in the fluids being mixed. Using a static mixer to blend two liquids is always improved if the injector for the secondary fluid has multiple injection points across the diameter of the pipe. A single injection point or a side tap will often put the additive on one side or the other of the first element and perhaps continue to be split through several of the following elements. The more similar the fluid properties of the bulk flow and the additive are, the easier the mixing is. Mixing low viscosity and high viscosity fluids, whatever the proportions, often causes problems in static mixers.

Beyond typical flow velocities, more accurate characteristics are needed to decide how many elements are needed and how much pressure is necessary to get the fluid through the mixer. The common characteristic of flow through a pipe, the pipe Reynolds number, still applies to a static mixer. The pipe Reynolds number is expressed in Eq. 12.12:

$$\mathrm{Re} = \frac{\rho V d}{\mu} = \frac{V d}{\nu} = \frac{\rho Q d}{\mu A} \tag{12.12}$$

The Reynolds number represents the ratio of inertial forces to viscous forces, large values describe turbulent flow and small values are characteristic of laminar or viscous flow. Turbulent flow occurs at a Reynolds number above 4000 and the transition to laminar flow develops rapidly below that number. The value of the Reynolds number can be used to decide how many twisted elements are needed for applications, see Table 12.4.

Table 12.4 Number of static mixer elements

Re	n_e
>5000	2
1000–5000	4
100–1000	6
10–100	12
<10	18

Most pressure drop calculations for static mixers begin with either equivalent length factors or valve coefficient methods. The specific design, size, and construction will affect the factors used to describe the pressure increase over an open pipe. Specific manufacturer information is necessary if a very accurate estimate of the pressure drop is needed. Many, especially low viscosity, applications do not cause a significant increase in pressure through the mixer, so most pumps have sufficient capacity to handle the additional pressure losses.

12.7 Challenges and Troubleshooting

Troubleshooting mixing problems requires an open mind. Do not start assuming that the mixer is the cause of all the process problems. Often, the lack of specific mixing performance criteria or requirements make mixing an unknown against which all problems can be assigned. Begin by defining what the mixer is expected to do. Remember that a mixer will not cause a reaction to take place. It only brings the reactants together and distributes them for uniformity or temperature control. Try to separate the effects of mixing from other possible influences, including raw materials, operator errors or procedures, and analytical problems.

12.7.1 Careful Observations

The first step in any mixer problem is to make careful observations. Sometimes, statistical analysis may be required to detect a problem or observe an improvement. In other cases, the problem and solution may be obvious. Anything that can be done to safely observe the mixing, may provide clues to the nature of the problem. If the surface of the liquid is not moving, or only moving in some locations, mixing is likely a part of the problem. If the surface is all moving in a circular pattern, with a deep vortex in the center, top-to-bottom motion may not be effective and mixing may be slow. The observations should be made both with the tank full and with the tank empty. Broken internals or missing impellers are obvious problems.

Many reasons can exist for changes in results. For the obvious, if the process is successful sometimes and the mixer is a fixed speed and mount, the problem is probably not the mixer operation. If the problem has developed suddenly, then something has changed. Of course, rule out the mixer by checking for broken parts or other significant equipment changes. Then review all of the possible changes that may have occurred with the process. Other changes may be more subtle or even misleading.

12.7.2 Process Problems

If the problem has developed slowly, heat transfer on the jacket side can become fouled over a period. However, unless the mixer has a variable speed drive, mixer speed is not likely to change unless modifications are made to the motor or drive. If the mixer is a portable mixer, the positioning could change gradually or because of a specific event. Although most pharmaceutical processes follow carefully specified procedures with weighed and checked ingredients, some steps may not be clearly specified in the instructions and may have been changed without being observed or reported.

Many process problems occur when a new product is brought from the laboratory or development. In the ideal case, the development test and production equipment selection are geometrically similar and have been tested to decide the proper scale-up method. A change in batch size or mixing equipment can cause problems associated with the design change. See the chapter on scale-up methods (Chapter 13). The development testing should cover a sufficient range of operating conditions to know what works and what does not. Unknowns can always enter the scale-up process, so additional development testing may be necessary to duplicate the production problems and find solutions. No single or certain scale-up method works for all applications and sometimes a critical variable is overlooked and not properly handled with scale-up.

If the issue becomes one of whether more intense mixing will improve the process, testing may be the best method for making such a determination. If the mixer operates at a fixed speed with given impeller type and tank, the question becomes: How can a different mixing intensity be tested? Testing with a smaller batch size will have the same effect as increasing the mixing intensity. The same mixer operating in a smaller batch, smaller by 10 or 20%, will increase the mixing intensity for characteristics such as power per volume or torque per volume. If impeller operation does not change the flow pattern significantly, less volume should have an effect similar to more intense mixing. If no change in process results is observed with a smaller batch, mixing intensity may be sufficient for the process and more intense mixing will be of little value. If the results of a smaller batch are better, then consideration should be giving to increasing the mixing, with either a higher speed or larger impeller. However, such a change may require a larger motor, drive, or even the shaft diameter. Critical speed also needs to be checked for such changes.

Nomenclature

D	impeller diameter [m]
d	pipe diameter [m]
d_s	shaft diameter for shear stress [m]
d_t	shaft diameter for tensile stress [m]
f_H	hydraulic force factor
L	shaft length (to impeller location) [m]
M	shaft bending moment [N•m]
N	rotational speed [s^{-1}]
n_e	number of static mixer elements
n_i	number of impellers
P	impeller power [W]
Q	volumetric flow rate [m^3/s]
T	tank diameter [m]
v	linear velocity [m/s]
V	volume [m^3]
v_{tip}	impeller tip speed [m/s]
Z	liquid level [m]
Dimensionless Groups	
$\mathbf{N}_\mathrm{P}$	impeller power number

N_{Re} impeller Reynolds number
$N_{\Theta 99\%}$ dimensionless blend time
Re pipe Reynolds number

Greek

ε energy dissipation rate [m^2/s^3]
μ fluid viscosity [Pa•s]
ν kinematic viscosity [m^2/s]
σ_s allowable shear stress [Pa]
σ_t allowable tensile stress [Pa]
ρ fluid density [kg/m^3]
τ shaft torque [N•m]

References

Amanullah, A., Buckland B.C., & Nienow, A.W. (2004). Mixing in the fermentation and cell culture industries, *Handbook of Industrial Mixing, Science and Practice*, Paul, E.L., Atiemo-Obeng, V.A., & Kresta, S.M. (eds), John Wiley & Sons, Inc., Hoboken, NJ.

Atiemo-Obeng, V.A., Penney, W.R., & Armenante, P. (2004). Solid-liquid mixing, *Handbook of Industrial Mixing, Science and Practice*, Paul, E.L., Atiemo-Obeng, V.A., & Kresta, S.M. (eds), John Wiley & Sons, Inc., Hoboken, NJ.

Benz, G.T. (2011) Bioreactor design for chemical engineers, *Chem. Eng. Prog.*, August, 21–26.

Couper, J.R., Penney, W.R., Fair, J.R., & Walas (2005) S.M., Mixing and agitation, in *Chemical Process Equipment, Selection and Design*, 2nd edn, Chapter 10, Gulf Professional Publishing, Elsevier, Burlington, MA.

Dickey, D.S. & Fasano, J.B. (2004). Mechanical design of mixing equipment, *Handbook of Industrial Mixing, Science and Practice*, Paul, E.L., Atiemo-Obeng, V.A., & Kresta, S.M. (eds), John Wiley & Sons, Inc., Hoboken, NJ.

Grenville, R.K. & Nienow, A.W. (2004). Blending of miscible liquids, *Handbook of Industrial Mixing, Science and Practice*, Paul, E.L., Atiemo-Obeng, V.A., & Kresta, S.M. (eds), John Wiley & Sons, Inc., Hoboken, NJ.

Hemrajani, R.R. & Tatterson, G.B. (2004). Mechanically stirred vessels, *Handbook of Industrial Mixing, Science and Practice*, Paul, E.L., Atiemo-Obeng, V.A., & Kresta, S.M. Editors, John Wiley & Sons, Inc., Hoboken, NJ.

Leng, D.E. & Calabrese, R.V. (2004). Immiscible liquid-liquid systems, *Handbook of Industrial Mixing, Science and Practice*, Paul, E.L., Atiemo-Obeng, V.A., & Kresta, S.M. (eds), John Wiley & Sons, Inc., Hoboken, NJ.

Middleton, J.C. & Smith, J.M. (2004). Gas-liquid mixing in turbulent systems, *Handbook of Industrial Mixing, Science and Practice*, Paul, E.L., Atiemo-Obeng, V.A., & Kresta, S.M. (eds), John Wiley & Sons, Inc., Hoboken, NJ.

Nienow, A.W., Wisdom, D.J., & Middleton, J.C., (1977), The effect of scale and geometry on Flooding, circulation and power in gassed stirred vessels, *Proc. 2nd Dureopean Mixing Conference*, Cambridge, pp. 17–34.

Ozcan-Taskin, G. & McGrath, G., (2001), Draw down of light particles in stirred tanks, *IChemE*, 79, Part A.

Ozcan-Taskin, G. (2006), Effect of scale on the drawdown of floating solids, *Chem. Eng. Sci.*, 60, 2871–2879.

Ozcan-Taskin, Gg. & Wei, H. (2003), The effect of impeller-to-tank diameter ratio on draw down of solids, *Chem. Eng. Sci.*, 58, 2011–2022

Paul, E.L., Midler, M., & Sun, Y. (2004), Mixing in the Fine Chemicals and Pharmaceuticals Industries, *Handbook of Industrial Mixing Science and Practice*, Paul, E.L., Atiemo-Obeng, V.A.m & Kresta, S.M. (eds), John Wiley & Sons, Inc., Hoboken, NJ.

Zhu, H., Nienow, A.W., Bujalski, W., & Simmons, M.J.H. (2009). Mixing studies in a model aerated bioreactor equipped with an up- and down-pumping 'Elephant Ear' agitator: Power, hold-up and aerated flow field measurements, *Chem. Eng. Res. & Des.*, 87, 307–317.

Zwietering, T.N. (1958), Suspending of solid particles in liquid by agitators, *Chem. Eng. Sci.*, 8, 244.

13
Scale-Up

David S. Dickey
MixTech, Inc., USA

13.1 Introduction

This chapter discusses the objectives and approaches to scale-up of fluid and powder blending applications. Included in the discussion are the inherent challenges of scaling up from lab scale (clinical trial phase 1 and 2) through to pilot scale (clinical trial phase 3) and to commercial scale. The need for consistent blending mechanisms during scale-up is often the key to success. The technical basis from dimensional analysis and similarity for scale-up analysis are put in perspective. Fluid properties like density and viscosity are related to aspects of mixing performance. Powder scale-up issues such as compaction problems and power cohesion are discussed with regard to both powder properties and geometry design.

Mixing scale up is an empirical process that should begin in the laboratory as active pharmaceutical ingredients (APIs) are being developed. Most pharmaceutical processes are limited and controlled by government and industrial standards; hence it is critical to establish the mixing and process conditions that will produce a quality product. The ideal situation is to be able to make process changes within an established range of mixing intensities to adapt or improve production process conditions.

The purpose of small-scale laboratory or development testing is to easily, quickly, and less expensively adjust conditions for successful processing. Then scale-up methods can be applied to the equipment design and operating conditions to duplicate results in production

Pharmaceutical Blending and Mixing, First Edition. Edited by P.J. Cullen, Rodolfo J. Romañach, Nicolas Abatzoglou and Chris D. Rielly.

equipment. Mixing scale-up should not be treated as an afterthought, but must be integral during the development process and support a Quality by Design paradigm.

Most of the guidance for mixing scale-up depends on the characteristics of the mixing process. As discussed throughout this book mixing equipment can be used to handle single phase liquids, multi-phase immiscible liquids for dispersions or emulsions, solid-liquid systems for suspensions or dissolution and dry or wet powder blending applications. Each type of application may have different requirements for scale-up and within each classification multiple scale-up options have to be considered. No matter how desirable, scale-up cannot duplicate all the characteristics of a small-scale development process in a large-scale process. Instead, development testing needs to establish the essential mixing characteristic and maintain that condition within an acceptable range. Usually some minimal level of mixing intensity is required for each of several process variables, so even if scale-up is not the same for each variable, a minimum effective intensity can be established. In other instances, a maximum mixing intensity may be established by testing.

13.2 Similarity and Scale-Up Concepts

Scale-up of fluid mixing applications has a theoretical basis in dimensional analysis and similarity. Fluid properties like density and viscosity can be directly related to aspects of mixing performance. The objective of scale-up is the duplication of a process result. Scale-up is different from either dimensional analysis or similarity, although those other methods can be used to guide scale-up decisions.

13.2.1 Dimensional Analysis

Dimensional analysis stems from the idea that physical quantities, related as a combination or equality, must have the same dimensions. Thus, a time and a velocity cannot be added to find a characteristic length. However, different types of forces can be added to represent the total force acting on an object. Physical quantities, such as density, velocity, or length, can be associated with the physical dimensions of mass, length, and time, which are typically represented by $\boldsymbol{M}$, $\boldsymbol{L}$, and $\boldsymbol{t}$. Thus a velocity has the dimensions of "length/time" ($\boldsymbol{L/t}$) and a force can be represented by "mass × acceleration" ($\boldsymbol{ML/t^2}$).

From the concept of dimensional consistency, comes the Buckingham $\boldsymbol{\Pi}$ theorem, which states that for every physically meaningful relationship involving n variables, there are $n - m$ independent dimensionless groups, where m is the number of fundamental dimensions. In physical processes, such as mixing, only three fundamental dimensions: mass, length, and time, are considered. Working from the Navier–Stokes equations describing the mass and momentum balance for a Newtonian fluid, three dimensionless groups can be developed for mixing applications, as described in Bird, et al. (1960, pp. 106–107).

Reynolds number

$$N_{\mathrm{Re}} \equiv \frac{D^2 N \rho}{\mu} \tag{13.1}$$

Froude number

$$N_{Fr} \equiv \frac{N^2 D}{g} \tag{13.2}$$

Power number

$$N_P \equiv \frac{P}{\rho N^3 D^5} \tag{13.3}$$

The Reynolds number is a ratio of inertial to viscous forces, which at large values correspond to turbulent flow and at small values relates to laminar or viscous flow. For mixing applications, the rotational speed, represented by *N,* is evaluated in revolutions per second, not radians per second. The Froude number is a ratio of inertial to gravitational forces, which may describe the size of surface waves or vortex depth in liquid mixing applications. Gravity has an observable effect on surface motion. The power number can be developed from dimensionless pressure and represented as a ratio of pressure forces to inertial forces. The power number provides a practical relationship between impeller power, impeller diameter, rotational speed, and fluid density. While these groups are not often held constant as a means to scale-up mixing, they do form the basis for empirical correlations that are scale independent. Empirical relationships between power number and Reynolds number have been developed for different types of geometrically similar impellers.

13.2.2 Similarity

Similarity is developed from physical models and can be extended to mathematical models. The simplest example of a physical model for mixing is a geometrically similar (scale) model of a mixed tank. For geometric similarity to exist, all of the linear dimensions of the small- and large-scale mixed tank are held to the same ratio between scales, as shown in Fig. 13.1. Geometric similarity simplifies scale-up for mixing applications, since the only remaining equipment variable is the rotational speed of the mixer.

Kinematic (motion) similarity is a form of mechanical similarity that exists when corresponding velocities are similar. With kinematic similarity a flow pattern can be described by dimensionless local velocities. Dimensionless velocity is the actual local velocity divided by a reference velocity. In liquid mixing equipment, that reference velocity is typically related to the impeller tip speed or peripheral velocity of an impeller. However, "tip speed" is commonly represented in dimensionless groups as simply the product of the rotational speed times the impeller diameter, ignoring the constant pi (π).

Dimensionless Velocity

$$N_v \equiv \frac{v}{ND} \tag{13.4}$$

While the details of local velocities or dimensionless velocities are rarely considered specifically for scale-up, they may be calculated by numerical methods, such as computational fluid dynamics (CFD). The flow patterns shown by computational methods can be useful in determining where high or low velocities exist and the direction of those

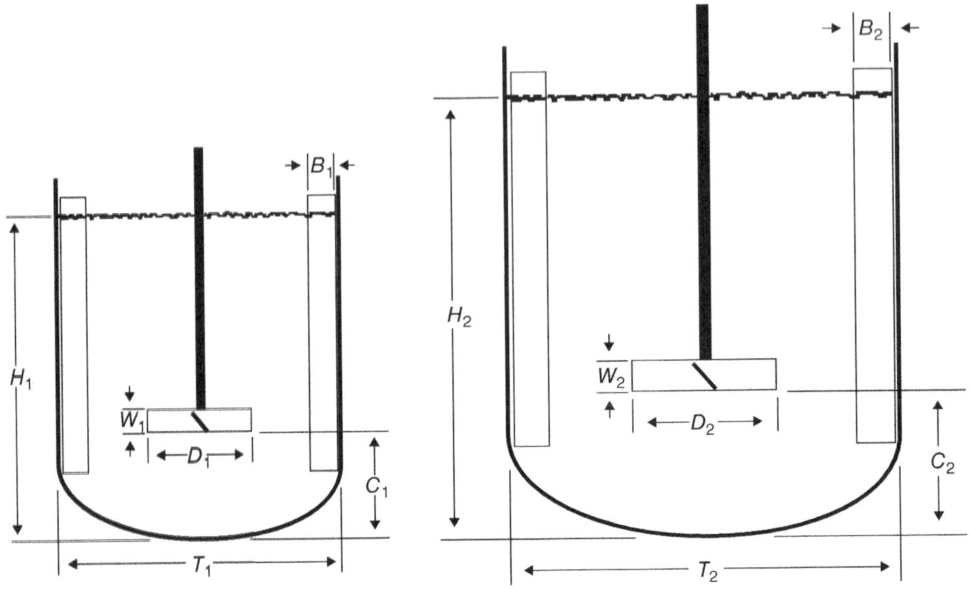

Figure 13.1 *Geometric similarity for mixed vessels*

velocities. However, local velocity values are difficult to interpret as successful or unsuccessful mixing intensity. The definition of intensity depends on the process objective, blending may be velocity dependent, while chemical reactions, solids suspension, or gas dispersion may have other intensity parameters.

The importance of kinematic similarity is less about the ability to estimate local velocities for a specific application and more about the understanding of how similarity can be applied in scale-up. Kinematic similarity exists for fully turbulent mixing in geometrically similar equipment. Thus, observing a flow pattern in a scale model mixing vessel will reveal the anticipated flow pattern in a large scale vessel. Additionally, kinematic similarity means that all local velocities are in the same proportion to the reference velocity. Doubling the impeller tip speed doubles all of the local velocities for a specific mixing vessel geometry. For scale-up of turbulent conditions, maintaining tip speed in geometrically similar systems will maintain corresponding local fluid velocities. Maintaining flow patterns and velocities can be an effective means of scale-up when liquid motion is the critical factor. Conditions, which result in effective mixing in a small scale vessel, may be duplicated by maintaining equal tip speed on scale-up. On a practical level, equal fluid velocities are what is typically seen as equal mixing intensity for many blending applications in different size vessels.

Kinematic similarity is not the only form of mechanical similarity that can be important in mixing studies. Dynamic similarity defines conditions where forces are defined with respect to a reference force. Fluid forces can be caused by the pressure differential between the front and back of an impeller blade as it moves through a turbulent fluid. Other forces on an impeller blade may be caused by viscous drag. The relative importance of pressure or viscous forces depends on the operating conditions for a mixing impeller. Under turbulent conditions, inertial forces or pressure forces dominate. While under laminar conditions, viscous drag forces dominate. The relative dominance of these forces can be defined by the Reynolds number. The ranges for mixing Reynolds numbers are shown in Eq. 13.5.

$$\begin{aligned}&\text{Turbulent mixing}: N_{Re} > 20{,}000\\&\text{Transitional mixing}: 20{,}000 > N_{Re} > 10\\&\text{Laminar mixing}: N_{Re} < 10\end{aligned} \tag{13.5}$$

13.2.3 Applied Scale-Up

The important differences between dimensional analysis, similarity, and scale-up are their respective purposes. Dimensional analysis may help identify how different variables interact with respect to each other. For instance, Reynolds number shows that tradeoffs exist between impeller diameter and rotational speed with respect to fluid density and viscosity. Also, dynamic viscosity and fluid density have opposite effects on the relative magnitudes of inertial and viscous forces. Conditions showing similarity may exist over a range of operating conditions. For instance, the flow pattern in a mixing vessel remains effectively unchanged for fully turbulent conditions at different velocity magnitudes. The flow pattern, represented by the relative magnitude of velocities, remains unchanged, although the absolute magnitudes of the velocities can all change in direct proportion for turbulent conditions. By comparison, scale-up typically has a specific objective. Certain conditions are expected to remain unchanged for scale-up. Maintaining a specific velocity, as characterized by an impeller tip speed, is a practical objective for scale-up. Local fluid velocities remain in constant proportion to other fluid velocities due to kinematic similarity, thus all corresponding fluid velocities are the same at constant tip speed with geometric similarity for fully turbulent conditions. Scale-up can use similarity and/or dimensional analysis, but not for a specific condition.

Perhaps the best way to explain these differences is by analogy to a graph. Dimensional analysis is like defining the axes of the graphs. Similarity may be for a given geometry or other system variable and defines a line on the graph. Scale-up takes a specific value, usually for a dimensional variable, and keeps it constant, perhaps taking a value off the curve (similarity) on the graph (dimensional analysis), see Fig. 13.2.

A graph of power number as a function of Reynolds number is based on dimensional analysis and similarity. The dimensional analysis defines the independent and dependent variables, such as Reynolds number and power number. Impeller power number results are typically reported as a function of Reynolds number. Because Reynolds number describes the relative importance of inertial and viscous forces and power number shows the impeller response to those forces resisting rotation through the fluid, similarity is like a curve on the graph. For a given impeller geometry in a baffled tank, the impeller power number is an empirical function of the impeller Reynolds number. The empirical value of the power number is established by testing of an impeller type (geometry) at different speeds in different fluids over a range of Reynolds numbers. For scale-up a specific value on the graph is used to predict or maintain a required characteristic for scale-up. Although a constant Reynolds number is never an effective requirement for scale-up, a Reynolds number for any size impeller may be used to find the corresponding power number at those conditions, Fig. 12.12.

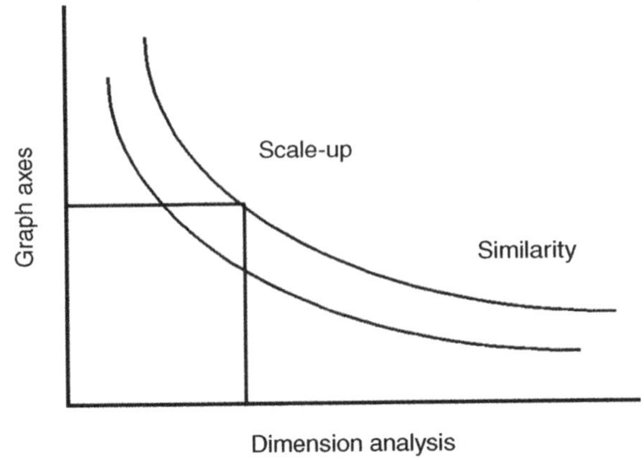

Figure 13.2 *Graphical analogy for dimensional analysis, similarity, and scale-up*

As mentioned, scale-up of a geometrically similar stirred vessel simplifies the process because all of the length dimensions of the large-scale vessel are in direct proportion to the dimensions of the small-scale vessel. The only remaining equipment variable for scale-up is the rotational speed of the mixer. Conducting development tests in a vessel that is geometrically similar to the production-scale vessel greatly simplifies many aspects of scale-up. With fully turbulent conditions in the small scale, scale-up will result in the same flow pattern in the large scale. Using a geometrically similar vessel for development, especially using a similar impeller avoids many problems caused by significant changes in mixing between development and production. Starting with or having a geometrically similar vessel in which to do development presumes knowledge about the production vessel size and geometry or should influence the selection of a production vessel and impeller. Although geometric similarity is not always possible, it is an important simplification for scale-up

13.3 Testing Methods

Perhaps the single most important aspect of mixing tests is variation. Without testing a range of operating conditions, little can be known about the effect mixing has on the process results. Further, without testing the limits for effective mixing, the potential for and characteristics of mixing problems may never be known until they appear in larger equipment. The word that best describes testing methods for mixing is "empirical." All mixing "results" begin or began with an empirical study, which means the results were obtained by observation. Those observations must be conducted scientifically, so they can be reproduced under equivalent conditions. Computational or analytical methods applied to mixing are only enhancements based on previous empirical studies. Model validation is the process by which computational models, such as CFD, are compared with empirical (measured) mixing results.

When testing different mixer speeds, changes should be made in a series of small increments, no more than about a 10% speed change at a time. A 10% speed change in turbulent mixing represents a 33% change in power. Large speed changes, such as half or twice the mixer speed are likely to take the process from transition to turbulent flow, or the reverse. To see if mixing problems develop for an application, a series of speed reductions may identify a condition for insufficient mixing. Scale-up is often done simply to avoid the known failure, since most industrial mixing applications operate in a safe range away from a failure condition. Failure to investigate or record a failure condition may result in a similar failure in production.

While changes to the rotational speed of a mixer are the easiest and most common method for investigating the effects of mixing, they only provide limited information for scale-up. Increasing or decreasing the rotational speed of an impeller will simultaneously increase or decrease mixing intensity as referenced to power, torque, or tip speed. To get a more complete view of mixing effects, the impeller diameter or type should be changed, besides the rotational speed. Different size impellers operating at different speeds can be selected to operate at the same power, but different torque and tip speed, or other combinations of the same and different characteristics. Knowing which mixing variable most nearly represents equivalent results may be an indication of what characteristic should be maintained for scale-up.

Testing with different impeller types not only changes the comparative quantities of power, torque, and tip speed for different rotational speeds, but also changes the flow pattern. The difference between a pitched-blade and straight-blade impeller includes not only a different power number, but also a change from an axial or mixed flow to a radial flow pattern. Such a change may show how important bulk motion or local turbulence may be for a particular process. The difference between a pitched-blade and hydrofoil impeller may show how more axial flow may reduce torque or power requirements for similar results.

One of the biggest problems with conducting small-scale mixing tests is that intense mixing or short blend times are not only possible, but are easy to achieve. Typical lab mixers and blenders have the capability of extremely intense mixing when placed in small quantities of liquid. The maximum speed on some lab blenders is capable of at least 5 or 10 times the practical power per volume intensity of an industrial mixer and many times the capacity of most pharmaceutical mixers. Whatever the mixer type used for development, it should be at least generally similar to the plant equipment, if not exactly geometrically similar.

Given the small volume of a typical lab beaker or flask, the time required for blending is very short compared with a typical production, mixed tank. Even the nearly solid-body rotation of fluid in a beaker or flask mixed by a magnetic stirrer bar will give uniform blend times of only a few seconds. The blend time in flasks is difficult to measure because the time is so short, Ndonga and Tatterson (2006). Even the rate or location for addition of a reactive ingredient may alter totally the mixing in a small container.

Testing for mixing effects is not an easy task in the laboratory, but careful records of all that was preformed can be of immense benefit later when the product or process is in production. Scale-up from the laboratory to a pilot study or pilot study to production is not easy. The more that is known on the small scale, the less likely large failures will occur.

13.4 Observation and Measurement

The dimensions of the mixing vessel and impeller are critical measurements in any mixing study. The size of the vessel, be it a beaker, flask, or small tank, is usually a matter of choice, but most tests are conducted with a known weight or volume of chemicals. All direct comparative tests should be conducted in similar vessels, with notes about the diameter, liquid level, and any internals other than the stirrer bar or mixing impeller. Baffles, typically three or four vertical plates at the vessel wall, will have a large effect on mixing, especially the flow pattern, even in a glass beaker. The dimensions of an impeller or stirrer bar are critical. An increase of less than 5% in diameter will increase power input by more than 25% at turbulent conditions. Laboratory impeller or stirrer bar dimensions should be made to fractions of a millimeter and the same one used in all experiments if possible. The same applies to larger, pilot scale impellers. With multiple blades, the measurements should be made for each blade from the shaft bore to the blade tip or the maximum diameter and an average used to calculate the effective diameter.

The rotational speed of the mixer is the variable most often used to characterize changes in mixing performance, especially for geometrically similar tests. Yet measuring or observing the rotational speed is not always easy and sometimes overlooked. Many laboratory or small-scale mixers do not come with an accurate speed readout. The simplest and most flexible method of speed measurement is a strobe light or optical tachometer. The light can be focused on the impeller in a transparent vessel or on a marked shaft in a closed metal vessel. Measuring and/or calibrating a magnetic stirrer should be part of any laboratory testing. A rotational speed and stirrer-bar dimensions should be included as part of the experimental results. In addition to measuring speed, it needs to be controlled and monitored during a test. As the load on the mixer increases, due to a changing density or viscosity, the speed often decreases with laboratory mixers. Careful observation may provide not only useful information for scale-up, but also information that might help monitor production conditions.

Power or torque measurements are often even more of a challenge in small equipment. While small-scale mixers can be adapted and instrumented to obtain torque or power readings, the safe operating range or process capabilities of such mixers may be severely limited. Torque or power measurements are best done with specific purpose equipment using load cells, strain gages, or sensitive electronic sensors. Most laboratory mixers with a torque or power display have low impeller loads compared with bearing friction or motor efficiency. As a result the mixer must be recalibrated for each operating speed. A proportionate speed increase in turbulent mixing should result in a squared increase in torque or a cubed increase in power, which is rarely observed in lightly loaded laboratory or pilot mixers. A more practical method for power analysis is a calculation from a known power number for an impeller. Literature references contain some power number values. Power requirements for impellers used in gas dispersion are even more complicated, because gas significantly reduces power and is different for different impeller types.

Some geometric characteristics, such as common length ratios, can help visualize the mixer. Length ratios, such as impeller-to-tank diameter ratio and blade-width-to-impeller diameter ratio, generalize the description of the mixer. Other characteristics, such as Reynolds number, power, torque, and tip speed can describe aspects of the mixing. For scale-up, volume related quantities, such as power per volume and torque per volume, can describe mixing even on different scales. For practical calculations, using convenient units of measure, correction factors are needed for dimensionless and dimensional results.

For example, taking tests run in a vessel with a 0.105 m diameter impeller, turning at 22 rps with a fluid having a density of 1150 kg/m^3 and a viscosity of 0.053 Pa•s. The Reynolds number would be:

$$N_{Re} = \left(\frac{D^2 N\rho}{\mu}\right) = \frac{(0.105)^2(22)(1150)}{0.053} = 5263 \tag{13.6}$$

The Reynolds number of 5263 in the bench scale is not fully turbulent, as described in Eq. 13.5. For Reynolds numbers greater than about 900, the effect of viscosity on power for a pitched-blade turbine is negligible, see Bates, et al. (1963) and Fig. 12.12.

A calculation for power, P, in watts [W] can be developed by rearranging the power number, $\mathbf{N}_P$, in Eq. 13.3. Assuming the example test was conducted with a pitched-blade turbine having a power number of 1.37, the impeller power would be:

$$P = N_P \rho N^3 D^5 = (1.37)(1150)(22)^3(0.105)^5 = 214\,\text{W} \tag{13.7}$$

A higher viscosity resulting in a lower Reynolds number would have increased the power number according to empirical correlations.

While power is commonly understood to represent information necessary to size the motor for a mixer, torque is often a better representation of mixing intensity for blending applications. Obviously, mixing a tank of liquid with a small impeller operating at a high speed can be expected to give similar mixing intensity compared with a large impeller operating at a low speed. When observed with respect to the characteristics commonly viewed as mixing intensity, typically fluid velocity, equal torque appears to give nearly equal results for different size impellers in the same tank. Thus torque, τ, in units such as Newton•meters [N•m] can be calculated with the example values:

$$\tau = \frac{P}{2\pi N} = \frac{(214)}{2\pi(22)} = 15.3\,\text{N•m} \tag{13.8}$$

Another variable of potential interest, especially related to drop or particle size in dispersions, is impeller tip speed, v_t, in units like meters per second [m/s]:

$$v_t = \pi N D = \pi(22)(0.105) = 7.26\,\text{m/s} \tag{13.9}$$

As mentioned, mixing has many different process objectives, such as blending, solids suspension, liquid dispersion, powder incorporation, and many other possible influences and combinations, consequently no single characteristic can be used to quantify mixing performance. Often the most useful understanding of a mixing problem can be achieved by simply observing flow patterns or blend time in a transparent vessel. A glass or clear plastic vessel can be a highly effective laboratory or bench-scale tool in developing and understand a mixing application. Depending on the desired or specified process result, the appropriate measurement must be applied. For liquid blending the time to uniformity, even local uniformity, may be critical, especially for rapid chemical reactions. Powder addition, solids suspension, and dissolution may all be factors in solid-liquid systems. Processes involving gas-liquid mass transfer and liquid-liquid dispersion can be more complicated for both measurement and scale-up since many factors may be involved.

13.5 Scale-Up Methods

13.5.1 Scale-Up with Geometric Similarity

Scale-up of a geometrically similar stirred vessel is simplified because all of the length dimensions of the large-scale vessel are in direct proportion to the small-scale vessel. The only remaining equipment variable for geometrically similar scale-up is the rotational speed of the mixer. Conducting development tests in a vessel that is geometrically similar to the production-scale vessel also provides good information about fluid motion. With fully turbulent conditions in the small scale, scale-up will result in the same flow pattern in the large scale. Using a geometrically similar vessel for development, especially using a similar impeller avoids many problems caused by significant changes in mixing between development and production. Starting with or having a geometrically similar vessel in which to do development presumes knowledge about the existing production vessel size and geometry or should influence the selection of a new production vessel. The scale-up methods associated with non-geometric similarity will be discussed later in this chapter.

Geometric similarity scale-up can be reduced to a simple expression of a correction factor with the inverse scale ratio, raised to an exponent, and applied to the successful, small-scale speed.

$$N_2 = N_1 \left(\frac{D_2}{D_1} \right)^n \tag{13.10}$$

The value of the exponent, n, depends on the scale-up characteristic that is to be held constant. This speed relationship only applies to geometrically similar scale-up.

Equal power per volume is a practical, although a conservative scale-up criterion. For geometric similarity and turbulent conditions, the scale-up exponent on the inverse length ratio is two-thirds:

$$N_2 = N_1 \left(\frac{D_1}{D_2} \right)^{2/3} \tag{13.11}$$

A power per volume scale-up might be used for equal mass transfer or other critical interfacial and chemical reaction applications.

The derivation of the exponent for power per volume serves as an example of how a constant characteristic can be reduced to a speed correction like Eq. 13.10. For turbulent conditions, mixer power is proportional to fluid density, rotational speed cubed, and impeller diameter to the fifth power. Dividing by volume is a practical way of increasing power in proportion to the quantity of fluid being mixed, see Eq. 13.12.

$$\frac{\rho N_1^3 D_1^5}{V_1} = \frac{\rho N_2^3 D_2^5}{V_2}$$

$$\frac{\rho N_1^3 D_1^5}{T_1^3} = \frac{\rho N_2^3 D_2^5}{T_2^3}$$

$$N_1^3 D_1^2 = N_2^3 D_2^2$$

$$N_2 = N_1 \left(\frac{D_1}{D_2} \right)^{2/3} \tag{13.12}$$

Volume for a cylindrical tank is proportional to the tank diameter cubed and impeller diameter can be substituted for tank diameter with geometric similarity.

Scale-up for equal tip speed has an exponent of one on the inverse scale ratio, which with geometric similarity also results in scale-up for equal fluid velocity in turbulent conditions.

$$N_2 = N_1 \left(\frac{D_1}{D_2} \right)^1 \tag{13.13}$$

With equal tip speed the product of rotational speed, N, times impeller diameter, D, remain equal in both scales. Equal fluid velocity has the effect of what is typically observed in different scale tanks as equal mixing intensity. The velocity of the fluid conveys an appearance of fluid motion and mixing intensity. This intensity does not equate to equal blend time, but rather the type of motion characteristic of adequate mixing for most blending applications. In other words, fluid motion occurs throughout the small scale tank in much the same way motion does in the large scale tank. Equal fluid velocity, or a scale-up exponent of one, also results in equal torque per volume with geometric similarity. Torque is proportional to power divided by rotational speed. Thus torque per volume, when rearranged like power per volume in Eq. 13.14 results in an exponent of two halves or one. Equal torque per volume and equal tip speed are not the same for non-geometric similarity as will be shown later in this chapter.

Scale-up for solids suspension should be done in the small scale with the same solids as expected in the large scale. Only the mixer and tank are kept in geometric similarity, not the particle size. Changes in particle size will alter the mechanism for settling and therefore the settling velocity. Small particles will settle according to Stokes Law with a laminar wake. Larger particles will settle with either a transitional or turbulent wake. So the exponent for equal suspension is a variable, Corpstein, et al. (1994).

$$N_2 = N_1 \left(\frac{D_1}{D_2} \right)^m \tag{13.14}$$

$$1 > m > 0.5$$

Slowly settling particles are likely to follow the flow of the fluid and may scale-up based on equal velocity, $m = 1$. Rapidly settling particles will require a smaller exponent, approaching power per volume or even equal Froude number in extreme cases. Values for the solids suspension, scale-up exponent are shown in Fig. 13.3, Corpstein, et al. (1994).

The design settling velocity is the terminal settling velocity for the solids times the density difference (Corpstein et al., 1994).

$$u_d = \left(\frac{\rho_p - \rho}{\rho}\right) u_t \tag{13.15}$$

As a rule-of-thumb, for a particle size distribution the settling velocity of the largest 90th-percentile particle can be used for an estimate of the terminal settling velocity in the design settling velocity.

For an equal Froude number, geometric similarity scale-up has an exponent of one half on the scale ratio.

$$N_2 = N_1 \left(\frac{D_1}{D_2}\right)^{1/2} \tag{13.16}$$

Because Froude number relates inertial to gravitational forces, it may represent vortex depth or wave height on the surface of an agitated liquid. For instance, to maintain a vortex depth one quarter of the liquid level from the lab scale to the plant scale would require equal Froude number with geometric similarity. This scale-up is also extremely severe and nearly impossible for large scale changes. The practical result is that ripple height and vortex depth, compared with the tank diameter, are typically less in larger tanks. Liquid that might splash out of a container in the lab may be handled properly in production with

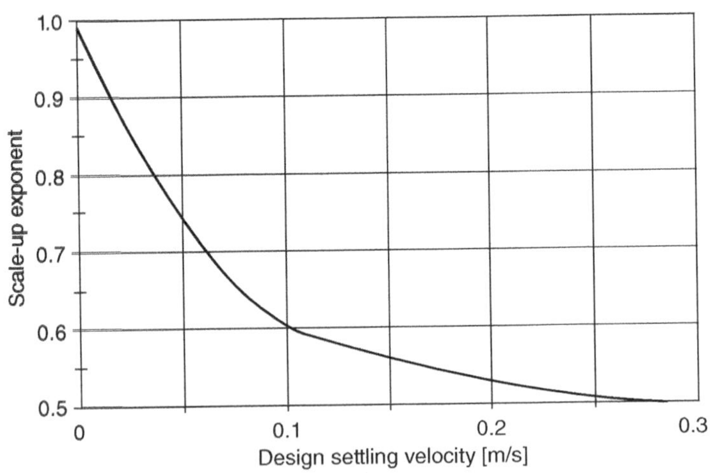

Figure 13.3 *Solids suspension scale-up exponent*

geometric similarity and a scale-up based on equal tip speed or power per volume, both of which result in a lower Froude number.

To hold the blend time constant with geometric similarity, the exponent is zero, so the speed remains constant.

$$N_2 = N_1\left(\frac{D_1}{D_2}\right)^0 = N_1 \tag{13.17}$$

While often interpreted from the constant value of the dimensionless blend time at turbulent conditions, this relationship is also understood from "grandma's" baking as the number of strokes with the spoon required to accomplish a degree of uniformity. A certain number of rotations of the impeller is required for a specific batch geometry to be blended. Whatever the rotational speed in turbulent conditions, or at the same Reynolds number in the transition range. The dimensionless blend time for a pitched-blade turbine is usually written to include the effect of impeller-to-tank diameter ratio and the liquid-level-to-tank-diameter ratio.

$$\mathbf{N}_{\Theta_{99\%}} = \Theta_{99\%}\ N\left(\frac{D}{\mathrm{T}}\right)^{2.3}\left(\frac{H}{T}\right)^{-0.5} \tag{13.18}$$

A correlation for dimensionless blend time as a function of Reynolds number shows how dimensionless blend time becomes essentially constant in the turbulent range and increases in the transition range as shown in Fig. 13.4.

The dimensionless blend time shows that the same number of rotations results in the same degree of uniformity.

Equal blend time is an extremely severe, and usually an impossible scale-up criterion, since for turbulent conditions, power increases with the impeller diameter to the fifth power. A tank with twice the volume contains eight times the liquid, but requires 32 times the power or four times the power per volume for equal blend time. The result of more practical scale-up rules is, as reasonably expected, that the larger tank takes longer to mix than the smaller tank.

Equal Reynolds number would result if the scale-up exponent were set at two.

$$N_2 = N_1\left(\frac{D_1}{D_2}\right)^2 \tag{13.19}$$

While equal Reynolds number seems to result in a similar level of turbulence, it does not provide sufficient fluid motion to assure uniform mixing with any significant scale change. An equal Reynolds number is not a practical scale-up criterion. The practical result from an increasing Reynolds number with scale-up is that the effect of viscosity decreases.

All of the practical scale-up rules for geometric similarity scale-up fall between equal tip speed and equal power per volume. Within that range, the reduction in speed that occurs between the small scale and large scale is largest for tip speed and smallest for power per

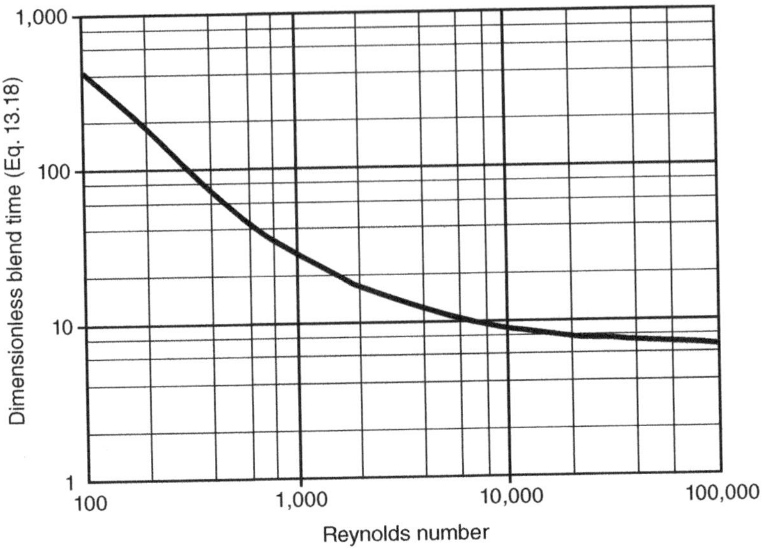

Figure 13.4 *Dimensionless blend time correlation for a pitched-blade turbine*

volume. The larger reduction in rotational speed, by holding tip speed constant, will result in a smaller large scale mixer than the smaller reduction in speed for power per volume. However, an added degree of conservatism for the tip speed scale-up occurs because the Reynolds number increases. An increased Reynolds number would be equivalent to the capability of handling a higher viscosity, in proportion to the scale change. However, this effect is of little consequence for fully turbulent conditions and only significant when the small-scale tests are conducted at conditions in the transition or viscous range. Table 13.1 summarizes and compares the different geometric similarity scale-up rules and the corresponding inverse, scale-ratio exponents. The reasons and results describe briefly some uses and consequences for the different rules.

13.5.2 Example of Geometric Similarity Scale-Up

As shown in Eq. 13.11 for equal power per volume and Eq. 13.13 for equal tip speed, scale-up for geometric similarity requires only an appropriate adjustment in mixer speed, at least for turbulent mixing. The following example will show the differences between tip speed and power per volume as scale-up criteria, and how calculations can be made to understand the effects on mixer performance.

Suppose we have a simple blending problem and have conducted a bench scale test. The bench-scale vessel is a vertical cylinder, with a flat bottom, and four standard baffles. The baffles are vertical plates mounted at the wall of the vessel to prevent uncontrolled swirling of the contents and to help create top-to-bottom motion with a pitched-blade turbine impeller. The bench-scale vessel is 250 mm in diameter with a 250 mm straight side. The bench test was successfully run with a ten-liter batch, approximately 204 mm liquid level, and a single, 85 mm diameter, pitched-blade turbine impeller running at 450 rpm. The pitched-blade turbine

Table 13.1 Scale-exponents

Scale-up method	Exponent on scale ratio	Typical scale-up reason or result
Equal blend time	0	Too intense – not practical
Equal Froude number	1/2	Too intense – not practical
Equal power per volume	2/3	For chemical reactions
Equal solids suspension	1/2 < n < 1	Equal solids suspension
Equal tip speed	1	Equal fluid velocity
Equal torque per volume	1	Equal fluid velocity
Equal Reynolds number	2	Insufficient fluid motion

had four-blades, mounted at a 45° angle, and a blade width one-fifth the diameter of the impeller. The power number for such an impeller is 1.37 (Bates, et al., 1963). The liquid in the batch had a viscosity of 10 cP = 0.01 Pa s and a density of 1100 kg/m^3. A summary of the mixing dimensions and characteristics (described in the section on Observation and Measurement) for the bench-scale test conditions are shown in the labeled column in Table 13.2.

Scale-up with geometric similarity to a 1500 mm diameter production-scale tank, requires the application of a 6:1 factor to all of the linear dimensions. Thus the tank straight side also becomes 1500 mm and the baffle width becomes 120 mm. The impeller diameter goes from 85 mm on the bench scale to 510 mm in production. With all of the plant-scale equipment dimensions defined by geometric similarity, the remaining variable, rotational speed, is selected to maintain some basic characteristic of mixing, such as tip speed or power per volume. For equal tip speed, the bench-scale rotational speed of 450 rpm is multiplied by the inverse length ratio, Eq. 13.13, to obtain a production-scale speed of 75 rpm. The other operating variables, power, power per volume, torque, torque per volume, and tip speed can be calculated in the same way they were for the bench-scale conditions. These values also appear in Table 13.2. Note that for an equal tip speed of 2.01 m/s, the torque per volume of 0.0060 N m/l is also the same for the bench and plant scales. Tip speed and torque per volume are the same with geometric similarity scale-up, but not with non-geometric scale-up.

Practical, but more conservative, scale-up results can be achieved by changing speed to hold power per volume constant, Eq. 13.11. In this case, the inverse scale ratio raised to the two-thirds power is multiplied times the bench-scale speed. Thus, 450 rpm is reduced to 136 rpm, as shown in Table 13.2. With equal power per volume, the torque per volume and tip speed both increase compared with the equal tip speed results, along with the Reynolds number and rotational speed. Although, a significant safety margin was used in suggesting a motor size in Table 13.2, the equal power per volume scale-up would require a larger motor, drive, shaft, and almost every other mixer component, including the price. As a rough guide to mixer cost, torque is closely related to the capital cost of the mixer, while the power is related to the operating cost.

13.5.3 Scale-Up Without Geometric Similarity

Geometric similarity means strict geometric similarity, especially for a critical variable like impeller diameter as represented by the impeller diameter-to-tank diameter ratio. Even small changes in the impeller diameter make large differences in the mixing intensity,

Table 13.2 *Geometric similarity scale-up example*

Dimensions and results	Bench scale test conditions	Tip speed scale-up	Power/volume scale-up
Tank diameter [mm]	250	1500	1500
Scale ratio	1:1	6:1	6:1
Liquid level [mm]	204	1222	1222
Fluid volume [l]	10	2160	2160
Baffle width [mm]	20	120	120
Fluid viscosity [cp]	10	10	10
Fluid density [kg/m^3]	1100	1100	1100
Mixer speed [rpm]	450	75	136
Impeller type	Pitched blade	Pitched blade	Pitched blade
Number of blades on impeller	4	4	4
Blade angle [degrees]	45	45	45
Power number	1.37	1.37	1.37
Impeller diameter [mm]	85	510	510
Impeller-to-tank diameter ratio	0.34	0.34	0.34
Blade width [mm]	17	102	102
Blade width to impeller diam. ratio	0.2	0.2	0.2
Off-bottom [mm]	100	600	600
Reynolds number	5961	35,764	64,987
Power [W]	2.82	102	609
Power/volume [W/l]	0.282	0.047	0.282
Torque [N•m]	0.060	13.0	42.8
Torque/volume [N•m/l]	0.0060	0.0060	0.0198
Tip speed [m/s]	2.01	2.01	3.64
Motor power [W]	200	750	1100

especially when the only compensation is the speed change by the rules for geometric similarity. The lower limit for geometric similarity is often defined by the available impeller sizes. Very small scale tests may require some interpretation of the impeller type, including magnetic stir bars, but with records kept for accurate dimensions and rotational speeds. These limitations do not mean that non-geometric scale-up is impossible, only that different methods and "rules" apply. The "rules" are not exact rules, but rather rules-of-thumb, which can be applied to calculated values for mixing characteristics.

While not essential always, a step-by-step method usually works best for scale-up with non-geometric similarity, Dickey (2004). The method may involve a couple of steps or several steps depending on the changes in mixer geometry. The method begins with a geometric similarity scale-up from the small-scale test vessel to an equivalent vessel with the proper large-scale tank diameter. This step assures a clear understanding of the resulting scale change. After the initial scale change, further changes are usually made in only one variable at a time, such as liquid level, impeller diameter, impeller type, or number of impellers, and so on. However, changing multiple geometry and operational variables may keep a combination of characteristics, such as tip speed and torque constant simultaneously. This one-step at a time method allows a check on the adequacy or appropriateness of each change. To explain and illustrate this step-by-step method an example problem will be used. The solution will involve more steps than absolutely necessary to achieve scale-up, but the steps also will show how either existing or new mixing equipment might be evaluated. Chemical reactions and formulations will not scale-up in the same way. Small scale experimental results should be used to help define the critical variable for the process.

13.5.4 Example of Non-Geometric Scale-Up

Suppose the application is the preparation of a typical water-based, liquid consumer product, such as cough syrup. The base is pure, deionized water, with some high-fructose corn syrup added for sweetness. Additional flavors and colors are added for the desired consumer product characteristics. A combination of active ingredients (APIs), typically powders, must be added and dissolved in the final batch. All of the minor and active ingredients are pre-weighed and added to the blended batch.

The bench-scale vessel is 250 mm in diameter with a 250 mm straight side for the 10-liter batch. The production tank is 2135 mm (84 inches) in diameter with a 2593 mm (102-inch) straight side for the 9465-liter (2500-gal.) batch. The bench-scale mixer has a single, 120-mm diameter pitched-blade turbine impeller. The production tank has a mixer with two 865-mm (34-inch) diameter pitched-blade turbine impellers. Thus, the impeller-to-tank-diameter ratio in the bench-scale vessel is 0.48, while the impeller-to-tank-diameter ratio in the production tank is 0.41. These geometry differences mean that the simple relationships for speed change do not apply for appropriate for scale-up. The process objective will depend on the process and the test results.

13.5.4.1 The First Step

The first step for non-geometric scale-up is with geometric similarity from the bench scale mixing results to the plant-scale tank diameter. This scale-up step will not account for the actual production tank volume, number of impellers, or impeller sizes. Those other adjustments will be made in the following steps, with evaluation of several mixing characteristics for each case. The first column in Table 13.3 shows the bench scale, 250 mm vessel diameter, conditions for the syrup recipe, which has a viscosity of about 15 mPa•s and a density of 1090 kg/m^3. The single pitched-blade turbine in the bench scale requires 4.64 W of power for 0.464 W/l power per volume. That power translates into 0.148 N•m of torque or 0.0148 N•m/l torque per volume, at a tip speed of 1.88 m/s.

Geometric similarity scale-up to a tank diameter of 2135 mm diameter involves a scale factor of 2135 to 250 or 8.54:1. For geometric similarity, the volume is only 6228 liter. The volume will be adjusted in the next step. For equal tip speed, the production scale-speed will be 35.13 rpm with the geometrically similar 1025 mm diameter impeller. The computed mixing characteristics are shown in the second column of Table 13.3.

13.5.4.2 The Second Step

The second step involves increasing the volume in the production-scale tank to the desired 9465 liter. The large-scale tank has a larger height-to-diameter ratio than the bench-scale vessel, which is common for larger tanks. Without changing the impeller diameter or operating speed, the mixing power, torque, and tip speed remain unchanged, but the per-volume

Table 13.3 Non-geometric scale-up example – single impeller steps

Dimensions and results	Bench scale conditions	Geometric scale-up	Increased volume
Tank diameter [mm]	250	2135	2135
Liquid level [mm]	204	1740	2644
Fluid volume [l]	10	6228	9465
Fluid viscosity [cp]	15	15	15
Fluid density [kg/m^3]	1090	1090	1090
Mixer speed [rpm]	300	35.13	35.13
Number of impellers	1	1	1
Impeller type	Pitched blade	Pitched blade	Pitched blade
Power number (each impeller)	1.37	1.37	1.37
Impeller diameter [mm]	120	1025	1025
Impeller-to-tank diameter ratio	0.48	0.48	0.48
Blade width [mm]	24	205	205
Blade width to impeller diam. ratio	0.2	0.2	0.2
Off-Bottom [mm]	120	1025	1025
Reynolds number (either impeller)	5232	44,681	44,681
Total power [W]	4.64	339	339
Total power/volume [W/l]	0.464	0.054	0.036
Total torque [N•m]	0.148	92.1	92.1
Total torque/volume [N•m/l]	0.0148	0.0148	0.0097
Tip speed [m/s]	1.88	1.88	1.88
Motor power [W]	200	1100	1100

quantities are reduced, Table 13.3. If the mixing requirements were related to some dispersion characteristic, then the tip-speed might be the correct characteristic to hold constant. However, if mixing intensity is more important, then equal torque per volume may be appropriate for the volume adjustment.

13.5.4.3 The Third Step

The third step will add a second impeller to the mixer shaft. This step will account for the two impellers in the actual production-scale mixer and compensate for the loss in the per-volume values of the previous step. When the two impellers are identical in size and type, the power and torque are effectively doubled from the single impeller case. However, to handle all cases, including different impellers, each impeller calculation should be done separately and the results added. The results of the dual impeller case are shown in Table 13.4. In this step, the rotational speed has been kept the same for equal tip speed, but all of the power and torque related quantities have doubled from the previous step.

13.5.4.4 The Fourth Step

The fourth step changes from the geometrically similar impeller diameters, at 1025 mm, to the actual production scale impeller diameters, at 865 mm. In this step, the tip speed is again held constant, so the smaller impellers require a higher rotational speed, 41.63 rpm. While equal tip speed is often a reasonable and practical scale-up criteria for geometric similarity, it may be less acceptable for non-geometric similarity. Often the equal tip speed for geometric similarity is effective because the mixing intensity remains constant with equal torque per volume. Thus, for non-geometric scale-up, equal torque per volume may be the better scale-up requirement.

13.5.4.5 A Fifth Step

A fifth step sets the actual dual impeller system in the production-scale tank to equal torque per volume by increasing the rotational speed from 41.63 to 46.78 rpm, see Table 13.4. At this rotational speed, the production-scale mixer is operating at a torque per volume level of 0.0148 N• m/l, the same torque per volume level that achieved successful results in the bench-scale syrup development.

13.5.4.6 A Sixth Step

A sixth step involves a practical consideration about the production-scale mixer. Rarely are mixing processes or mixing equipment so sensitive as to require speed settings like 35.13 rpm, 41.62 rpm, or 46.75 rpm. If a process is so sensitive as to require a highly restrictive rotational speed, a variable speed drive would be needed if the process were to work at all. Commonly, especially in production situations, mixers operate at nominal fixed speeds corresponding to standard gear reductions and motor speeds. Thus, the production-scale mixer in this example might have been operating at a standard speed, such as 56 rpm. The first column in Table 13.3 shows the mixing characteristics for the production mixer operating at 56 rpm. In most mixing applications, the required intensity is some minimum amount, above which a plateau is reached where a little more intensity does not adversely affect the product or production

13.5.4.7 A Seventh Step

A possible seventh step would be to scale-down from the production-scale conditions at the standard speed of 56 rpm to an equivalent torque per volume in the bench-scale vessel. These conditions are represented in the second column of Table 13.5. For equal torque per volume in both the production and bench scales, the bench scale mixer needs to operate at 360 rpm. Operating and applying the bench-scale mixer at these conditions is likely to duplicate many successful or problem characteristics associated with moving a new recipe from the bench to production. Any effort to duplicate production conditions on the bench before going into production, will reduce the number of problems and failures later.

13.5.4.8 Alternate Impeller Design

Another consideration might be the effect of changing to a different type of impeller. For this example, a more efficient hydrofoil design may be considered to replace the pitched-blade turbines in the production-scale tank. For this case, direct replacement of only the impellers means that the rotational speed remains unchanged. However, because of the lower power number for the hydrofoil impellers, $\mathbf{N}_P = 0.27$ compared with $\mathbf{N}_P = 1.37$ for the pitched-blade, the hydrofoil impellers must be larger. Because hydrofoil impellers are better at creating axial flow, only half the torque may be required to duplicate the process results obtained with pitched-blade turbines. For the same formulation application at 56 rpm, half the torque can be

Table 13.4 *Non-geometric scale-up example – dual impeller steps*

Dimensions and results	Dual impeller's actual volume	Actual impeller's equal tip speed	Actual impeller's equal torque/volume
Tank diameter [mm]	2135	2135	2135
Liquid level [mm]	2644	2644	2644
Fluid volume [l]	9465	9465	9465
Fluid viscosity [cp]	15	15	15
Fluid density [kg/m^3]	1090	1090	1090
Mixer speed [rpm]	35.13	41.63	46.78
Number of impellers	2	2	2
Impeller type	Pitched blade	Pitched blade	Pitched blade
Power number (each impeller)	1.37	1.37	1.37
Impeller diameter [mm]	1025	865	865
Impeller-to-tank diameter ratio	0.48	0.41	0.41
Blade width [mm]	205	173	173
Blade width to impeller diam. ratio	0.2	0.2	0.2
Off-bottom – upper impeller [mm]	1930	1930	1930
Off-bottom – lower impeller [mm]	1025	1025	1025
Reynolds number (either impeller)	44,699	37,721	42,393
Total power [W]	678	483	686
Total power/volume [W/l]	0.0716	0.0510	0.0724
Total torque [N•m]	184	111	140
Total torque/volume [N•m/l]	0.0195	0.0117	0.0148
Tip speed [m/s]	1.89	1.89	2.12
Motor power [W]	1,100	1,100	2,250

applied in the production tank with 1042 mm diameter hydrofoil impellers. These impellers have a 0.49 impeller-to-tank diameter ratio, which is still practical for this application.

If a change in impeller type is a serious consideration for production equipment, then the small-scale batch mixer should also be changed and tested. A direct comparison between results obtained with two different impeller types may also aid in deciding which variable must be held constant for scale-up. The systematic and step-by-step analysis of a scale-up or any mixing modification is helped by the constant evaluation of changes in mixing variables like torque per volume, tip speed, even power per volume and Reynolds number, tracking these mixing characteristics may offer insight into the mixer performance. The selection of the scale-up criteria will depend on the desired results for the process.

The preceding step-by-step method for non-geometric scale-up can be used for scale-up to a known equipment design, for the design of new mixing equipment, or for evaluation of alternate mixer modifications. The evaluation of equipment changes should be based on some degree of experience, ideally gained from some development testing or scale-up of similar applications.

13.5.5 Scale-Up for Powder Mixing

Scale-up for dry powder mixing is much more art than the perceived science of liquid mixing. By the very nature of powders, they do not have the consistent properties of an incompressible fluid, as for liquid mixing. Of major importance in the scale-up of powder mixing is the

Table 13.5 *Non-geometric scale-up example – alternate impeller design*

Dimensions and results	Actual impeller's nominal speed	Bench-scale equal torque nominal speed	Hydrofoil impeller's half torque/volume
Tank diameter [mm]	2135	250	2135
Liquid level [mm]	2644	204	2644
Fluid volume [l]	9465	10	9465
Fluid viscosity [cp]	15	15	15
Fluid density [kg/m^3]	1090	1090	1090
Mixer speed [rpm]	56	360	56
Number of impellers	2	1	2
Impeller type	Pitched blade	Pitched blade	Hydrofoil
Power number (each impeller)	1.37	1.37	0.27
Impeller diameter [mm]	865	120	1,042
Impeller-to-tank diameter ratio	0.41	0.48	0.49
Blade width [mm]	173	24	156
Blade width to impeller diam. ratio	0.2	0.2	0.15
Off-bottom – upper impeller [mm]	1930		1930
Off-bottom – lower impeller [mm]	1025	120	1025
Reynolds number (either impeller)	50,746	6278	73,639
Total power [W]	1176	8.03	588
Total Power/Volume [W/liter]	0.124	0.803	0.0621
Total Torque [N•m]	201	0.213	100
Total Torque/Volume [N•m/liter]	0.0212	0.0213	0.0106
Tip Speed [m/s]	2.54	2.26	3.06
Motor Power [W]	2250	200	1100

simple fact that powders can be compressed and that as a result, the flow characteristics can change drastically. With scale-up in powder systems, as the powder depth increases, the forces exerted on the powder at the bottom increase, often to the point of changing the bulk density and flow characteristics of the compacted powder. Recognizing this problem with powder mixing scale-up is often the first step in understanding potential problems.

While scale-up of powder mixing is more difficult and less consistent than scale-up of liquid mixing some same basic rules still apply. The first rule is geometry. Scale-up is usually best done when the same type of small-scale mixer as the large-scale mixer. Details of geometry are less critical in powder mixing because of changes in the powder characteristics with scale. Where the impeller-to-tank diameter ratio is very important in liquid mixing, the clearance between the ribbon and shell of a ribbon blender is not as critical in powder mixing. At the same time, the gap between the ribbon and the shell can have different effects on powder mixing scale-up depending on how much of the powder blend sticks to the sides of the blender shell. Sometimes a minor ingredient, such as an active pharmaceutical ingredient (API), becomes trapped in the layer of powder on a mixer surface. Again, the characteristics of the powder can make all the difference in the success or failure of a mixing scale-up.

With respect to powder mixing geometry, tumble blender applications should be tested and developed in small-scale tumble blenders. Ribbon blender applications should be developed in small ribbon blenders and so on. Sometimes testing in a small-scale ribbon blender might be applied to a large-scale paddle blender, since the paddle blender is less susceptible to some compaction problems encountered in large ribbon blenders. Because of the many different types of powder, blender scale-up is best done from a similar mixer with the actual powder. For new mixing equipment, most manufactures offer laboratory testing or a rental mixer for development before purchasing a mixer.

Rotational speed is the second major issue with the scale-up of powder mixing equipment. Again, one fundamental of mixing still holds most often and should always be a guide for scale-up of powder blending. The degree of uniformity of a blend depends more strongly on the number of revolutions made by the blender than the speed of the revolutions. As is typical with all large-scale mixing equipment, and for several practical reasons, the speed of revolution decreases. Thus, if it takes three minutes to blend a batch in a small-scale mixer and the large-scale mixer turns at 60% (3/5) of the small-scale speed, then the expected blend time for the large-scale mixer would be five thirds (5/3) of 3 min or 5 min.

Perhaps the most difficult judgment to make with powder blending scale-up is how critical rotational speed really is. Most powder blending equipment runs at a constant speed, most often set by the equipment manufacturer and characteristic of standard size mixers. The most common and practical scale-up rotational speed is likely to achieve an equal peripheral velocity for the rotating element of the mixer, whether it is a tumble blender or a ribbon blender. This effect is the same as the equal tip-speed scale-up, Eq. 13.18, for liquid blending. However, practical considerations, such as available gear reductions or standard chain drives may cause several different size mixers to run at the same speed, even from the same manufacturer

Special purpose equipment, such as bowl granulators or fluidized-bed granulators are designed along some basic principles that rely heavily on similar characteristics for the excipients. Many pharmaceutical products use the same or similar excipients, each with known handling characteristics. The addition of the minor quantities of active pharmaceutical ingredients (APIs) may not affect the bulk handling and processing characteristics. Similarly, the addition of liquid binders may behave similarly. The net result is that equipment design and process conditions are based more on empirical design methods than scale-up methods. With high-speed bowl granulators the tip speed and time for blending are carefully observed and controlled for consistent results.

Just as with liquid mixing scale-up, testing and development should concentrate on the important issues with a specific product or application. Considerations such as order of addition of ingredients can be important, especially if one ingredient is a fragile crystal or agglomerate. In which case, the fragile ingredient might be added late in the process to avoid excessive mixing and damage to the ingredient. In other cases, the addition rate of a liquid might be critical in an application where rapid addition may cause excessive wetting of parts of the batch and uneven moisture in the final product. Powder agglomeration is often accomplished by the addition of a liquid. Other practical considerations may be involved in scale-up, such as loading procedures. In the small-scale, a scoop may be used to load the mixer. In the large-scale, the same ingredient may be added in 100 lb. bags or even tote sack quantities. Rate, order, and location of addition need to be considered during development to be sure that a scale-up will work in large-scale production.

While peripheral velocity may work well for general scale-up of many mixer types, other criteria may apply where process conditions need to be duplicated. If a paddle blender or ploughshare blender is expected to lift and fluidize the powder, then equal Froude number, Eq. 13.12, or rotational speed squared times impeller diameter may be held constant for an appropriate scale-up criterion. This criterion causes the peripheral speed of the rotating equipment to increase more than equal peripheral velocity. As with liquid mixing, equal speed is rarely practical for significant changes in mixer size.

Because of the uncertainty in the response of different powders, the rules and methods for powder blending scale-up are less well-organized than for liquids. The effects of geometry differences are less significant in powder blending as all size differences can have adverse or positive effects. Often both with liquids and powders, avoiding failures should be the most important consideration. When a failure occurs in the small scale, note should be taken of the conditions and the evident mode of failure to avoid similar or related problems in the large scale. The failure mode is often represented by some minimum level of mixing necessary to achieve satisfactory mixing. Only in the extreme is greater mixing intensity a problem for most applications: Although many mixers provide more intense or longer blending than is needed for effective results.

All scale-up begins with the deciding of which test condition and what scale are most likely to produce useable results. Observing the effects of mixing intensity and procedures is an integral part of developing scale-up rules or limits. Only by careful observation can common problems be avoided and successful scale-up achieved.

13.6 Summary

Scale-up is more than just applying a "rule" to a satisfactory small-scale result. The more general the "rule," such as power per volume, the more care should be considered when applying it. Most of the common scale-up "rules" were developed and tested with geometrically similar conditions. The change of a simple geometric characteristic, such as the liquid-level-to-tank-diameter ratio, can invalidate a scale-up "rule," such as equal tip speed. Test result should investigate both the mechanisms of mixing and the limits of success. Some test results may be indicative of a mechanism for the mixing result. Scale-up begins with testing and that testing should be conducted to find the limits, minimum and maximum, for mixing intensity. Successful scale-up is often just a matter of avoiding failure conditions.

Nomenclature

- B baffle width
- C impeller off-bottom clearance
- D impeller diameter
- g acceleration of gravity
- H liquid level
- L length dimension

m number of dimensions
m exponent on solids suspension scale-up
$\boldsymbol{M}$ mass dimension
n number of variables
n exponent on geometric similarity scale-up
N rotational speed
$\mathbf{N}_{\mathrm{Fr}}$ Froude number
$\mathbf{N}_{\mathrm{P}}$ impeller power number
$\mathbf{N}_{\mathrm{Re}}$ Reynolds number
$\mathbf{N}_{\Theta}$ dimensionless blend time
T tank diameter
t time dimension
u_d design settling velocity
u_t terminal settling velocity
v_t impeller tip speed (note to editor - character is the italic letter vee, not Greek nu)
W blade width

Greek

Θ blend time
μ fluid viscosity (dynamic)
π pi
ρ fluid density
ρ_p particle density

References

Bates, R.L., Fondy, P.L., and Corpstein, R.R. (1963) An examination of some geometric parameters of impeller power, *I&EC Process Design and Development*, **2**, 4, 310–314.
Corpstein, R.R., Fasano, J.B., and Myers, K.J. (1994), The High-Efficiency Road to Liquid-Solid Agitation, *Chem. Eng.*, October, 138–116.
Dickey, D. S. (2004), Liquid agitation, in *Handbook of Chemical Engineering Calculations*, 3rd edn, Chapter 12. Chopey, N.P. (ed.), McGraw-Hill, New York.
Ndonga, M. and Tatterson, G. (2006), Characterization of mixing in flat-bottomed spherical flasks agitated with magnetic stirrers, *Chem. Eng. Comm.*, **193**,114–1421.

14

Equipment Qualification, Process and Cleaning Validation

Ian Jones[1] *and Chris Smalley*[2]
[1]*Innopharmalabs, Ireland*
[2]*Merck Sharp and Dohme, USA*

14.1 Introduction

The purpose of equipment commissioning, qualification, process validation and cleaning validation is to demonstrate operational control and integrity of dosage preparation, thereby assuring the health of the patient. Various approaches to demonstrating this control can be applied over the life of pharmaceutical manufacture. The goal of this chapter is to give the reader an appreciation for where the qualification and validation processes have originated from and where they will position themselves over the coming years. There is no standard approach to equipment commissioning, qualification, process validation or cleaning validation within the pharmaceutical industry. Consequently the approaches defined within this chapter are sometimes subjective and personal.

The chapter is divided into three sections – equipment qualification, blending process validation and cleaning validation. A common theme running through the chapter is the future vision for qualification and process validation activities. This theme is the application of Quality Risk Management tools to redesign our approach to validation. Quality Risk Management is an approach that has existed in other industries such as the nuclear, aeronautical and space industries for decades. Several recent guidance documents have been developed to facilitate the implementation of Quality Risk Management in the

Pharmaceutical Blending and Mixing, First Edition. Edited by P.J. Cullen, Rodolfo J. Romañach, Nicolas Abatzoglou and Chris D. Rielly.

pharmaceutical industry. In 2003 the International Conference for Harmonization formed an expert working group to develop guidelines on quality risk management. Its goal was to develop a harmonized pharmaceutical quality system applicable across the lifecycle of the product emphasizing an integrated approach to quality risk management and science. In 2005 their guidance documents ICH Q8 on Pharmaceutical Development and Q9 on Quality Risk Management were published. In 2008 the FDA published their guidance documents 'Pharmaceutical cGMPs for the 21st Century – A Risk Based Approach' (FDA, 2008). These documents have formed the backbone of numerous other direction documents on pharmaceutical quality systems, for example GAMP 5 and ISPE baseline guide on commissioning and qualification.

14.2 Blending Equipment Commissioning and Qualification

Equipment commissioning and qualification are essential to confirm that the equipment is working correctly and within the expectations pre-defined by the equipment user.

Figure 14.1 will be familiar to those involved in equipment commissioning and qualification over the past 15 years. This flowchart defines the lifecycle of commissioning and qualification from user requirement specification – where the customer defines their requirements, through to validation maintenance – continually confirming that the equipment and process are still operating in a state of control. This process was sequential and involved the duplication of many tests due to the qualification of the personnel or controls present at various stages. This traditional approach to validation projects had been focussed towards the V-model approach (an iterative approach) so that system performance qualification can easily be matched up one for one. This approach can often become very detailed and cover a wide range of requirements well beyond those necessary to assure product quality and patient safety. In many cases this duplication was not 'value adding' and only led to complacency by those executing the tests because they knew that the tests would be repeated again later in the qualification process. ASTM E2500 is a Standard Guide for Specification, Design and Verification of Pharmaceutical and Biopharmaceutical Manufacturing Systems and Equipment. ASTM E2500 focuses on what one could call process requirements, those that are relevant to product and process safety, and which are based on scientific understanding of the product and processes. This is consistent with ICH guidelines where an alternative 'Verification Approach' was generated. This is the process that will drive equipment commissioning and qualification over the coming years.

14.2.1 Outline of the Verification Approach

The verification approach is outlined in Figure 14.2. It consists of a core model of a four step lifecycle: requirements, specification and design, verification, acceptance and release. These four steps are followed by operation and continuous improvement. Four supporting activities utilized in the process are Good Engineering Practice, Risk Management, Design Review, and Change Management.

The ASTM E2500 guide describes a science and risk-based approach to the specification, design and verification of manufacturing systems and equipment that have the potential to affect product quality and patient safety.

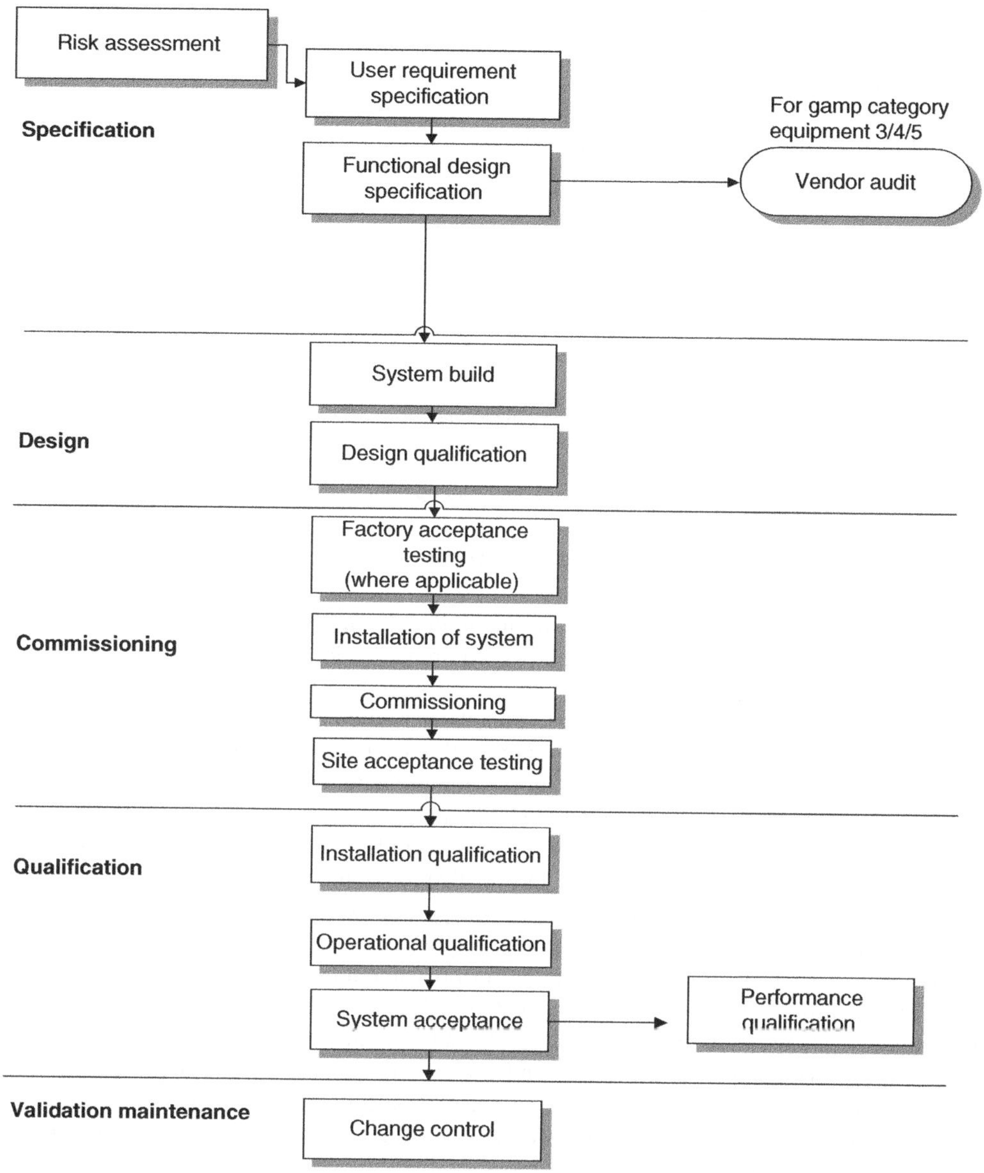

Figure 14.1 *Historical approach to Equipment Commissioning and Qualification*

14.2.2 Requirements Phase

The verification process proposed begins with identification of the requirements. Before the design of a system may commence, product and process requirements are shared with the designers. The requirements document contains the user requirements and lists the attributes that are critical to the functionality of the process. The design will determine how to meet that functionality. Two separate requirement documents may be created,

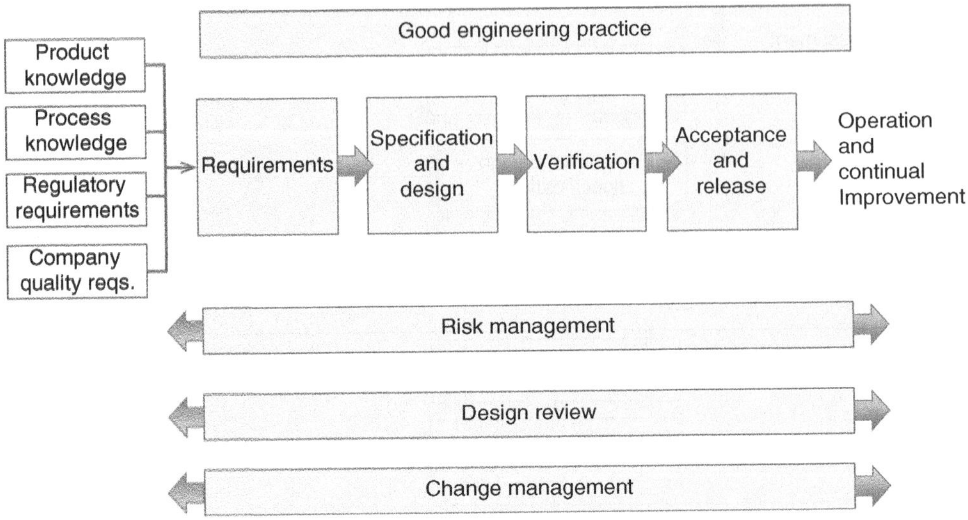

Figure 14.2 *The Specification, Design, and Verification Process, from ASTM E2500-07*

a Product/Process & Regulatory Requirement document that feeds directly into the Verification Quality Strategy, and a business requirements document, depending upon the complexity of the equipment/system.

A Project Verification plan is created to plan the activities. The Requirements document forms the fundamental basis for all subsequent activities. By focusing on the product attributes, the risk to the patient and regulatory requirements this approach provides clear direction in the subsequent activities and results in an efficient and effective verification. ASTM E2500 states that 'Specific requirements should be identified and should provide the basis of further specification, design and verification of the manufacturing system.' And that 'Specific requirements should be based on product knowledge, process knowledge, regulatory requirements and company quality requirements'. The Requirements document focuses on what is needed, without being prescriptive about how the requirements are to be met. The Requirements documents focus on Critical Aspects of the manufacturing systems that are related to product quality, patient safety and regulatory compliance. Critical aspects are identified based on sound product and process understanding and are documented. These requirements will then provide the basis for the specification, design and verification of manufacturing systems. The Product/Process & Regulatory Requirement document is approved by the quality authority.

All individual requirements should be uniquely numbered, indicating a sequential requirement statement number. Requirement statements should be verifiable and should meet the following criteria:

- Be stated in such a way that it can be verified by inspection, analysis, or demonstration.
- They should be clear and concise making it possible to evaluate whether the design meets the requirement.

The quality by design road map for equipment is to define desired performance attributes CQAs (Critical to Quality Attributes) upfront. Design the equipment to meet these CQAs, understand the impact CPPs (Critical Process Parameters) have on the CQAs, identify and control critical attributes, continually monitor and update the process in a controlled manner to assure consistent quality.

14.2.3 Specifications and Design Review Phase

The design review stage of the verification process begins when the preliminary requirements document is created. The verification approach uses Quality by Design (QbD) concepts and these are applied to ensure that critical aspects are designed into systems during the specification and design process. ASTM E2500 describes design reviews as the 'planned and systematic reviews of specifications, design, design development and continuous improvement changes performed as appropriate throughout the life-cycle of the manufacturing system. Design reviews evaluate deliverables against standards and requirements, identify problems, and propose required corrective actions'.

The design review activities follow the progress of the project and the project's main deliverables are reviewed by a team of identified SMEs including members from the quality unit. There is a special focus on where risk can be mitigated and this forms the focus point for the risk management. The design review meetings are cross-functional and cross-disciplinary to ensure that all critical aspects are addressed. The meetings focus on the technical solutions as well as on the risk aspect and thus every design review contains a risk assessment update.

The Design Review process should be an ongoing activity through the design phases, and appropriate in relation to the projects complexity, history, and especially risk to the patient. The aim is to reduce or eliminate risk to CQAs and CPPs by design, control or monitoring.

Design reviews are employed to assure that product and process requirements are satisfied by the design. The design review ensures that all critical manufacturing system aspects are appropriately addressed. Risks to product quality and patient safety are identified; and unacceptable risks are mitigated by design or by other means. Certain factors such as the quality risk, size of the project, knowledge of technologies to be used and so on, affect the review process and stages that may need to be adjusted. In small projects with few and small changes, the Design Review can be implicit during the approval of the Change Request and the updated design documents by the involved stakeholders.

The conceptual design is used, where necessary to generate various alternatives for evaluation in response to the demands of the User Requirements Specifications for individual systems. Suitable time and resources should be committed to the development, documentation and communication of those user requirements. This will ensure greater understanding of the project goals and definition.

During design review, the process steps and operating parameters are studied. The sources of variability that each unit operation is likely to encounter are identified. The possible range of variability for each input into the operation is considered. The process steps and operating parameters for potential criticality are evaluated. A mechanism to limit or control variability based on experimental data is established. It is important to understand the sources of variation, detect the presence and measure degree of possible variation, understand its impact on the process and ultimately product attributes and manage it in a manner commensurate with the risk it represents to the process and product. The mechanisms for managing variability is part of the control strategy and this might include employing advanced manufacturing technologies to detect, analyse and control feedback loops to react to input variability. Wherever feasible, the Design Review should evaluate implementation of Process Analytical Technology (PAT) to detect, analyse the data, and optimally provide automated process adjustments for those sources of variation that have been identified as critical to the process (FDA, 2004).

In the case of new equipment the design review documents may be used as the basis for assessment. These assessments can be used to assist in establishing preventative and predictive maintenance requirements, and should be periodically reviewed against results obtained and the manufacturer's recommendations.

The Verification approach is driven by Risk Management during the design review and relies on supporting activities including GEP, Engineering Change Management and Good Documentation Practices. The broad involvement of Subject Matter Experts (SMEs) facilitates a lean approach with application of technical design documents that are necessary from an engineering and construction perspective. With the focus on risk mitigation and risk management combined with technical expertise from the SMEs, the Verification approach ensures that quality is built in, controlled and documented without having overly extensive documentation requirements.

The issued for comments draft ISPE baseline guide states that 'Specification and design activities should focus on those aspects that have been identified as being critical to product quality and patient safety. These critical aspects of the manufacturing system should be identified and documented by Subject Matter Experts'.

It is during the design phase of the system lifecycle that defined business needs and system requirements are analysed and specific engineering solutions are developed in response to those requirements. Good Engineering Practices should be applied to ensure the approved design specification and conditions are appropriately managed, controlled and executed.

Each phase of design completes a different layer of design information and level of detail extending from facility level architecture to detailed specification of components within the system.

The draft issued for comments ISPE draft baseline guide states that 'Strategic planning for verification testing, project delivery processes, and system owner maintenance program concepts should be initiated early in the conceptual design process'.

An engineering change management program should be in practice following schematic design to effectively manage significant changes in scope, budget, schedule or design intent.

Detailed design, component level design specifications & engineering drawings are developed and approved during detail design, providing the basis for equipment purchase and defining requirements for fabrications and installation.

Approved design specifications provide the technical basis for issuance of purchase orders for equipment and instrument components. Suppliers and Fabricators supporting process-critical systems or other systems that represent a risk to the project should be audited or evaluated prior to purchase agreements being finalized.

When equipment is installed on site a design review should be conducted to confirm that systems & equipment are properly installed and that engineering drawings correctly reflect the 'as built' configuration of the system and system boundaries.

A risk based data and documentation requirements definition process should be conducted to streamline the information deliverables while supporting minimum information needs.

The project team should have a formal system for reviewing the design at different stages, against objectives to ensure that adequate quality is delivered at optimum cost.

All Design Review meetings should be documented. Documentation should include what was reviewed, design discrepancies, action items, their resolution and inclusion of any other explanatory comments. When the Design Review process is finalized, the results of the Design Review must be summarized. For large projects it should be in a Design Review Summary Report.

If the design review process provides suggestions for design corrections, the final statement must state that the proposed corrections are implemented and include documents, drawings and so on, affected by the changes, revisions or assessments required and how they will be managed.

The design review if conducted properly and documented, provides verification that the critical product quality attributes as identified during the risk assessment, have been adequately represented by the intent of the design documentation. By continually reviewing the design in order to assess the risks, the project team can mitigate the probability of failures during execution.

14.2.4 Verification Phase

14.2.4.1 Verification Quality Strategy

The Verification Quality Strategy (VQS) provides a single-source document that identifies the Critical Aspects of a system necessary for a product/manufacturing process related directly to Quality and Patient Safety and the intended design solution and/or method of control of the Critical Aspects (as an output of the Design Review). The Verification Quality Strategy is used to document the intended verification testing (including directly or by reference to the testing methods or document location where the testing was conducted), which will require Quality review and approval. This would provide a means of traceability of these test methods back to the requirements. The Verification Quality Strategy is the main lifecycle document, it is approved at the finalization of the design before any verification testing takes place and is updated again at the end of testing. The VQS identifies and documents the Critical Aspects based on product and process information (C/KPPs, CQAs, cGMP, regulatory requirements) and acceptance criteria relating to the product(s) and/or process(es) within the project scope.

The Verification Quality Strategy is consistent with the principles of Risk Management as outlined in ICHQ9 (ICH, 2009). The majority of verification activities are typically addressed by Good Engineering Practice (GEP) and this testing does not require Quality review and approval. The scope of this document is to summarize the risks assessed outputs from the Requirements Definition, Design Basis and Design Review activities to focus the verification on Critical Aspects.

The Verification Quality Strategy is a part of the overall risk management activity and is intended to document the verification activities for critical aspects that must be reviewed and approved by the relevant Quality Authority. The development of the VQS is started early in the project, it links the requirements to associated system elements via critical aspects. It focuses QA attention and effort, it provides the basis for asset criticality post project, it defines the critical aspects test strategy and acceptance criteria, it gains agreement among all key parties on items critical to product quality.

The output of the VQS feeds into the Project Verification Plan defining critical aspects verification test strategy and acceptance criteria.

It is important that the VQS is done top-down from the product and process understanding, not bottom-up from the manufacturing system equipment or functions side. This should be ensured by following the top down approach linking down from Critical Quality Attributes to Key/Critical Process Parameters and then to Critical Aspects of the manufacturing system.

Early in the project the Verification engineer reviews the need for any quality risk assessments with the project Quality Authority. The risk assessment(s) would be identified in the Project Verification plan and would be included within/as part of the Verification Quality Strategy documentation.

Besides the Critical Quality Attributes and Process Parameters, there may be some critical GMP controls associated with the manufacturing processes that should also be identified and approved by the Quality Authority and demonstrated as part of the overall Quality system in the VQS.

These GMP controls are typically incorporated into site Quality Systems and can include but are not limited to: Calibration, Preventative Maintenance, Sterilization/Sanitization, Change Control among others. These GMP controls are considered during system design and should be incorporated into the design, turn over packages, ongoing maintenance, and general operation. Typically the Quality Authority will want to ensure that they are in place before the final turn-over of the manufacturing system after completed Verification.

14.2.4.2 Verification Planning

The core planning document for verification execution is the Project Verification Plan (PVP). The PVP defines the verification approach to be utilized for the project, describing responsibilities for verification testing (for example system vendors, contractors/consultants, etc.). The Project Verification Plan defines the scope of work, what will be done, who will do it, how it is done, when it is done and will define how the process is documented and reported.

14.2.4.3 Verification Testing

Verification testing refers to a planned and documented method for performing test activities that demonstrate fitness for use of manufacturing equipment, systems and facilities, prior to the handover of the manufacturing systems for Process Validation. Verification includes all the relevant engineering activities traditionally associated with static/dynamic testing and integrated functional testing. Verification testing is based on Good Engineering Practice (GEP) to ensure that the identified requirements are met including any quality, regulatory, environmental, health, and safety or business requirements. ASTM E2500 states that 'The extent of verification and the level of detail of documentation should be based on risk, including those associated with product quality and patient safety, and the complexity and novelty of the manufacturing system'.

Upon completion of the design and design review process, verification testing requirements can be determined and are defined in the project specific Verification Quality Strategy and the finalized Project Verification Plan, which are completed prior to the start of testing. The level of verification testing and related documentation should be commensurate with the criticality level of the aspects identified.

The Verification Test Plans are developed by Engineering with involvement of the appropriate SMEs. The ASTM guide delegates quality control of installation and operational verification to appropriate SMEs (personnel with appropriate education, training and experience).

Verification testing demonstrates that all identified critical and non-critical requirements for a manufacturing system are met. Critical Aspects and the associated acceptance criteria are identified in the Verification Quality Strategy and addressed during the design review process. Non-critical aspects will typically be verified but may consist more of a recording of the 'as found' field conditions.

The verification approach sees the traditional activities undertaken during the qualification phase, which are deemed necessary through the risk assessment process, executed within the verification process using Good Engineering Practices and engineering change management.

Verification testing must, at a minimum, demonstrate that the equipment/systems are installed and functioning correctly. Testing verifies that the system adequately controls Critical Aspects (CAs) to ensure consistent product quality. Verification testing also ensures that all other identified regulatory, environmental, health, safety or business requirements are met. The verification testing identifies activities to be performed to verify the proper system installation, start-up, and functional testing. It defines the inspection or test methods, and data collection requirements. It may include acceptance criteria, recorded results, and observations. The principle of verification strategy is that comprehensive testing is performed and documented only once in the qualification lifecycle.

By focusing on the risk to the patient and leveraging the expertise of the supplier and subject matter experts based on Good Engineering Practices, verification is considered as a set of integrated activities that can replace the activities previously known as commissioning, IQ and OQ. Regulated company commissioning, IQ and OQ activities may then be omitted or limited to an assessment of the suppliers activities and documentation, and if necessary performing mitigation activities to close gaps. This eliminates much of the costly duplicated testing that does little or nothing to protect the patient.

The procedural steps of inspection or testing should be described and documented in a manner that a person technically familiar with the system could execute them. Verification testing includes all type of testing; static, dynamic and integrated/functional testing. For large projects a Verification Test per manufacturing system would be expected. The breakdown of the tests would be established based on the project design and procurement approach. The test document would include all relevant testing associated with that equipment/system to provide assurance that the system operates as per design specifications. The extent of verification and the level of detail of documentation should be based on risk, including those associated with product quality and patient safety, and the complexity and novelty of the manufacturing system. The approach for leveraging vendor documentation is defined in the project verification plan and suitable vendor testing is leveraged and not repeated during Verification Testing. Leveraging of Critical Aspect testing from vendors is dependent on confidence in the vendor based on an audit or vendor assessment. Vendor testing for Critical Aspects that will be leveraged requires Quality Authority pre-approved acceptance criteria. For critical tests an independent SME review of completed test activities is required.

Commissioning testing as well as other forms of engineering testing including FAT, SAT and pre-functional testing fall under the umbrella of verification testing. The issued for comments ISPE draft baseline guide defines commissioning as 'a well defined, documented and managed engineering approach to the start up and turnover of facilities, systems and equipment to the end user that meets established design requirements and stakeholder expectations'. Verification testing confirms that the equipment and manufacturing system is installed as per the project specifications and engineering design criteria. Where possible, the expectation is that the Contractor(s) installing the system would provide the test documentation completed at the end of the construction phase and would be included in the hand-over from Construction. Typical Verification documentation includes: Construction Mechanical/Electrical Completion Hand-over with punch list of any pending items, Material of Construction (MOC) certifications and verification (as needed), Instrument/ Electrical Wiring checks, Pump alignment/rotation check Regulation, Adjustment and Setting to Work (Parameter setting), and Automation system hardware installation testing.

The issued for comments ISPE draft Baseline guide volume 12 provides guidance to produce lifecycle evidence, which verifies that the as-installed implementation of the design meets the process requirements and the control of risk to the patient is documented. By focusing on risk resources are prioritized to focus on issues critical to quality.

A Project or Engineering Change Management System (ECM) must be in place for the project during Verification testing. It is important that the ECM system ensures that changes are evaluated for possible impact on Verification tests already performed, and that any of the corrective actions deemed necessary are taken. Any proposed changes affecting Critical Aspects of manufacturing systems must obtain prior Quality review and approval. Changes affecting critical environmental, health, safety or business aspects must be communicated to the appropriate SMEs.

Project change management should be applied to all engineering changes to follow established good engineering practices. Recognizing the difference between process performance requirements and engineering solutions, and the frequent need to adjust and adapt or change those engineering solutions as knowledge is gained from process pilot studies, equipment start up and initial operations changes may occur during installation and operational verification. Changes to design (once it has been approved), installation, or operation should be planned, documented and approved by SMEs following the risk based approach. If the change is to a document approved by the quality unit this change needs to be approved by the quality unit up front. If a critical element cannot meet the pre-established acceptance criteria, the quality unit should be notified, the impact assessed and appropriate corrective actions or alternative approved. If a change affects a system that contained or contains product intended for distribution this change needs to be approved before implementation of the change.

Further Verification testing verifies that the equipment or system operates and performs as per its intended purpose and specifications. The establishment of a consistent calibration program does more than prescribe what is to be done to produce a quality product the right way every time. A calibration program satisfies regulatory requirements, reduces quality costs through early detection of non-conforming products and processes with the use of measuring equipment of known accuracy. Measuring equipment should be calibrated as often as necessary to maintain accuracies necessary to meet product and process tolerances.

For certain systems user requirements may dictate verification testing to verify that the system performs according to process/product requirements, while integrated with associated systems in the final production and/or validation test environment. Examples of this testing include, engineering batch runs, wet runs, recipe testing, Purified Water sampling, and so on. The Project Verification Plan will identify if any performance testing will be included in Verification testing and is summarized in the SARR.

The Verification Quality Strategy and Design Review define the identification and risk control of Critical Aspects, in addition to the test strategy. Verification testing of critical aspects is included in the test plan and requires the appropriate level of detail in the writing of the test, appropriate SME involvement in the approval of the test plan, test execution and review of test results.

In the case where acceptance criteria of Critical Aspects are not met there should be a clear path forward of how to handle this discrepancy, with Quality Authority involvement. During the verification phase, inspections should be conducted both at the vendors factory (FAT), where applicable, and after installation on-site. Integrated testing is typically performed after mechanical completion including controls and include integrated testing of the system (i.e. with the automation (controls) or combined with other equipment/systems such as a packaging line), along with any additional tests still required for verification of the identified Critical Aspects.

The most cost and time effective method is to incorporate the verification test activities in the vendor's FAT/SAT directly. This requires extended cooperation with the vendors to ensure the Critical Aspects are incorporated into the vendor test documentation. The Verification test document and test activities for Critical Aspects should be approved by the appropriate SMEs prior to test execution.

For all verification, the procedural steps and test results should be documented in a manner permitting objective pass/fail decisions to be reached. The degree to which these are documented should be based on the criticality of the aspect being tested. All documentation methods may be utilized as long as the methodology is defined and provides unambiguous results that the acceptance criteria, as agreed upon in the Design Review, have been met.

All verification testing requires good documentation practices including identification of the tester and recording of the date the test was conducted. Testing of non-critical aspects does not always need to include verification against established acceptance criteria but may rather be a recording of as-found conditions. Examples could include check sheets, drawing walk downs, vendor certification, materials of construction, and so on. Testing of Critical and non-critical Aspects can rely solely on vendor verification and documentation provided that a satisfactory vendor assessment has been performed. Confirmation that the manufacturing system is fit for intended use is documented in the System Acceptance and Release Report that includes a review or overview of the results, along with a review of any non-conformances with stated acceptance criteria of Critical Aspects.

A formal lessons-learned process should be in place for evaluating the project for different stages and agree on what went well and what did not go well. The report from lessons learned would be available for future reference and continuous improvement purposes.

Suitable qualified and independent subject matter expert(s) who did not perform the verification should review all completed inspection or test documentation. The review authority should have appropriate responsibility for the delivery or verification of conformance to specifications.

Process understanding (especially for new processes) is never perfect, and the initial engineering design specifications and drawing for increasingly sophisticated equipment and control systems are also never perfect, the provision for learning and adjustment should be included and expected during installation through facility start-up. Items that cannot be readily corrected or that might impact other inspections or tests, should be handled using the discrepancy/punch list or change management procedures as appropriate.

14.2.4.4 Site Acceptance and Release Report

A Site Acceptance Release Report (SARR) is written to provide documented Subject Matter Expert (SME) confirmation that the manufacturing system is fit for its intended use. SARRs should include a review or overview of the verification results, and a review of any non-conformances. The SARR should also identify the Final Design Review Summary Report (DRSR) and Final Verification Quality Strategy (VQS) documents and reference their storage locations. The Turn Over Package (TOP), if utilized, should also be identified and its storage location referenced. SARRs should contain a clear statement as to whether or not the manufacturing system is fit for its intended use. Such documentation should be prepared and approved by Subject Matter Experts. Such documentation for systems with Critical Aspects should be approved by the Quality Authority.

A successful verification proves the identified residual risks to be in control, thus the system being acceptable and fit for use.

The completed tests should be referenced and document IDs provided.

The ASTM E2500 guide states that 'All completed verification documentation should be reviewed by suitable qualified and independent subject matter expert(s), who did not execute the verification test.'

Non-conformances from verification plans should be addressed and resolved by the reviewer and other appropriate Subject Matter Experts as part of verification testing. A review of non-conformances with stated acceptance criteria of Critical Aspects (CAs) must be included in the SARR. The Test Plan Non-Conformance Log and Test Plan Non-Conformance Form(s) may be attached or summarized.

Once the System Acceptance and Release Report (SARR) is completed and approved, 'Change Control' via the Quality Authority change control procedure takes over from the project or engineering change management process that was in effect through the Verification Testing. In this regard, physical system and control/software changes that could affect Critical Aspects, must be made in accordance with approved Quality Authority procedures governing change control.

Continuous Equipment Reviews. All equipment should form part of a periodic review of their performance. The frequency of these reviews should be determined based on the criticality of the equipment using a risk based approach.

14.3 Blending and Mixing Validation

This section introduces the history of process validation (in particular of blend validation), the reasons for blend validation, approaches to carrying out validation of a blend and sources of information, both from industry best practices and from a regulatory perspective.

The Food and Drug Administration (FDA) in 1987 defined validation as 'Establishing documented evidence which provides a high degree of assurance that a specific process will consistently produce a product meeting its pre-determined specifications and quality attributes'. In addition the act of process validation was defined as, 'establishing documented evidence which provides a high degree of assurance that a specific process will consistently produce a product meeting its pre-determined specifications and quality characteristics'.

This was not the first time such a definition had been published, The Kefauver-Harris Amendments of 1962, which were as a result of the thalidomide tragedy in Europe (the FDA's vigilance prevented the drug's marketing in the United States), strengthened the rules for drug safety and required manufacturers to prove their drugs' effectiveness. Prior to then, cGMP and process validation were not required by law.

During the following two decades the FDA's attention was on process inspections. Major content uniformity problems were discovered during the Formulator-Oriented Rx Drug Study (FORDS) Program following complaints of clinical failures of such significant marketed products such as digoxin. 20 of the 32 digoxin firms sampled, as part of this FDA programme, produced batches that failed the USP content uniformity test.

In 1971 significant content uniformity failures were also revealed in a study on ethinylestradiol tablets. Of 15 batches sampled, 4, or 27% failed to meet requirements. This involved 4 of the 7 firms sampled. Analysis of 90 tablets from one batch showed a range from 35 to 252% of declared, with an average of 99.4% of declared. Eleven of the 90 tablets contained less than 50% of declared and 15 contained more than 150%. Poorly controlled manufacturing processes were the major contributing factors in most of these nonconformances, and certainly the results were accentuated in products containing high potency actives such as digoxin and ethinylestradiol, where the active is a small percentage of the total tablet weight. These types of observations continued well into the 1980s and beyond, until in 1993 the most infamous of modern cases.

The Barr ruling of February 1993 by Judge Alfred M. Wolin (United States of America vs Barr Laboratories, Civil Action No. 92–1744) was a watershed in the pharmaceutical landscape. Judge Wolin declared that blend testing is necessary to increase the likelihood of detecting inferior batches. It also declared that the appropriate sample size for blend and content uniformity in both validation and ordinary production batches is three times the active ingredient dosage size. Prior to this ruling, no specifics were universally accepted for this practise. Large samples akin to today's assay samples were routinely used as proof of not only potency, but of uniformity of dosage. Judge Wolin also ruled against the practice of compositing samples for the purpose of content uniformity, the averaging of results and ensuring adequate investigation of failing results.

In August 1999 the FDA issued a Draft Abbreviated New Drug Application (ANDA) Guidance for Industry titled 'ANDA's: Blend Uniformity Analysis' that detailed blend uniformity sampling and acceptance criteria for the determination of final blend uniformity for generic drug products. Although this guidance was written specifically to address ANDA's, the guidance was also adopted as standard practice in the development of NDA's (New Drug Applications). The proposed release criteria established for blend uniformity were to be used in addition to, and independent from, the USP finished product uniformity release requirements. Based on the Blend Uniformity Guidance, batches that failed to meet the blend uniformity acceptance criteria should be rejected regardless of the products ability to demonstrate final product uniformity. Application of such acceptance/rejection criteria proved troublesome for many pharmaceutical processes where sample thieving of cohesive mixes resulted in non-conforming results.

In 2000 The Product Quality Research Institute (PQRI), a collaborative process involving FDA's Center for Drug Evaluation and Research (CDER), Industry, and Academia, formed a blend uniformity working group that in 2002 issued a proposal to the FDA with respect to both ANDAs and NDAs. This proposal recommended the use of stratified sampling for final blend and in-process dosage units. The proposal recommended the use of final blend uniformity and dosage unit uniformity to demonstrate overall batch uniformity, with the possibility of using dosage unit uniformity in lieu of blend uniformity during routine commercial production. In May of 2002 the draft ANDA's: 'Blend Uniformity Analysis' was withdrawn by the FDA. As a result of the PQRI proposal, the FDA issued a Draft Guidance for Industry titled 'Powder Blends and Finished Dosage Units – Stratified In-Process Dosage Unit Sampling Assessment' in October 2003 that detailed the criteria for the use of stratified sampling and acceptance criteria to demonstrate batch uniformity.

Most recently in 2008, the FDA published their Process Validation draft guidance for industry, 'Process Validation: General Principles and Practices' , which specifically defines process validation as 'as the collection and evaluation of data, from the process design stage throughout production, which establishes scientific evidence that a process is capable of consistently delivering quality products'.

This revised guidance document was approved in January 2011 and conveys the FDA's current thinking on process validation and is consistent with the basic principles first introduced in the 1987 guidance.

Process validation is not just an FDA or a U.S. requirement. Similar requirements are included in the World Health Organization (WHO) Technical Report Series (e.g. 908 and 937), where the following definitions apply: 'Action of proving, in accordance with the principles of GMP, that any procedure, process, equipment, material, activity or system actually leads to the expected results' and 'Documented evidence which provides a high degree of assurance that a specific process will consistently result in a product that meets its predetermined specifications and quality characteristics.'

The Pharmaceutical Inspection Co-operation Scheme (PIC/S), 'The documented evidence that the process, operated within established parameters, can perform effectively and reproducibly to produce a medicinal product meeting its predetermined specifications and quality attributes' (June 2006). Similar definitions and expectations are present in the European Union (EU) requirements, Australia, Canada, Japan, and other international authorities. Figure 14.3 depicts some of the major events in the evolution of process validation with an emphasis on pharmaceutical blending.

14.3.1 Why do You Need to Validate Pharmaceutical Blends/Mixes?

So why do pharmaceutical blending/mixing activities need to validated? Quality is assured by end product testing, it is not enough to ensure the quality of the finished capsule or tablet? There are three primary answers to this question.

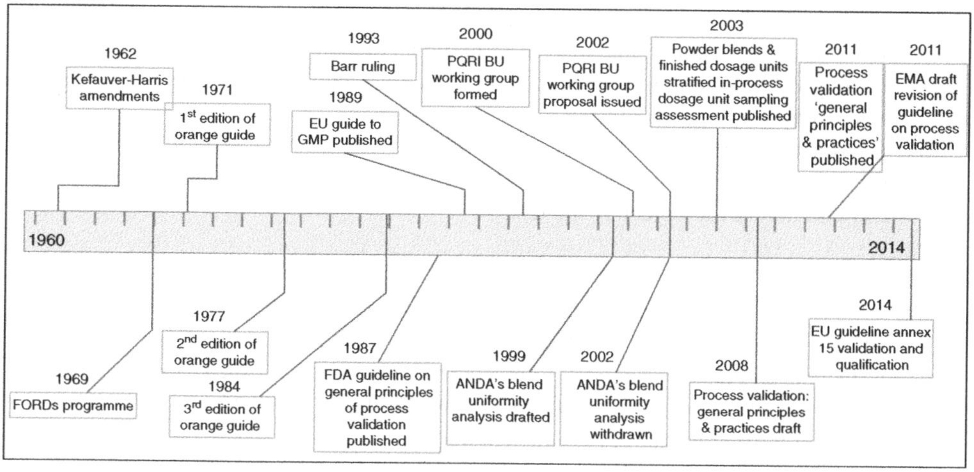

Figure 14.3 *Evolution of Process Validation, emphasis on blending*

1. It is an essential part of cGMP.
2. It is a legal requirement.
3. It saves money.

The introduction to this piece has briefly outlined the legal and regulatory evolution of expectations and requirements for the validation of pharmaceutical blends/mixes. Validation activities are considered fundamentally critical to the assurance of quality during manufacture of pharmaceuticals, and as we have seen, the emphasis from agencies has increased over time (Lindboe, 2008).

This provides a vindication to answers 1 and 2, however, how does the labour intensive and time consuming practise of validation improve the financial position of pharmaceutical companies? Historically process validation studies in general and validation of blending in particular had been considered tantamount to a drain on resources. However, consider the GMP-related recalls associated with finished product of sub-optimal uniformity. Inadequately defined and poorly understood manufacturing processes cannot be said to be in true control or capable of twenty-first century validation criteria.

Consider Judge Wolin's rulings for America vs Barr Laboratories (Civil Action No. 92–1744); Barr Laboratories was ordered to cease distribution until such a time as they had conducted concurrent or prospective validation studies on 24 named products, in addition, 15 other products required concurrent or prospective validation studies. The government also asked the Court to recall 15 batches of 10 different drug products; Barr vigorously contested each of these recall requests, but the court upheld the requests in 12 of the cases.

The court ordered a recall of one batch of product on the basis of an initial content uniformity failure and no basis to invalidate the test result and on a history of content uniformity problems with the product. The court ordered the recall of one batch of product after having concluded that a successful resample result alone cannot invalidate an initial OOS result. The court ruled that the firm must recall a batch that was released for content uniformity on the basis of averaged test results. On the basis of an initial content uniformity failure and no basis to invalidate the test result and on a history of content uniformity problems with the product, the court ordered another batch recalled. The financial burden of such recalls can be very significant.

The court ruled that sample size influences ultimate blend test results and that the sample size should resemble the dosage size. Any other practice would blur differences in portions of the blend and defeat the object of the test.

> Blend testing is necessary to increase the likelihood of detecting inferior batches.
>
> Blend content uniformity testing cannot be waived in favor of total reliance on finished product testing because finished product testing is limited.
>
> Multiple individual samples taken from different areas cannot be composited. However, when variation testing is not the object of assay testing, compositing is permitted.
>
> Firms must demonstrate through validation that their sampling technique is representative of all portions and concentrations of the blend. This means that the samples must be taken from places that might be problems, weak or hot spots in the blend.

Unless otherwise specified in the individual monograph, the requirements for dosage uniformity are met if the amount of the active ingredient in each of the 10 dosage units as determined from the Weight Variation or the Content Uniformity method lies within the range of 85.0–115.0% of the label claim and the relative standard deviation (RSD) is less than or equal to 6.0%.

If 1 unit is outside the range of 85.0–115.0% of label claim and no unit is outside the range of 75.0–125.0% of label claim, or if the Relative standard deviation is greater than 6.0%, or if both conditions prevail, test 20 additional units. The requirements are met if not more than 1 unit of the 30 is outside the range of 85.0–115.0% of label claim and no unit is outside the range of 75.0–125.0% of label claim and the Relative standard deviation of the 30 dosage units does not exceed 7.8% (USP29 <905>).

14.3.2 When do You Need to Validate Blending/Mixing?

There are two mandatory times when blending/mixing must be validated;

1. When an entirely new product or a new method of blending/mixing of an existing product is introduced. Steps should then be taken to demonstrate its suitability for routine processing, that is, validation. The defined blending/mixing process, using the materials and equipment specified, should be shown to yield a product consistently of the required quality and uniformity.
2. Significant amendments to the blending/mixing process, particularly any change to equipment or raw materials, which may affect product quality and/or the reproducibility of the process, should be always be validated.

   There are times when a third requirement for blend validation studies also exists, particularly in an industry that is moving more and more towards superior lifecycle management:
3. Processes and procedures should undergo periodic critical revalidation to ensure that they remain capable of achieving the intended results. This may or may not include the blending/mixing unit operations. A drug product with a historically strong performance,

and extensive blend/mixing data available from initial development and previous process validation may not require such extensive analysis at the blending/mixing unit operation stages.

14.3.3 Components of Blending/Mixing Validation

Previously we have looked at why we validate our blending and when should we validate; now we turn our attention to the how of executing a blending/mixing validation study.

14.3.3.1 Process Development

Validation of a blending/mixing process utilizes information generated during the entire development sequence that produced the final process. It is supported by all phases of development from the product concept.

As a potential product moves through the various developmental stages, blending/mixing information is continually generated and incorporated into a master documentation file.

When the validation runs are planned for the final blending/mixing process they are based on the master documentation file contents that define the Design Space. The information generated during the validation runs is usually the last major item to go into the master documentation file.

Though blending/mixing validation may seem to be a stand-alone item, it actually is an integral portion of the entire product/process development sequence.

It logically follows on from process development work on blending/mixing in stages I–3; that is, Product Design and Development, Pilot Laboratory (Clinical) and Pilot Scale production.

The objectives of blending/mixing development trials at stage III (100 kg pilot production) is to qualify and optimize the process in full-scale production equipment and facilities. Rushing through the first (100 kg) pilot-production batch in order to proceed with formal validation should be discouraged. Small problems that often arise during (100 kg) scale-up should be addressed immediately and not ignored. Such problems are often best addressed by returning to the laboratories (10 kg) for supplemental process characterization and qualification studies. The opportunity for developing a deeper understanding of the product and its process cannot be overstated. It is during process development when a robust process can be found through resolving problems encountered.

14.3.3.2 The Protocol

When we are validating a blending/mixing process we typically are generating documented proof that when you take predetermined quantities of specific raw materials (ingredients) mix/blend them according to an identified and predetermined recipe, using identified and confirmed (qualified) equipment that a final blend will be consistently produced that meets predetermined acceptance criteria.

This is a planned activity, this is not an evaluation of process parameters, the expected results, in the form of acceptance criteria, is agreed in writing in advance. Acceptance criteria are intended to ensure the quality, safety and efficacy of the final product and are a crucial part of any validation.

The master document that contains the statement of intent is known as the *protocol.* It should be written by an appropriately qualified and experienced individual, also it should at a minimum contain;

- a full process description
- the quantities of each raw material (including overages) required,
- the exact pieces of equipment that can be used, their respective qualification and calibration status'
- the recipe (including defined Critical Process Parameters, CPPs)
- the sampling requirements
- the level of testing to be performed and the test methods to use
- acceptance criteria and justification of same
- methods of analysis of test results
- references to applicable procedures, policies and guidelines both internal to the organization and regulatory bodies including what procedure to follow in the event of an out of specification result or a deviation from the protocol.
- roles and responsibilities of all parties involved in the study
- approval by the Quality Unit.

The World Health Organisation (WHO) in its Expert Working Group (EWG) technical reports on process validation declare that protocols must

> ...include significant background information, explain the rationale for and the objective of the study, give a full description of the procedures to be followed, set out the parameters to be measured, describe how the results will be analyzed, and provide pre-determined acceptance criteria for making conclusions.

14.3.4 What to Validate

The mixing or blending unit operation may occur once or several times during tablet manufacture. For example, a direct compression formulation may involve one blending step in which the drug and the excipients are blended together prior to compression. A wet granulation formulation may require two mixing/blending steps:

1. prior to granulating to have a uniform drug/excipient mixture, and
2. after milling the dried granulation to add other excipients, such as the lubricant.

Some or all the items provided in this section may therefore be pertinent for validation, depending on the mixing or blending objective.

The following physical properties of the drug and excipients are typical properties in creating a uniform mix or blend, other formulation specific properties should have been identified and quantified during development:

- Bulk density
- Free moisture content
- Particle shape

- Particle size distribution
- Surface area

Materials that have similar physical properties will be easier to form a uniform mix or blend and will not segregate as readily as materials with large differences.

- Acicular needle-shaped
- Angular sharp-edged or having a rough polyhedral shape
- Crystalline freely developed in a fluid medium of geometric shape
- Dentritic having a branched crystalline shape
- Fibrous regularly or irregularly thread-like
- Flaky plate-like
- Granular having approximately an equi-dimensional irregular shape
- Irregular lacking any symmetry
- Modular having rounded, irregular shape
- Spherical global shape

14.3.4.1 Items to Consider

Mixing or Blending Technique. Diffusion (tumble), convection (planetary or high intensity), or pneumatic (fluid bed) techniques can be used to mix or blend materials. Determine the technique that is required for the formulation or process objective. It may be different, depending on whether you are mixing the drug and excipients for a direct compression formulation or adding the lubricant (e.g. magnesium stearate) to the granulation.

Mixing or Blending Speed. Determine the intensity (low/high shear) and/or speed (rpm) of the mixing or blending. Mixing the drug and excipient will require more intense mixing than adding the lubricant to the final blend.

Mixing or Blending Time. How much mixing or blending is required to obtain a uniform mixture? The mixing or blending time will be dependent on the mixing or blending technique and speed.

Experiments done to determine if the materials can be overmixed, resulting in demixing or segregation of the materials. Demixing can occur due to the physical property differences (e.g. particle size distribution and density). For example, demixing can occur in a direct compression formulation in which the drug substance is micronized (5 μm) and the excipients are granular (500–1000 μm).

Drug Uniformity. Blend uniformity is usually performed to determine the uniformity of drug throughout the mix or blend. Representative samples should be taken throughout the mix or blend.

The sampling technique and handling of the materials are key in obtaining valid blend uniformity results. Segregation of the sample can occur by overhandling, resulting in inaccurate results. For the final blend (blend prior to compression), the sample taken should be equivalent to the weight of a single tablet, but in no circumstance should exceed three times the weight of a single tablet.

Excipient Uniformity. Besides drug uniformity, excipients need to be uniform in the granulation or blend. Two key excipients are:

Lubricant: The lubricant needs to be distributed uniformly in the mixture/granulation for the high-speed compression operation. Uneven distribution of the lubricant can result in picking and sticky problems during compression. It can also lead to tablet performance problems (low dissolution due to excessive lubricant in some tablets).

Colour: The colorant(s) need(s) to be evenly distributed in the mixture so that the tablets have a uniform appearance (e.g. colour, hue and intensity). The colouring agent may need to be pre-screened or more uniformally dispersed in the blend prior to compression to avoid speckling or shading of the colour.

Equipment Capacity/Load. The bulk density of materials or granules will affect the capacity of the equipment. If an excipient in the formulation affects the density of the final blend to a greater extent than any other ingredient, then a well-controlled density specification for that excipient may be warranted.

Test different-sized loads in the mixer/blender (e.g. 30, 50 and 70% of working volume) for optimal mixing or blending. Undercharging or overcharging a blender can result in poor drug or tablet lubricant distribution.

Continued Process Verification. In 2008 the FDA (2008) published their Process Validation draft guidance for industry, 'Process Validation: General Principles and Practices' that specifically defined process validation as 'the collection and evaluation of data, from the process design stage throughout production, which establishes scientific evidence that a process is capable of consistently delivering quality products.'

This revised guidance document (FDA, 2011) was approved in January 2011 and conveys the FDA's current thinking on process validation and is consistent with the basic principles first introduced in the 1987 guidance.

This guidance describes process validation activities in three stages: (1) Process Design: The commercial manufacturing process is defined during this stage based on knowledge gained through the development and scale-up activities, (2) Process Qualification: The process design is evaluated to determine if the process is capable of reproducible commercial manufacturing and (3) Continued Process Verification: Ongoing assurance is gained during routine production that the process remains in a state of control.

The benefits of PAT analysers are clear and referred to in the above 'guidance for industry' in stages 1, 2 and 3. Stage 1 can use PAT analysers while 'building and capturing process knowledge and understanding in addition to establishing a strategy for process control'. Stage 2 may use PAT analysers during Process Performance Qualification in confirmation of process design and demonstration that the commercial manufacturing process performs as expected.

However, they are of most importance during stage 3, during the establishment and maintenance of an ongoing programme to collect and analyse product and process data that relate to product quality. The 'Guidance for Industry' notes that 'scrutiny of intra-batch as well as inter-batch variation is part of a comprehensive continued process verification

A thorough understanding of the process will also provide a means to continuously verify the robustness of the process. Certainly there will be other factors that impact the ultimate content uniformity of the dosage form, including transport and storage of the blend, however, the blend will be the predominant factor. Understanding the impact of the discharge of the blend into intermediate containers, how it flows or is placed into the tablet compression equipment, encapsulation equipment, or other dosage preparation method, among other factors that impact the quality of the blend will enable knowledge of the content uniformity to provide monitoring of the success of the blending process.

14.4 Blending Cleaning Validation

The purpose of this section is to describe the program for performing cleaning development studies for new or existing products for their removal from blending equipment. Cleaning development studies determine cleaning feasibility, or 'cleanability', which cleaning procedures will adequately remove process soils from product-contact equipment surfaces associated with the blending processes. Following development of a cleaning procedure, validation and controls to assure that the developed and validated procedure is employed will need to be instituted (Le Blanc 2010).

14.4.1 Cleaning Development Studies

The understanding of soils and the development of cleaning chemistries are fundamental in delivering successful and appropriate cleaning processes. What follows describes methods regularly employed to identify, build and enhance the scientific basis of cleaning processes, procedures and criteria.

14.4.1.1 Soil Characterization

The understanding of any soil is crucial to its proper cleaning and removal from process equipment. By gathering information such as soil formulation, dissolution characteristics, degradation characteristics and a method detection and recovery, a more complete picture of the necessary chemistry and energies required for an acceptable cleaning procedure of pharmacological dosage forms is understood. Furthermore, by conducting a risk assessment on all soils in a process or contacting a particular piece or style of blending equipment, attention and efforts can be focused on the most challenging soils. The risk assessment must be documented, with the conclusion/action plan defining which soils will be evaluated. The following tools should be applied where appropriate to facilitate proper development of cleaning processes. This should minimally include evaluation of potentially worst-case soils, which frequently is the API.

General Information. Pertinent information on materials contacting blending process equipment should be gathered and documented. Information on said materials should include formulation identity, quantity, component concentration, Material of Construction (MOC) interactions, solubility characteristics, toxicity and safety information of each component. For components, such as new drug products, where the information is not available the following suggested studies below should be conducted.

Dissolution. The partition of a soil from a surface material of construction may be evaluated in the presence of the intended cleaning chemistries. These studies will seek to understand and document the process by which an analyte is caused to desorb and/or dissociate from a surface or matrix upon which it has previously adhered.

Degradation. The rate at which a soil is made more soluble by disruption of its many structural layers may be evaluated in the presence of the intended cleaning chemistries. These studies will seek to understand and document the cleaning chemistry introduced as well as the known degradation products of the API.

Detection. In order to assure that all of the analytical assays employed to detect residual product or process components or cleaning agents after cleaning are appropriate, the detection of representative process soils should be demonstrated. Limits of detection or quantification should be considered when demonstrating the suitability of the assay to the soil as it relates to cleaning acceptance criteria.

Recovery. The recovery efficiency of sampling methods should be evaluated to demonstrate appropriateness of the technique for the soils under consideration. There are two general types of sampling methods employed that should be considered for a given process soil. Those methods are surface sampling and rinse sampling.

Surface: Surface recovery swabbing for residual Total Organic Carbon (TOC) should be performed for direct product contact equipment materials of construction prior to any cleaning to prove that residual product or process solution is detectable on the surface of blending equipment. This swabbing method must be evaluated for its effectiveness on each product and cleaning chemical. This method may be affected by surface material, therefore all MOCs used in a process should be considered for their effect on soil recovery.

Rinse: Rinse recovery studies may be performed to evaluate the removability of a product or process solution from the surface of process equipment via aqueous rinses. This may be tested by lab-scale, closed system studies with the introduction of a known amount of soil then collection and appropriate analysis of the final rinse effluent.

Theoretical Matrix Analysis. Soils should be evaluated to determine which theoretically possess the greatest risk in terms of ability to clean, or 'clean-ability.' A matrix of chemical groupings, solubility, concentrations and other properties of the current commercial blending process should be employed in this analysis. This exercise should be procedural based, logical and reproducible, indicating the theoretical difficulty of any process solution or soil to be efficiently cleaned using current cleaning procedures. By theoretically ranking soils in terms of cleanability, the potentially most challenging soils may be identified. This theoretical matrix may make allowances for exceptional components with characteristics such as highly hydrophobic, highly toxic or potent, strong oxidizing and reducing agents and any other under-characterized blend components. The most challenging soils should be used in cleaning qualification studies where applicable.

14.4.1.2 Documentation of Soil Characterization

It is important to document each of these elements of soil characterization, from the risk assessment through rinse recovery studies. These documents then form the basis for demonstrating knowledge of the cleaning process and justification for subsequent validation. The objective of each evaluation, test plan, and results must be included in this documentation.

In-Use Process Parameters. During the development of an effective and efficient cleaning procedure several items need to be considered. These items include soil(s) type, concentration and delivery, in-use times, soiled hold times, use temperature, steam or chemical decontamination, dry compressed air, sparging and other potential process specifics. The challenge posed by a soiling blend may be affected by these and other required manufacturing parameters. Therefore an accurate or worst-case model of the blending process should be used during the development process to increase the probability of success when applied to the actual blending equipment.

Cleaning Chemistry Selection. The chemistry or agent employed to clean soiled equipment surfaces should be based on the soil characteristics and in-use process parameters as described previously. Cleaning agents used for blending equipment should not only address soil removal, but also should be detectable, free rinsing and low foaming (for agitated applications, such as CIP). These cleaning agents are considered raw materials for the cleaning process and are controlled and released. During the cleaning chemistry development, consideration must be given to the types of cleaning agents, their characteristics, and their delivery with regards to operator safety. These are described next.

Cleaning Chemical Delivery. Where possible, chemicals suitable for delivery via an automated, centralized system to the cleaning system should be used.

In situations where the automated chemical distribution system will not deliver the cleaning chemical to the target equipment, the choice, concentration and manual manipulation procedure of said chemical should be made with operator safety in mind.

Small-Scale Cleaning Development. The small-scale development activities are intended to determine fundamental parameters and standard operating procedures. In order to gain increased efficiencies and fundamental cleaning cycle understanding, discrete laboratory scale analyses should be performed. This development work may be done both at a bench (coupon studies) scale as well as at laboratory (small volume test equipment) scale. In bench scale testing an input of no prior experience of soils with cleaning solutions may lead to an output of a proposed cleaning chemistry, time and temperature for a cleaning solution. These studies are typically rapid, multivariable and conducted under a conservative (seeking to be less robust than the actual cleaning process) approach. In a lab scale-modelling situation the input may be a problematic soil that requires greater solution flow and action. The output of such modelling may include a CIP cycle tested at semi-scale providing confidence in the cleaning solution moving forward to the manufacturing scale. These risk assessment activities reduce in equipment down time for cycle development as well as provide the basic cleaning information elements necessary for a successful and optimized cleaning cycle validation.

These activities may continue to be documented as described in Section 14.1.1.7, or they may be documented using a developmental protocol and report. At this stage a protocol would not have pre-approved acceptance criteria for the tests. The risk assessment begun in Section 14.1.1 will be updated to reflect the soil characterization and in-use process parameters that have become inputs to this cycle development.

Modelling of In-Process Operations
In order to conservatively challenge a bench or laboratory scale cleaning development process, the parameters posed by the blending process that negatively impact the cleanability need to be replicated in a meaningful way.

Empirical Cleanability Assessment
Much like the way the in-use process parameters should be accurately modelled during development, the cleaning process parameters should be accurately or conservatively modelled using Design of Experiments (DOE), where experiments are designed to evaluate cleaning process response to the manipulation of selected parameters. Cleanability assessments should be performed where possible. By utilizing cleaning process modelling, the initial determination of cleaning cycle parameters should provide an effective cleanability technology transfer for use in the subsequent full-scale development, commissioning and qualifying activities.

The four basic elements essential in every proposed cleaning cycle include: Time; Action (physical contact of cleaning solution to soils); Chemistry and Concentration;

Temperature
Cleaning cycle modelling and development will employ either accurate process modelling (applying in-use process conditions and actual cleaning parameters) or a conservative modelling approach necessary to propose effective cleaning cycle elements. This modelling approach may include methods (or combinations) such as:

Static soaks; Agitated soaks; Ultrasonic soaks; Cascading action; Spray delivery/coverage (including assessment of spray ball trajectory).

Full-Scale Cleaning Cycle Development. Though small-scale development activities are intended to determine fundamental parameters and standard operating procedures, the details of delivering the cleaning solutions via cleaning equipment may need to be developed at full scale on the actual blending equipment. In certain situations, such as a new or refurbished manufacturing facility, central CIP equipment start-ups or new process equipment, full-scale cycle development may be necessary to ascertain cleaning system operational parameters. Full-scale cleaning cycle development may be performed concurrent with commissioning or GMP manufacturing activities. For full-scale cleaning cycle development, a developmental protocol is appropriate. Acceptance criteria will now be included, however, failure to achieve acceptance criteria would result not in a deviation as it would in a validation protocol, but rather would result in changes made to the process parameters and the test re-executed.

The following are items that should be considered during full-scale development:

Typical Cycles
The cleaning cycles employed may include:

- Water Rinse(s), Water Wash, Water Rinse(s)
- Water Rinse(s), Caustic Wash, Water Rinse(s) (preferred or most commonly used cycle)

- Water Rinse(s), Caustic Wash, Water Rinse, Acid Wash, Water Rinse(s), bearing in mind that the final rinse should be as good as or better than the solvent quality used for manufacturing, and will influence the microbial residual in the equipment.

Pre-Cleaning Activities

Certain pre-cleaning activities that may be detrimental or inefficient to a successful cleaning cycle include:

- Pre-cleaning Steam decontamination – This activity may increase the difficulty of soil removal.
- Pre-cleaning Soak – This activity greatly reduces efficiency with minimal improvement in cleaning process, so long as the 'soiled hold time' is appropriately controlled.

Blending Equipment Minimum Working Volumes

The equipment minimum working volumes required allowing for continuous pump and agitator operation will be determined and set. With the use of cavitation free pumps working volumes or heals should be minimized. Cleaning system attributes that may affect the minimum working volume are supply and return piping hold up volumes and volume loss due to system valve pulsing.

Path Hydraulics Sequence Timing

In order to ensure proper cleaning solution flow with no dead ends, hold up areas or return pump cavitation, the following automated cycle items should be set and adjusted until an uneventful cycle can be completed.

- Valve sequencing
  - Prime pumps prior to wash and rinse cycles.
  - Path and drain valve actuation during wash and rinse cycles
  - Condensate valve actuation during rinsing
- Return pump delay times
- Instrumentation timing
- Alarms and interlocks.

System Draining

The system must be configured to fully drain at the end of a wash or rinse step with nothing more than water droplets adhered to interior wetted surfaces. The system may be forced to drain by either a timed air blow down or gravity drain. Air blow downs may also be used to reduce humidity post final rinse.

Cleaning Agent Contact and Recirculation Times

The cleaning agent contact and recirculation times should be set based on those modelled during small-scale development. For process lines and blending equipment that see increased cleaning action relative to the conservative model used during small-scale development (e.g., turbulent flow), reduced contact times may be indicated. Under these conditions, a way to gauge reduced contact times may be through the use of line exchange volumes (one exchange volume equals volume to flood said pipe), which should take into account only the volume of the process lines soiled and equipment (not CIP supply and return lines). Exchange volumes are for use on piping only. Minimally, the contact time for any given circuit will be at least one minute. The following minimum line exchange volumes should be used when setting reduced path contact or recirculation times:

- ≥6 line exchange volumes for pre-rinses
- ≥14 line exchange volumes for once through caustic
- ≥6 line exchange volumes for once through acid
- ≥8 line exchange volumes for rinses post chemical wash
- ≥8 line exchange volumes for the final rinse.

Spray Coverage Development

- Development of Spray Device(s)

  The spray device should be positioned and modified as necessary to provide complete coverage of equipment internal wetted surfaces. Note that typically only the top 1/3 of the blending equipment is contacted by direct spray coverage, the remaining internal wetted surface area is covered via corresponding cascading action of the solution.

  The flow rate of fluid at the spray device should be set as necessary to achieve complete spray coverage. A fluid flow rate of either 0.1 to 0.3 gallons per minute per square foot of internal surface area, or 2.5 to 3.0 times the circumference of the blending equipment in gallons per minute should be considered as a starting point for spray device development. The spray device flow rate should correspond to a fluid velocity of ≥5 Feet Per Second (FPS) in the spray device circuit piping to provide optimal cleaning action of the included piping. Though, the influent flowrate through the spray device should not exceed the maximum effluent flowrate through the drain of the equipment to avoid solution accumulation in the equipment during cleaning operations.
- Ensuring Continued Use of Spray Device(s) as Developed

  Orientation of the spray device (and location if more than one is used) at the completion of successful development should be visibly and permanently marked at connection points, and have mechanical interlocks for identical placement/orientation.
- The flow rate and pressure found to be successful during development should be permanently stamped on the spray device.

Flow Rates, Pressure and Temperature

Flow rates for process lines should be set to ≥5 FPS. If ≥5 FPS is not achievable, then a reduced flowrate that insures flooded lines or turbulent flow should be set. Lines should be identified and documented in the commissioning test plan where a flowrate of ≥5 FPS is not achieved.

The supply pressure of cleaning agents during wash and rinse steps should be equal to or greater than the minimum pressure required by the spray device.

The system should be set to operate at or above the cleaning agent temperature recommended in the small-scale development (i.e., the lower temperature alarm limit with appropriate system response should be set at the temperature proposed in the development study).

The system should maintain the above minimum flow rates, pressures and temperatures for the times specified in the cleaning cycle parameters.

Cycle Optimization

A full scale cleaning challenge with actual or worst case process soils may be needed to provide a risk reducing opportunity to gauge cleaning chemistry, and cycle efficiency, including optimizing cycle time. This activity should look for uneventful completion of the cycle and confirm cleaning cycle appropriateness. This confirmation run should include a visual inspection and may include additional analytical testing of the surfaces cleaned.

Documentation

At the completion of full-scale cleaning cycle development, a comprehensive development report is needed to document the parameters and procedures developed and confirmed as part of this activity. This report will contain, or reference as appropriate:

- Cleaning process description
- Procedures utilized that must be in at least draft form and from this point forward maintained under a change control process
- Cycle parameters and settings used to achieve satisfactory results
- Sampling plan and test methods used
- Test results
- Review of the Risk Assessment and further definition of the Risk Plan
- This developmental report now becomes the basis for writing the cleaning validation protocol.

14.4.2 Cleaning Validation

Cleaning validation is performed to assure that production materials that come into contact with the blending equipment (including utensils) surfaces are not contaminated or adulterated.

A cleaning validation study typically requires a minimum of three (3) consecutive, successful verification runs. In the absence of three (3) batches or other unique circumstances, cleaning verification is performed to assure the equipment is suitable prior to the next use, however, validation using at least three consecutive, successful verification runs is eventually necessary. Cleaning validation for cross-contamination will rely upon validated analytical methods for the API or selected marker(s). These will be the core elements of the cleaning validation protocol. This protocol continues to implement the Risk Assessment Action Plan and will contain:

- A full description of the cleaning process
- The quantities of each material needed,
- The exact pieces of equipment and utilities that can be used, confirmation of their respective qualification and calibration statuses
- The recipe (including defined Critical Process Parameters, CPPs)
- The sampling plan including directions for swabbing or rinse collection
- Acceptance criteria and justification of same
- Methods of analysis of test results
- References to applicable procedures, policies and guidelines both internal to the organization and regulatory bodies including what procedure to follow in the event of an out of specification result or a deviation from the protocol.

- Roles and responsibilities of all parties involved in the study
- Approval by the Quality Unit.

In general, the requirement for residual detergent analysis and/or the microbial analysis is cleaning process related, and requires at least one validation study (i.e. three runs) for each cleaning process. The validation study shall address possible variations in microbiological flora, using a risk-based assessment considering route of administration (i.e. oral, parenteral, topical) and nature of the product.

The use profile of the equipment shall be determined, documented, and categorized into one of the following:

1. Dedicated product/product family equipment.
   Cleaning occurs between a predetermined number of batches and/or lapsed period of time. This would need to be validated. Validation shall address the worst-case situation, which may entail circumstances in addition to or in *lieu* of drug substance cleaning.
2. Multi-product equipment.
   This equipment is used to manufacture a variety of different products. Cleaning occurs between products.
   Equipment for campaigns shall be handled as dedicated equipment during the campaign and as multi-product equipment between the campaigns of different products.

Hold Times

Equipment shall be cleaned as soon as practical after use. Maximum holding times needs to be set between use and cleaning, and cleaning and sampling. The cleaning validation study needs to incorporate three runs at the maximum holding time.

For equipment used in the manufacture of parenteral dosage forms, maximum holding times must be validated from cleaning to sterilization.

SOPs need to be in place to assure that cleaned equipment is stored properly.

Determination of Chemical Residual Limits for Cleaning Validation Acceptance Criteria.

Identify the API or marker to be tested for removal.

The following approaches are recommended for multi-product equipment used for manufacturing dosage forms unless special toxicological concerns have been established. The 1/1000 approach may not be suitable for API manufacture, so the 10 ppm approach, or visual determination if that is more conservative, can be substituted. Refer to the decision tree that follows.

1. The 1/1000 approach
   Not more than 1/1000 of the total minimum daily dose for a 70-kg adult will appear in the maximum daily dose of the next product, except for equipment utilized for paediatric dosage for which a weight adjustment needs to be made accordingly. Refer to the appropriate regulatory guidance for paediatric dosage.
2. The 10 ppm approach (except for highly potent product)
   Not more than 10 ppm of the product being cleaned will appear in the next product.
   Visual determination with criteria should also be performed in addition to 1/1000 approach or 10ppm approach.
3. Highly potent product (special toxicological consideration)
   For highly potent products the approach shall be individually considered and limits set and justified. Dedicated equipment may be called for.

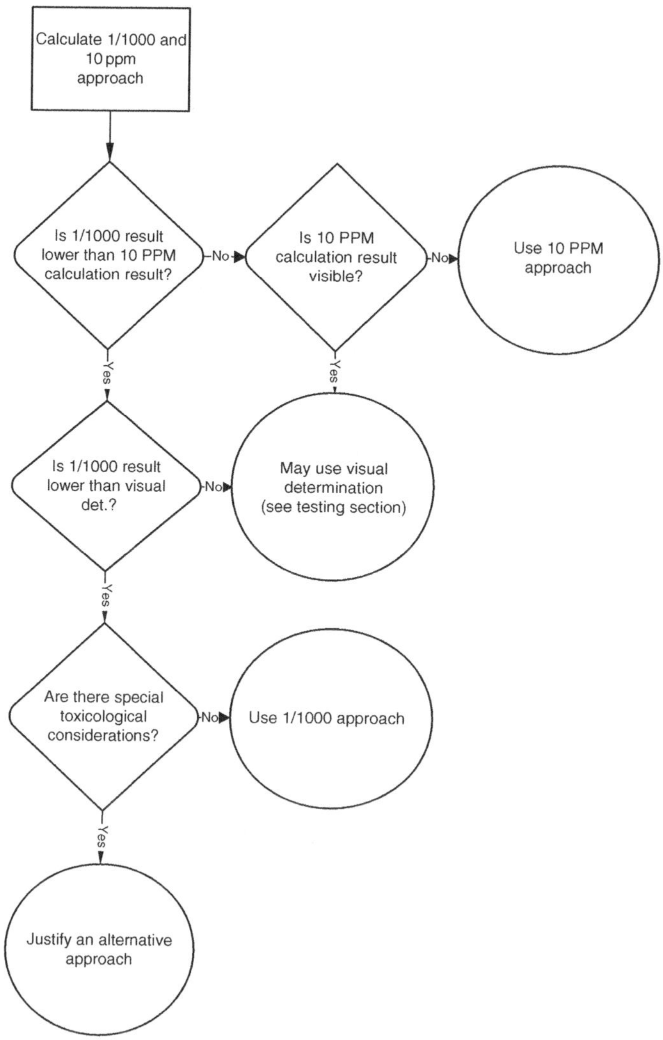

Figure 14.4 *Decision tree for determination of acceptance criteria*

The decision tree depicted in Figure 14.4 may be used to assist in worse case justification.

For cleaning agent residue limits no more than 1/10,000 of the LD_{50} value for a 70-kg adult will appear in the maximum daily dose of the next product for all cleaning agents except for equipment utilized for paediatric dosage for which a weight adjustment needs to be made accordingly. Notice that if cleaning development studies demonstrate that water alone is capable of satisfactorily cleaning blending equipment, not only is the cleaning process simplified, but also the validation.

4. *Visual Cleanliness*

A Visual inspection of equipment shall be performed to align the validation of the cleaning process with the routine inspection of equipment after cleaning.

For some products, a visual determination of cleanliness during validation shall be justified when calculations of acceptance criteria for the residual marker(s) is higher than a visual residue determination. The surfaces shall be readily inspectable. A visual determination method shall be developed using objective criteria. This is frequently used for less toxic compounds and especially where an opacifier, such as titanium dioxide, is part of the blend.

Documentation:
Site Acceptance and Release Report
A Site Acceptance Release Report (SARR) is written to provide documented Subject Matter Expert (SME) confirmation that the cleaning process is fit for its intended use. SARRs should include a review of the test results and any non-conformances. The SARR will review the Risk Assessment to assure that all of the assumptions have been verified, or that lessons learned resulted in changes to the cleaning process as part of continuous improvement. The SARR will be prepared and reviewed by the SMEs, and approved by the Quality Unit.

Maintenance of the Validated State
At the completion of a validation study, the following activities shall be in place:

- Review of SOPs to assure that they conform to the validated parameters, and inclusion in the equipment status control system.
- Recording of routine cleaning operations.
- Implementation of change control for the validated equipment and product.
- Inclusion in the Validation Master Plan.
- Controls over cleaning utensils.
- Control over cleaning agents including release by the Quality Unit.
- An ongoing monitoring program of the effectiveness of the cleaning program shall be considered, including periodic verification studies. Special consideration shall be given to highly potent products and microbial cleanliness after storage. Alternately, a means of continuous monitoring, such as PAT, may be employed. Frequently, the final rinsate is tested for conductivity/resistance/light induced fluorescence techniques to determine if the blending equipment cleaning was satisfactory. The level and sensitivity of the testing of final rinsate may depend upon the quality of the water used for that final rinse. As the pharmaceutical manufacturing industry transitions towards continued cleaning process verification philosophies the requirement for rapid mobile analytical technologies may become essential in order to sustain robust and lean equipment cleaning processes. Analytical techniques such as NIR Chemical Imaging may prove useful in meeting these needs (Jones *et al.*, 2012).

14.5 Conclusion

This chapter has attempted to provide the reader with an appreciation for the history, current status and future approaches to commissioning, qualification, blending process validation and cleaning validation. It is clear that the pharmaceutical industry needs to bring greater control to the manufacturing processes while at the same time not incurring more costs.

This may be achieved by delivering on more effective commissioning, qualification, process validation and continuous verification management. The application of Quality Risk Management tools will assist in restructuring our approach to equipment commissioning, qualification and process validation activities.

14.6 Acknowledgements

The authors would like to thank John Costello and Philip Ennis for their opinions and industry expertise in preparing this chapter.

References

ASTM (2007). *Standard Guide for Specification, Design and Verification of Pharmaceutical and Biopharmaceutical Manufacturing Systems and Equipment.* ASTM International Standard Designation E 2500–07, published August 2007, ASTM, West Conshohocken, PA, www.astm.org.

Food and Drug Administration (FDA) (2004), Guidance for Industry: PAT – A Framework for Innovative Pharmaceutical Development, Manufacturing and Quality Assurance, September 2004, Washington, D.C., U. S. Government Printing Office.

Food and Drug Administration (FDA) (2009), Pharmaceutical CGMPs for the 21st Century – A Risk-Based Approach, Final Report September 2008, Washington, D.C., U. S. Government Printing Office.

Food and Drug Administration (FDA) (2008), Guidance for Industry: Process Validation, General Principles and Practices, Draft November 2008, Washington, D.C., U. S. Government Printing Office.

Food and Drug Administration (FDA) (2011) Guidance for Industry 'Process Validation: General Principles and Practices' Washington, D.C., U. S. Government Printing Office.

International Conference on Harmonisation (ICH) (2009) Technical Requirements for Registration of Pharmaceuticals for Human Use, *ICH Harmonised Tripartite Guideline, Pharmaceutical Development* Q8(R2), Step 4, August 2009.

International Conference on Harmonisation (ICH) (2005)Technical Requirements for Registration of Pharmaceuticals for Human Use, *ICH Harmonised Tripartite Guideline, Quality Risk Management* Q9, Step 4, November 2005.

Jones, I., Cullen, P.J., Greene, A. (2012) Using PAT to support the transition from cleaning process validation to continued cleaning process verification. *Journal of Validation Technology*, **18**, 50–56.

Le Blanc, D.A. (2010), Cleaning Validation – Practical Compliance Solutions for Pharmaceutical Manufacturing, Volume 2, Destin A. LeBlanc, March 2010, ISBN 1-933722401, PDA/DHI Books, Bethesda, MD.

Lindboe, W.G. (2008), Validation of solid dosage finished goods, Chapter 30, in *Validation of Pharmaceutical Processes*, 3rd Edn, J. Agalloco and F.J. Carlton, (eds), Informa Healthcare USA, New York.

Part IV
Optimization and Control

15

Process Analytical Technology for Blending

Nicolas Abatzoglou
Chemical Engineering and Biotechnological Engineering, Université de Sherbrooke, Canada

This chapter discusses the objectives of the process analytical technology (PAT) initiative and how it may be incorporated into the blending process. Perspectives on PAT adoption from both regulatory agencies, such as the European Medicines Agency (EMEA) and the U.S. Food and Drug Administration (FDA), as well as from the International Conference on Harmonization are detailed. Novel, non-evasive, real-time techniques, such as single point spectrometry and chemical imaging, are assessed. The chapter introduces statistical tools, such as chemometrics, to manage data-rich measurements.

15.1 Introduction

This section covers the actual role of process analytical technology (PAT) in pharmaceutical manufacturing and development, particularly in pharmaceutical blending. It also makes the link between PAT and good manufacturing procedures (GMP), and outlines how PAT is helping to enable the evolution of quality systems.

The U.S. Food and Drug Administration (FDA) and the European Medicines Agency (EMEA) are in agreement on the following definition of PAT: "A system for designing, analysing, and controlling manufacturing through timely measurements (i.e., during processing)

Pharmaceutical Blending and Mixing, First Edition. Edited by P.J. Cullen, Rodolfo J. Romañach, Nicolas Abatzoglou and Chris D. Rielly.

of critical quality and performance attributes of raw and in-process materials and processes, with the goal of ensuring final product quality" [1].

15.1.1 The Role of PAT in Pharmaceutical Manufacturing: Is PAT Really New?

PAT is a mature, well-advanced field in process engineering by the chemical industry. The reason this fact is not well known is that the chemical industry use the term Process Control instead of PAT. The latter includes the analytical tools allowing for in-line monitoring, signal acquisition and signal treatment/use in simple and sophisticated control systems. Both batch and continuous process monitoring and control benefit from the development and application of in-line, on-line and at-line, old and new, physical (i.e., temperature, pressure, flow rate), and chemical (pH, gas and liquid flow composition) analysis technologies. However, PAT in the pharmaceutical industry is a rather new field, clearly demonstrated by the fact that the FDA, although it has started talking openly about this need since 2001 by means of the work of the Advisory Committee for Pharmaceutical Science [1], has officially adopted the PAT concept and produced a directive on it in 2004 [2]. The reasons for this "lag" are numerous, but it is of interest to understand the most influential ones because the future development and deployment of PAT in pharmaceutical manufacturing is highly dependent on them. I propose to divide these reasons into three main categories as follows: (1) inertial, (2) scientific/technical, and (3) financial. I will try to analyze them in the following text:

1. Inertial reasons: This category covers all roadblocks associated with the prevailing quasi-worldwide pharmaceutical manufacturing culture. It is well known, and not worth detailing here, that regulatory approval of pharmaceutical product commercialization is a lengthy and risky process. Regulatory agency approval of a substance – in its final formulation – as a drug that can be administered to patients does not mean that the owner/producer has the license to put the drug on the market. The latter necessitates an official audit of its manufacturing protocol and product quality control (QC). When PAT was proposed as the most promising and efficient means of improving process and product quality, pharmaceutical companies understood that resource-intensive procedures for all running production processes had to be re-thought in an even more intensive way. When they expressed their concerns, nobody had a satisfactory answer. Moreover, process understanding based on first scientific principles had already been attempted without success because of intended process complexity. Pharmaceutical practitioners were certain that stochastic modeling of such processes was doomed to fail because it would be unable to provide the requested precision. Another crucial point was the lack of an "engineering" way of thinking: process improvement through understanding of physico-chemical characteristics and prevailing process steps rather than through purely empirical-phenomenological methods relying on the statistical design of experiments (DoE).
2. Scientific/technical reasons: In-line analytical technologies developed for the chemical/petrochemical industries perform well when applied to classical fluids, whether gas or liquid. Although these streams are not ideal, there are well known and reliable thermodynamic and fluid mechanical models that are highly robust. This is not the case with mixed (solid-fluid) flows, either solid-liquid or solid-gas. When solid-state phases,

mainly divided solids in the form of granules or powders, are present, the number of variables and parameters upon which phenomena depend increase dramatically. Thus, mathematical problems become prohibitively difficult. In the vast majority of pharmaceutical manufacturing, both upstream and downstream, the processes are multi-phase and complex, rendering it arduous to study prevailing mechanisms and their modeling.

3. Financial reasons: The investment of pharmaceutical companies in the development of new drugs and formulations is usually the biggest part of their capital expenditures. Once a substance qualifies as a commercial drug, the patent is usually already quite old, and the company involved has to speed-up its entry into the marketplace. Since pharmaceutical companies have personnel well trained and experienced in setting-up statistical process optimization and QC, they are very reticent to engage in understanding all mechanistic process steps with the hope of being able to deliver as rapidly as in the case of their well-established procedures.

15.1.2 Why PAT is Feasible

In [2], it is explained that in FDA's PAT definition, the term "analytical" includes all chemical, physical and microbiological techniques as well as mathematics and risk analyses. In pharmaceutical manufacturing, in-line analytical tools for real-time measurement must be non-destructive and non-invasive. The FDA proposes four types of PAT tools (PAT tool box) to measure, understand, track, and control a process:

- Analyzers measuring critical process parameters, that is, spectrometers quantifying mixture composition over time.
- Statistics engaged in DoE.
- Process control through really functional knowledge transfer or mainly based on multivariate statistical analysis and strategies.
- Knowledge management and continuous improvement, that is, mathematical models and protocols.

A PAT application is defined as the combination of two or more of these four tools to ensure proper monitoring and control of processes.

This means that it is not always necessary to develop full process understanding – in the academic sense of the term – but rather to find an efficient combination of science and empirical knowledge to improve existing quality. As an example, it is unnecessary to understand all underlying mechanisms during dry particulate mixing to be able to follow the efficacy and efficiency of the process step and decide whether its product must advance to the next process of the manufacturing chain. Nevertheless, if sufficient information on particle segregation and agglomeration tendency is available, the latter can be (1) used to avoid undesired outputs, and (2) introduced in analytical tools to avert the resulting biases, improving measurement precision and, more generally, reliability.

Although there has been an initial "lag phase," considerable growth of PAT applications in pharmaceutical manufacturing has been observed during the last 10 years. Pharmaceutical companies that invested internally in the field and other that established collaborations with academia [3] state that there has been considerable growth, mostly driven by technological advances and regulatory encouragement, demonstrated returns from effective PAT implementation and business strategies focused on reducing the cost of manufacturing. This growth has been accompanied by significant publication of scientific and technical papers as well as the organization of PAT-specific national and international workshops, symposia, colloquia, and conferences.

15.1.3 Where PAT can be Applied in Pharmaceutical Manufacturing

Although the focus is on blending, it is important to provide the reader with more general information regarding the utility of PAT in the pharmaceutical industry [2].

In pharmaceutical product QC there is growing interest in the application of continuous quality verification (CQV) and real time release (RTR) as part of evolving quality manufacturing systems. RTR testing (RTRt) is the ability to evaluate and ensure the acceptable quality of the operational modules and final products in pharmaceutical production processes based on process data; a typical valid RTRt relies on a combination of measured physico-chemical attributes and efficient process control (ICH Q8R1). CQV and RTR are techno-economically feasible only whenever reliable PAT systems are available.

PAT systems can provide the initial process understanding (and, consequently, define the critical attributes of a process). Such knowledge helps in both qualitatively and quantitatively defining the role of the process critical attributes in quality aspects during manufacturing. Based on process understanding, it may be possible to adjust and adopt more efficient manufacturing protocols and monitor corresponding manufacturing processes during operation; the latter ensures that critical process elements are within the desired range and that product features are within specifications. Product release can be based on a combination of process parameters and real time material attributes in lieu of finished product (FP) testing.

PAT-based advanced process control (APC): PAT provides a significant advantage in traditional process control in terms of monitoring unit progression or batch maturity and determining the process or batch end-point. PAT-based (usually statistical) APC (APC-SPC) is of even greater potential benefit to optimally control process outcomes in terms of both product quality, such as improved potency and reduced impurities, as well as business attributes, such as yield, batch time, and processing costs.

15.1.4 The Regulatory Framework

15.1.4.1 US FDA

The FDA PAT guidance of 2001 and the subsequent presentations in 2001 and 2002 found easily in the www space [1] is more encouraging than enforcing. This is because its primary objective is to "motivate" companies to understand the advantages that might accrue in the future in innovation, development, production, and quality assurance. It can be done, namely by improving their quality, lowering capital losses due to failures, and anticipating technical and regulatory constraints that might be roadblocks to innovation.

In September 2004, the FDA released another PAT-driven guidance for industry under the title: *PAT – A Framework for Innovative Pharmaceutical Development, Manufacturing, and Quality Assurance* [1]. It complemented the previous guidance in that it described a strategy for regulatory implementation of PAT by the FDA. This PAT framework guidance became a foundation stone for the creation of more advanced life cycle-oriented quality systems, incorporating quality by design (QbD) (ICH Q8) and quality risk management (QRM) (ICH Q9).

15.1.4.2 EMEA

An EMEA PAT team was appointed in November 2003 to establish a forum for creating dialogue and understanding the European regulatory framework around PAT, especially for filing applications and review processes. The EMEA PAT team believes the current regulatory framework in Europe supports PAT implementation. The team produced a "Reflection Paper" in March 2006 under the title: "Chemical, pharmaceutical and biological information to be included in dossiers when Process Analytical Technology (PAT) is employed." It provides succinct recommendations about how PAT-related information should be presented in marketing authorizations applications or variations. The reflection paper incorporated commentary about QRM and QbD elements (design space and DoE), in alignment with ICH Q8 and Q9. In response to the increasing application of near-infrared spectroscopy (NIRS) PAT in the pharmaceutical industry, the EMEA prepared a *Note on the Use of Near-Infrared Spectroscopy by the Pharmaceutical Industry and the Data Requirements for New Submissions and Variations CPMP/QWP/3309/01 and EMEA/CVMP/961/01.*

15.1.4.3 Other Regulatory Perspectives

The National Institute of Health Science (NIHS) of Japan formed a working group with representation from industry and the NIHS, to discuss analytical technical innovations along with the regulatory aspects of PAT activities. The NIHS, as a participant in the International Conference on Harmonisation of Technical Requirements for the Registration of Pharmaceuticals for Human Use (ICH), is actively involved in the development of ICH Quality Guidelines, including ICH Q8, Q9 and Q10.

The Therapeutic Goods Administration of Australia has been working with industry on PAT application as an alternative to laboratory testing.

Scientific justification and demonstration of the benefits of PAT have been significant in the progressive regulatory acceptance of PAT in many countries.

American Standards of Testing and Materials (ASTM): In tandem with its current good manufacturing procedures (cGMPs) as twenty-first century initiatives, the FDA liaised with the ASTM in 2003 to constitute ASTM Committee E55 on the Manufacture of Pharmaceutical Products. As of 2009, ASTM Committee E55 is composed of three sub-committees, two of which support PAT application:

- E55.01 – PAT System Management
- E55.02 – PAT System Implementation and Practice.

These sub-committees are focused on developing consensus standards, in coordination with all stakeholders (including manufacturers, regulators, and professional trade associations), that facilitate implementation of PAT by industry and clarify FDA expectations. Currently-approved standards, specifically for PAT, include:

- *E2474–06 Standard Practice for Pharmaceutical Process Design Utilizing Process Analytical Technology.*
- *E2363–06a Standard Terminology Relating to Process Analytical Technology in the Pharmaceutical Industry.*

Additional PAT-related standards are under development. The current status of these and other activities covering the manufacture of pharmaceutical products can be found at the link to the ASTM Committee E55 website: www.astm.org/COMMIT/COMMITTEE/E55.htm.

15.1.4.4 Pharmacopoeia Guidance

PAT-related guidance within the United States pharmacopeia (USP) and European pharmacopeia (EP) is captured in monographs for specific analytical techniques such as NIRS. The most notable are USP <1119> Near-Infrared Spectroscopy (NIRS), USP <1120> Raman Spectroscopy (RS), and EP 2.2.40 Near-Infrared Spectrophotometry. These monographs provide details about instrument capabilities, diagnostic system suitability, method validation, and other scientific practices for associated techniques.

15.1.4.5 PAT in Divided Solids Mixing

In this chapter, the term "divided solids" is preferred to its quasi-equivalents (i.e., "granular systems," "particulate systems," and "powders"), because it is more general and includes all categories expressed by the preceding terms. The term incorporates all uni- and multi-component systems made up of particles whose moisture is such that their appearance is dry. Uni- and multi-component systems containing significant quantities of water and presenting a rather pasty or muddy appearance are termed "semi-solid systems."

The principal reason for the lack of knowledge on processes involving the handling of divided solids is their complexity. Depending on the particle size distribution (PSD), these systems (mixtures) are non-homogeneous at the microscopic and sometimes macroscopic levels. Their behavior depends on a significant number of parameters, such as purity, crystallinity, surface energy, electrostatic load, elasticity (Young's modulus), density, PSD, surface specificity, porosity, morphology, true, loose and packed density, moisture, geometry of their container, and wall-particle interactions. This complexity is responsible for the sometimes chaotic and counter-intuitive behavior of divided solids. Efforts, mainly phenomenological, to measure and predict these phenomena are reported in the literature [4, 5, 6, 7]. In all cases, the greatest difficulty is the lack of robust in-line analysis methods aimed at developing process understanding. Pursuant to the development of the first PAT tools, constant efforts were made by the pharmaceutical industry and researchers in the field of analytical techniques, for example, measurement of PSD [8], NIRS [9], Fourier-transformed mid-IR [10], RS [11,12], laser- or light-induced fluorescence (LIF) [13], nuclear magnetic resonance (NMR) [14] and data-mining/exploitation mathematical methods (Chemometrics) [15,16].

15.2 Chemometrics and Data Management

Chemometrics can be defined as: " . . . the chemical discipline that uses mathematical, statistical and other methods employing formal logic to design or select optimal measurement procedures and experiments and to provide maximum relevant chemical information by analyzing chemical data" – North American Chapter of the International Chemometrics Society (www.namics.nysaes.cornell.edu/chem_info.html).

Chemometrics is the science of extracting information from chemical systems. It is a highly interfacial discipline incorporating methods frequently included in core data-analytical disciplines, such as multivariate statistics, applied mathematics, and computer science, as well as chemistry, physics, biological sciences, and chemical/biotechnological engineering.

Although even the earliest analytical experiments in chemistry involved a form of chemometrics, the field is generally recognized to have emerged in the 1970s as computing power increased exponentially, becoming widely available and time- and cost-efficient for scientific investigation. The term "chemometrics" was coined by Svante Wold in 1974, and the International Chemometrics Society was formed shortly thereafter by Wold and Bruce Kowalski, both pioneers in the field. Wold was Professor of Organic Chemistry at Umea University in Sweden, and Kowalski was Professor of Analytical Chemistry at the University of Washington in Seattle.

Multivariate analysis is the most critical "building block" of chemometrics. The data resulting from infrared and ultraviolet (UV)/visible spectroscopy are voluminous and number in the thousands of measurements per sample. Mass spectroscopy, NMR, atomic emission/absorption and chromatography experiments are all by nature also highly multivariate. Techniques, such as principal components analysis (PCA) and partial least squares (PLS), are deployed the most for (a) extracting practical, structured information from these data, and (b) building realistic and efficient process simulation and prediction models. PCA and PLS have proven to be very effective at empirically modeling usually complex and more chemically-interesting information, exploiting the interrelationships or "latent variables" in data, and providing the basis for further numerical analysis, such as regression, clustering, and pattern recognition. In particular, the PLS method was heavily engaged in chemometric applications for many years before it began to find regular use in other fields.

In the 1980s, three dedicated journals made their appearance: *Journal of Chemometrics* (from John Wiley & Sons, Ltd), *Chemometrics and Intelligent Laboratory Systems* (from Elsevier), and *Journal of Chemical Information and Modelling* (from the American Chemical Society). These journals continue to cover both fundamental and methodological research in chemometrics. At present, most routine applications of existing chemometric methods are commonly published in application-oriented journals (e.g., *Applied Spectroscopy, Analytical Chemistry, Analytica Chimica Acta, Talanta, American Pharmaceutical Review*, and *European Pharmaceutical Review*). Several important books/monographs on chemometrics were also first published in the 1980s and more recently.

15.2.1 PAT Data Management and Interpretation

Multiple algorithms exist for the analysis of PAT data; they can be broadly divided into two categories: (1) those used for data pre-processing and (2) those applied for interpretation. Finally, after validation these algorithms may be used to monitor a critical process parameter.

15.2.1.1 Data Pre-Processing

Pre-processing algorithms are adopted for untreated data to assist in interpretation, for example, by increasing the signal/noise ratio or improving the resolution of a signal related to a specific analyte. In all cases, the role of a pre-processing function must be understood, and its use in a particular situation justified. Moreover, no careful pre-processing can result in loss of useful chemical information, thus disabling considerably the efficacy of the subsequently derived predictive model.

15.2.1.2 Data Interpretation

PAT data interpretation is the establishment of scientifically and technically sound relationships between the process and product attributes and the available. It frequently involves the generation of a mathematical model for the prediction of these attributes in future datasets.

15.2.1.3 Validation of PAT Methods

The validation of PAT methods should be considered in a manner similar to the validation of conventional analytical methods, to confirm consistency of method performance and facilitate regulatory approval. In this respect, the validation of PAT methods should comply with ICH Q2R1 – Validation of Analytical Procedures: Text and Methodology, pertaining to method validation as well as applicable cGMP requirements.

The extent of PAT method validation depends on its intended use and should be commensurate with the criticality and assessed risk to product quality and compliance.

PAT method validation frequently involves comparison with conventional analytical techniques and evaluation of their relative performance. In all cases, validation must demonstrate that the PAT method is robust and fit for its intended purpose.

15.2.1.4 PAT Data Management

Data management is an important aspect of PAT, particularly when for product/process monitoring and control or as replacement for registered in-process or end-product testing (i.e. RTR). Typically, PAT data differ in many ways from those obtained by conventional process or laboratory instruments. For example, many PAT analyzers generate multidimensional data, for example a spectrum consisting of wavelength versus absorbance data for several hundreds or thousands of points per spectrum. Moreover, chemometrics/statistics often need to be applied to convert the raw signal into a value or "information" associated with the process parameter(s) or attribute of interest. Frequently PAT data are collected in a continuous or semi-continuous fashion. The combination of these factors results in the potential for having significantly larger and more complex datasets associated with a process compared with processes that do not utilize PAT.

The fact that most manufacturers of PAT analyzers utilize proprietary data formats, and instrument drivers further complicates data analysis, storage, and post-manufacturing review.

Ultimately, large amounts of PAT data have to be collected, analyzed, displayed, transmitted, processed, and stored in a manner that provides timely information about manufacturing process variables.

Therefore, an appropriate data management system is a key aspect of PAT deployment and use, to accommodate all these factors.

Retention requirements for data need to comply with cGMP requirements applicable to particular PAT applications.

15.2.1.5 PAT Applications

PAT tools are intended for various applications in industrial pharmaceutical production. Their extents of use or development advancements are provided in Table 15.1. This table is compiled by the author based on literature and personal knowledge in this field. It is

Table 15.1 PAT realistic opportunities in pharmaceutical production "unit operations"

Processes / In-line PAT tools	Raw materials handling	Reactors	Solid-liquid separation	Drying	Size reduction granulation	Powders blending	Tableting	Coating
Particles size	+++	+	+++	++	++	++	–	–
NIR	+	+	++	+++	+	+++	++	++
MIR(*)	–	++	+/–	–	–	–	–	–
UV	–	++	+	–	–	–	–	–
Raman	+	++	++	–	–	+	++	++
LIF	++	++	+	+/–	+	+	+	–
Imaging	+	+/–	+/–	+/–	+	+/–	+	–
Effusivity	+/–	–	–	+/–	+/–	+/–	–	–

Notes:
+++: Available technology
++: Very probable technology
+: Promising technology
+/–: Not yet tested or tested but not conclusive yet
–: Rather improbable technology

possible that some of the PAT presented in Table 15.1 have other applications or that some of them are better developed but not yet reported by corporate R&D activities.

15.3 Near-Infrared Spectroscopy (NIRS)

NIRS, a vibrational spectroscopy technique, provides qualitative and quantitative analyses. It may also serve as PAT for monitoring and controlling drug substance synthesis and FP manufacturing processes. Actually, NIRS is the most exploited PAT tool in pharmaceutical blending. The particular importance of NIRS as a PAT is related to the following characteristics:

- NIRS is neither destructive nor invasive;
- C–H, N–H and O–H chemical bonds, which are found in almost all pharmaceutical formulations, absorb strongly at NIRS wavelength range. Moreover, the overtones of these links are a function of their relative position within molecules and, consequently, each chemical compound has its own NIRS signature;
- NIRS can be applied to all types of physical states, including solids and divided solids (powders and granules);
- NIRS is humidity-sensitive;
- NIRS does not require particular sample preparation;
- NIRS spectra can be acquired within fractions of a second.

The EMEA is actually working on producing new guidelines on this analytical technique, which is the most advanced and frequently encountered in all PAT efforts. According to the prevailing glossary:

- A NIRS method is referred to as a primary method when it is part of a final QC and release protocol to market a finished pharmaceutical product. Usually, when NIRS becomes the release method, it is used off-line for conventional release protocols or at-line for RTR.
- A NIRS method is referred to as an alternative when it is employed instead of a conventional (reference) method (e.g., chromatography, UV-Vis spectroscopy).
- A NIRS method is referred to as an in-process control when it is part of a feed-forward or in-line control strategy. It may be a part of RTRt.
- A NIRS method may also be applied for data-mining purposes (process knowledge), if it is linked to elements of a PAT concept. In this case, NIRS only serves to enhance process understanding.

Although a significant number of publications on NIRS and data analysis/interpretation by chemometrics are available, the technique is quite recent in pharmaceutical blending. Ciurczak and Drennen [17], followed by Hailey et al. [18], Wargo and Drennen [19] and Sekulic et al. [20,21], took the first significant steps in this direction.

Sekulic et al. [20,21] modified a miniature Flobin blender to enable the incorporation of a fiber optic probe for on-line NIR spectral data collection. The experiments were successful in detecting spectral changes, the target being the production of a qualitative model able to predict the mixing end-point. The results led to a number of helpful conclusions, namely:

- NIRS data pre-treatment was necessary to produce a successful chemometric model, but there was no clear advantage among the various methods; only the second derivative, Savitsky–Golay transformation, appeared to be more sensitive to noise.
- The model developed was able to predict a similar end-point for additional runs of the same composition.

Although these results were very promising, the qualitative nature of chemometrics did not provide proof that the model could be applied as efficiently to other final compositions and to other production scales. In fact, it was expected that all these (scale parameters, final composition and, of course, nature of the ingredients) would play a very important role.

Ufret and Morris [22] developed a theoretical mathematical model on the kinetics of mixing in pharmaceutical operations. The model code is called "additive volume mixing"; to calculate the model intrinsic parameter (called "characteristic fraction of mixing") and to prove its validity as well as utility, they tested two different size bin blenders (1.5 and 14.8 ft^3) and on-line NIR diffuse reflectance (DR-NIRS) analysis to follow the blending process. Although the main focus of the paper was not in- or on-line NIRS analysis (which was rather employed as a validation tool), and there is not really enough information regarding the way the NIR technique was calibrated, this study has proven more scientifically that the speculated influence of parameters, such as formulation properties, mixer geometry, and process scale on the mixing behavior of a system is a reality.

El-Hagrasy et al. [23] investigated NIRS as a tool to monitor powder blend homogeneity. Testing was done with salicylic acid (SA) and Fast-Flo lactose in an 8-qt V-blender. Optical ports were installed at six positions on the blender, allowing spectral collection by fiber optics. A traditional thief probe retrieved samples for UV reference analysis. The blender was stopped at pre-selected time points for NIR and UV data collection. Several algorithms and sampling protocols were studied to identify an optimum methodology for blend homogeneity determination. The blending process was also monitored with an (Indium-Antimony (InSb) imaging camera for comparison with traditional NIRS and UV reference data. Both qualitative and quantitative models were developed. The main new information derived from was:

- Environmental conditions and component concentration had an impact on the blending process. This was rather expected and the conclusion could be reached even without NIRS, meaning also that in-line monitoring is necessary on each blending run.
- Multiple sampling points were essential for accurate and precise estimation of mixing end-points.

Although the contribution of this work was significant, the conclusions were somehow discouraging because it has shown that significant investment was needed (many sampling ports and the development of new models whenever changes were made) to ensure the requested QC. Moreover, if environmental conditions were not stable, the validity of the model could not be taken for granted.

Blanco et al. [24] performed similar experiments in parallel. They reported all previous related investigations in tabular form containing the following data: APIs analyzed, excipients, NIR spectral mode, and methods for monitoring homogeneity (namely, chemometrics). However, the utility of the results was relatively low because the experimental blending process was small lab-scale (total mass of the mixture below 50 g) and blending (with an intermittent propeller) was not representative of any industrial-scale pharmaceutical process.

El-Hagrasy et al. [25, 26] published their efforts to develop qualitative and quantitative models for the prediction of blend homogeneity and the characterization of powder mixing kinetics by in-line (real time) NIRS. The models were built for binary mixtures of SA, as representative of an API, and Fast-Flo lactose, as representative of an excipient; the tests were conducted in an 8-qt (7.6 l) PK V-blender. The three main variables tested were: environmental conditions (humidity levels of 20 and 60%), API level (3–11%) and blender rotation speed (12.8–20.3 rpm). The D-optimal experimental design resulted in a sufficiently robust model. Real time NIR spectra were obtained through 12 sapphire windows. Reference sampling was undertaken at 10 different blender locations with an in-house-built multi-compartment thief probe. The reference analytical method was API quantification through UV spectroscopy. Although thief sampling can introduce a bias due to local segregation phenomena (invasive sampling), enhanced by the fact that the binary mixture is rather non-cohesive (quite free-flowing), NIR calibration was done on the same samples and, consequently, systematic error was averted. The rough spectral data were pre-treated by a second derivative, which proved to be more efficient than standard normal variate and multiplicative scatter correction. The authors discovered that principal components regression (PCR) and PLS models were not very efficient. This conclusion was attributed to a systematic NIRS error from the difference in powder compaction between the calibration samples and real time data acquisition (DR). It is well known that both PSD and powder bed void space have a significant impact on NIR spectra. Multi-term linear regression (MLR) and a significant decrease in the number of wavelengths taken into consideration have significantly improved these models; thus, they reported that from the initial seven wavelengths chosen only one seemed to be significant. Finally, these authors determined (without giving more details) that the models over-predicted potency (API concentration). They attributed this positive bias to the difference between off-line (samples scanned outside the blender for calibration) and in-line (through sapphire ports) NIRS. They also adopted the method to evaluate the intensity of intra-shell vs inter-shell mixing kinetics. They divided the optical ports into five groups with the assumption that ports ranging horizontally showed the intra-shell while those arranged vertically disclosed inter-shell mixing characteristics. The results revealed that intra-shell was significantly faster that inter-shell mixing kinetics, leading to the conclusion that it was precarious to trust single-port NIRS data monitoring to decide the blending end-point. They also demonstrated that it was preferable to load the ingredients to be blended equally in the two V-blender arms. Although these studies were very useful, they were only an incremental effort and indicated, more clearly, the way to go. The conclusions were indicative of the following:

- Even for binary mixtures, the building of a sufficiently reliable and robust model was difficult.
- The relative mobility of ingredients within the mixture (cohesiveness) was an important factor to consider.
- In-line DR-NIRS data-mining could be successful, but NIR calibration with external samples was a source of error (compaction).
- V-blenders were anisotropic in terms of mixing kinetics, and the extent of this behavior may be affected by the nature of the powder mixtures and operating conditions.

Since powder mixing kinetics is of importance, Portillo et al. [27] worked on producing a new method, called the "compartments model." Recognizing that a deterministic model relying on discrete elements (particles) dynamics simulation was not yet possible because of intensive calculation needs, they proposed a compartment modeling approach. They were inspired by the effort to model fluid mixing in reactors, incorporating micro-mixing mechanisms, including turbulence. Compartment modeling relies on the assumption that the solid blender can be spatially discretized to a number of compartments (subsections), which are assumed to be perfectly mixed. Over time, flow occurs between these compartments, allowing the exchange of particles. This flow represents convective/dispersive mixing components in opposition to the diffusive component encountered exclusively within the boundaries of each compartment. The model was built on sampling within five pre-defined (rather arbitrarily) compartments that lay vertical to the rotation axis and slightly tilted with regard to rotation direction. Thus, each compartment had only two boundaries with adjacent compartments, and there were no triple boundary points. The model was a binary mixture composed of monodisperse particles with different sizes, chemical identities, and colors. The paper provided information on the effects of sampling location, number and size of samples, size of particles, and sampling time on model efficiency. This work was interesting academically but the produced model cannot yet be directly applied in monitoring industrial pharmaceutical blending. It is ideal because the particles used have ideal forms and are monodisperse. There is insufficient information on the nature of the particles and the sampling technique. It is also curious that the study does not make reference to the endeavor of El-Hagrasy et al. [26] to calculate mixing kinetics. It would be interesting to examine the compartment model by relying on the kinetic observations of this paper.

Zhang et al. [28] implemented the hidden Markov model (HMM) to recognize patterns in pharmaceutical blending from in-line NIRS. A binary, rather cohesive mixture, composed of 65%w/w wheat and 35%w/w corn powders, was tested. The experiments were performed in a custom-made blender (stirred tank) not well described in the paper. Although it is understood that the target was data-mining and analysis rather than process, the fact that the set-up was not used industrially was quite limiting. The authors compared the more conventional moving block of standard deviation (MBSD) technique to the proposed HMM. Derived from the Markov chain, the HMM holds that the output of a process is a function of the immediately previous state and that history of the event does not play any role. It should be noted that, in time-series phenomena, time increment size is crucial. A HMM is different in that the previous states are not observable, but rather derived (estimated) by observations. A HMM is characterized by two probabilities: transition, which gives the probability of transit to another state, and output, the probability of reaching one of the known output states. The reported results are satisfactory and lead to the main conclusion that random (unmodeled) noise is essentially eliminated; however, this is replaced by a much more intensive model training and calculation effort. Moreover, due to its nature, an HMM model for one mixing condition is independent from the others. Finally, as expected, the model's efficiency relies on the two main model parameters, N and M, where N are the hidden states, and M, the number of observation symbols. The latter require optimization every time the model is to be used. The utility of this model – which is based on an assumption that is slightly more realistic than that of the Markov chain in the case of pharmaceutical blending – depends upon the successfulness of its optimization.

Wu and Khan [29] of the FDA published incremental work in the area of NIRS in an effort to propose an integrated strategy for evaluating powder blending process end-point and kinetics within the actually-prevailing QbD-driven pharmaceutical engineering environment. They tested a multi-component mixture made up of three excipients; Microcristalline cellulose (MCC); Hydroxy Propyl Methyl Cellulose (HPMC), and Eudragit L 100–55 with ibuprofen as API. The mixing runs were performed in a Turbula-Shaker mixer (www.wab.ch/en/mischer.html) operated at 72 rpm at very low scale (5 g batch run). NIR measurements were done by stopping the mixer at pre-defined time points and taking NIR scans by inserting an NIR transflectance probe inside the turbula vial. The authors say that their work demonstrated the possibility of an integrated QbD approach to understanding blending processes but unfortunately, at their process scale, the only useful point was the feasibility of following blending evolution with a specific probe in an environment with none of the problems and error sources encountered in real industrial scale.

Lapointe-Garant et al. [30] attempted to derive qualitative chemometric models to predict pharmaceutical blending end-points. Their work provided valuable data because it was one of the most realistic, the reason being that a Wyeth, now Pfizer, proprietary vitamin formulation, containing 16 different ingredients, was studied. Their NIRS system was a Micro electro-mechanical system (MEMS)-based spectrometer, giving spectral coverage of 1350–1800 nm and an acquisition time of less than 100 ms. The measuring probe provided 40-mm spot size, and penetration of the sample was estimated to be about 1 mm. The instrument was installed directly on the V-blender, and a sapphire window was mounted on the cover of the blender at the spot where the NIR probe made the NIR reflectance measurement. The system communicated with a laptop computer through a Wi-Fi wireless connection and could be trigger-operated to automatically acquire a NIR spectrum at a specified point in rotation time-space. The trigger activated NIR acquisition when the blender was upside down with powder fully blanketing the V-blender's cover. The powder was considered to be in a static state when powder analysis was performed. Each rotation triggered an acquisition, and each acquisition generated four NIR spectra averaged in a single spectrum for a total acquisition time of 400 ms, excluding software integration. This averaging helped in increasing the signal-to-noise ratio. To best model a typical production batch, 1-ft^3 (28.5 l) laboratory-scale batches in the study underwent the same manufacturing procedure as production batches except that there was no side-mixing. In other words, entire vitamin formula ingredients were added to the V-blender separately, creating a maximum state of segregation before any mixing.

Two types of blend homogeneity analyses were presented in the study, each having its own strengths and weaknesses.

The first method relied on Mean block standard deviation (MBSD), but when variance calculation (Eq. 15.1) was replaced by Eq. 15.2, the MBSD gave significantly improved results. Note that σ^2 of Eq. 15.2 is always higher that σ^2 of Eq. 15.1.

$$\sigma^2 = \frac{\sum_{i=1}^{N}\left(A_i^{t_i} - A_i^{t_{i-1}}\right)^2}{N} \tag{15.1}$$

Conventional formula for variance

$$\delta^2 = \frac{\sum_{i=1}^{N}\left|A_i^{t_i 2} - A_i^{t_0 2}\right|}{N} \tag{15.2}$$

Modified variance formula: σ^2

The second method, termed "distance analysis," relies on the comparison of every newly-acquired spectrum during a batch with a reference group of spectra. The reference group must be carefully chosen to represent a homogeneous state of the studied formula. A dimension less distance value is then computed between the newly-acquired spectrum and the reference group. When that distance is less than a pre-defined limit value, the blend is homogeneous and the mixing process can be stopped. Many types of mathematical tools can compute the distance between the reference group and the newly-acquired spectrum. For instance, the Mahalanobis distance is such a mathematical tool; it was first introduced in 1936. The tool assigns a different weight to every variable; in our case, every wavelength. The reference group is first described in vector space, and variables with the most significant variations are assigned a weight of greater magnitude in the analysis. The Hotelling T^2 distance investigated in this study is similar to the Mahalanobis distance but does not use a covariance matrix. It performs best when applied to scores of variables after PCA. The two methods have proven to be efficient, and each one has advantages and disadvantages that are described in columns 1 and 2 of Table 15.2.

Abatzoglou et al. [31] added a quantitative model for 8 among 16 ingredients of the mixture system reported in Lapointe-Garant et al. [30]. Quantification model building required very meticulous development because of the high complexity level. The large number of ingredients and the low concentration of some of them increased model complexity and may lead to significant errors. The process for model development is highlighted in Figure 15.1.

Table 15.2 *Comparative study of NIR blend analysis. Reprinted with permission from* EPR, Real-Time NIR Monitoring of Pharmaceutical Blending Process with Multivariate Quantitative Models *by N. Abatzoglou et al., 5, 57–67. Copyright (2005) Russell Publishing Co.*

Qualitative study		Quantitative study
Variance study	Distance study	PLS
Pros • Quick implementation for every formula. • Lower error due to reference selection. • Spectral pre-process less critical.	**Pros** • Precise information about blending state. • Can detect wrong components or wrong concentrations. • Moderate modeling effort required.	**Pros** • Detailed information about the blending state of each component quantified. • Precise evaluation of mixing time. • Monitoring of individual components.
Cons • No information about component concentrations. • No information about types of components. • Can slightly underestimate blending time. • Should be used with statistical process control rules.	**Cons** • No information about component concentrations. • Spectral pre-process is critical. • Reference is critical.	**Cons** • Heavy modeling effort required. • Spectral pre-process is critical. • No information about the entire formula unless every ingredient is quantified (which may be problematic in complex formulations). • Difficult to assess true model error when scale changes (i.e. scale-up at production level).

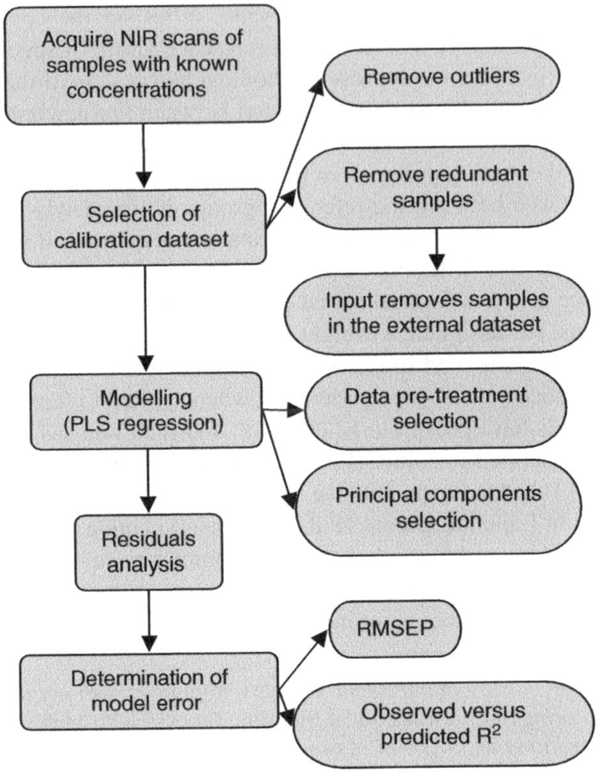

Figure 15.1 *Model development process. Reprinted with permission from* EPR, Real-Time NIR Monitoring of Pharmaceutical Blending Process with Multivariate Quantitative Models *by N. Abatzoglou et al., 5, 57–67. Copyright (2005) Russell Publishing Co.*

The authors also proceeded to a scale-up of the method. A multivariate model developed in lab-scale experiments may perform well in laboratory trials, but scale-up of the model is not always straightforward. Ideally, a model should be developed with NIR spectra acquired during a full-scale production batch so that every possible noise is taken into account in model-building, knowing it is plausible that noises are a function of the unit operation scale. Thus, the same MEMS-based NIR system was fitted on a full-scale production V-blender with 125 ft^3 of working volume. The probe of the system employed to acquire NIR spectra was fixed to a specially-modified V-blender's cover equipped with a sapphire window. Trigger acquisition was set for four spectra per turn averaged as one.

The batch monitored followed the regular manufacturing process of Wyeth Pharmaceuticals, now Pfizer, for the targeted formula. It included two mixing steps in the V-blender, an initial mixing step of 20 min for every vitamin and mineral, and a second mixing step for lubricant addition. Note that the full-scale production process comprised several pre-mix operations performed in smaller blenders to better disperse low-concentration ingredients.

Scale-up of the model seemed adequate although it was unfeasible to compare actual production NIR scans with lab references. Only few of the ingredients actually stabilized around 100% of the theoretical input value. Even though model scale-up was adequate, the actual error of measurement was higher than the relative mean standard error of prediction (RMSEP) values obtained in the lab-scale study. This error was not measurable in the production-scale study. Moreover, the same kind of correlation was observed for low-concentration ingredients.

Recently the potential of multiple point NIR spectroscopy has emerged and tested for pharmaceutical blending applications [31]. The spatial nature of the approach helped detecting good and poor mixing positions inside the blender that are affected by convective and diffusive mixing. A commercial offering that does not require switching between the probes has been developed (MultiEye™, Innopharmalabs, Ireland).

Although NIRS spectra are complex, owing to the lack of peak specificity, the technique is becoming increasingly interesting because of these promises. The elements responsible for this attractiveness are:

- Recent technical advances.
- The availability of many MEMS-based in-line and wireless data acquisition NIRS apparatuses in the market.
- Multi-point NIR spectroscopy technology for spatial analysis
- Progress in chemometrics and software on the market that make data-mining, NIRS calibration, statistical modeling and statistical process control easier.

Recently, Anderson et al. [33] have published a quite comprehensive chapter in the *Handbook of NIR Spectroscopy* describing the Pharmaceutical applications of NIR spectroscopy. They include the measurement of blend uniformity in both dry formulation and wet granulation processes.

15.4 Raman Spectroscopy (RS)

The Raman phenomenon was observed and reported by Raman in the 1930s. When photons excite a vibrational molecule to a high energy level there are three outcomes: (1) drop back to the initial energy level by emitting a photon of equal frequency as the incident excitation photon (scattering); (2) fall back but to slightly higher energy than the initial level with synchronous emission of a red-shifted (lower than the initial) photon, and (3) fall back but at slightly lower energy than the initial level with the synchronous emission of a blue-shifted (higher than the initial) photon. Case (2) is called the Stokes shift, and case (3), the anti-Stokes shift. The reason why scattering was known earlier was that cases (2) and (3) were characterized by very low probability (1 out of 10^7 photons were so shifted), and their detection was initially impossible. RS relies on the Stokes shift. Since the shift is a function of chemical bond nature and intensity is a function of molecule concentration, RS can be both a qualitative and quantitative analytical technique [34, 35, 36].

RS is based on monochromatic incident light usually from a laser source in the visible, NIR or near-UV range. The rich literature in the field defines all types of RS modes and possible applications. The pharmaceutical applications of RS have been gathered and presented by Šašić [37] in his homonymous book. Although RS can be exploited in various pharmaceutical engineering fields, the target here is blending and we report on it.

Vergote et al. [38] studied Fourier transform-RS to monitor an in-line blending process of diltiazem hydrochloride pellets and paraffinic wax beads in a 4-l planetary SS-bowl mixer equipped with a K-shaped mixer arm. A fiber optic Raman probe was attached to a 20-mm diameter glass window positioned at the wall, 10 cm from the bottom of the mixer bowl. A conventional end-sampling thief probe collected samples and analyzed them off-line by high performance/pressure liquid chromatography (HPLC). Mean square of differences between two consecutive spectra served to evaluate the evolution of the mixing process over time. These relatively simple experiments depicted an interesting potential for RS, but since they were performed in an apparatus of much lower than industrial-scale processes, it would be highly risky to pretend that they are extendable to that scale.

Hausman et al. [39] applied 785-nm on-line RS to study blend uniformity in a pharmaceutical formulation composed of a "low-dose" API (1%w/w azimilide dihydrochloride) in spray-dried lactose, crospovidone and magnesium stearate. They used a variable-speed 8-qt transparent PK V-blender. Azimilide was added to the bottom of the blender, followed by lactose, crospovidone and magnesium stearate. The components were mixed at 6.75 rpm until the end-point for the experiment was reached. Blender content was monitored in-line by RS. The fiber optic probe was inserted into the blender through the I-bar port. Raman spectra were collected every 20 s. The 20-s sampling interval allowed for averaging of two rotations, considered as representative sampling of the entire blend. Sample size probed by RS during these experiments was calculated to be approximately 1 mg, based on an estimated number of particles exposed to the laser during acquisition time. The results were analyzed by both univariate (peak corresponding to the API) and multivariate chemometrics; both delivered successful API predictions, even at API concentrations as low as 0.1%w/w, attributed to the particular sensitivity of RS for this API. The data indicate that RS is as efficient as end-point determination by thief sampling and off-line HPLC analysis. Although the authors concluded that the method could be extended (scaled-up) to automatically control the blending end-point, it remains unknown whether this has been done.

Šašić [37] reported that LaPlant and Romero (2005) also applied RS to study blending via a lab-scale bin blender and a non-contact 785 nm RS probe interfaced with samples via a sapphire window. Conventional chemometrics were undertaken (PCA), and the end-point was monitored by calculating the most significant PC score value over time (or blender rotation); thus, a PC1 equal to zero meant that the blending end-point was reached.

Jayawickrama et al. [40] published their results on the potential of RS application in various pharmaceutical manufacturing processes, among which blend uniformity in a tablet press conduit. A non-contact Raman probe (785 nm, 6-mm spot size, 250-mm focal length, with a 7" extension tube) was mounted onto a Teflon holder, which, in turn, was mounted on a clear plexiglass feed conduit before tablet compression. The Raman probe was located outside the feeder just below the level sensor. The Raman data were recorded continuously during tablet compression with 30-s exposure time and two accumulations. The method assured the in-line evaluation of 1 dose unit per analysis, the sought scrutiny level. A two principal components (PCs) partial least squares-type 1 (PLS1) multivariate calibration model was developed for laboratory-prepared samples to obtain predicted quantitative blend uniformity values from Raman data. The results were in good agreement with off-line HPLC analysis, demonstrating good potential for scale-up and industrial application. We are not aware of such scale-up and adoption of the method for real industrial manufacturing time.

De Beer et al. [41] set out to propose a strategy for implementing a PAT system in the blending step of pharmaceutical production processes. In fact, the real output of their work was the evaluation of a 785-nm Raman spectrometer as an in-line non-invasive technique to monitor pharmaceutical formulation blending as well as its comparison with a similar but NIR-based technique. These authors tested diltiazem HCl as API, with Avicel PH 102, lactose DCL 21, and SiO_2 as additives/excipients. The probable reason is that the high Raman signal of diltiazem HCl renders its RS analysis easy. The mixing equipment in the RS study was a Gral™ 10 high shear mixer from GEA-Collette, and the Raman signal was acquired through a fiber optic immersion probe attached to the wall of the mixer bowl. NIR-RS comparison was performed in a larger mixer (Gral™ 75 high shear mixer from GEA-Collette) and without an API (diltiazem HCl). NIR and RS spectra were acquired simultaneously, but the NIR probe was inserted from the top of the blender and the RS probe at the side. This introduced an obvious bias, but since the target was to evaluate the end-point of the mixing process, with a statistical tool (i.e., comparison of the mean standard deviation (MSD) between consecutive spectra), the method was appropriate. The conclusions were very positive. RS proved to be efficient, and NIR and RS were equivalent in predicting the mixing end-point. Although the methodology was well-described and valid, the results were just confirming previous knowledge, and their utility was limited in that the RS equipment was efficient. Since these systems are multivariate and equipment-specific, direct industrial scale-up is not possible if the mixer type is changed.

Recently, Salvas et al. [42] worked on RS to evaluate the possibility of replacing actually-used QC of the final solid dosage forms (pharmaceutical tablets) by an at least as efficient but faster and less cost-intensive technique. Although their work did not address blending issues, the conclusions can be helpful in future works in this field and they are briefly reported here. The study tried to determine the influence that calibration parameters have on multivariate predictive model performance, and as an output, to render such a method more generalized and less case-specific. In previous literature, the only paper related to the subject was by Blanco et al. [43], who investigated the effects that two-sample preparation procedures had on NIRS performance in quantitative pharmaceutical analyses. Huang et al. [44] compared the robustness of NIRS-based predictive models elaborated by different multivariate techniques. They studied least square regression, ridge regression and various PLS regressions (–2, 3 and 4) in the context of varying dataset size. They demonstrated "that the relative performance of calibration methods depends on calibration data size for a given dataset." This work, while addressing the topic of calibration data size, did not cover calibration itself. Salvas et al. [42] evaluated the effect of 8 independent parameters on the performance of the predictive model developed. The parameters were not examined separately but rather in relation to one another, so any potential interaction could be investigated. The main advantage and contribution of this approach is that the whole development protocol is assessed at once, and the resulting, optimized recommendations are applicable to most future situations. More specifically, it was found that the number and, most importantly, the possibility of selecting an adequate set of calibration points among the total number had a very significant influence on model performance. Using more replicates of the same points did not contribute to the final performance and, hence, savings could be achieved by acquiring less PAT measurements. The contribution is original because the most frequently-encountered recommendation regarding calibration samples is "the more the better," but producing more points is more costly and more time-consuming, so if no tangible gain is made, it is not that much better. The conclusions obtained from this work are, hence, a good basis to take a reasonable decision regarding the total number of samples to be manufactured for calibration purposes. Moreover, reference measurements, which are usually considered as an "absolute must," were found not to contribute significantly to model performance. Also, it has been proven that the manufacturing method for development samples does not have a significant impact on model performance as long as it allows homogenous samples to be obtained.

Ten years ago, RS was considered to be a capital and operating cost-intensive technique. Moreover, there were few and not very reliable probes with real time in-line analytical capabilities. Recent technical advances led to less expensive and reliable hardware, and techno-economic feasibility is nowadays relying on precision, accuracy and sensitivity. RS is expected to become a successful PAT tool for at least a part of solids-blending operations.

15.5 Image Analysis

Image analysis is not a new technique; however, advances in computer science and, consequently, in calculation capacity, have improved its possibilities considerably. Since solids and, in our case, particularly pharmaceutical solids, are complex micro-heterogeneous systems whose behavior depends, namely, upon their morphology, micro-imaging is seen more and more as an interesting method. But how could this technique be linked with these mixing systems? In pharmaceutical manufacturing, the size distribution of mixed solids is pre-defined because it can affect various organoleptic and pharmacokinetic properties and, consequently, it is not really a physical parameter to be followed during the mixing step. This prevails unless the parameter changes over the duration of mixing to an extent that can be detrimental to the marketed final product. However, there are specific cases where the technique can provide PAT-sensitive and highly valuable information. These cases are:

- When mixed materials have significant size distribution differences.
- When in-line, non-invasive PAT is to be used for the evaluation of chemical composition of the blend over time as well as the prediction and determination of end-points, and since they are size-sensitive (i.e., NIRS, LIF), their combination with imaging can provide interesting solutions.

Visual characterization in pharmaceutical powders is not a well-developed field and is never reported in the literature as a technology for in-line blending evaluation, either quantitatively or qualitatively. However, for the reasons cited previously, we will describe some efforts made concerning other pharmaceutical particulate systems image analysis. Laitinen et al. [45] applied surface image analysis aimed at the in-line evaluation of PSD in two processes involved in granulation: spraying and drying. The method is presented as part of the PAT context. Surface images were taken under controlled illumination conditions (a light source and a monochrome CCD camera). The procedure, from the pictures to the calculation of PSD, encompasses the following steps:

- Two images of each sample are taken by illuminating the sample once from its left and then from its right.
- This produces two digital images with matrices, of which pixels belong to grayscale.
- The difference in the two digital images is then calculated based on grayscale whose resolution is pre-defined. For the theoretical (blank), completely smooth surface, the

difference is a matrix with zeros. In this work, for real images, the scale ranges between −255 and +255.

- The same sample is analyzed with sieving, which gives PSD.
- The procedure allows the development of a multivariate PLS model. In fact, in the PLS model, X was the gray scale difference matrix and Y was the sieve analysis result.

The technique has also been successful in correlating the PSD of a sample with the properties of tablets produced from the sample. Thus, normalized, successful image analysis could predict the specifications of a pharmaceutical tablet.

Realpe and Velázquez [46] described an image processing and analysis technique named "invariant image moments" that is able to characterize pharmaceutical powder morphology and size. Since some critical pharmaceutical product specifications are a function of these two characteristics, they propose the technique as a PAT tool.

Previously, in 2003, the same authors [47] had published their work on image processing and analysis for the determination of concentrations in powder mixtures. They undertook NIR in parallel to develop and validate their univariate and multivariate prediction models. This is perhaps the only known work able to be used in blending. However, it has a serious limitation: the method functions only if the components to be measured have significantly different colors.

Recently a real-time stereoscopic imaging approach has been developed specifically for the pharmaceutical industry (EyeconTM, Innopharmalabs, Dublin, Ireland). The technology consists of a fast and sensitive camera synchronized with illumination from a ring of five red, five green and five blue pulsed LEDs. The illumination is based on the principle of photometric stereo imaging and the color distribution on the sample employed to provide topological information, which, in turn permits the identification of particle edges for size determination [48]. The approach has been assessed against reference techniques [48] and for monitoring of particle size during twin screw granulation [49]. Figure 15.2 shows the technology integrated into a spheronization process.

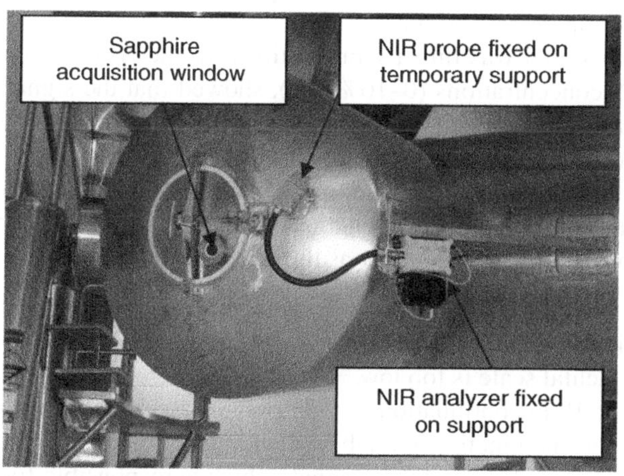

Figure 15.2 *NIR installed on the 125-ft^3 V-blender. Reprinted with permission from* EPR, Real-Time NIR Monitoring of Pharmaceutical Blending Process with Multivariate Quantitative Models *by N. Abatzoglou et al., 5, 57–67. Copyright (2005) Russell Publishing Co.*

15.6 LIF Spectroscopy

LIF is another non-invasive technique whose potential to monitor on- or in-line pharmaceutical blending processes has been assessed during the last 10 years. A significant number of molecules in pharmaceutical formulations, both APIs and excipients, have the possibility of being excited when irradiated at a suitable wavelength and emitted at another wavelength, a phenomenon called fluorescence. The theory of fluorescence is well described in [50].

LIF has very interesting properties because it is compound-specific and presents no hysteresis. It is also characterized by a high signal/noise ratio. This phenomenon causes problems to other methods, such as RS, because sometimes the emitted fluorescence hides Raman scattering. Nevertheless, this characteristic gives LIF the possibility to be used in the case of highly potent drugs in which the active ingredients to be measured are found in very low concentrations.

Lai et al. [51] presented a first R&D note in the area of LIF use in monitoring powder blending. Previous publications proved its successful application in monitoring liquids and gases in the automotive and biomedical sectors (Beer, 1995 and Alfano, 1998 in [51]). More academically, Unger and Muzzio in [51] employed the technique to monitor liquid mixing in impinging jets.

In this work, the authors tested triamterene as an API because of its very high fluorescence properties. Testing was done at small lab-scale: a 20-ml glass micro-blender filled to 60% capacity (8 g) with a binary mixture containing 0–10%w/w triamterene in an anhydrous lactose excipient (100–90%w/w). The LIF Ar 488-nm laser beam was directed at a single fixed position (1/3 from the top or the bottom of the powder level) for 20 min at a rotation speed of 20 rpm. The main results from this work were:

- Powder bulk density had a directly proportional effect on LIF signals. The tested density range was 0.45–0.8 kg/l.
- Blending end-point (time to reach homogeneity) was not affected by the loading mode: triamterene at the top or the bottom.
- Although the LIF signal was directly proportional to the API concentration, the tests, with various API concentrations (0–10%w/w), showed that the signal vs concentration function was not linear. Linearity was only obtained at low concentrations (0–1%). This was attributed to saturation of the output signal detector and constitutes an important finding because if LIF is used for quantitative monitoring, all parameters (i.e., source laser power intensity, excitation wavelength, detector sensitivity) must be optimized with non-saturation of the available detector as the criterion.

It was not clear in this paper which and how standard deviation was calculated. Finally, it is difficult to decide whether the technique would be of interest at the industrial level because the experimental scale is too low.

Lai and Cooney [52], in continuation of their previous work, reported on a portable LIF system to monitor on-line kinetics in a lab-scale, tumbler-type blender. They still worked with triamterene because of its high LIF signal, which is responsible for its low detection limit (0.02%w/w). Anhydrous lactose was still used as principal excipient and a small dose (0.1%w/w) of Carbosil was added as flow enhancer. The LIF probe was operated at 480 nm, which was found to be optimally strong/weak for this highly fluorescent API. Higher excitation was obtained at 400 nm (16 times stronger than at 480 nm), but had to be used only for API concentration typically lower than 1%w/w. The two blenders were still small (minibins), made from poly-ethylene-terephthalate (PET). They were cylinders of 130-ml and 400-ml total volume respectively, and they had the same shape ratio. They were harnessed at 50% working volume. Moreover, to check feasibility with other formulations, they also tested the method on Amoxicillin (a fluorescent API) in a mixture with Orlistat (a non-fluorescent excipient). Another mixture, made of an undisclosed API in spray-dried lactose monohydrate and microcrystalline cellulose, was finally LIF-tested in a 50-ml V blender at also 50% working volume. The LIF measurements (concentrations) were validated by thief sampling and UV spectroscopy after sample dilution in methanol. These observations and results, although difficult to extrapolate directly to higher scale, are very interesting because they give numerous indications regarding the characteristics and the main attributes of this method of analysis. The most important are:

- It is essential to have precise information about LIF excitation wavelengths as well as fluorescence wavelengths for each compound.
- The method can be applied only if the components emit fluorescence at distinct wavelengths. The authors do not mention if there is still a possibility, in this restrictive case, of applying multivariate instead of univariate statistical analysis and modeling.
- This work provided information on the penetration depth of LIF in powders and showed that the emission signal's intensity decreased exponentially over depth, but there was a point where the decrease (first derivative of the signal over depth) levelled off, most probably because of random photon migration. Of course, these data changed for each packing density, wavelength and particle distribution. All developers in the field have to take these details into consideration.
- Testing with three different API concentrations distinguished the three mixing mechanisms (1: convective; 2: shear; 3: diffusive), but this was expected, and the only useful observation was that LIF worked appropriately for qualitative estimation of the end-point.
- The two different volume bin blenders gave similar results, but since the scale between them was only 2:1 and their working volume was small, definite conclusions were not possible.
- As with all in-line, non-invasive, spectroscopic techniques, the quality of the reading windows is critical. Thus, sticky material that can adhere to the window prevents the LIF technique from being efficient, and additional measures must be taken to clean it continuously or periodically.

In a very recent paper Karumanchi et al. [53] have tested LIF as a PAT tool and established a relationship between LIF and HPLC analysis to determine mixing profiles and end-point in pharmaceutical powder blending. All blending was done at the facilities of a pharmaceutical company (GSK) using a Metolift post blender and a 124 L intermediate bulk container. Fluorescence detection was accomplished using a Honeywell on-purpose built LIF sensor with a xenon strobe light source and photomultiplier tube style detector. The strobe had an adjustable energy range of 100–180 mJ at 1–20 Hz. The wavelength range was 190–650 nm and was configured with excitation and emission filters appropriate to the API used. Although the work is rather factual and targeted in evaluating the feasibility of monitoring powder blending evolution with an LIF-based methodology, it reports results allowing for the determination of local blending efficiency by identifying locations in the 124 L mixing tote as potential dead spots.

15.7 Effusivity

Effusivity of a body is defined as the square root of the product of thermal conductivity (k), density (ρ) and heat capacity (C_p). It macroscopically describes the body's capacity to receive and transmit a quantity of heat to its environment. Since each substance has its known effusivity, the latter was employed by Mathews et al. [54] to monitor the degree of homogeneity of powder mixtures by measuring mixture effusivity at different locations in a V-blender. As effusivity can be monitored in-line, it has been proposed as a PAT.

Léonard et al.[55] investigated effusivity, density, and UV spectroscopy in an attempt to evaluate the technical feasibility of effusivity as a PAT tool in pharmaceutical powder blending. The main conclusion is that density (both bulk and real) of the mixture and its components is a critical attribute.

15.8 Other Potential Sensor Technologies

Terahertz spectroscopy (TS) and Terahertz pulsed spectroscopy (TPS) are other non-destructive spectroscopic methods proposed recently as having the potential to become PAT tools. TS uses the far-infrared radiation of the electromagnetic spectrum, extending from 60 GHz to 4 THz (2–130 cm^{-1}). The energy contained in such radiation is lower than most internal vibrations of the molecules, but it is absorbed by intermolecular vibration modes. This property enables TS to detect and differentiate the crystalline properties of solid materials. Regarding Terahertz radiation, the best known way of producing it [56] is by exploiting sources of incoherent blackbody radiation, such as mercury arc lamps. However, it can be generated by femtosecond lasers and special photoconductive semiconductor antenna switches, even at room temperatures. Detection is achieved through a time-gated, coherent detection scheme using electro-optic sampling.

Taday [57] evaluated TS as a PAT tool, studying potency levels in paracetamol (4-acetamidophenol) and aspirin (ASA) test tablets by chemometrics and, more specifically, PLS models. They demonstrated its high potential but mainly high cost, and the absence of most systematically-driven studies has not yet permitted greater TS application. Zeitler et al. [58] undertook TPS for the physical characterization of pharmaceuticals (carbamazepine as API). This possibility arises from the fact that these techniques are able to quantify crystalline forms (physical characteristics).

Ho et al. [59] analyzed the coating quality of pharmaceutical tablets by Terahertz pulsed imaging (TPI). Terahertz radiation (2–120 cm^{-1}) is particularly interesting for coating analysis as it has the capability of penetrating most pharmaceutical excipients, and, hence, allows non-destructive coating analysis. TPS was employed to determine Terahertz refractive indexes on the sustained-release excipients used in this study. Moreover, Zeitler et al. [60] published a review on TPS and TPI for the physical characterization of pharmaceutical drug materials and final solid dosage forms. Their review focused on the development and performance of pharmaceutical applications of Terahertz technology compared with other tools for physical characterization.

So far, there are no studies on the application of TS techniques in pharmaceutical mixing. However, we report it because quantifying crystalline forms is possible in some mixing operations when the blend contains TS-recognizable crystalline materials and follows their presence as a function of mixing time.

15.9 Comments on PAT in Liquid Formulation Mixing

Liquid mixing is a much easier and highly-studied area. Its full development would fall outside the scope of this book. However, in-line QC of such a pharmaceutical operation is rather difficult, and almost all existing manufacturing procedures rely on statistical QC. There is no available information on in-line analysis (PAT) techniques for liquid mixing in the pharmaceutical industry. Wyeth Montreal – now a Pfizer company – announced the first PAT in 2008 in the field by implementing physical analysis based on in-line monitoring of the refractive index of the blend over time. The results were impressive and cut cycle time by a factor of at least three-fold. Although the author contributed in this endeavor, so far no permission has been granted to make the method and the results publicly available.

Although other pre-cited spectrometric techniques could be evaluated, the fact that liquid is under continuous movement is problematic. This is not the case with tumbling blenders where powder at the bottom profits from some quasi-immobility for a brief but sufficient time for spectrometric analysis. Nevertheless, if the effects of various types of movement (process understanding) are known, chemometrics could be deployed efficiently to quantitatively evaluate side-effects and attain high quality in-line chemical and/or physical analysis of liquid mixtures.

References

[1] Food and Drug Administration, *Advisory Committee for Pharmaceutical Science*, November 28; available online at http://www.fda.gov/ohrms/dockets/ac/01/slides/3804s1.htm (accessed January 9, 2015) (2001).

[2] *Guidance for Industry PAT — A Framework for Innovative Pharmaceutical Development, Manufacturing, and Quality Assurance*, U.S. Department of Health and Human Services Food and Drug Administration, Center for Drug Evaluation and Research (CDER), Center for Veterinary Medicine (CVM), Office of Regulatory Affairs (ORA), Pharmaceutical CGMPs, http://www.fda.gov/cvm/guidance/published.html, September (2004).

[3] N. Abatzoglou, Pharmaceutical Industry/University collaboration R&D on Process Analytical Technologies, *Eur Pharm Rev.*, **2**, 42–45 (2010).

[4] N. Abatzoglou and J.S. Simard, Prediction of segregation tendency occurrence in dry particulate pharmaceutical mixtures: development of a mathematical tool adapted for granular systems application, *Pharm Dev Technol.*, **10**(1), 59–70 (2005).

[5] S.R. de Silva, A. Duroy, and G.G. Enstad, Segregation mechanisms and their quantification using segregation testers, in *IUTAM Symposium on Segregation in Granular Flows*, Kluwer Academic Publishers, Netherlands, p. 11–29 (2000).

[6] J.R. Johanson, Smooth out solids blending problems, *Chemical Engineering Progress*, **96**(4), 21–37 (2000).

[7] L.H. Cartilier and A.J. Moës, Effect of drug agglomerates upon the kinetics of mixing of low dosage cohesive powder mixtures, *Drug Dev. Ind. Pharm.*, **15**(12), 1911–1931 (1989).

[8] BMS PAT Team, *PAT for Drug Substance Particle Size Monitoring – A Process Development Case Study*, Presentation of October 23, 2003.

[9] J.C. Soto, C.P. Mez, W. Caraballo, C. Conde, T. Li, K.R. Morris, and R.J. Romanach, On line non-destructive determination of drug content in moving tablets using near infrared spectroscopy, *PAT The Journal of Process Analytical Technology*, **2**(5), 8–15 (2005).

[10] K. Pollanen, A. Hakkinen, S.P. Reinikainen, J. Rantanen, M. Karjalainen, M. Louhi-Kultanen, and L. Nystrom, IR spectroscopy together with multivariate data analysis as a process analytical tool for in-line monitoring of crystallization process and solid-state analysis of crystalline product, *Journal of Pharmaceutical and Biomedical Analysis*, **38**(2), 275–284 (2005).

[11] M.T. Islam, N. Rodriguez-Hornedo, S. Ciotti, and C. Ackermann, The potential of Raman spectroscopy as a process analytical technique during formulations of topical gels and emulsions, *Pharmaceutical Research*, **21**(10), 1844–1851 (2004).

[12] E.W. Ciurczak, Molecular Spectroscopy Workbench: Report from the 19th IFPAC/PAT Initiative Conference, *Spectroscopy*, **20**(3), 40–42 (2005).

[13] The Consortium for the Advancement of Manufacturing of Pharmaceuticals (CAMP), http://web.mit.edu/pharmi/Web_pages/CAMP.html (accessed January 13, 2015), *Light Induced Fluorescence for Pharmaceutical Products*, Final Report, MIT, December 31, 2000.

[14] E.J. Draheim and A.J. Ragauskas, NMR studies. II. Investigation of process analytical NMR techniques for the pulp and paper industry, *Journal of Wood Chemistry and Technology*, **17**(3), 287–296 (1997).

[15] T. Kourti, Multivariate dynamic data modeling for analysis and statistical process control for batch processes, start-ups and grade transitions, *J. of Chemom.*, **17**(1), 93–109 (2003).

[16] J.A. Lopes, P.F. Costa, T.P. Alves, and J.C. Menezes, Chemometrics in bioprocess engineering: process analytical technology (PAT) applications, *Chemometrics and Intelligent Laboratory Systems*, **74**(2), 269–275 (2004).

[17] E.W. Ciurczak and J.K. Drennen, Applications of near-IR spectroscopy in the pharmaceutical industry, *Spectroscopy*, **7**(6), 12–14 (1992).

[18] P.A. Hailey, P. Doherty, P. Tapsell, T. Oliver, and P.K. Aldridge, Automated system for the on-line monitoring of powder blending processes using near-infrared spectroscopy. Part I. System development and control, *Journal of Pharmaceutical and Biomedical Analysis*, **14**(5), 551–559 (1996).

[19] D.J. Wargo and J.K. Drennen, Near-infrared spectroscopic characterization of pharmaceutical powder blends, *Journal of Pharmaceutical and Biomedical Analysis*, **14**, 1415–1423 (1996).

[20] S.S. Sekulic, H.W. Ward II, D.R. Brannegan, E.D. Stanley, C.L. Evans, S.T. Sciavolino, P.A. Hailey, and P.K. Aldridge, On-Line monitoring of powder blend homogeneity by near-infrared spectroscopy, *Anal. Chem.*, **68**(3), 509–513 (1996).

[21] S.S. Sekulic, J. Wakeman, P. Doherty, and P.A. Hailey, Automated system for the on-line monitoring of powder blending processes using near-infrared spectroscopy Part II. Qualitative approaches to blend evaluation, *Journal of Pharmaceutical and Biomedical Analysis*, **17**, 1285–1309 (1998).

[22] C. Ufret and K. Morris, Modeling of powder blending using one-line near-infrared measurements, *Drug Development and Industrial Pharmacy*, **27**(7), 719–729 (2001).

[23] A.S. El-Hagrasy, H.R. Morris, F. D'Amico, R.A. Lodder, and J.K. Drennen III, Near-infrared spectroscopy and imaging for the monitoring of powder blend homogeneity, near-infrared spectroscopy and imaging for the monitoring of powder blend homogeneity, *Journal of Pharmaceutical Sciences*, **90**(9), 1298–1307 (2001).

[24] M. Blanco, R.G. Bano, and E. Bertran, Monitoring powder blending in pharmaceutical processes by use of near infrared spectroscopy, *Talanta*, **56**, 203–212 (2002).

[25] A.S. El-Hagrasy, F. D'Amico, and J.K. Drennen III, A process analytical technology approach to near-infrared process control of pharmaceutical powder blending. Part I: D-optimal design for characterization of powder mixing and preliminary spectral data evaluation, *Journal of Pharmaceutical Sciences*, **95**(2), 392–406 (2006).

[26] A.S. El-Hagrasy and J.K. Drennen III, A process analytical technology approach to near-infrared process control of pharmaceutical powder blending. Part III: Quantitative near-infrared calibration for prediction of blend homogeneity ond characterization of powder mixing kinetics, *Journal of Pharmaceutical Sciences*, **95**(2), 422–434 (2006).

[27] P.M. Portillo, F.J. Muzzio, and M.G. Ierapetritou, Characterizing powder mixing processes utilizing compartment model, *International Journal of Pharmaceutics*, **320**, 14–22 (2006).

[28] H. Zhang, Z. Jiang, J.Y. Pi, H.K. Xu, and R. Du, On-line monitoring of pharmaceutical production processes using hidden Markov model, *Journal of Pharmaceutical Sciences*, **98**(4), 1487–1498 (2009).

[29] H. Wu and M.A. Khan, Quality-By-Design (QbD): An integrated approach for evaluation of powder blending process kinetics and determination of powder blending end-point, *Journal of Pharmaceutical Sciences*, **98**(8), 2784–2798 (2009).

[30] P.-Ph. Lapointe-Garant, S. Simard and N. Abatzoglou, Real-time NIR monitoring of a pharmaceutical blending process through multivariate analysis-derived models, invited plenary lecture, *1st WSEAS International Conference on Multivariate Analysis and its Application in Science and Engineering (MAASE'08)*, Istanbul, Turkey, May 27–29 (2008), ISBN: 978–960–6766–68–8.

[31] N. Abatzoglou, P.-Ph. Lapointe-Garant, and J.-S. Simard, Real-time NIR monitoring of pharmaceutical blending processes with multivariate quantitative models, *European Pharmaceutical Review*, **5**, 57–67 (2009).

[32] O. Scheibelhofer, N. Balak, P.R. Wahl, D.M. Koller, B.J. Glasser, and J.G. Khinast. Monitoring blending of pharmaceutical powders with multipoint NIR spectroscopy. AAPS PharmSciTech, **14**, (1) (2013)

[33] C.A. Anderson, J.K. Drennen, and E.W. Ciurczak, Pharmaceutical applications of near-infrared spectroscopy, Chapter 30, in *Handbook of Near-Infrared Analysis*, M. Dekker (ed.), New York, **35**, 585–611 (2008), ISBN 084937393X.

[34] M. Schmitt and J. Popp, Raman spectroscopy at the beginning of the twenty-first century, *Journal of Raman Spectroscopy*, **37**(1–3), 20–28 (2006).

[35] E. Smith and G. Dent, *Modern Raman Spectroscopy – A Practical Approach*, John Wiley & Sons, Inc., Hoboken, 210p (2005).

[36] K.A. Bakeev, *Process Analytical Technology*, Blackwell Publishing, Oxford, 451p. (2005).

[37] S. Šašić (ed.), *Pharmaceutical Applications of Raman Spectroscopy,* S. Šašić, Wiley Series on Technologies for the Pharmaceutical Industry, S. Ekins, Series Editor, ISBN 978–0-8138–1013–3 (2008).

[38] G.J. Vergote, T.R.M. De Beer, and C. Vervaet et al. In-line monitoring of a pharmaceutical blending process using FT-Raman spectroscopy, *European Journal of Pharmaceutical Sciences*, **21**, 479–485 (2004).

[39] D.S. Hausman, R.T. Cambron, and A. Sakr, A. Application of Raman spectroscopy for on-line monitoring of low dose blend uniformity, *International Journal of Pharmaceutics*, **298**(1), 80–90 (2005).

[40] D. Jayawickrama, A. El Hagrasy, and S.Y. Chang, Raman applications in drug manufacturing processes, *American Pharmaceutical Review*, **9**(7), 10–17 (2006).

[41] T.R.M. De Beer, C. Bodson, B. Dejaegher, B. Walczak, P. Vercruyss, A. Burggraev, et al., Raman spectroscopy as a process analytical technology (PAT) tool for the in-line monitoring and understanding of a powder blending process, *Journal of Pharmaceutical and Biomedical Analysis*, **48**, 772–779 (2008).

[42] J. Salvas, J.-S. Simard, and N. Abatzoglou, Raman spectroscopy to analyze intact pharmaceutical tablets: Factors influencing MVPM-based PAT methods, *American Pharmaceutical Review,* **April**, 46–53 (2010).

[43] M. Blanco, J. Coello, H. Iturriaga, S. Maspoch, and N. Pou, Influence of the procedure used to prepare the calibration sample set on the performance of near infrared spectroscopy in quantitative pharmaceutical analyses, *The Analyst*, **126**(7), 1129–1134 (2001).

[44] J. Huang, D. Brennan, L. Sattler, J. Alderman, B. Lane, and C. O'Mathuna, A comparison of calibration methods based on calibration data size and robustness. *Chemometrics and intelligent laboratory systems*, **62**(1), 25–35 (2002).

[45] N. Laitinen, O. Antikainen, J. Rantanen, and J. Yliruusi, New perspectives for visual characterization of pharmaceutical solids, *Journal of Pharmaceutical Sciences*, **93**(1), 165–176 (2004).

[46] A. Realpe and C. Velázquez, Pattern recognition for characterization of pharmaceutical powders, *Powder Technology*, **169**, 108–113 (2006).

[47] A. Realpe and C. Velázquez, Image processing and analysis for determination of concentrations of powder mixtures, *Powder Technology*, **134**, 193–200 (2003).

[48] A. Silva. A. Burggraeve, Q. Denon, P. Van der Meeren, N. Sandler, T. Van Den Kerkhof, et al.. Particle sizing measurements in pharmaceutical applications: Comparison of in-process methods versus off-line methods. *European Journal of Pharmaceutics and Biopharmaceutics*, **85**(3) 1006–1018, (2013).

[49] A.S. El Hagrasy, P. Cruise, I. Jones, and J.D. Litster. In-line size monitoring of a twin screw granulation process using high-speed imaging. *J Pharm Innov.*, **8**(2), 90–98 (2013).
[50] C. Kaminski, *Planar Laser Induced Fluorescence*, University of Cambridge, Department of Chemical Engineering, 2002, June 24; available online at http://laser.cheng.cam.ac.uk/wiki/images/4/4e/MI_4.pdf (accessed January 9, 2015).
[51] C.K. Lai, D. Holt, J.C. Leung, C.L. Cooney, G.K. Raju, and P. Hansen, Real time and non-invasive monitoring of dry powder blend homogeneity, *AICHE Journal*, **47**(11), 2618–2622 (2001).
[52] C.K. Lai and C.C. Cooney, Application of a fluorescence sensor for mini-scale on-line monitoring of powder mixing kinetics, *Journal of Pharmaceutical Sciences*, **93**(1), 60–70 (2004).
[53] V. Karumanchi, M.K. Taylor, K.J. Ely, and W.C. Stagner, Monitoring powder blend homogeneity using light-induced fluorescence, *AAPS PharmSciTech*, **12**(4), 1031–1037 (2011).
[54] L. Mathews, C. Chandler, S. Dipali, P. Adusumilli, S. Lech, S. Daskalakis, and N. Mathis, Monitoring blend uniformity with effusivity, *Pharmaceutical Technology North America*, **26**(4), 80–84 (2002).
[55] G. Léonard, F. Bertrand, J. Chaouki, and P.M. Gosselin, An experimental investigation of effusivity as an indicator of powder blend uniformity, *Powder Technology*, **181**, 149–159 (2008).
[56] Ph.F. Taday and D.A. Newnham, Technological advances in terahertz pulsed systems bring far-infrared spectroscopy into the spotlight, *Spectroscopy Europe*, **16**(5), 20–24 (2004).
[57] Ph.F. Taday, Applications of terahertz spectroscopy to pharmaceutical sciences, *Philosophical Transactions of the Royal Society of London, Series A: Mathematical, Physical and Engineering Sciences*, **362**(1815), 351–364 (2004).
[58] J.A. Zeitler, Ph.F. Taday, M. Pepper, and T. Rades, Relaxation and crystallization of amorphous carbamazepine studied by terahertz pulsed spectroscopy, *Journal of Pharmaceutical Sciences*, **96**(10), 2703–2709 (2007).
[59] L. Ho, R. Mueller, M. Roemer, K.C. Gordon, J. Heinaemaeki, P. Kleinebudde, et al., Analysis of sustained-release tablet film coats using terahertz pulsed imaging, *Journal of Controlled Release*, **119**(3), 253–261 (2007).
[60] J.A. Zeitler, Ph.F. Taday, D.A. Newnham, M. Pepper, K.C. Gordon, and T. Rades, Terahertz pulsed spectroscopy and imaging in the pharmaceutical setting: A review, *Journal of Pharmacy and Pharmacology*, **59**(2), 209–223 (2007).

16
Imaging Fluid Mixing

Mi Wang
Institute of Particle Science and Engineering, School of Chemical and Process Engineering, University of Leeds, UK

16.1 Introduction

Flow visualization is one of most effective tools for understanding and characterizing complex, unsteady mixing processes. Over recent years, flow visualization technologies have undergone great advancement, which has changed our concept of vision from photographic-based 'seeing is believing' (Mann et al. 1995) to computer-based seeing 'without eyes' (Mann 2005). Typically, this progress can be demonstrated representatively by the development and application of Particle Image Velocimetry and Process Tomography.

Reflecting on the history of Process Analytical Technology (PAT) development, the techniques of imaging and point measurement have always progressed in conjunction. However, the application of imaging techniques in industry has somewhat lagged behind the status achieved in the field of medicine. Part of the reason may be the maturity of these technologies from the perspective of industrial users, including the lack of quantitative imaging and difficulty in image interpretation. Another explanation may stem from economic considerations and marketing demands. In recent years, flow visualization techniques have shifted the concept from qualitative picture to fully quantitative visualization based on multi-dimensional measurements, which are offering information of a type and level of detail that was previously associated only with numerical simulations. This shift has been, to a significant extent, a consequence of advances in computers and

Pharmaceutical Blending and Mixing, First Edition. Edited by P.J. Cullen, Rodolfo J. Romañach, Nicolas Abatzoglou and Chris D. Rielly.

related technologies during the same period. It has produced a revolution of sorts in the ability to experimentally visualize and analyse fluid flow in pipelines and process reactors, and allow on-line access to quantitative information on the three-dimensional spatial structure and temporal dynamics of complex flows, which had been almost unimaginable previously (Dahm and Southerland 2000). Facing the challenges presented by market globalization, PAT has been recognized as a framework for innovative process manufacturing and quality assurance of present and future industries. There is no doubt that advanced flow visualization techniques, as a part of PAT, will play an important role in modern process manufacture (Dahm and Southerland 2000), particularly, in mixing processes (Mavros 2001, Fagan et al. 2009).

Considering the important role of point measurement and visualization based on multiple points in the characterization of mixing processes, as well as in the evaluation of imaging results, a few conventional point measurement techniques are described briefly in this chapter, including the Pitot tube, conductivity cell, hot-wire anemometry and Laser Doppler anemometry. The greater part of the chapter describes non-invasive imaging techniques, including photographic imaging, digital particle image velocimetry and process tomography. Applications of process tomography, a promising novel technology, in mixing processes are described in outline, including magnetic resonance imaging, positron emission particle tracking imaging and electrical process tomography, mainly in the guise of electrical impedance tomography.

In this chapter, we try to avoid involving the complication of deep theories and electronic engineering but to provide typical examples and illustrations of applications. Extensive references for theories, techniques and applications are given for more detailed study. It should be pointed out that given the complex nature of fluid flowing in a mixing process, no universal visualization technique can cover its broad dynamic range and specific physical and chemical environments. Every visualization technique has limits in its application. At the end of the description for each technique, the limitations are addressed to aid readers in selecting a suitable technique to avoid any over-expectation for their particular application.

At the present time, a broad range of flow visualization techniques are available, which continue to be in a state of rapid development during very recent years, for example, mass vibration imaging, spectroscopic imaging and photo acoustic imaging. It has become clear during the preparation of this chapter that we could not include all these techniques in a single chapter. The techniques described may be treated as typical rather than exhaustive. Considering the practicability of the techniques in their current forms for application in process manufacture environment, some techniques are not covered in this chapter. For example, ultrasound Doppler velocimetry and the more recently developed ultrasound Doppler velocity profiler are not included due to their limitations for turbulent flows although they present successful velocity measurements in pipeline flows (Takeda 1995, Ihejirika and Ein-Mozaffari 2007).

Vision has sometimes been considered peripheral to a numerical engineering solution, but today's imaging technologies can provide a mass of quantitative information. The size of data increases in proportion to the speed demanded for data acquisition. Typically, for an image data set collected within just one minute, with an imaging speed of 1 ms per frame, it may take approximately 50 minutes to review if these images are replayed at a speed of 20 frames per second and the size of the data could amount to several Gigabytes!

The challenge remaining is how to extract information and reduce it to a few simple numbers for process analyses and control in mixing processes. It is obvious that the key to the solution should be in the hands of researchers, scientists and engineers in the areas of process engineering. We hope that the knowledge of fluid imaging technologies, as described in this chapter, provide useful information to those working in these fields, as well as other readers who have interest in the area.

16.2 Point Measurement Techniques

The concept of point measurements is not new but it was an important step change from visualizing with the eye to measuring by numbers. Even though two-dimensional (2D) or three-dimensional (3D) imaging techniques are now available for modern industry, point measurement techniques are still playing a significant role in the monitoring of fluid mixing processes, evaluation and calibration of computational fluid dynamic modelling (CFD) or imaging results.

The earliest point measurement techniques for measuring fluid mixture velocity and concentration include the measurement of differential pressures with a Pitot tube (Pitot 1732, Darcy 1858) and conductivity with a conductivity cell (Maxwell 1891), respectively. With a Pitot tube, the fluid velocity at the point inside a mixing vessel can be deduced using a simplified Bernoulli equation. Mavros (2001) reviewed its applications in stirred vessels (Jaworski and Fořt 1991, Nikiforaki et al. 1999, Wolf and Manning 1966).

Particle concentration (expressed as the volume fraction, α_c) can be converted from the conductivity distributions by use of Maxwell's relationship (Maxwell 1891) as given here:

$$\alpha_c = \frac{2\sigma_1 + \sigma_2 - 2\sigma_{mc} - \sigma_{mc}(\sigma_2/\sigma_1)}{\sigma_{mc} - \sigma_{mc}(\sigma_2/\sigma_1) + 2(\sigma_1 - \sigma_2)} \tag{16.1}$$

where σ_1 is the conductivity of the first phase or water, σ_2 is the conductivity of the second phase or particles, σ_{mc} is the local mixture's conductivity. The equation can be simplified if the second phase is assumed to be non-conductive material, for example, air:

$$\alpha_c = \frac{2\sigma_1 - 2\sigma_{mc}}{\sigma_{mc} + 2\sigma_1} \tag{16.2}$$

The same conversion has been widely used in electrical resistance tomography (Wang et al. 2006). The conductivity cell technique has also been extended for measurement of fluid velocity in both two- and three-dimensions (Lucas et al. 2004, Li et al. 2009). The technique is simple and the probe can be made to the scale of a few millimetres with a responding time of sub-milliseconds, which can be made in the laboratory, as well as being obtained from commercial suppliers (Millipore 2007).

Comparing these two techniques, the hot-wire anemometer (HWA) meets the frequency and length scale requirements more easily. The bandwidth is normally 20 kHz or more and probes can be made with sensor lengths down to 0.5 mm or even smaller (Jørgensen et al. 2003). HWA is predominantly used for the measurement of fluid velocity based on the principle of convective heat transfer from an electrically heated wire in a fluid flow (Bruun 1995). The wire is usually made of tungsten, platinum, or platinum-iridium with a diameter of typically 5 μm and a length of 1–2 mm. By combination of several wires on the same probe, it is possible to measure simultaneously all three components of the velocity vector (Mavros 2001). Recently, with the assistance of micro-electromechanical systems (MEMS), the sensor can be made of thin hot-film on a solid base (Lőfdahl and Gad-el-Hak 1999). The basic measurement principle can be expressed using King's Law (King 1914) and King's later works (King 1915, 1916).

$$E^2 = A + BV^n \tag{16.3}$$

where E is the voltage across the wire; V is the velocity; A, B and n are constants determined through the calibration, which depend on fluid physical properties such as viscosity, density and specific heat, as well as the temperature difference between the sensor and the fluid (Jørgensen 1996). Extensive development in techniques (Khoo et al. 1999, Buder et al. 2007, Berson et al. 2009) and applications in the mixing process (Lu and Ju 1987, Jourdan et al. 2001) are reported (Mavros 2001, Fagan et al. 2009).

Laser Doppler anemometry (LDA) is an optical technique with an important advantage over previous point measurement techniques – its probe lies outside the stirred vessel. Therefore, it does not disturb the fluid flow in the vessel. In principle, a laser beam is split into two coherent beams crossing at a point inside the stirred vessel. Parallel interference fringes interleaved with high and low intensities are formed in an intersection volume around the point. When the frequency of one of beams is slightly shifted using a 'Bragg' cell, it will cause the fringe pattern to pulsate at a steady frequency (Mavros 2001, Fagan et al. 2009). The fringe separation (d) is determined by,

$$d = \frac{\lambda}{2 sin\,(\theta / 2)} \tag{16.4}$$

where λ is the wavelength and θ is the angle between the two beams. When a particle passes through this volume, it changes this pulsation frequency, known as the Doppler effect. Particle velocity (u) can be determined from the Doppler frequency shift (f_D) and the fringe separation (d).

$$u = f_D d \tag{16.5}$$

LDA has been extensively used for characterizing the fluid flow inside stirred vessels (Chen 1988, Jahangiri 2005, Fagan et al. 2009).

With an additional detector to LDA, it becomes possible to simultaneously measure both the particle velocity and the size, which is known as phase Doppler anemometry (PDA). The second detector also receives the Doppler frequency shift but with a phase difference from that of the original detector, which is proportional to the angular position of these two detectors. The phase shift in the presence of a particle is proportional to the diameter of the particle. Applications on mixing processes in an agitated vessel were reported (Guiraud et al. 1997, Ljungqvist and Rasmuson 2004, Laakkonen et al. 2006).

It should be noted that all measurement techniques have their limitations. Their suitability to a specific application should be carefully considered. The inserted probes, such as a Pitot tube, conductivity cell and hot-wire anemometry, may affect the fluid flow. Furthermore, results are normally affected by physical and chemical properties of fluid in mixing, for example, the conductivity cell can well handle the concentration measurement from gas-in-water or solid-in-water mixtures. However, its measurement is also a function of temperature and pH value of the fluid in process. Therefore, they have to be calibrated with the assistance of other sensors or relevant information. In addition, both Pitot and hot-wire anemometry are unsuitable for solid-liquid mixing due to the risks of blockage and damage. A conductivity cell cannot be used for the fluids whose continuous phase is non-conductive. Most optical-based techniques have the non-intrusive advantage and an inconsequential interference from physical and chemical properties of fluids in processes. However, the fluid must be optically transparent; therefore, they can only be applied to a solid-liquid mixing process with a very low concentration, typically, less than 1% of solids or with a transparent stimulant having similar physical properties to that of the process fluid. It will not be applicable for opaque fluids and may not be practical in a large-scale vessel.

16.3 Photographic Imaging

Quantitative visualization of chemical processes and the consequent incorporation of images into process control loops was an idea that many scientists and engineers developed for various chemical reactors and flow rigs. Stirred vessels used as chemical reactors have the same potential to benefit from quantitative imaging, although in this case, not just for control purposes but also as a powerful adjunct to model development and validation. Photographic imaging is a classical technique which provides direct 'seeing is believing' in many chemical processes. It has seen tremendous evolution due to recent progress in optical physics and hardware engineering, including the pulsed laser sheet illumination technique and fast charge-coupled device (CCD) imaging equipment. It still plays an important role in laboratory-scale research, process monitoring and validation.

To clearly visualize turbulent convective mixing, a visible inert tracer is used as a pulsed injection into a stirred vessel. Under the illumination of a structured light source, the mixing process inside a stirred vessel is recorded in space and time using photographic equipment, which may be further processed to produce either qualitative or quantitative two-dimensional images of the mixing process.

Mann et al. (1995) used an acid pulse injected into a stirred alkaline fluid in a 30 dm^3 glass vessel utilized for the inert tracer experiments, using methyl red as an indicator, showing acid as red in colour and alkali as a deep yellow. A sequence of views at a stirred speed of 100 rpm was recorded by a video camera after the acid pulse was injected. The unsteady interrogation of the mixing was labelled by change of fluid colour reporting the acid pulse spread outwards and downwards towards the impeller in time sequence. These images then were used for validation of computational fluid dynamic modelling through larger three-dimensional networks-of-zones to computational fluid dynamics predictions in full three dimensions (Mann et al. 1993, 1995, Rahimi et al. 1999). A miscible liquid mixing in a large-scale stirred vessel ($H = T$ in $2.3\,m^3$) was conducted and video images were used for validation of the three-dimensional visualization reconstructed by electrical resistance tomography (Stanley et al. 2001). The experiments consisted of short-duration injection of 1 dm^3 of a mixture of nigrosine dye and concentrated brine. The convection and turbulence inside the stirred vessel caused the injection pulse of tracer to mix into the fluid in the vessel. Figure 16.1 shows the simultaneous video captured images following the injection at $t = 0$ of the miscible nigrosine blue-dye/concentrated brine pulse. The surface

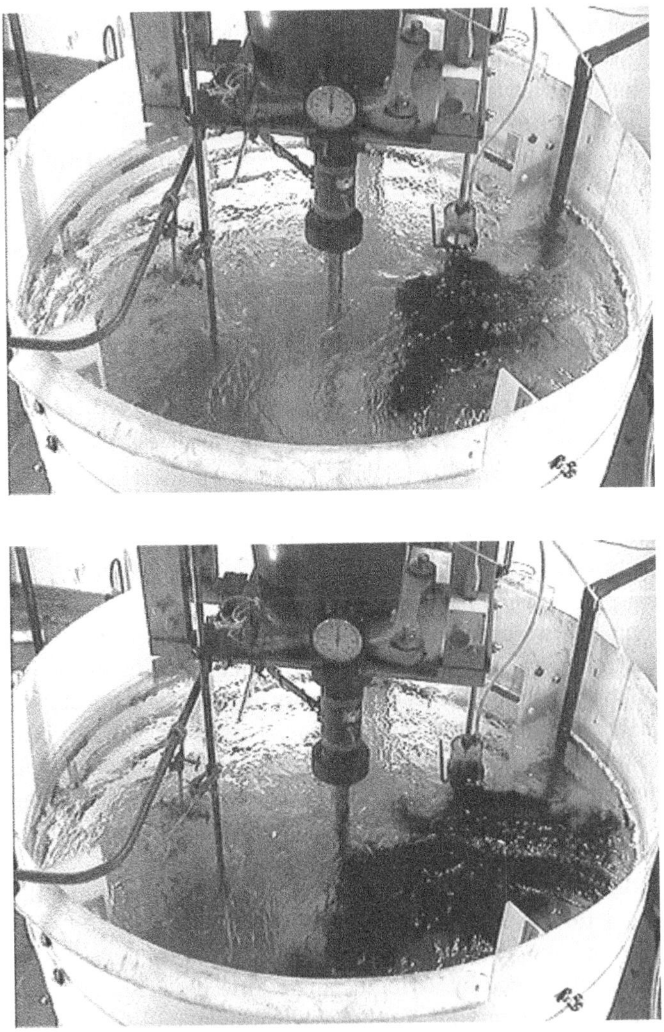

Figure 16.1 *Real video images (at 1 s intervals) of the dye/brine mixing. Reprinted with permission from NNL, S.J. Stanley, E. Wabo, R. Mann and K. Primrose, Dual-validation of miscible liquid mixing in a stirred vessel imaged by electrical resistance tomography (ERT),* 2nd World Congress on Industrial Process Tomography, Hannover, Germany, *151–158. Copyright (2001) NNL*

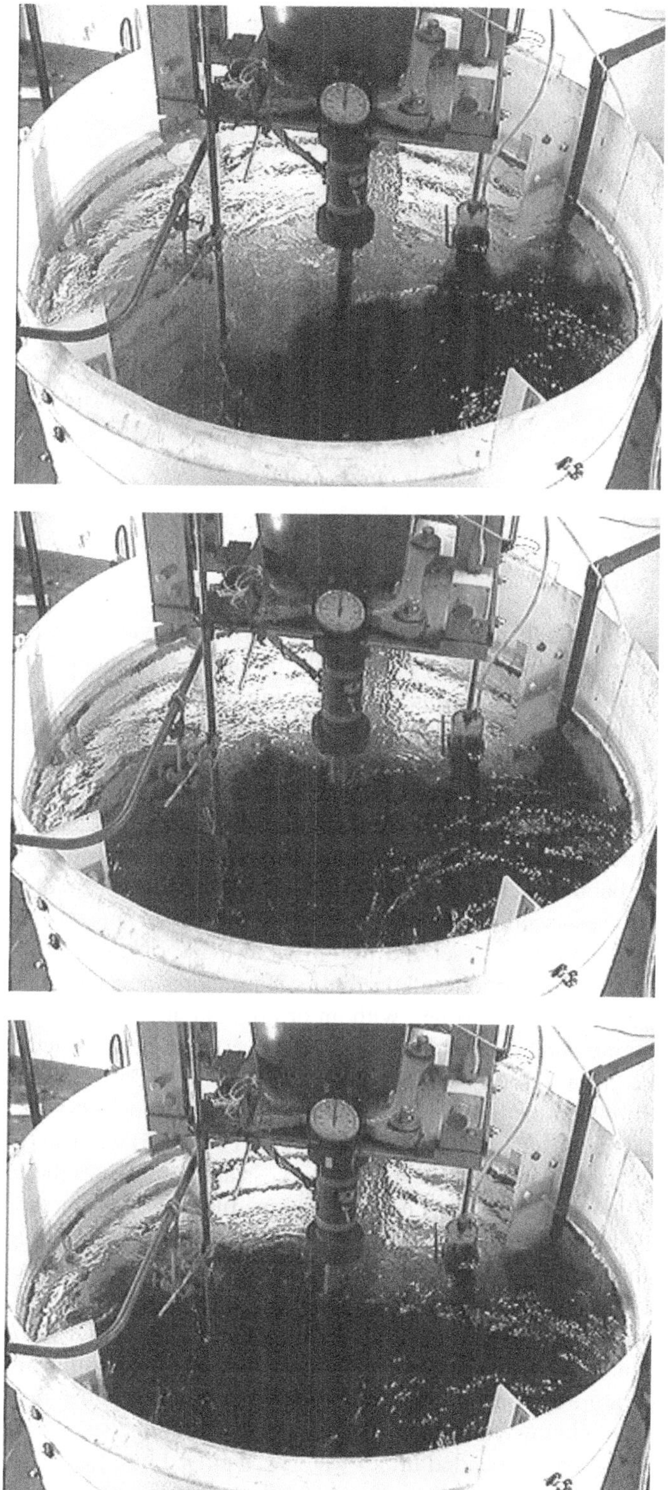

Figure 16.1 (*continued*)

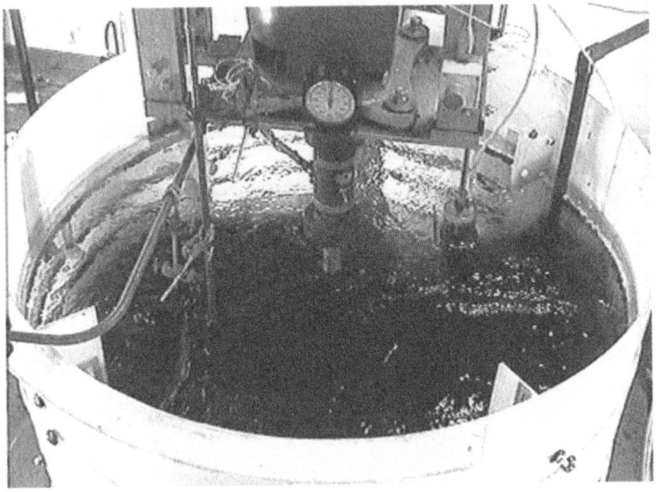

Figure 16.1 *(continued)*

of the stirred vessel is roughened by the turbulence, which provides a somewhat less clear view of the vessel interior. However, in spite of this surface roughness, the outline of the tracer cloud is readily distinguishable by eye (being assisted by the use of bright lights clustered around the far side of the cylindrical vessel). The visualization however only captures the observable boundary of the spreading tracer.

A photographic technique, referred to as streak photography, was also widely used for visualization of solid-liquid mixing in stirred vessels (Sachs and Rushton 1954), in which small amounts of transparent particles with a specific gravity, for example, acrylic DIAKON beads and tiny air bubbles, served as flow tracers. The vessel was normally installed inside a trough of square cross-section and the gap between the vessel and trough was filled with water. The walls of both the vessel and trough were made of transparent acrylic plastic material (Perspex). The directions of the light illumination and the image recorder are applied to two flat-sides of the trough with an orthogonal angle. By adjusting the shutter speed of the imaging camera, the trajectories of tracers can be recorded. Then, the flow patterns as well as flow velocity can be visualized (Figure 16.2), where the length of the streaks is proportional to the liquid velocity (Bakker and Fasano 1994).

A liquid crystal thermographic technique (Cooper et al. 1975) was used to determine the transient mixing characteristics of the mixing process and to measure the mixing time in a cylindrical unbaffled vessel (D = 0.1 m, H = 0.12 m) filled with water and agitated by an axial flow impeller (Lee and Yianneskis 1994). The vessel and a square trough had a similar arrangement to those used in streak photography. The liquid crystals in microcapsule form used in the work have a mean diameter of approximately 10 μm and a specific gravity of about 1.0. The colour displayed by the liquid crystals could be visually observed for temperatures between 24 and 29°C with a response time of 3 ms. Within this range, small changes in temperature can be recorded by a CCD video camera with a unique value of hue that is calibrated with known temperature of the water bath in the vessel over 24 and 29°C. A tracer of liquid crystal suspended in hot water was pulsed into the vessel. A collimated 2 mm thick sheet of white light produced by a 1 kW mercury lamp was used to illustrate the

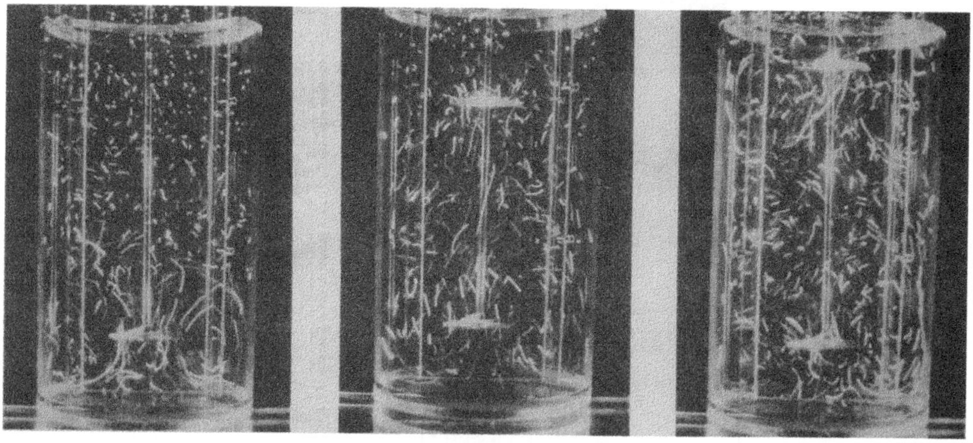

Figure 16.2 Streak photographs of different arrangements of axial impellers with three blades, D/T (the impeller bottom clearance to vessel diameter) = 0.35. The length of the streaks is proportional to the liquid velocity. Reprinted with permission from IChemE, A. Bakker and J.B. Fasano, Effects of flow pattern on the solid distribution in a stirred tank, Eighth European Conference on Mixing, IChemE Symposium Series 136, 1–8. Copyright (1994) IChemE

liquid crystals from one flat-side of the trough. The heat generated by the light source was dissipated by the water placed in the gap between the vessel and the trough. Hence the effect on hue display was negligible. The images were recorded with the CCD video camera from the other side of the trough which had an orthogonal angle to the plate of illumination. The results (Figure 16.3) showed that the state of mixing of passive scalar pulsed into the vessel (temperature) can be accurately determined during the mixing process (Lee and Yianneskis 1994).

The concentration (in colour) and velocity (in streak) images obtained using photographic techniques directly links with the sight-knowledge of the images and therefore provides an easy understanding of the mixing process. However, it only responds to a narrow mixing dynamic range and is limited to information on either the surface or a relevant thick slot of the cross section of the mixing vessel. It also has difficulty from the quantitative interpretation of images.

16.4 Digital Particle Image Velocimetry

The name, *Particle Image Velocimetry* (PIV), first appeared in the literature in the early eighties. Adrian (1984) and Pickering and Halliwell (1984) were amongst the first to point out that the seeding densities as high as those required in the speckle mode for Laser Speckle Velocimetry (LSV) are rarely achieved in practice (Chan 2008). They therefore argued that the low seeding density mode of LSV should be more appropriately classified as PIV. The photographic principle of PIV is the same as that addressed in the previous section but a more capable laser source and sensitive CCD camera are used as the photographic equipment. Adrian (1991) extensively reviewed the history and early development of the PIV technique and its applications, which provides an excellent reference for the

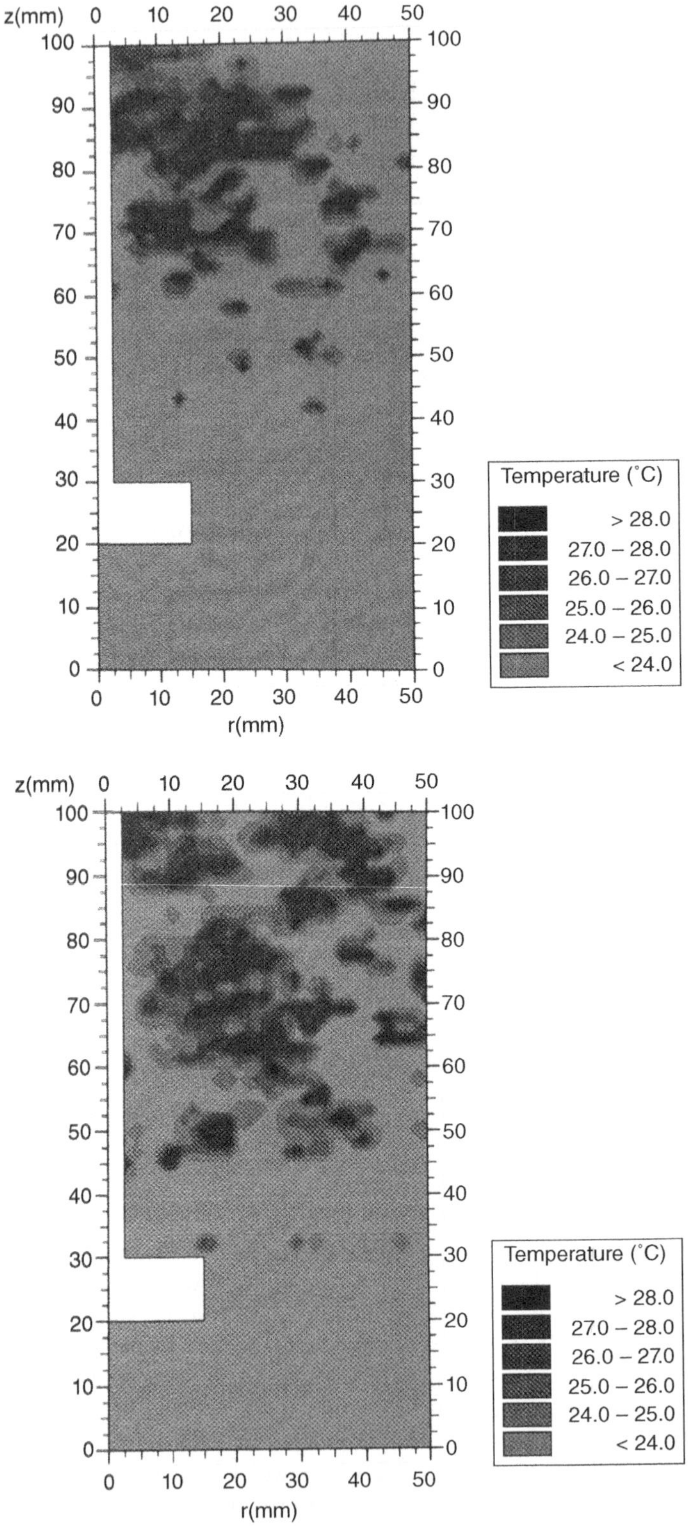

Figure 16.3 *Temperature contours of the flow field at 1, 2 and 5 s after pulsing the liquid crystal tracer. Reprinted with permission from* IChemE, *K.C. Lee and M. Yianneskis, Mixing characterisation of s stirred reactor with an axial flow impeller, Eighth* European Conference on Mixing, IChemE Symposium Series *136, 503–509 Copyright (1994) IChemE*

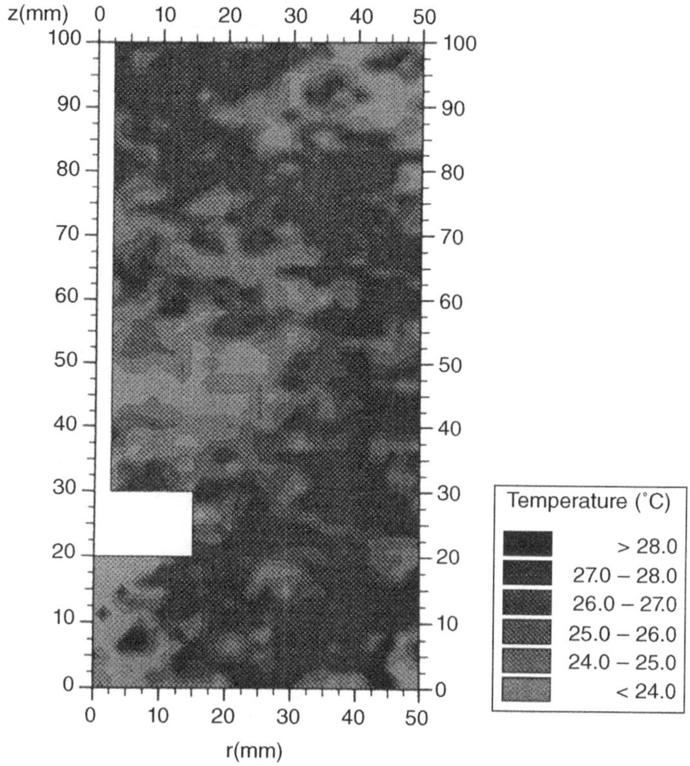

Figure 16.3 *(continued)*

technique. The implementation of the PIV technique in a digital mode by Willert and Gharib (1991) provided a dramatic reduction in image processing time, but at the cost of spatial resolution. Willert and Gharib (1991) and Westerweel et al. (1991) demonstrated that measurement accuracy is not adversely affected by a switch to digital processing (Dooley 2005). It was proposed to produce a two-dimensional (2D) velocity map from the cross-correlation of sequential images with a precise time interval.

PIV is a non-invasive planar optical measurement technique which provides a means of measuring the velocity of seeded particles (or tracers) in the flow of interest over a plane illuminated by a thin fan of laser light. The 2D velocity map is deduced from a cross-correlation process of sequential images recorded at precise time intervals by a highly sensitive, rapid CCD camera. The camera is normally located orthogonally to the laser light source. A square water-trough containing the target vessel is normally required and the walls of the vessel and trough must be light transparent, similar to those used in conventional photographic techniques. To maximize the signal-to-noise ratio, the operation is normally conducted in a dark room. The position and physical dimensions of the imaging plane of the flow field are defined by the laser source. With the illumination of two laser flashes on the imaging plane, a pair of digital photographic images of the flow field is recorded on computer. The velocity map is deduced from a cross-correlation analysis applying to a group of neighbouring imaging pixels within an estimated maximum interrogation region/window

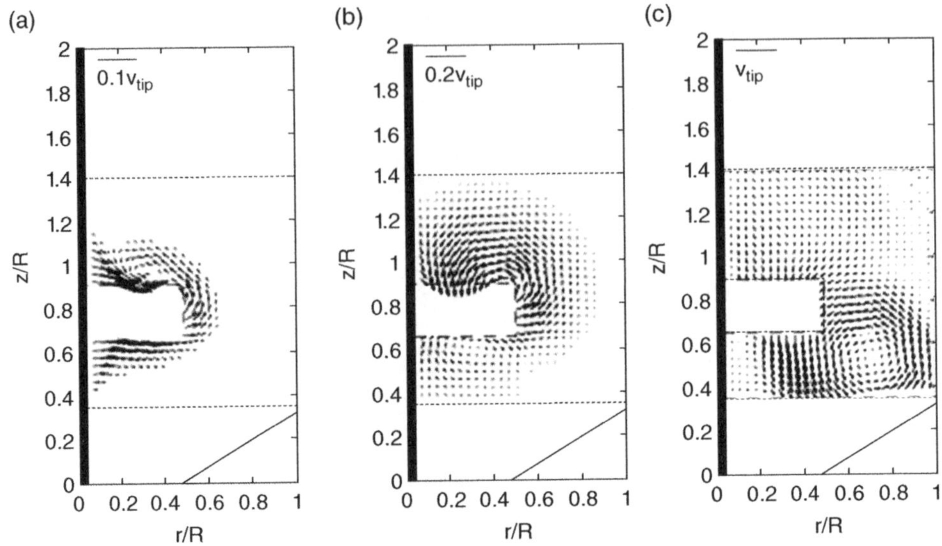

Figure 16.4 *Experimental flow patterns on an axial-radial plane for different impeller rotation rates. (a) N = 1 s⁻¹. (b) N = 2 s⁻¹ and (c) N = 8 s⁻¹. Reprinted with permission from* Chem. Eng. Research and Design, *Courbe et al. 2008, 86, 545–553. Copyright (2008) Elsevier*

between the two images. The cross-correlation process is repeated until all the required velocity information is extracted from the captured record. Nowadays, the PIV technique demonstrates its capability of measuring the fluid velocity field in a tank almost instantaneously, making it possible to study large-scale, time-dependent phenomena in the tank, which is responsible for much of the mixing process.

PIV is now regarded as the method of choice in measuring velocity data as quantitative flow visualization for the imaging mixing process and for code validation in computational fluid mixing (CFM). Maheo (1998) used the PIV technique to characterize free surface wakes and mixing layers in terms of Reynolds decomposition – mean and fluctuating velocity components – by processing thousands of consecutively-recorded particle images (Dooley 2005). Couerbe et al. (2008) investigated the yield stress due to the agitation of a thixotropic shear-thinning fluid. Both experimental approaches using PIV and numerical simulation via CFD were carried out. Steady-state experiments were conducted at three impeller rotation speeds (1, 2 and 8 s^{-1}) for a stirred vessel. The material was a 3 wt.% suspension of laponite in distilled water. PIV measurements were performed in a conical-bottomed cylindrical vessel of diameter T = 0.19 m. A three-blade Mixel TT agitator (Mixel, Dardilly, France), with a diameter D = 0.5T, was mounted on a vertical shaft. The impeller clearance from the vessel bottom to the lowest horizontal plane was C = 0.33 T. Figure 16.4 shows the two-dimensional velocity fields determined for N = 1 s^{-1}, N = 2 s^{-1} and N = 8 s^{-1}. Results from the experiment and simulation were compared.

Recent advances in the PIV technique have been extended to measure all three velocity components in a plane or in a volume simultaneously to allow application of the PIV technique to more complex flow phenomena, which is known as Stereoscopic PIV. The method of stereoscopic PIV for extracting the third, out-of-plane, velocity component is based on the principle of parallax with two cameras. In PIV, by placing two cameras so that they observe the light-sheet plane from two different angles, the parallax effect means that slightly different two-velocity component vector maps from each camera are obtained (Dantec Dynamics Ltd.). However, the conventional stereoscopic PIV measurement results within one single plane often do not yield enough information to determine all velocity-based terms in the fluid governing equations (such as Navier–Stokes equations). Kaehler and Kompenhans (1999) proposed a dual-plane stereoscopic PIV by using two sets of double-pulsed Nd:Yag lasers with additional optics to illuminate the objective fluid flow with two orthogonal linearly polarized laser sheets at two spatially separated planes. A dual-plane system stereoscopic PIV was set-up and its application to a lobed jet mixing flow was reported (Hu et al. 2001). The measurement results were obtained using the dual-plane stereoscopic PIV system to provide all three components of the velocity and vorticity fields of the lobed jet mixing flows instantaneously and simultaneously. For the ensemble-averaged values of the out-plane velocity component, the differences between the stereoscopic PIV and LDV measurement results were found to be less than 2%.

In order to record the concentration distribution with the velocity simultaneously, a combined digital PIV and planar laser induced fluorescence technique was also developed for measurement of mixing processes (Wing-Keung Law and Wang 2000, Dantec Dynamics Ltd 2010, Fagan et al. 2009). Some chemical substances become fluorescent when they are explored under particular light sources, which are termed *photochromic dyes*. The light intensity of photochromic dye in the mixing process is recorded and then interpreted to the concentration of the dye. The method of recording the fluorescent effect at a point of fluid under a laser beam illumination is called Laser-Induced Fluorescence (LIF) or Planar Laser-Induced Fluorescence (PLIF) if the photochromic effect on a two-dimensional plane is illuminated by a plane laser source. The combination of PIV and PLIF provided extremely useful information for instantaneously visualizing both concentration and velocity distributions of complex fluid flow in the mixing process (Houcine et al. 1996, Lemoine et al. 1996, Unger and Muzzio 1999).

The major limitation of PIV is that it can only function for light-transparent fluid mediums and cannot be applied on concentrated fields (Wing-Keung Law and Wang 2000, Dooley 2005). The optical systems in their current forms are delicate. Therefore, they are rarely applied as an on-line visualization tool to most industrial processes.

16.5 Magnetic Resonance Imaging

Magnetic resonance imaging (MRI), or nuclear magnetic resonance imaging (NMRI), was originally used as a mode of medical imaging in radiology to visualize detailed internal structures and limited functions of the body. Magnetic resonance imaging is a development of nuclear magnetic resonance. Originally, the technique was referred to as nuclear magnetic resonance imaging (NMRI). However, because the word nuclear was associated in the public's minds with ionizing radiation exposure, it is generally now referred to simply as MRI. Scientists still use the term NMRI when discussing non-medical devices operating using the same principles. The term magnetic resonance tomography (MRT) is also occasionally used (Wikipedia 2010).

MRI provides much more refined characterization of different soft tissues of the body than X-ray tomography. Unlike X-ray tomography, MRI uses no ionizing radiation. Rather, it uses a powerful magnetic field to align the nuclear magnetization of (usually) hydrogen atoms in water in the body. Radio frequency (RF) fields are used to systematically alter the alignment of this magnetization. This causes the hydrogen nuclei to produce a rotating magnetic field detectable by the scanner. This signal can be manipulated by additional magnetic fields to build up sufficient information to construct an image of the body (Squire and Novelline 1997). Modern fundamentals of MRI are introduced in recent monographs (Callaghan 1993, Blumich 1999, Kimmich 1997, Levitt 2002). The first MR image was published in 1973 (Lauterbur 1973, Filler 2010) and the first cross-sectional image of a living mouse was published in January 1974 (Lauterbur 1974). The first studies performed on humans were published in 1977 (Damadian et al. 1977, Hinshaw 1977). By comparison, applying MRI to chemical and materials science and engineering only gained significant interest over the past 10–15 years (Mantle and Sederman 2003) due to it being non-intrusive and also its capability to 'see' through an opaque medium in the process. These developments have been comprehensively reviewed by some researchers, for example, as a tool to study materials science (Eidmann et al. 1996; Blumich and Kuhn 1992), flow (Fukushima 1999) and food science (Belton et al. 1999). Dynamic MRI investigations of chemical processes and reaction phenomena have appeared in the literature in the last 5–6 years (Mantle and Sederman 2003).

Gladden and Alexander (1996) highlighted a number of MRI applications in process engineering. One of the earliest MRI studies of particulate suspensions investigated the slip casting process of an Al2O3 þ 30wt% water suspension into a plaster of Paris mould (Hayashi et al. 1988). With MRI data, numerical simulations were evaluated for batch sedimentation and viscous re-suspension in a Couette cell containing non-neutrally buoyant PMMA particles of diameter 0.0794 cm in 96% glycerol solution (Rao et al. 2002). MRI was also used to characterize the kinematics of mixing and size segregation of dry binary mixtures and filling level in a Turbula shaker-mixer (Porion et al. 2004, Sommier et al. 2001). They concluded that MRI can be used for studying the kinematics of mixing and segregation of dry binary granular mixtures but it requires either preparing the grain by coating it with oil or to work with oil-containing particles such as seeds in this application. A study of the mixing of solids in gas-fluidized beds was reported (Fennel et al. 2005). An ultra-fast MRI with an imaging rate of 12 ms was used to measure the rate of axial mixing in a vertical direction of a small batch of poppy seeds suddenly added to the upper surface of a bed of sugar crystals fluidized by air. The extent of a model system for mixing with a fluid and particle batch system using MRI was quantified (Lee et al. 2001).

Magnetic resonance imaging is a power visualization technique to provide excellent resolutions in both spatial and temporal dimensions. It is also regarded as 'green' technology without radioactive emission. It has approved successes in laboratory-based research and applications. However, the current status of the technique still has difficulties for on-line visualization of industrial processes due to the high cost of devices and complex in its installation.

16.6 Positron Emission Particle Tracking Imaging

Positron emission tomography (PET) and positron emission particle tracking (PEPT) have recently been widely used in scientific and engineering research to optimize the design, operational conditions and to evaluate modelling and simulation work. PET has been used

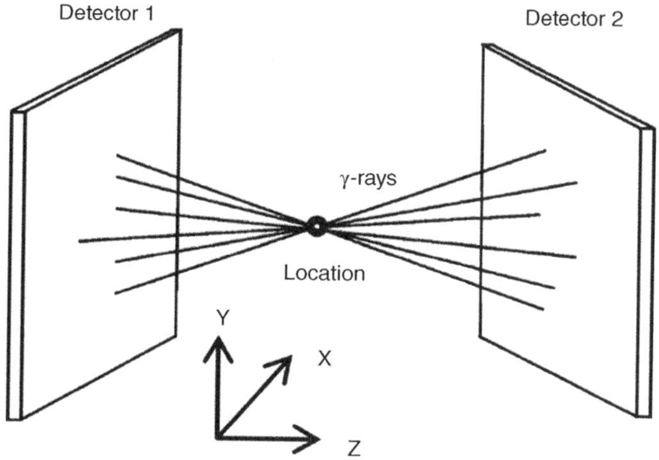

Figure 16.5 *Schematic diagram of PEPT for a single particle. Reprinted with permission from Particuology, 6, 16–23. Copyright (2008) Elsevier*

for mapping a liquid flow, for example: observation of lubricant distribution in aeronautical engines, tracking fluids in rock cracks, chemical reactors, food processors, diagnosis and treatment of tumours and so on (Parker and McNeil 1996). It provides the recording of radioactivity distribution for building up a three-dimensional image of the tracers. The PEPT technique allows up to three positron-emitting particles to be accurately and non-invasively tracked in opaque vessels for mapping granular flows in engineering applications. For example, dynamic behaviour of catalysts in chemical reactors, mixing and segregation in mixers, dryers, rotating kilns, solid–liquid slip velocity in ball mills, particle rotation, solid flow structure, bubble flow pattern in fluidized beds and granulators, solid motion in food processors and so on (Cox et al. 2003, Barigou et al. 2003, Kuo et al. 2005, Parker and Fan 2008).

Parker and Fan (2008) described the PEPT systems developed at the University of Birmingham, which involved a labelled tracer particle, a positron camera and a location algorithm for calculating the tracer location and speed. The tracer particle was labelled with a radio-nuclide, which decays by β^+ decay with the emission of a positron. Each positron rapidly annihilated with an electron, giving rise to a pair of 511 keV γ-rays which were emitted almost exactly back-to-back. The camera consisted of two position-sensitive detectors, each with an active area of 590 × 470 mm, mounted on either side of the field of view, and was used to detect pairs of 511 keV γ-rays. The two γ- rays were simultaneously detected in the two detectors, which defined a trajectory passing close to the source. Then, the location of the tracer particle was calculated using a specific location algorithm based on the fact that all the uncorrupted γ-ray trajectories for a given set of events should meet (to within the resolution of the camera) at a point in space, as shown in Figure 16.5.

Conway-Baker et al. (2002) used PEPT to study the motion of media in a stirred grinding mill and identified the main differences between this media motion and the classical theory of motion within fluid mixing (Figure 16.6). Three regions have been classified within the mill and it was found that the impeller speed altered the relative position of these

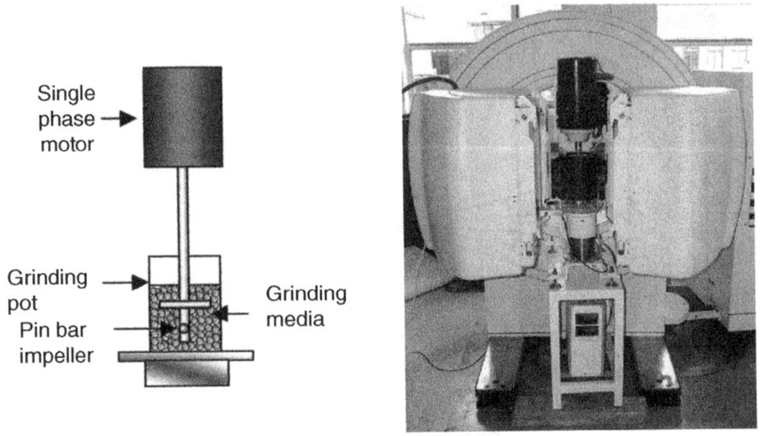

Figure 16.6 Photograph of mill in position in the PEPT rig. Reprinted with permission from Minerals Engineering, 15, 53–59 Copyright (2002) Elsevier

regions. Three different impellers were also studied which gave different forms of motion (Figure 16.7).

PET and PEPT imaging are all based on radioactive tracer emissions presenting an excellent resolution at the demanded destination or areas. Due to its radioactive nature, the limits of the installation flexibility and cost of equipment, it is only suitable for laboratory investigation. In addition, both techniques have a slow responding time therefore not being able to provide instantaneous imaging of mixing dynamics.

16.7 Electrical Process Tomography

Electrical process tomography is a relatively new technology, which is based on measurements of electrical properties of materials by applying a low frequency (from DC up to few MHz) electric field (e.g. current or voltage) or a magnetic field. A low frequency electromagnetic field can penetrate most process materials which are opaque to the light. The electrical techniques also avoid the hazards of ionizing radiation generated from nuclear emission techniques, for example, X-ray or γ-ray based techniques. They are inexpensive and relatively straightforward to implement with the potential for sub-millisecond temporal resolution. Due to the limited number of measurements and the propagation nature of low frequency electromagnetic waves, they normally provide images with a spatial resolution around 5% (the diameter of the object to the diameter of the vessel) and a homogeneity resolution better than 1% (e.g. the mean concentration of gas in water). Electrical process tomography was recognized as a highly capable technology to provide an on-line macro-view of fluid processes in both academic research and Industry (Dyakowski 1996, Mann and Wang 1997, York 2001, Tapp et al. 2003, Bolton and Primrose 2005, Stanley and Bolton 2008, Sharifi and Young 2013).

Electrical process tomography, including electrical capacitance tomography (ECT), electrical impedance tomography (EIT) and electromagnetic induction tomography (EMT), is based on the specific properties of materials principally sensed by each technique.

ECT senses the permittivity distribution of dispersed materials in a fluid process with a non-conductive continuous phase; EIT is specified for a process that has a conductive continuous phase; EMT is mainly applied for high conductive fluids, which can induce measurable current under a magnetic field. Electrical resistance tomography (ERT) is a particular case of electrical impedance tomography when the real component of electrical impedance is the dominant property of materials in an EIT process application. The

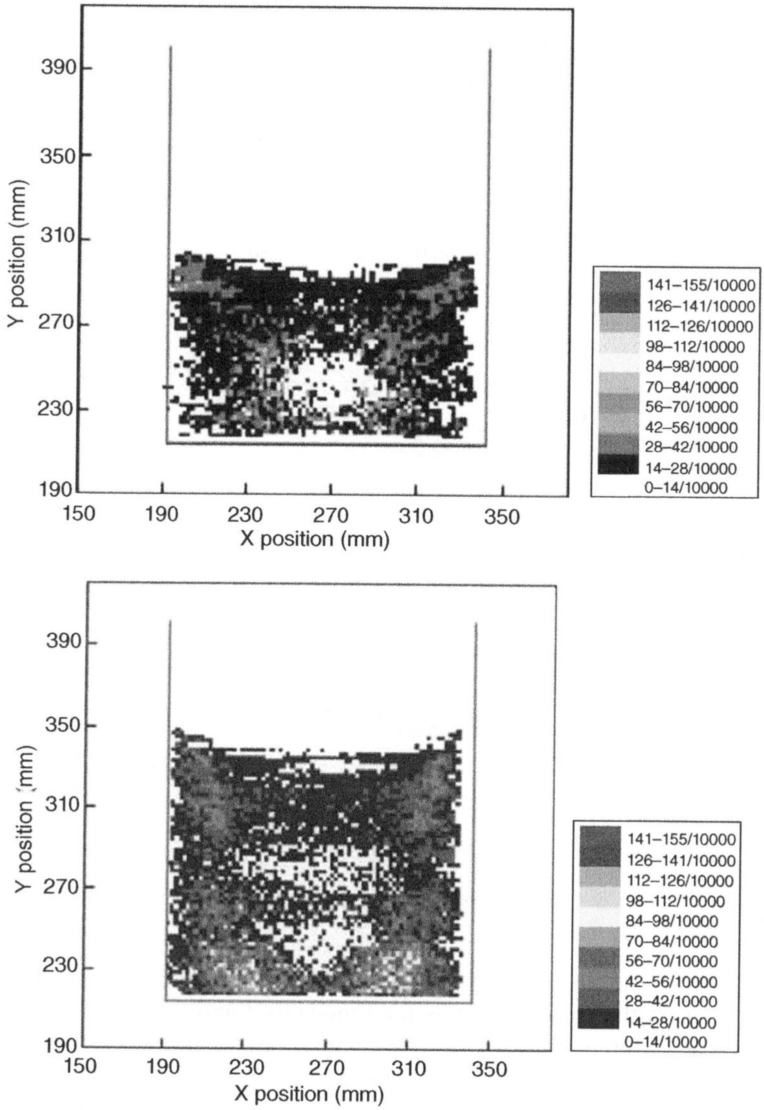

Figure 16.7 *Occupancy plots for various impeller speeds indicated by number of events at position per 10 000 events. Reprinted with permission from* Minerals Engineering, *15, 53–59. Copyright (2002) Elsevier*

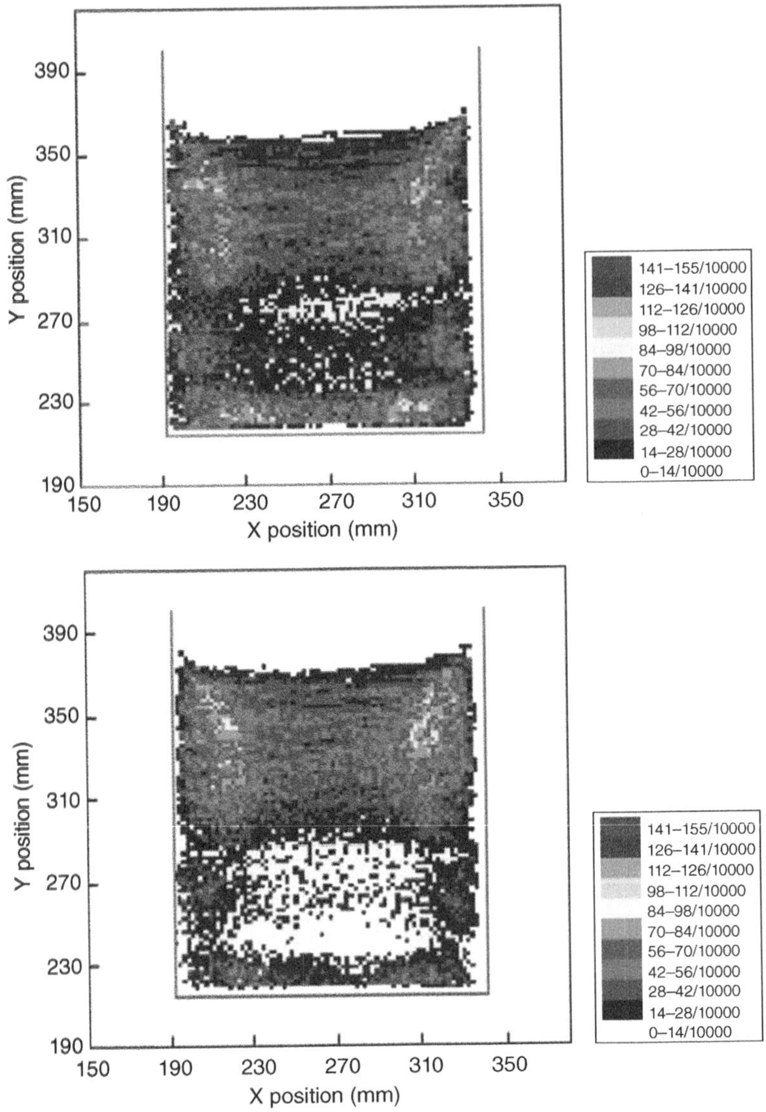

Figure 16.7 *(continued)*

combination of two of these three modes, for example, ECT+ERT, may extend the measurement range, therefore named as multimodality tomography. In the case of EIT, the sensor is made from multiple electrodes arranged around the periphery of the internal wall of the process vessel or pipeline, in contact with the process medium but not intrusive to the medium. An alternating current is applied to some electrodes and voltages are measured from the remaining electrodes, according to a predefined sensing strategy. Then these voltage measurements are used to reconstruct the impedance distribution inside the vessel with a specific inverse algorithm. Both early and more recent developments can be found

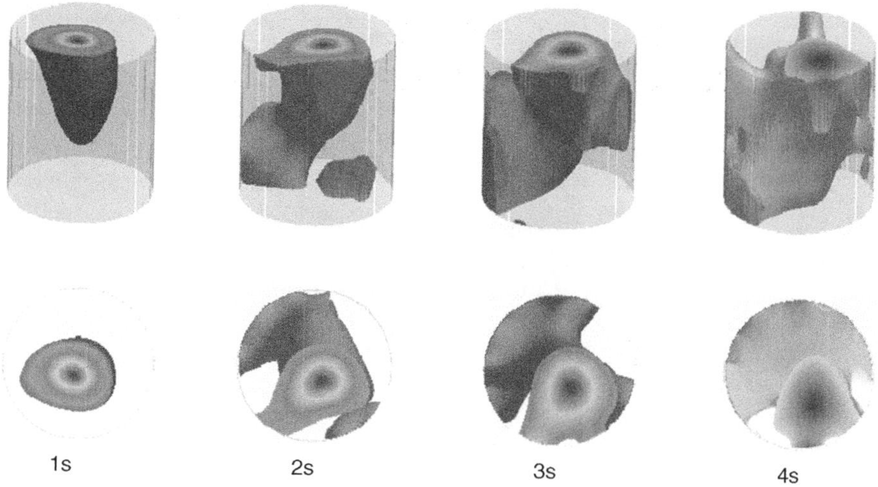

Figure 16.8 *Monitoring a dynamic miscible liquid mixing in a baffled 2.7 m³ mixing tank using ERT (mixing index: 0.16 mS cm⁻¹) (conductivity of pulse brine: 13.5 mS cm⁻¹ in volume 10 dm³, speed of Rushton stirrer: 100 rpm). Based on Stirred vessel mixing in 3-D using electrical resistance tomography, M. Wang, R. Mann, A.E. Forrest, P.J. Holden, F.J. Dickin, T. Dyakowski, R.B. Edwards, 11 (A),* CIE Beijing, *650–653 (1997)*

from many articles (ECT: Huang et al. 1988; Xie et al. 1993; Reinecke and Mewes 1996; Yang et al. 1999; Marashdeh et al. 2008; EIT: Wang et al. 1993, 1995, 2002, 2004, 2005b; Dickin et al. 1996; Pinheiro et al. 1998; Wilkinson et al. 2006; Murphy et al. 2006; EMT: Yu et al. 1993; Peyton et al. 1996; Ma et al. 2005; Dual modality: Qiu et al. 2007).

The non-intrusive measurement of mixing inside a stirred vessel in three-dimensions, using electrical resistance tomography, provides powerful opportunities for characterizing and quantifying the process complexities of the non-stationary behaviour and air-core vortex profile in mixing processes (Mann et al. 1997), the mixing index of mixing of a pulp suspension and chlorine dioxide (Yenjaichon et al. 2011), the flow and velocity profile of various milk solutions in various pipelines (Sharifi and Young, 2012a) and milk total solids and fat content in a stirred tank (Sharifi and Young, 2012b). An early study reported an application of EIT for 3D imaging of the concentration of solids in a slurry mixer as a function of key process variables (particle size, impeller type, agitation speed) (McKee 1994, Williams et al. 1996). It was demonstrated as to how EIT can provide a wealth of detailed data to allow model development. On-line 2D imaging of miscible liquid/liquid mixing and gas-liquid mixing in a large scale baffled mixing vessel ($2.3\,m^3$) fitted with eight planes of EIT sensor was reported in 1996 (Dickin and Wang 1996, Mann et al. 1996). 3D imaging of an air-core vortex and mixing performances of a gas-liquid and miscible liquid mixing in the same vessel was reported (Mann et al. 1996; Wang et al. 1997). Figure 16.8 shows a typical set of resistivity contours interpolated from a stack of eight-plane 2D images, rendered as a solid body isometric image. Results are presented from times of 1, 2, 3 and 4 s following the surface addition of 10 dm^3 of concentrated brine (conductivity of $13.5\,mS\ cm^{-1}$) into a background conductivity of $0.1\,mS\ cm^{-1}$ at $t = 0$. The stirrer speed was 100 rpm generating an estimated internal flow of $0.686\,m^3\ s^{-1}$. The mixing time were estimated using a

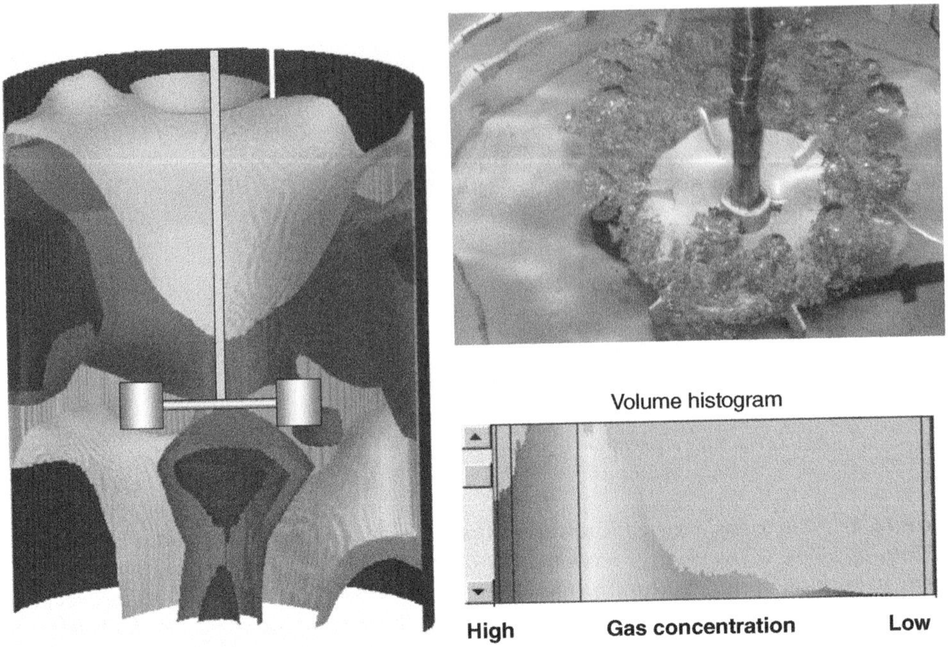

Figure 16.9 *Pseudo-stationary gas-liquid mixing. Based on Stirred vessel mixing in 3-D using electrical resistance tomography, M. Wang, R. Mann, A.E. Forrest, P.J. Holden, F.J. Dickin, T. Dyakowski, R.B. Edwards, 11 (A),* CIE Beijing, *650–653 (1997)*

colorimeter probe and was approximately 14 s. High conductivity is presented by red regions and low conductivity as blue regions (cut off by the isosurface). The conductivity at the isosurface, as a mixing index, is 0.16 mS cm^{-1}, which was adopted from the final conductivity of the liquids after mixing was completed. Further studies of a gas-liquid system (air-water) have allowed tomographic gas distribution to be compared with established characteristic flow patterns (Wang et al. 2000). A multi-isosurface 3D gas concentration distribution was produced from stack of eight-plane 2D images, which presented gas equal-concentration contours (Figure 16.9). In the experiment, gas was sparged from a pipe beneath a six-blade Rushton turbine at 3.5 litre sec^{-1} with agitation at 73 rpm.

Holden et al. (1998) quantitatively characterized the gas-liquid and miscible liquid mixing behaviour with ERT. Based on the time resolved 3D ERT results, the centroid and variance of the concentration distribution in three dimensions can be obtained as a time series to track the movement, dispersion, stretch and rotation of the concentration distribution in the tank. Several analytical methods were applied to the 3D electrical resistance tomography image of the stirred-vessel experiments (Li and Wei 1999). By sampling at different scales and locations, the ratios of standard deviation to mean and the entropy of corresponding volumes can be calculated to examine the degrees of uniformity. The 3D wavelet decomposition was applied to digital images, which provides an effective method of analysing the mixing process at various scales (Li and Wei 1999). ERT was also applied to detect mixing pathologies inside a stirred vessel ERT (Holden et al. 1999). Stanley et al. (2002) reported a tomographic imaging of fluid mixing in three dimensions for single-feed semi-batch operation of a stirred vessel. He also presented an application of ERT for interrogation of a barium sulphate precipitation with two

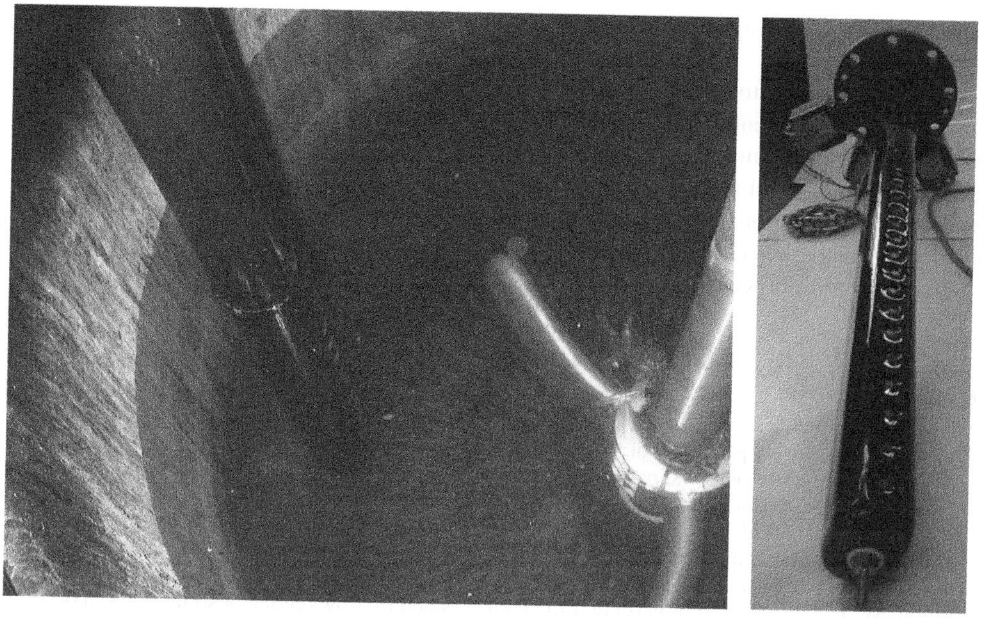

Figure 16.10 *Photograph of a linear sensor located within an industrial reactor. Reprinted with permission from cidic and radioactive environment,* Chemical Engineering Journal, *130, 165–169. Copyright (2007) Elsevier*

different semi-batch processes (Stanley et al. 2005). Specific regional analyses have been highlighted during such a process reflecting the complex reaction and precipitation kinetics. A number of investigations of using ERT for evaluation of computational fluid dynamic (CFD) model were reported, including the performance of a batch stirred vessel (Wabo et al. 2004), a Lightnin A310 in a gas sparged mixing tank (Robert and Doblin 2003) and the rinsing step of yoghurt in a dairy plant (Henningsson et al. 2007). Further research on measurement of miscible liquids mixing in a stirred vessel with electrical resistance tomography was also reported (Kim et al. 2006), the mixing time in the agitation of non-Newtonian fluids through a four-sensing plane ERT (Pakzad et al. 2008), a true three-dimensional electrical impedance tomography was for investigating a miscible liquid mixing in a semi-tech scale stirred tank (Stephenson et al. 2009), an evaluation of the mixing times estimated by a correlation model with that predicted by ERT for the Rushton turbine surface feed (Grenville and Nienow 2004). Bolton et al. (2002) developed and applied a linear electrical tomography sensor for monitoring the phase distribution in industrial reactors in both laboratory and pilot-scale stirred vessels. Measurement of solids concentration and distribution were demonstrated in the article. Bolton et al. (2007) also applied an EIT system with a linear electrode array for monitoring of stirred mixing operation in a remote, acidic and radioactive nuclear industrial environment. Murphy et al. (2006) used linear arrays of electrodes in conjunction with electrical impedance tomography to spatially interrogate industrial processes that have only limited access for sensor placement. These compromises are expected using a small number of vertically positioned linear arrays to facilitate 3D imaging using electrical tomography.

It was concluded that the sensor (Figure 16.10) is suitable for one-off trouble-shooting and process optimization studies of industrial process vessels and also suitable for retrofitting to industrial process vessels for on-line measurement of phase distribution.

Electrical process tomography has an excellent response time and good adaptability to industrial environments, as well as low costs in both installation and maintenance. However, due to the non-linear nature of the low frequency electric field distribution and the limited number of measurements it presents a low spatial resolution and non-uniform sensitivity distribution over the domain interested. Therefore, it is regarded as a highly available macro visualization technique for both laboratory-scale investigation and industrial mixing process.

References

Adrian, R.J., Scattering particle characteristics and their effect on pulsed laser measurements of fluid flow: speckle velocimetry vs. particle image velocimetry. *Appl. Optics*, **23**, 1690–1691 (1984).

Adrian, R.J., P.W. Offutt, C.C. Landreth, Z. Liu and T.J. Hanratty (eds), *Applications of Laser Anemometry in Fluid Mechanics*. Springer, Berlin (1991).

Bakker, A. and J.B. Fasano, Effects of flow pattern on the solid distribution in a stirred tank, *Eighth European Conference on Mixing*, IChemE Symposium Series **136**, 1–8 (1994).

Barigou, M., P.G. Fairhurst, P.J. Fryer and J.P. Pain, Concentric flow regime of solid–liquid food suspensions: Theory and experiment. *Chemical Engineering Science*, **58**(9), 1671–1686 (2003).

Belton, P.S., B.P. Hills and G.A. Webb (eds), *Advances in Magnetic Resonance in Food Science*, Royal Society of Chemistry, Cambridge (1999).

Berson, A., P. Blanc-Benon and G. Comte-Bellot, A strategy to eliminate all nonlinear effects in constant-voltage hot-wire anemometry, *Review of Scientific Instruments*, American Institute of Physics, **80**(045102), 1–7 (2009).

Blumich, B. and W. Kuhn (eds), Magnetic resonance microscopy: methods and applications, in *Materials science, Agriculture and Biomedicine*, VCH, Cambridge (1992).

Blumich, B., *NMR Imaging of Materials*, Oxford University Press, Cambridge (1999).

Bolton, G.T., C.H. Qiu and M. Wang, A novel electrical tomography sensor for monitoring the phase distribution in industrial reactors, *Fluid Mixing* **7**, IChemEng, University of Bradford (2002).

Bolton, G.T. and K.M. Primrose, An overview of electrical tomography measurements in pharmaceutical and related application areas, *AAPS Pharm. Sci. Tech.*, **6**(2), Article **21**, 137–143 (2005).

Bolton, G.T., M. Bennett, M. Wang, C. Qiu, M. Wright, K. Primrose, S.J. Stanley and D. Rhodes, Development of an electrical tomographic system for operation in a remote, acidic and radioactive environment, *Chemical Engineering Journal*, **130**, 165–169 (2007).

Bruun, H.H., *Hot-Wire Anemometry: Principles and Signal Analysis*. Oxford University Press, New York (1995).

Buder, U., A. Berns, R. Petz, W. Nitsche and E. Obermeier, AeroMEMS wall hot-wire anemometer on polyimide substrate featuring top side or bottom side bondpads, *IEEE Sensors Journal*, **7**(8), 1095–1101 (2007).

Callaghan, P.T., *Principles of Nuclear Magnetic Resonance Microscopy*, Oxford University Press, New York (1993).

Chan, V., *The Art of Laser Velocimetry*, available at: www.holomap.com/ (accessed 10 January, 2015) (2008).

Chen, K. Laser-Doppler Anemometry in a baffled mixing tank, *Chem. Eng. Comm.*, **72**, 141–157 (1988).

Conway-Baker, J., R.W. Barley, R.A. Williams, X. Jia, J. Kostuch, B. McLoughlin and D.J. Parker, Measurement of the motion of grinding media in a vertically stirred mill using positron emission particle tracking (PEPT), *Minerals Engineering*, **15**, 53–59 (2002).

Cooper, T.E., R.J. Woolf and J.F. Meyer, Liquid crystal thermography and its application to the study of convective heat transfer, *Journal of Heat Transfer, Transactions of the ASME*, 442–450 (1975).

Couerbe, G., D.F. Fletcher, C. Xuereb and M. Poux, Impact of thixotropy on flow patterns induced in a stirred tank: Numerical and experimental studies, *Chem. Eng. Research and Design*, **86**, 545–553 (2008).

Cox, P.W., S. Bakalis, H. Ismail, R. Forster, D.J. Parker and P.J. Fryer, Visualisation of three-dimensional flows in rotating cans using positron emission particle tracking (PEPT). *Journal of Food Engineering*, **60**(3), 229–240 (2003).

Dahm, W.J.A. and K.B. Southerland, Quantitative flow visualisation via fully-reserved four-dimensional imaging, in *Flow Visualization: techniques and examples*, A. J. Smits and T. T. Lim (eds), Imperial College Press (2000).

Damadian, R., M. Goldsmith and L. Minkoff, NMR in cancer: XVI, Fonar image of the live human body. *Physiological Chemistry and Physics*, **9**, 97–100 (1977).

Dantec Dynamics Limited, Bristol, UK, available at: www.dantecdynamics.com/ (accessed 10 January, 2015) (2010).

Darcy, H., Relative à quelques modifications à introduire dans le tube de Pitot, *Annales des Ponts et Chaussées*, Series 3; **15**, 351–359 (in French), (1858).

Dickin, F.J. and M. Wang, Electrical resistance tomography for process applications, *Meas. Sci. and Technol.*, IOP, **7**, 247–260 (1996).

Dooley, B.S., *Stereo digital particle image velocimetry investigation of a free surface mixing layer*, PhD Thesis, California Institute of Technology, Pasadena, California, US (2005).

Dyakowski, T., Process tomography applied to multi-phase flow measurement, *Meas. Sci. Technol.*, **7**, 343–353 (1996).

Eidmann, G., R. Savelsberg, P. Blümler and B. Blümich, The NMR MOUSE, a mobile universal surface explorer, *J. Magn. Reson. Ser. A*, **122**, 104, (1996).

Fagan, C.C., P.J. Cullen and C.P. O'Donnell, Monitoring and control of mixing operations, in *Food Mixing Principles and Applications*, P.J. Cullen (ed.), Wiley-Blackwell (2009).

Fennell, P.S., J.F. Davidson, J.S. Dennis, L.F. Gladden, A.N. Hayhurst, M.D. Mantle, C.R. Müller, A.C. Rees, S.A. Scott and A.J. Sederman, A study of the mixing of solids in gas-fluidized beds, using ultra-fast MRI, *Chemical Engineering Science*, **60**, 2085–2088 (2005).

Filler, A.G. The history, development, and impact of computed imaging in neurological diagnosis and neurosurgery: CT, MRI, DTI, *Internet Journal of Neurosurgery*, **7**(1) (2010).

Fukushima, E., Nuclear magnetic resonance as a tool to study flow, *Annu. Rev. Fluid Mech.*, **31**, 95–123 (1999).

Gladden, L.F. and P. Alexander, Applications of nuclear magnetic resonance imaging in process engineering, *Meas. Sci. Technol.*, **7**, 423–435 (1996).

Grenville, R.K. and A.W. Nienow, Blending of miscible liquids, in *Handbook of Industrial Mixing: Science and Practice*, Paul, E.L., Atiemo-Obeng, V.A., and Kresta, S.M. (eds), Chapter 9, John Wiley & Sons, Inc., New Jersey (2004).

Guiraud, P., J. Costes and J. Bertrand, Local measurements of fluid and particle velocities in a stirred suspension, *Chemical Eng. J.*, **68**(2–3), 75–86 (1997).

Hayashi, K., K. Kawashima, K. Kose and T. Inouye, NMR imaging of advanced ceramics during the slip casting process *J. Phys. D-Appl. Phys.*, **21**, 1037–1039, (1988).

Henningsson, M., M. Regner, K. O¨stergren, C. Tragardh and P. Dejmek, CFD simulation and ERT visualization of the displacement of yoghurt by water on industrial scale, *Journal of Food Engineering*, **80**, 166–175 (2007).

Hinshaw, D.S., P.A. Bottomley, G.N. Holland, Radiographic thin-section image of the human wrist by nuclear magnetic resonance, *Nature*, **270**, 722–723 (1977).

Holden, P., M. Wang, R. Mann, F.J. Dickin, Macromixing using electrical resistance tomography, *AIChE Journal*, **44**(4), 780–790 (1998).

Holden, P.J., M. Wang, R. Mann, F.J. Dickin and R.B. Edwards, On detecting mixing pathologies inside a stirred vessel using electrical resistance tomography, *Trans IChemE*, **77**, Part A, 709–712 (1999).

Houcine, I., H. Vivier, E. Plasari, R. David and J. Villermaux, Planar laser induced fluorescence for measurements of concentration fields in continuous stirred tank reactors, *Experiments in Fluids*, **22**, 95–102 (1996).

Hu, H., T. Saga, T. Kobayashi, N. Taniguchi and M. Yasuki, Dual-plane stereoscopic particle image velocimetry: system set-up and its application on a lobed jet mixing flow. *Experiments in Fluids*, **31**, 277–293 (2001)

Huang, S.M., A. Plaskowski, X.G. Xie and M.S. Beck, Capacitance-based tomographic flow imaging system, *Electronics Letters*, **24**(7), 418–419, (1988).

Ihejirika, I. and F. Ein-Mozaffari, Using CFD and ultrasonic velocimetry to study the mixing of pseudoplastic fluids with a helical ribbon impeller, *Chem. Eng. Technol.* **30**(5), 606–614 (2007).

Jahangiri, M., A laser Doppler anemometry study of the Rushton turbine velocity profile for mixing of polymeric liquid, *Iranian Polymer Journal*, **14**(6), 521–530 (2005).

Jaworski, Z. and I. Fořt, Energy dissipation rate in a baffled vessel with pitched blade turbine impeller, *Collect Czech Chem Commun*, **56**, 1856–1867 (1991).

Jørgensen, F.E., The computer-controlled constant-temperature anemometer. Aspects of set-up, probe calibration, data acquisition and data conversion. *Meas. Sci. & Technol.*, **7**(10), 1378–1387 (1996).

Jørgensen, F.E., V.G. Chernoray, A.A. Bakchinov, L. Lőfdahl, A multi-sensor hot-wire anemometer system for investigation of wall-bounded flow structures, *Experimental Thermal and Fluid Science*, **27**, 207–214 (2003).

Jourdan, G., L. Schwaederlé, L. Houas, J.F. Haas, A.N. Aleshin, S.V. Sergeev and S.G. Zaytsev, Hot-wire method for measurements of turbulent mixing induced by Richtmyer–Meshkov instability in shock tube, *Shock Waves*, **11**, 189–197 (2001).

Kaehler, C.J. and J. Kompenhans, Multiple plane stereo PIV: technical realization and fluid-mechanical significance, in *Proceedings of the 3rd International Workshop on PIV*, Santa Barbara (1999).

Khoo, B.C., Y.T. Chew, C.J. Teo and C.P. Lim, The dynamic response of a hot-wire anemometer: III. Voltage-perturbation versus velocity perturbation testing for near-wall hot-wire/film probes, *Meas. Sci. Technol.*, **10**, 152–169 (1999).

Kim, S., B. Ngansib Nkaya and T. Dyakowski, Measurement of mixing of two miscible liquids in a stirred vessel with electrical resistance tomography, *International Communications in Heat and Mass Transfer*, **33**, 1088–1095 (2006).

Kimmich, R., *NMR Tomography, Diffusion, Relaxametry*, Spinger, Berlin (1997).

King, L.V., On the convection of heat from small cylinders in a stream of fluid: determination of the convection constants of small platinum wires, with applications to hot-wire anemometry, *Philos Trans Roy Soc London,* A, **214**, 373–432 (1914).

King, L.V., On the precision measurement of air velocity by means of the linear hot-wire anemometer, *Philos Mag J Sci*, Sixth Series, **29**, 556–77 (1915).

King, L.V., The linear hot-wire anemometer and its applications, *Technical Physics J. Franklin Inst.*, **181**, 1–25 (1916).

Kuo, H.P., P.C. Knight, D.J. Parker and J.P.K. Seville, Solids circulation and axial dispersion of cohesionless particles in a V-mixer, *Powder Technology*, **152**, 133–140 (2005).

Laakkonen, M., V. Alopaeus and J. Aittamaa, Validation of bubble breakage, coalescence and mass transfer models for gas-liquid dispersion in agitated vessel, *Chemical Engineering Science*, **61**(1), 218–228 (2006).

Lauterbur, P.C., Image formation by induced local interactions: examples of employing nuclear magnetic resonance, *Nature*, **242**, 190–191 (1973).

Lauterbur, P.C., Magnetic resonance zeugmatography, *Pure and Applied Chemistry*, **40**, 149–157 (1974).

Lee, K.C. and M. Yianneskis, Mixing characterisation of s stirred reactor with an axial flow impeller, *Eighth European Conference on Mixing*, IChemE Symposium Series **136**, 503–509 (1994).

Lee, Y., M.J. McCarthy and K.L. McCarthy, Extent of mixing in a two-component batch system measured using MRI, *J Food Engineering*, **50**, 167–174 (2001).

Lemoine, F., M. Wolff and M. Lebouché, Simultaneous concentration and velocity-measurements using combined laser-induced fluorescence and laser-Doppler velocimetry – Application to turbulent transport, *Experiment in Fluids*, **20**, 319–327 (1996).

Levitt, M.H., *Spin Dynamics*, John Wiley & Sons, Ltd, Chichester (2002).

Li, H., M. Wang, Y. Wu and G. Lucas, Volume flow rate measurement in vertical oil-in-water pipe flow using electrical impedance tomography and a local probe, *MultScienTechn.* **21**(i1–2.70), 81–93 (2009)

Li, L. and J. Wei, Three-dimensional image analysis of mixing in stirred vessels, *AIChE Journal*, **45**(9), 1855–1865 (1999).

Ljungqvist, M. and A. Rasmuson, The two-phase flow in an axially stirred vessel investigated using phase-Doppler anemometry, *Canadian Journal of Chemical Eng.* **82**(2), 275–288 (2004).

Lőfdahl, L. and M. Gad-el-Gak, MEMS applications in turbulent and flow control, *Progress in Aerospace Sciences*, **35**, 101–203 (1999).

Lu, W.M. and S.J. Ju, Application of hot-film anemometry to air-water flow in aerated stirred tanks, *Chem Eng Commun*, **56**, 57–75 (1987).

Lucas, G.P., R. Mishra and N. Panayotopoulos, Power law approximations to gas volume fraction and velocity profiles in low void fraction vertical gas-liquid flows, *Flow Meas. Instrum.*, **15**, 271 (2004).

Ma, X., S.R. Higson, A. Lyons and A.J. Peyton, Development of a fast electromagnetic induction tomography system for metal process applications, *Proceedings for 4th World Congress on Industrial Process Tomography*, Aizu, Japan, VCIPT, 196–201 (2005).

Maheo, P.M., *Free-surface turbulent shear flows*, PhD Thesis, California Institute of Technology, (1998).

Mann, R., P. Ying and R.B. Edwards, Application of a 3D networks-of-zones mixing model to a stirred vessel, *Eighth European Conference on Mixing*, IChemE Symposium Series **136**, 317–324 (1993).

Mann, R., S.K. Oillai, A.M. El-Hamouz, P. Ying, A. Togatorop and R.B. Edwards, Computational fluid mixing for stirred vessel: progress from seeing to believing, *Chem. Engineering Journal*, **59**, 39–50 (1995).

Mann, R., F.J. Dickin, M. Wang, T. Dyakowski, R.A. Williams, R.B. Edwards, A.E. Forrest and P.J. Holden, Application of electrical resistance tomography to interrogate mixing processes at plant scale, *Chem. Eng. Sci.*, **52**, 2087–2097 (1997).

Mann, R. and M. Wang, Electrical process tomography: Simple and inexpensive techniques for process imaging, *Measurement + Control*, **30**, 206–211 (1997).

Mann, R., Electrical process tomography: seeing 'without eyes' inside stirred vessels, *J Zhejiang Univ. Science*, **6A**(12), 1379–1385 (2005).

Mann, R., M. Wang, F.J. Dickin, T. Dyakowski and P.J. Holden, Resistance tomography imaging of stirred vessel mixing at plant scale, *IChemE Symposium Series, IChemE*, **140**, 155–167 (1996).

Mantle, M.D. and A.J. Sederman, Dynamic MRI in chemical process and reaction engineering, *Progress in Nuclear Magnetic Resonance Spectroscopy* **43**, 3–60 (2003).

Marashdeh, Q., L.-S. Fan, B. Du and W. Warsito, Electrical capacitance tomography - A perspective, *Ind. Eng. Chem. Res.*, **47**, 3708–3719 (2008).

Mavros, P., Flow visualization in stirred vessels, *Trans IChemE*, **79**, Par A, 113–120 (2001).

Maxwell, J.C., *A Treatise on Electricity and Magnetism*, 3rd edn, Clarendon Press, Oxford, p. 440 (1891).

McKee, S.L., *Tomographic measurements of solid–liquid mixing*, PhD Thesis, UMIST (1994).

Millipore Corporation, Billerica, MA, www.millipore.com. (2010)

Murphy, S.C., S.J. Stanley, D. Rhodes and T.A. York, 3D electrical tomographic imaging using vertical arrays of electrodes, *Meas. Sci. Technol.* **17**, 3053–3065 (2006).

Nikiforaki, L., K.C. Lee and M. Yianneskis, Circulation time measurements with miniature radio frequency identification devices, in Benkreira, H. (ed.), *Fluid Mixing 6,* IChemE Symp. Ser. no. **146**, 47–57 (1999).

Pakzad, L., F. Ein-Mozaffari, P. Chan, Measuring mixing time in the agitation of non-Newtonian fluids through electrical resistance tomography, *Chem. Eng. Technol.*, **31**(12), 1838–1845 (2008).

Parker, D.J. and P.A. McNeil, Positron emission tomography for process applications, *Meas. Sci. Technol.*, **7,** 287–296 (1996).

Parker, D.J. and X. Fan, Positron emission particle tracking – Application and labelling techniques, *Particuology*, **6**, 16–23 (2008).

Peyton, A.J., Z.Z. Yu, G. Lyon, S. Al-Zeibak, J. Ferreira, J. Velez, et al., An overview of electromagnetic inductance tomography: description of three different systems, *Meas. Sci. & Technol.*, **7**(3), 261–271 (1996).

Pickering, C.J.D. and N.A. Halliwell, Speckle photography in fluid flows: signal recovery with two-step processing, *Appl. Optics*, **23**, 1128–1129 (1984).

Pinheiro, P.A.T., W.W. Loh and F.J. Dickin, Three-dimensional reconstruction algorithm for electrical resistance tomography, *IEE Proc.-Sci. Meas. Technol.*, **145**(3), 85–95 (1998).

Pitot, H., Description d'une machine pour mesurer la vitesse des eaux courantes et le sillage des vaisseaux, *Mémoires de L'Académie,* November (in French) (1732).

Porion, P., N. Sommier, A.-M. Fauge're and P. Evesque, Dynamics of size segregation and mixing of granular materials in a 3D-blender by NMR imaging investigation, *Powder Technology*, **141**, 55–68 (2004).

Qiu, C., B.S. Hoyle and F.J.W. Podd, Engineering and application of a dual-modality process tomography system, *Flow Measurement and Instrumentation*, **18**, 247–254 (2007).

Rahimi, M., P.R. Senior and R. Mann, Image-reconstruction 3D visual modelling of stirred vessel mixing for an inclined-blade impeller, *Fluid Mixing*, IChemE Symposium Series, **146**, 135–145 (1999).

Rao, R., L. Mondy, A. Sun, S. Altobelli, A numerical and experimental study of batch sedimentation and viscous resuspension, *Int. J. Numer. Meth. Fluids*, **39**(6), 465–483, (2002).

Reinecke, N. and D. Mewes, Recent developments and industrial/research applications of capacitance tomography, *Meas. Sci. Technol.*, **7**, 233–246 (1996).

Robert, B. and C. Doblin, An investigation of sparged mixing tank using electrical impedance tomography and computational fluid dynamics, *3rd International Conference on CFD in the Minerals and Process Industries*, CSIRO, Melbourne, Australia, 593–598 (2003).

Sachs, P. and J.H. Rushton, Discharge flow from turbine type mixing impellers, *Chem. Eng. Prog.*, **50**(12), 597–603, (1954).

Sharifi, M. and B. Young, Qualitative visualization and quantitative analysis of milk flow using electrical resistance tomography, *Journal of Food Engineering*, **112**, 227–242 (2012a)

Sharifi, M. and B. Young, Milk total solids and fat content soft sensing via electrical resistance tomography and temperature measurement, *Food and Bioproducts Processing*, **90**, 659–666 (2012b).

Sharifi, M. and B. Young, Electrical resistance tomography (ERT) applications to chemical engineering, *Chemical Engineering Research and Design*, **91**(9), 1624–1645 (2013).

Sommier, N., P. Porion, P. Evesque, B. Leclerc, P. Tchoreloff and G. Couarraze, Magnetic resonance imaging investigation of the mixing-segregation process in a pharmaceutical blender, *International Journal of Pharmaceutics*, **222**, 243–258 (2001).

Squire, L.F. and R.A. Novelline, *Squire's Fundamentals of Radiology*, 5th edn, Harvard University Press (1997).

Stanley, S.J. and G. Bolton, A review of recent electrical resistance tomography (ERT) applications for wet particulate processing, *Part. Part. Sys. Charact.*, **25**, 207–215 (2008).

Stanley, S.J., E. Wabo, R. Mann and K. Primrose, Dual-validation of miscible liquid mixing in a stirred vessel imaged by electrical resistance tomography (ERT), *2nd World Congress on Industrial Process Tomography*, Hannover, Germany, pp. 151–158 (2001).

Stanley, S.J., R. Mann and K. Primrose, Tomographic imaging of fluid mixing in three dimensions for single-feed semi-batch operation of a stirred vessel, *Trans, I. Chem. E.*, **80**, Part A, 903–909 (2002).

Stanley, S.J., R. Mann and K. Primrose, Interrogation of a precipitation reaction by Electrical Resistance Tomography (ERT), *AIChE Journal*, **51**(2), 607 (2005).

Stephenson, D.R., T.L. Rodgers, R. Mann and T.A. York, Application of three-dimensional electrical impedance tomography to investigate fluid mixing in a stirred vessel, in *13th European Conference on Mixing*, London, pp. 14–17 (2009).

Takeda, Y., Instantaneous velocity profile measurement by ultrasonic Doppler method, *JSME International Journal of Fluid and Thermal Engineering*, **38**, 8–16 (1995)

Tapp, H.S., A.J. Peyton, E.K. Kemsley and R.H. Wilson, Chemical engineering applications of electrical process tomography, *Sensors and Actuators*, **B**(92), 17–14 (2003).

Unger, D.R. and F.J. Muzzio, Laser-induced fluorescence techniques for the quantification of mixing in impinging jets, *AIChE J.*, **45**(12), 2477–2486 (1999).

Wabo, E., M. Kagoshima and R. Mann, Batch stirred vessel mixing evaluated by visualized reactive tracers and electrical tomography, *Chemical Engineering Research and Design*, **82**(A9), 1229–1236 (2004).

Wang, M., F.J. Dickin and M.S. Beck, Improved electrical impedance tomography data collection system and measurement protocols, in *Tomography Technique and Process Design and Operation*, M.S. Beck, E. Campogrande, M. Morris, R.A. Williams and R.C. Waterfall (eds), Computational Mechanics Publications, pp. 75–88 (1993).

Wang, M., F.J. Dickin and R.A. Williams, Modelling and analysis of electrically conducting vessels and pipelines in electrical resistance process tomography, *IEE Proc. Sci. Meas. Technol.*, **142**(4), 313–322, (1995).

Wang, M., R. Mann, A.E. Forrest, P.J. Holden, F.J. Dickin, T. Dyakowski and R.B. Edwards, Stirred vessel mixing in 3D using electrical resistance tomography, *Electronic Measurement and Instrument Society*, **11**(A), CIE, Beijing, 650–653 (1997).

Wang, M., Inverse solutions for electrical impedance tomography based on conjugate gradients methods, *Meas. Sci. & Technol.*, **13**, 101–117 (2002).

Wang, M., A. Dorwood, D. Vlaev and R. Mann, Measurements of gas-liquid mixing in a stirred vessel using electrical resistance tomography, *Chem. Eng. Sci.*, **77**, 93–98 (2000).

Wang, M., Y. Ma, N. Holliday, Y. Dai, R.A. Williams and G. Lucas, A high performance EIT system, *IEEE Sensors Journal*, **5**(2), 289–299 (2004).

Wang, M., Seeing a new dimension – the past decade's developments on electrical impedance tomography, *Progress in Nature Science*, **15**(1), 1–13, (2005b).

Wang, M., G. Lucas, Y. Dai, N. Panayotopoulos and A. Williams, Visualisation of bubbly velocity distribution in a swirling flow using electrical resistance tomography, *Part. Part. Syst. Charact.*, **23**, 321–329 (2006)

Westerweel, J., J.B. Flör and F.T.M. Nieuwstadt, Measurement of dynamics of coherent flow structures using particle image velocimetry. In *Applications of Laser Anemometry in Fluid Mechanics*. R.J. Adrian, P.W. Offutt, C.C. Landreth, Z. Liu and T.J. Hanratty (eds), Springer, Berlin, pp. 476–499 (1991). Adrian, R.J., *A*

Wikipedia, http://en.wikipedia.org/wiki/Magnetic_resonance_imaging (2010).

Wilkinson, A.J., E.W. Randall, T.M. Long and A. Collins, The design of an ERT system for 3D data acquisition and a quantitative evaluation of its performance, *Meas. Sci. Technol.*, **17**, 2088–2096 (2006).

Willert, C.E. and M. Gharib, Digital particle image velocimetry, *Experiments in Fluids*, **10**, 181–193 (1991).

Williams, R.A., X. Jia and S.L. McKee, Development of slurry mixing models using resistance tomography. *Powder Technology*, **87**, 21–27 (1996).

Wing-Keung Law, A. and H. Wang, Measurement of mixing processes with combined digital particle image velocimetry and planar laser induced fluorescence, *Experimental Thermal and Fluid Science*, **22**(3–4), 213–229 (2000).

Wolf, D. and F.S. Manning, Impact tube measurement of flow patterns, velocity profiles and pumping capacities in mixing vessels, *Can. J. Chem Eng*, **44**, 137–142 (1996).

Xie, C.G., S.M. Huang, B.S. Hoyle, C.P. Lenn and M.S. Beck, Transputer-based electrical capacitance tomography for real-time imaging of oilfield flow pipelines, in *Tomography Technique and Process Design and Operation*, M.S. Beck, E. Campogrande, M. Morris, R.A. Williams and R.C. Waterfall (eds), Computational Mechanics Publications, pp. 333–346 (1993).

Yang, W.Q., D.M. Spink, T.A. York and H. McCann, An image reconstruction algorithm based on Landweber's iteration method for electrical capacitance tomography, *Meas. Sci. & Technol.*, **10**(11), 1095–1099 (1999).

Yenjaichon, W., G. Pageau and M. Bhole, C. Bennington and J. R. Grace, Assessment of mixing quality for an industrial pulp mixer using electrical resistance tomography, *The Canadian Journal of Chemical Engineering*, **9999**, 2–9 (2011).

York, T., Status of electrical tomography in industrial applications, *Journal of Electronic Imaging*, **10**(3), 608–619 (2001).

Yu, Z.Z., A.T. Peyton, M.S. Beck, W.F. Conway and L.A. Xu, Imaging system based on electromagnetic tomography (EMT), *Electronics Letters*, **29**(7), 625–626 (1993).

17

Discrete Element Method (DEM) Simulation of Powder Mixing Process

Ali Hassanpour and Mojtaba Ghadiri
Institute of Particle Science and Engineering, School of Chemical and Process Engineering, University of Leeds, UK

17.1 Introduction to DEM and its Application in Pharmaceutical Powder Processing

The analysis of the behaviour of particle assemblies encountered in many particulate processes is complex due to the heterogeneous nature of individual entities, resulting in a wide ranging interaction of primary particles under different applied operating conditions. Cundall (1971) developed a numerical method to simulate the mechanical response of particle assemblies subjected to forces and displacements. In this method the position, velocity, acceleration and contact forces of each element were calculated and updated with time in small time steps. Elements representing the particles in the assembly were either disks or spheres. The velocity and acceleration of the elements were calculated based on Newton's laws of motion and contact forces were obtained based on linear spring model. This method has become known as the *Discrete Element Method* (DEM) and has been used extensively for the simulation of mechanical behaviour of granular media.

There has been considerable progress in recent years on the application of the DEM to the analysis of the mechanics of granular media based on the TRUBAL computer code developed by Cundall and Strack (1979) and further extended by various researchers. The DEM has been used to simulate the behaviour of granular media for various engineering applications, such as fluidized bed (e.g. Tsuji, 1993 and di Renzo *et al.*, 2008), pneumatic

Pharmaceutical Blending and Mixing, First Edition. Edited by P.J. Cullen, Rodolfo J. Romañach, Nicolas Abatzoglou and Chris D. Rielly.

conveying (e.g. Chu and Yu, 2008; Kuang *et al.*, 2008), powder dispersion (e.g. Higashitani *et al.*, 2001; Calvert *et al.*, 2011), particle flow in various vessels (e.g. Wassgren *et al.*, 2002; Datta *et al.*, 2008; Hassanpour *et al.*, 2011) and granulation (e.g. Moreno *et al.*, 2006; Hassanpour *et al.*, 2013). A thorough review of application of DEM is provided by Zhu *et al.* (2008).

With increasing computer power and memory at affordable costs, new developments have embraced complex particle shapes, computationally more efficient contact models, use of a large number of particles and moving to smaller particles and particle breakage and wear. For particle shape a variety of approaches have been developed ranging from clumped-spheres (Favier *et al.*, 1999), polyhedra shapes (Potapov and Campbell, 1997; Hogue, 1998), mathematical shape functions, for example super-quadrics (Delaney and Cleary, 2009), to digital voxel packing (Jia *et al.*, 2007). The early developments of the contact models range from the simple linear spring and dash pot and Coulombic, first proposed by Cundall (1971) and by Walton and Brown (1986), to the more rigorous non-linear models. For normal deformation, Thornton and co-workers developed models based on Hertz analysis for elastic deformation, JKR model (Johnson *et al.*, 1971) for adhesion, and Thornton and Ning (1998) model for plastic deformation (see the recent review by Thornton *et al.*, 2013). For tangential deformation and sliding, the adhesive contact model of Savkoor and Briggs (1977) is rigorous, as it is based on the fracture mechanics of a crack extension, taking the adhesive contact geometry as a crack. However, these models are computationally very demanding and hence attempts have been made to develop simpler models (e.g. see Di Maio and Di Renzo, 2005). More recently, a number of simplified models have emerged to speed up the computations, particularly for very large number of small particles requiring short integration time step, but their accuracy and validity need yet to be more thoroughly checked (Tomas, 2007; Luding, 2008, Pasha *et al.*, 2014; Thakur *et al.*, 2014). Particle breakage and wear pose the greatest challenge to DEM for realistic and reliable simulations, as debris and fragments have irregular shapes and in turn influence the mechanics of flow and contact stress (Antonyuk *et al.*, 2006; Kalman *et al.*, 2009). The approach of using bonded spheres to form an agglomerate requires a reliable model of contact bond breakage, and this in turn depends on the failure mode of the bond itself, that is, ductile, semi- or fully brittle (see e.g. Golchert *et al.*, 2004). The early work of Potapov and Campbell (1997) by sticking polyhedra together enabled the simulation of breakage of non-spherical particles, but the failure rules were unrealistic as they had pre-determined crack planes. Obviously there is a lot yet to be done to address the limitations of the DEM in modelling the interactions of a large number of irregular particles, as it occurs in the breakage process. Nevertheless there have also been notable successes, an account of which is given in the text that follows for mixing application.

One of the areas where the DEM has a great potential for predictive analysis is powder mixing. This is a key process operation in industrial sectors such as detergent, cosmetic, food and pharmaceutical manufacturing. A wide variety of mixers are used depending on specific application requirements, including batch and continuous mixers with a wide range in shear rates, residence times and specific energy inputs. Understanding, control and optimization of these processes are of strategic importance, but at the same time very challenging. To optimize these process operations, a key step is to understand powder kinematic behaviour (flow fields, mixing patterns etc.) to enable efficient process design and control. There has been considerable work reported in the literature on the characterization of the powder flow behaviour during mixing under various process conditions (e.g.

Bridgwater, 1976; Laurent and Bridgwater, 2000; Portillo *et al.*, 2007). However, it is difficult to obtain an insight to the internal flow field during mixing processes and to address the kinematic behaviour of powders using experimental approaches, particularly at large scales. Most experimental measurements of internal flow are based on Positron Emission Particle Tracking (PEPT), but this technique is suitable for laboratory and small scale mixers (Laurent and Bridgwater, 2000; Ng *et al.*, 2007). Therefore, the ability to model the mixing process in various larger mixers using the DEM has attracted attention and grown along with the computing power.

17.2 DEM Simulation of Powder Mixing

Various types of mixers have been simulated using DEM. Mixing equipment falls into two major categories: (1) rotating blenders and (2) internal blade mixers. Simulations of particle mixing have been carried out extensively for various types of mixers, such as rotating drums (Muguruma *et al.*, 1997; Chaudhuri *et al.*, 2006; Yang *et al.*, 2008; Xu *et al.*, 2010), V-blenders (Moakher *et al.*, 2000; Kuo *et al.*,2002; Lemieux *et al.*, 2008; Tahvildarian *et al.*, 2013), Tote blenders (e.g. Arratia *et al.*, 2006), double cone blenders (Moakher *et al.*, 2000) and complex moving mixers (Marigo *et al.*, 2011).

For the internal blade mixers, the work is mainly focused on helical mixers (2D simulation by Kaneko *et al.*, 2000 and 3D by Schutyser *et al.*, 2003), mixers with vertical axis blades (Stewart *et al.*, 2001; Zhou *et al.*, 2004; Sato *et al.*, 2008; Hassanpour *et al.*, 2013; Chandratilleke *et al.*, 2012), and horizontal axis blades (Hassanpour *et al.*, 2011; Li *et al.*, 2013; Sarkar and Wassgren, 2012). A recent review by Bridgwater (2012) suggests that the modelling studies so far have enhanced our knowledge of physical behaviour such as internal flow structure; however, modelling should be backed by experimental observations, and predictions should be made without adjustment of material properties in modelling.

Qualitative results are a quick way to understand how mixing devices operate, however, the data would be insufficient for the process control and design. DEM simulation results could be in the form of flow pattern observations (Figs 17.1 and 17.2) and qualitative mixing and segregation (Fig. 17.3). Qualitative comparison between simulation and experiments are usually based on observation of segregation/mixing using coloured particles.

An in depth understanding of the mixing mechanisms requires a quantitative analysis. Parameters such as particle velocity distribution (Fig. 17.4), circulation intensity (Fig. 17.5), and mixing/segregation index (Figs 17.6 and 17.7), are usually quantified under various process conditions such as fill ratio, number of revolutions and revolutions per minute (rpm). For example, Tahvildarian *et al.* (2013) have utilized the DEM simulations for the quantification of circulation intensity and axial dispersion of powders in V-blenders. Their study suggests the optimum operating conditions in terms of fill level and rpm for achieving better mixing efficiency for such type of mixers. In another study by Marigo *et al.* (2011), it is shown that for Turbula® mixer the mixing rate initially decreases with the rotational speed, but subsequently increases (Fig. 17.8). In their work DEM has been used to quantify the operating conditions for achieving the optimum mixing rate in a Turbula® mixer.

With the recent advances in computer hardware as well as optimization of DEM softwares, it is now possible to simulate complex equipment geometry, and moving components using different particle shapes. This can facilitate the design and optimization of complex equipment for mixing processes. However, computer power is still inadequate for

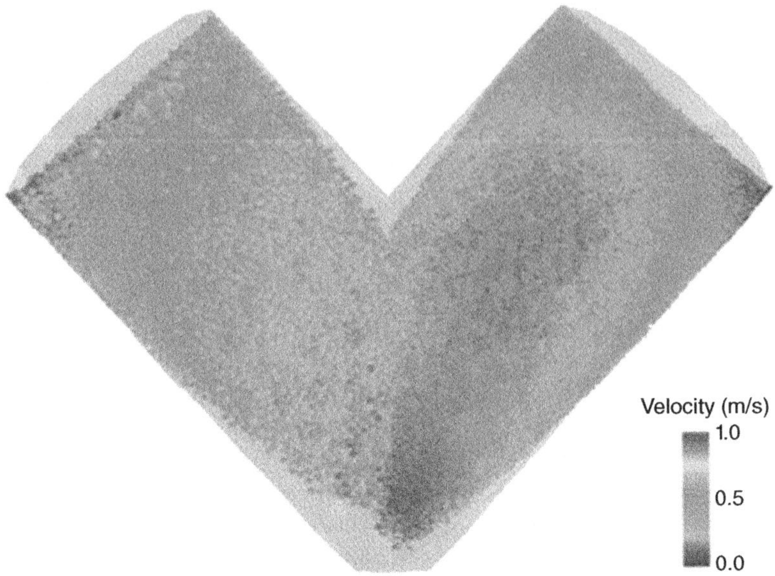

Figure 17.1 *Front-view illustration of the particle velocity field in a V-blender. Reprinted with permission from* Powder Technology, *Large-scale numerical investigation of solids mixing in a V-blender using the discrete element method by M. Lemieux, G. Léonard, J. Doucet, L.-A. Leclaire, F. Viens, J. Chaouki, F. Bertrand, 181, 2, 205–216. Copyright (2008) Elsevier*

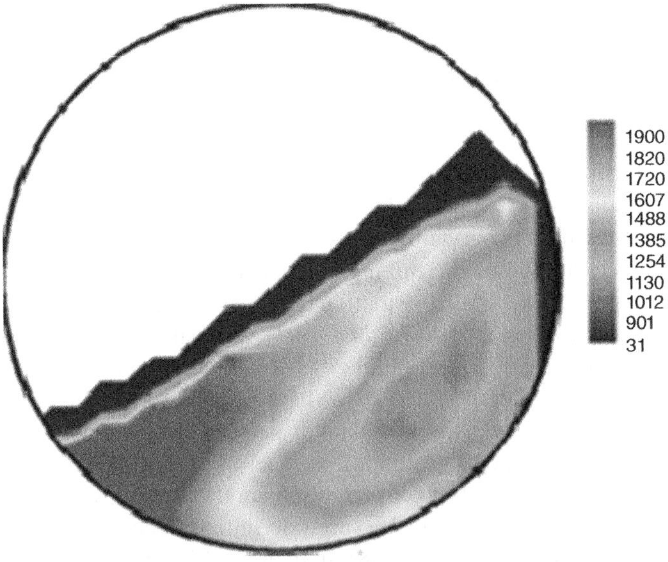

Figure 17.2 *DEM simulation of particle collision velocity (mm/s) in a cylindrical rotating drum. Reprinted with permission from* Powder Technology, *Experimentally validated computations of flow, mixing and segregation of non-cohesive grains in 3D tumbling blenders, Maher Moakher, Troy Shinbrot, Fernando J. Muzzio, 109, 1–3, 58–71. Copyright (2000) Elsevier*

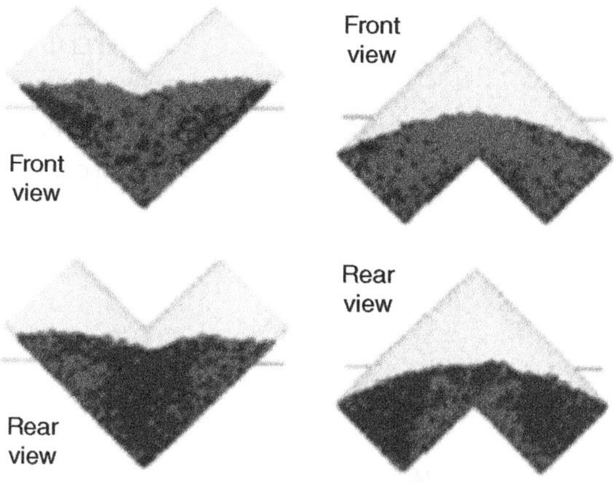

Figure 17.3 *Mixing/segregation patterns DEM simulation of V-blender after two revolutions viewed from different directions. Reprinted with permission from* Powder Technology, *Experimentally validated computations of flow, mixing and segregation of non-cohesive grains in 3D tumbling blenders, Maher Moakher, Troy Shinbrot, Fernando J. Muzzio, 109, 1–3, 58–71. Copyright (2000) Elsevier*

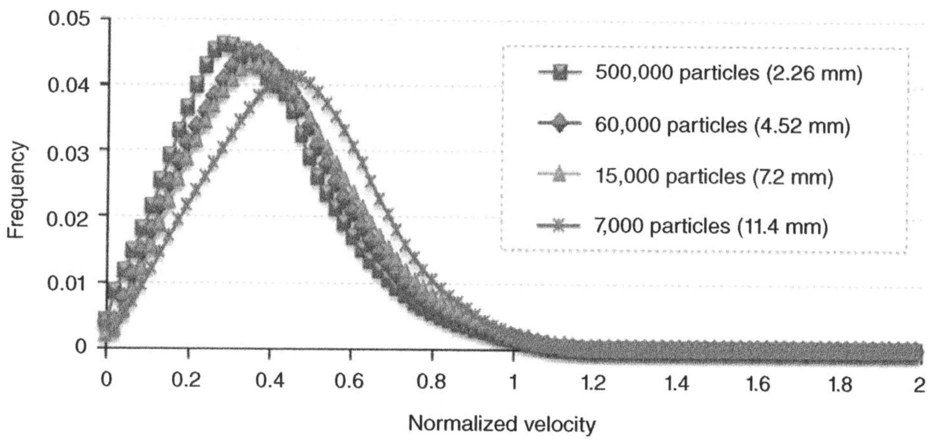

Figure 17.4 *Number based frequency distribution for particle velocity (normalized by the paddle tip speed) for different particles sizes in a Forberg mixer. Reprinted with permission from* Powder Technology, *Analysis of particle motion in a paddle mixer using Discrete Element Method (DEM), Ali Hassanpour, Hongsing Tan, Andrew Bayly, Prasad Gopalkrishnan, Boonho Ng, Mojtaba Ghadiri, 206, 1–2, 189–194. Copyright (2011) Elsevier*

simulating full populations of particles for real industrial scales (billions of particles). A number of researchers have considered the use of larger particles in the simulations to reduce the particle number and simulation time (Sato *et al.*, 2008 and Hassanpour *et al.*, 2009), whilst in some cases the properties of large particles have been calibrated (Hassanpour *et al.*, 2009 and 2011). However, reliability of this method in terms of predicting actual powder flow characteristics remains a fundamental question and needs to be addressed.

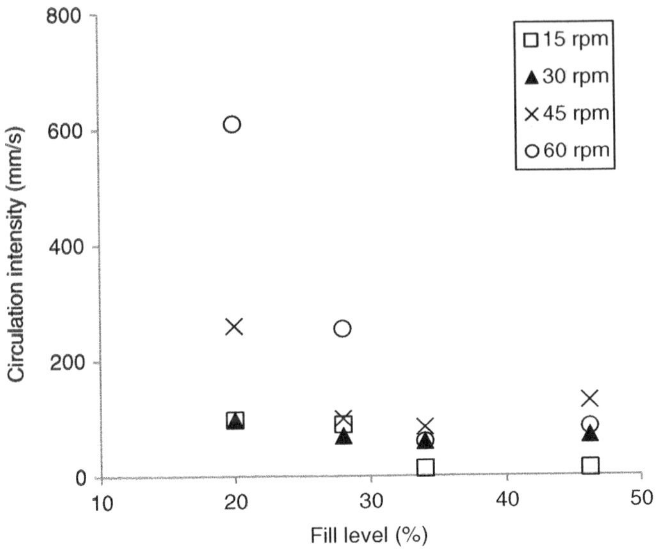

Figure 17.5 Circulation intensity of particles in a V-blender as a function of fill level at different rotational. Reprinted with permission from Particuology, Circulation intensity and axial dispersion of non-cohesive solid particles in a V-blender via DEM simulation, Parisa Tahvildarian, Farhad Ein-Mozaffari, Simant R. Upreti, 11, 6, 619–626. Copyright (2013) Elsevier

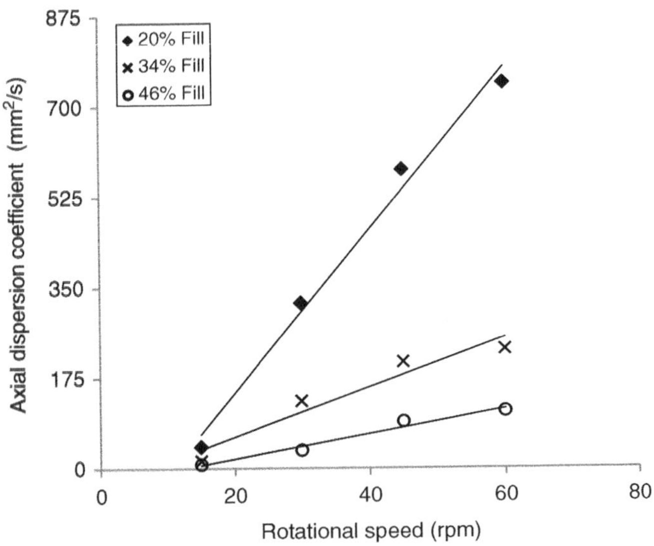

Figure 17.6 Axial dispersion coefficient of particles in a V-blender as a function of fill level at different rotational. Reprinted with permission from Particuology, Circulation intensity and axial dispersion of non-cohesive solid particles in a V-blender via DEM simulation, Parisa Tahvildarian, Farhad Ein-Mozaffari, Simant R. Upreti, 11, 6, 619–626. Copyright (2013) Elsevier

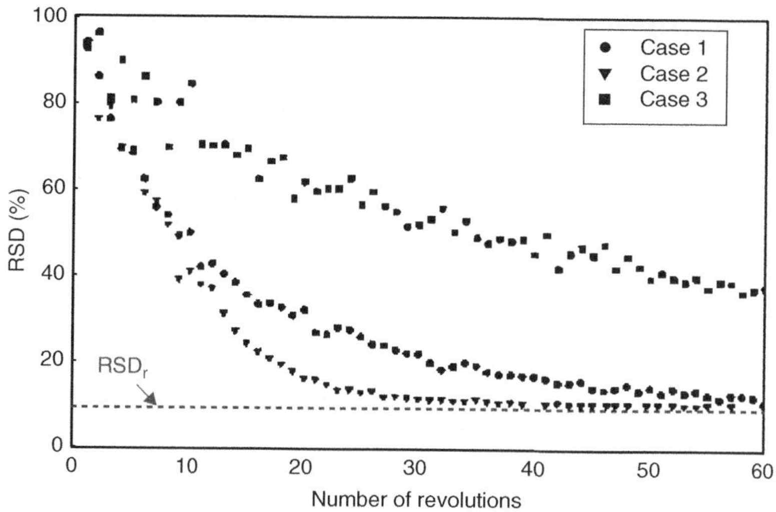

Figure 17.7 *Relative standard deviation (RSD) of particle concentration used to quantify the mixing tendency of particles in V-blenders. Reprinted with permission from* Powder Technology, *Large-scale numerical investigation of solids mixing in a V-blender using the discrete element method by M. Lemieux, G. Léonard, J. Doucet, L.-A. Leclaire, F. Viens, J. Chaouki, F. Bertrand, 181, 2, 205–216. Copyright (2008) Elsevier*

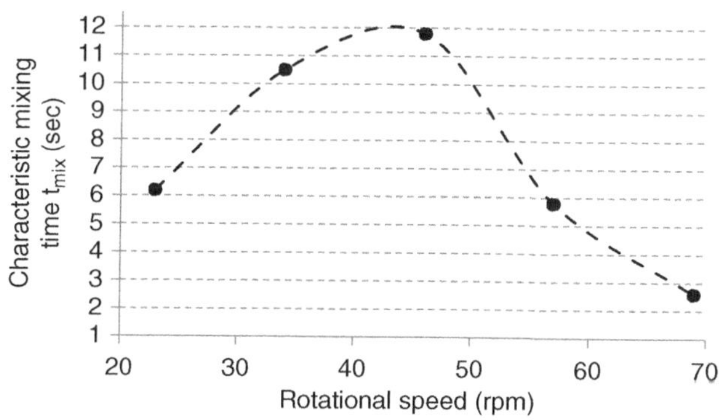

Figure 17.8 *Characteristic mixing time in Turbula® mixer as function of rotational speed. Reprinted with permission from* International Journal of Pharmaceutics, *Application of Positron Emission Particle Tracking (PEPT) to validate a Discrete Element Method (DEM) model of granular flow and mixing in the Turbula mixer, M. Marigo, M. Davies, T. Leadbeater, D.L. Cairns, A. Ingram, E.H. Stitt, 446, 1–2, 46–58. Copyright (2013) Elsevier*

A recent study by Hassanpour *et al.* (2011) focused on addressing the capability of DEM to simulate the powder flow pattern in a paddle mixer. In particular they investigated the effect of particle size on the dynamics of powder flow inside a horizontal mixer. For analysis of flow field of the mixer, the EDEM computer code developed by DEM-solutions was used. Particle motion in the mixer was analysed to determine the granular dynamics, and in particular the velocity field was identified.

Figure 17.9 shows the 3D representation of the Forberg commercial mixer used by Hassanpour *et al.* (2011) in the DEM computer code. The mixer consists of two intersected semi-cylinders of the same span and two counter-rotating impellers, each with 10 paddles positioned pair-wise along five axial positions. Hassanpour *et al.* (2011) considered the powders to be non-cohesive and the Hertz–Mindlin model was used for the normal and tangential interactions. The reason for this was stated to be for the comparison with the experimental work using PEPT, which were carried out on dry, free-flowing particles.

The simulation by Hassanpour *et al.* (2011) was carried out with a smaller number of larger particles, however, the sensitivity of powder dynamics to the particle size was analysed by simulation using various particles sizes (Table 17.1) but with similar mechanical properties. The particle number for each case was calculated based on a 100% fill level in the mixer and on all cases, the filling was carried out while the mixer impellers were stationary. All cases of simulations were carried out under the same operating conditions and for 10s of real time. The qualitative results in Fig. 17.10 (all snapshots at identical times) showed similar velocity and flow patterns for all simulations.

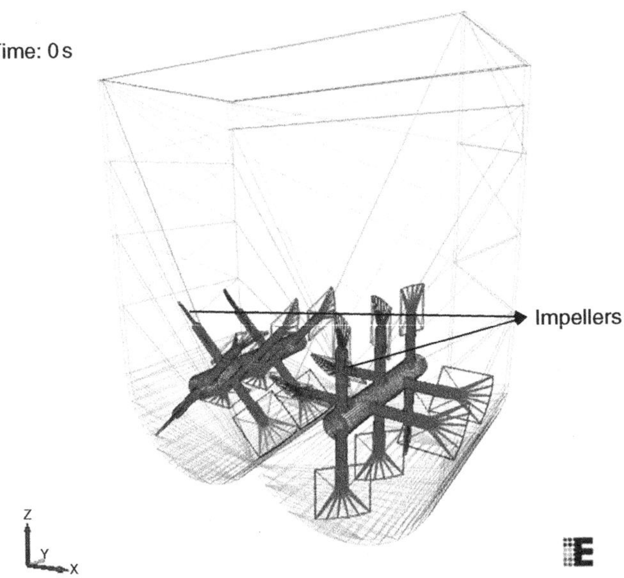

Figure 17.9 The imported geometry of the paddle mixer simulated by DEM. Reprinted with permission from Powder Technology, Analysis of particle motion in a paddle mixer using Discrete Element Method (DEM), Ali Hassanpour, Hongsing Tan, Andrew Bayly, Prasad Gopalkrishnan, Boonho Ng, Mojtaba Ghadiri, 206, 1–2, 189–194. Copyright (2011) Elsevier

Table 17.1 The modelling conditions for the sensitivity analysis on size using DEM simulation (Hassanpour et al., 2011)

Simulation Case	A	B	C	D
Particle diameter (mm)	11.40	7.20	4.52	2.26
Total particle number	7,000	15,000	60,000	500,000

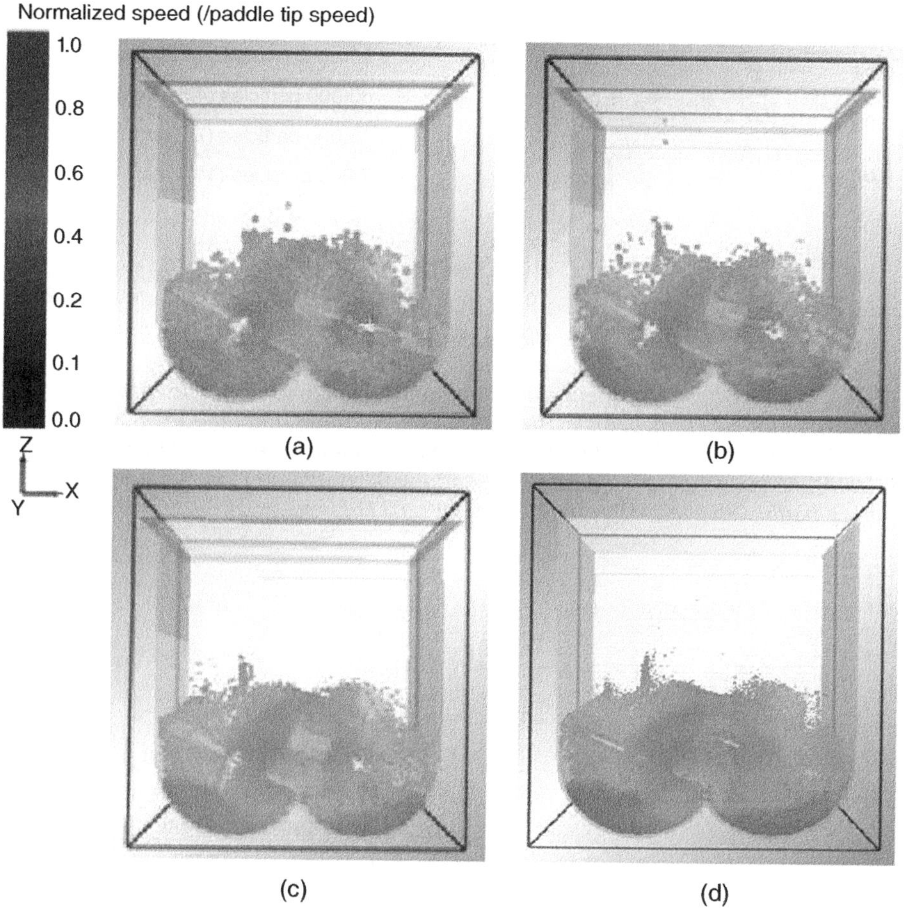

Figure 17.10 *The schematic flow fields inside the paddle mixer simulated by the DEM, where snapshots were taken at identical time for systems with various particle sizes (a: 11.40 mm, b: 7.20 mm, c: 4.5 mm and d: 2.26 mm). Reprinted with permission from* Powder Technology, *Analysis of particle motion in a paddle mixer using Discrete Element Method (DEM), Ali Hassanpour, Hongsing Tan, Andrew Bayly, Prasad Gopalkrishnan, Boonho Ng, Mojtaba Ghadiri, 206, 1–2, 189–194. Copyright (2011) Elsevier*

The quantitative results in terms of time averaged normalized velocity distributions (overall magnitude) in Fig. 17.11 have shown that a percentage of particles were stagnant (zero velocity) for all systems. It was observed that the mean average velocity magnitude of all particles rapidly increased with time and quickly reached a steady condition (Fig. 17.12). The steady state average velocity magnitude decreased only slightly as the particle size was reduced (Fig. 17.13). Therefore it was suggested that for the simulation of powder flow with given 'specific' conditions a modelling system with larger particles could safely be used.

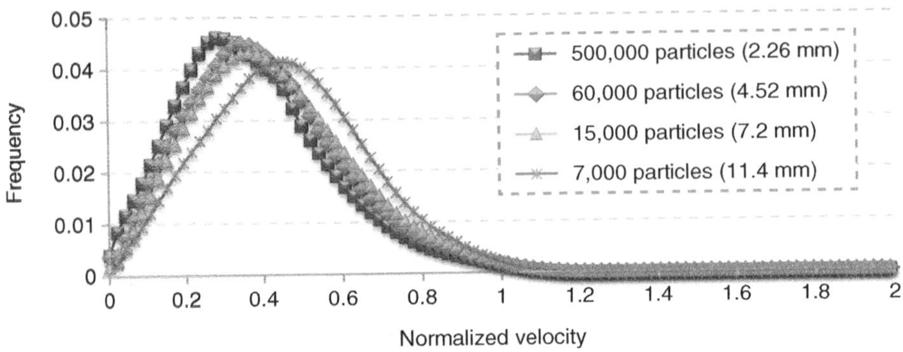

Figure 17.11 Number based frequency distribution for particle velocity (normalized by the paddle tip speed) for different particles sizes in a Forberg mixer. Reprinted with permission from Powder Technology, *Analysis of particle motion in a paddle mixer using Discrete Element Method (DEM), Ali Hassanpour, Hongsing Tan, Andrew Bayly, Prasad Gopalkrishnan, Boonho Ng, Mojtaba Ghadiri, 206, 1–2, 189–194. Copyright (2011) Elsevier*

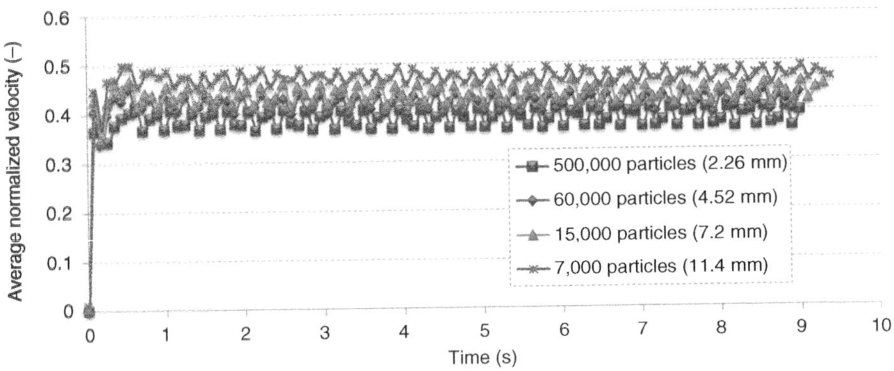

Figure 17.12 Evolution of mean particle velocity by time for different particles sizes in a Forberg mixer. Reprinted with permission from Powder Technology, *Analysis of particle motion in a paddle mixer using Discrete Element Method (DEM), Ali Hassanpour, Hongsing Tan, Andrew Bayly, Prasad Gopalkrishnan, Boonho Ng, Mojtaba Ghadiri, 206, 1–2, 189–194. Copyright (2011) Elsevier*

17.3 Validation and Comparison with the Experiments

Validation of DEM predictions is often carried out qualitatively or quantitatively by comparing results with identical experiments. Qualitative comparisons are usually based on visual methods for transparent vessels, such as particle image velocimetery (PIV) or image analysis of coloured particles. One of the shortcomings of these methods is that the results are more related to the behaviour of particles at the observable surface of the vessel rather than internal powder flow structure. In an investigation by Moakher *et al.* (2000) the

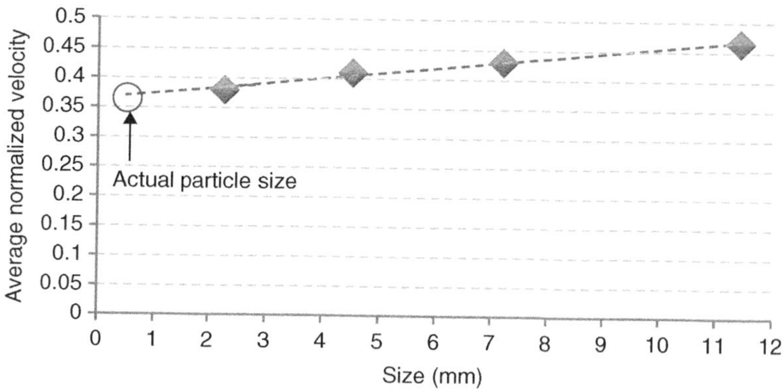

Figure 17.13 *Steady state mean particle velocity as a function of different particles sizes in a Forberg mixer. Reprinted with permission from* Powder Technology, *Analysis of particle motion in a paddle mixer using Discrete Element Method (DEM), Ali Hassanpour, Hongsing Tan, Andrew Bayly, Prasad Gopalkrishnan, Boonho Ng, Mojtaba Ghadiri, 206, 1–2, 189–194. Copyright (2011) Elsevier*

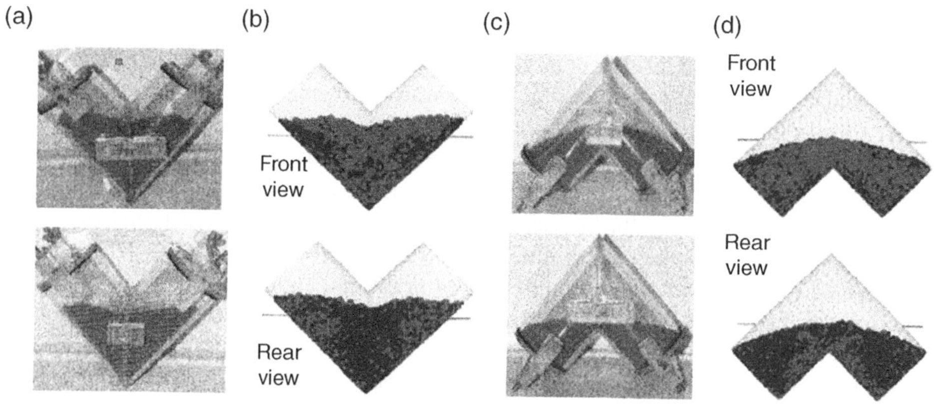

Figure 17.14 *Mixing/segregation patterns of different size particles (a) experiment in upright transparent V-blender; (b) corresponding simulation in upright vessel after two revolutions; (c) experiment in inverted orientation and (d) corresponding simulation in inverted orientation. Reprinted with permission from Powder Technology, Experimentally validated computations of flow, mixing and segregation of non-cohesive grains in 3D tumbling blenders, Maher Moakher, Troy Shinbrot, Fernando J. Muzzio, 109, 1–3, 58–71. Copyright (2000) Elsevier*

DEM simulation of different size particle mixing in a V-blender has been visually compared with the experiments. They used a transparent V-blender and examined the mixing and segregation pattern using coloured particles, viewed from different angles (Fig. 17.14). They reported a good agreement with the experimental mixing/segregation patterns at different revolutions and orientations.

One of the common approaches for quantitative validation is the comparison of internal solids motion in mixers with the data from PEPT experiments. PEPT works by tracking the position of one tracer particle over a long period of time (usually 10–20 min) to generate sufficiently accurate time averaged data. The time averaged velocity field inside the mixer can then be calculated and compared with the DEM simulation results of identical cases. Stewart *et al.* (2001) carried out a quantitative comparison between the time-averaged velocity profiles from PEPT measurements and corresponding DEM simulations for a bladed mixer (Fig. 17.15). The velocity fields were compared at different mixer heights for different particle friction coefficient and an acceptable agreement between the simulation and experiments was observed.

Marigo *et al.* (2013) used the PEPT data to calculate a dispersion coefficient of the particles for the Turbula mixer. They compared the results with the DEM simulations of the same mixer and found that the general qualitative trends of the dispersion coefficient were similar (Fig. 17.16). However, they reported that DEM quantitatively over-predicted the results. This was attributed to the choice of DEM input parameters.

Tahvildarian *et al.* (2013) have compared the axial dispersion of particles from DEM simulation of mixing in a V-blender with the experimental results from PEPT carried out by Kuo *et al.* (2005). A good agreement between predictions and experiments has been achieved for the effect of rotational speeds at different fill ratios (Fig. 17.17). Likewise, a comparison of particle circulation intensity obtained from DEM and PEPT results shows similar trends with the fill ratio at different rotational speeds (Fig. 17.18).

In the study by Hassanpour *et al.* (2011), the velocity fields from both DEM simulation and PEPT were compared inside a commercial paddle mixer. Both DEM and PEPT showed two vertical and horizontal (forward and backward movement) mixing patterns for the powder flow in the paddle mixer. The horizontal flow pattern was reported to be due to the manufacturer's design of tilted paddles. The work has shown that modelling could assist the design and modification of mixers to create desirable mixing patterns.

Hassanpour *et al.* (2011) further analysed the particle dynamics in terms of particle velocity distributions. In their work, due to the computational limitations, DEM simulations were carried out for a maximum of 10 s of real time, enough for at least 20 impeller revolutions in the mixer. Within this period, the data over one single particle did not produce enough information to be comparable to PEPT measurements; therefore, the data from all particles in DEM simulation were used in their calculation.

The time-averaged normalized velocity distribution obtained from DEM analysis predicted a smooth distribution of particle velocities while the PEPT data showed more scatter or fluctuation in the frequency plot (Fig. 17.19). Furthermore, it should be noted that DEM simulation predicted a small percentage of stagnant particles, while PEPT results did not show that. The reason for such discrepancies was attributed to the sampling method: PEPT analysis is based on data from only one particle, that is, the tracer, while the DEM results consider the velocity profiles of the full population of particles in the simulation.

The results of the average particle velocity normalized to paddle tip speed, across a range of process conditions including fill level, impeller speed, and particle density, both from DEM and PEPT in Fig. 17.20 showed a consistent trend. However, it was reported that the average speeds simulated in DEM were systematically lower than the PEPT measurements over the range of conditions tested. It should be noted that the conclusions are specific for the conditions of the cases studied by Hassanpour *et al.* (2011) and may not be appropriate to generalize for all cases of powder mixing. A sensitivity analysis is necessary to be carried out when powder mixing process is simulated using DEM.

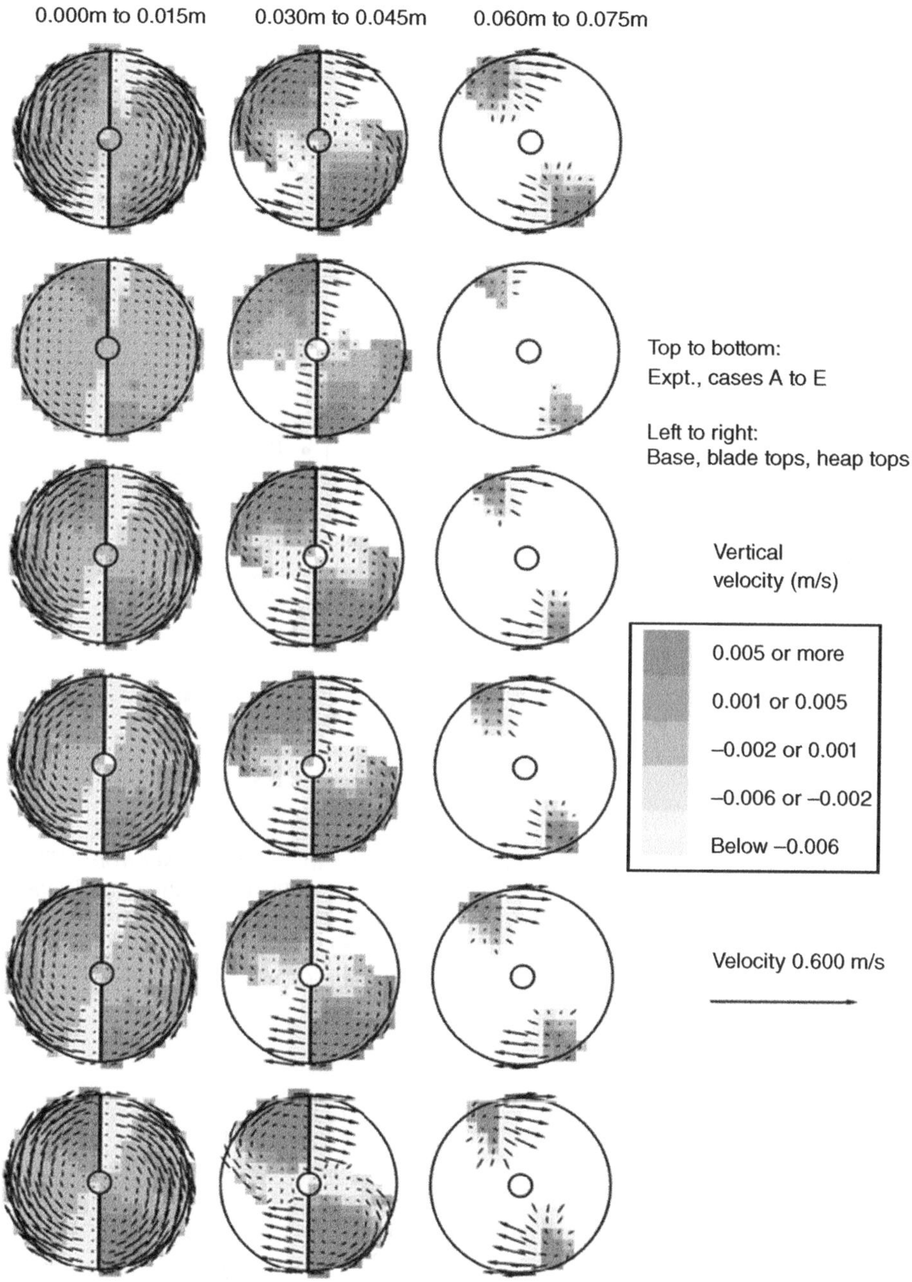

Figure 17.15 *Comparison of velocity fields of a bladed mixer at different heights from PEPT experiment and DEM simulations. The first row from the top represents the experimental results at different mixer height. Rows below the first one are the simulated results with different sliding and rolling friction coefficients: case A, 0.2 and 0.025 mm; case B, 0.3 and 0.0 mm; case C, 0.3 and 0.025 mm; case D, 0.3 and 0.05 mm and case E, 0.5 and 0.025 mm. The cell shade indicates the vertical velocity while the vectors show the horizontal velocity. Reprinted with permission from* Chemical Engineering Science, *Simulated and measured flow of granules in a bladed mixer – a detailed comparison by R.L. Stewart, J. Bridgwater, Y.C. Zhou, A.B. Yu, 56, 19, 5457–5471. Copyright (2001) Elsevier*

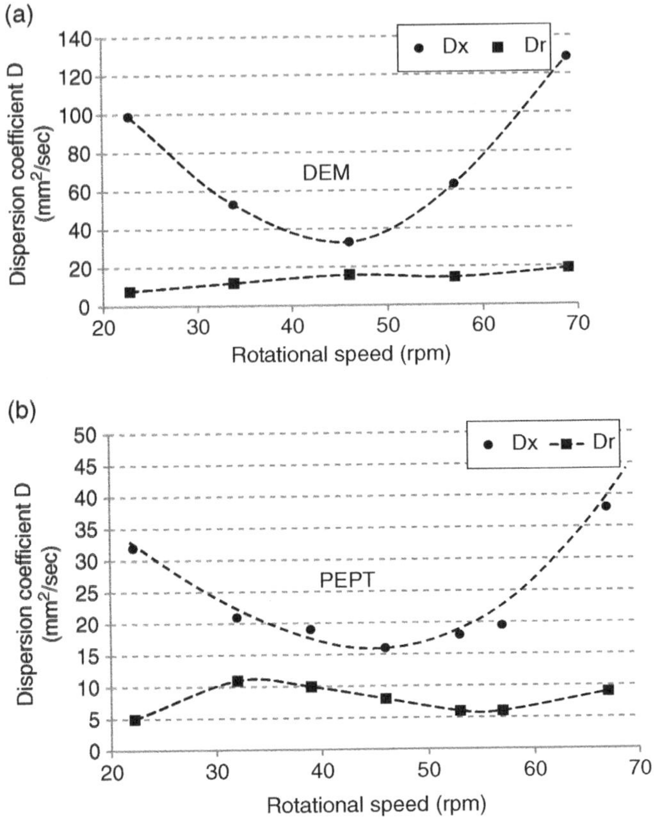

Figure 17.16 *Comparison of the dispersion coefficient for the Turbula mixer from DEM and PEPT. Reprinted with permission from* International Journal of Pharmaceutics, *Application of Positron Emission Particle Tracking (PEPT) to validate a Discrete Element Method (DEM) model of granular flow and mixing in the Turbula mixer, M. Marigo, M. Davies, T. Leadbeater, D.L. Cairns, A. Ingram, E.H. Stitt, 446, 1–2, 46–58. Copyright (2013) Elsevier*

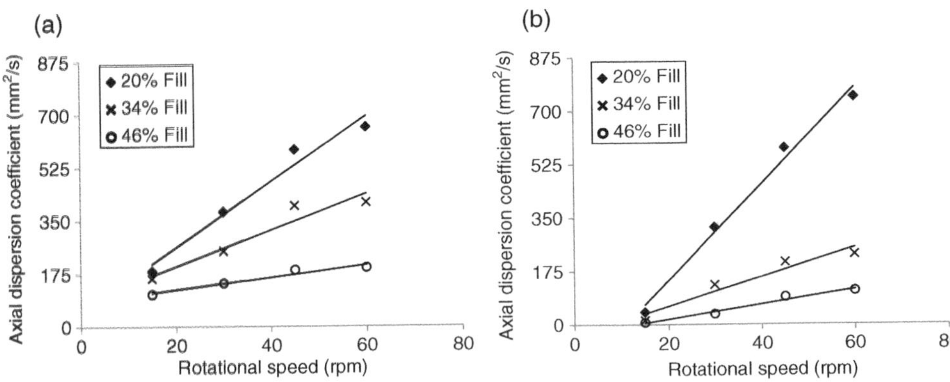

Figure 17.17 *Axial dispersion coefficient of particles in a V-blender as a function of fill level at different rotational speeds from PEPT measurements (a) and DEM simulation (b) (Tahvildarian et al., 2013). Reprinted with permission from* Particuology, *Circulation intensity and axial dispersion of non-cohesive solid particles in a V-blender via DEM simulation, Parisa Tahvildarian, Farhad Ein-Mozaffari, Simant R. Upreti, 11, 6, 619–626. Copyright (2013) Elsevier*

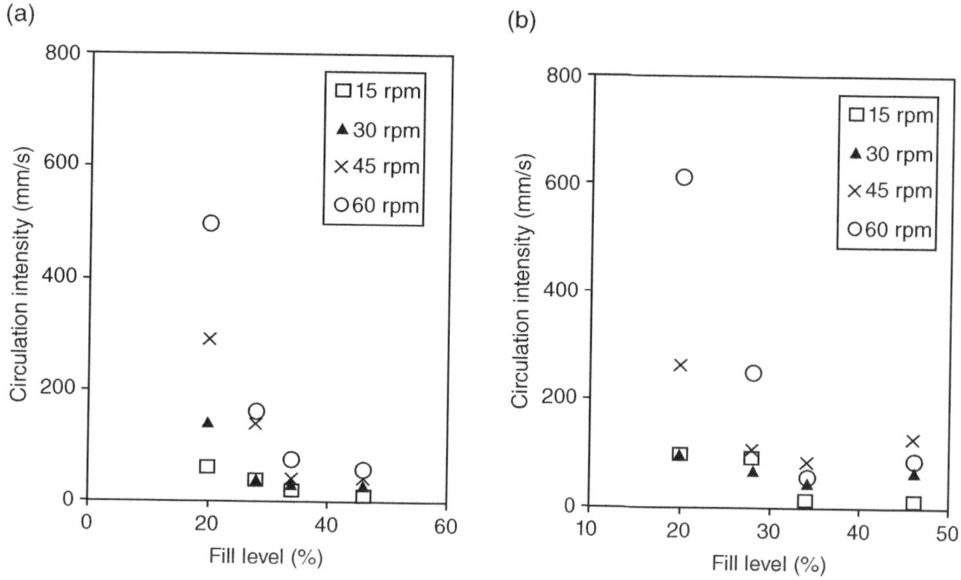

Figure 17.18 *Circulation intensity of particles in a V-blender as a function of fill level at different rotational speeds from PEPT measurements (a) and DEM simulation (b). Reprinted with permission from* Particuology, *Circulation intensity and axial dispersion of non-cohesive solid particles in a V-blender via DEM simulation, Parisa Tahvildarian, Farhad Ein-Mozaffari, Simant R. Upreti, 11, 6, 619–626. Copyright (2013) Elsevier*

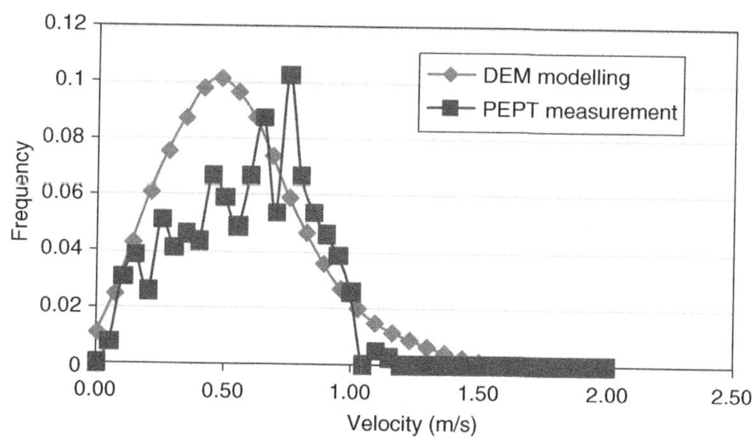

Figure 17.19 *Comparison of particle velocity distributions (normalized to the paddle tip speed) from DEM and PEPT. Reprinted with permission from* Powder Technology, *Analysis of particle motion in a paddle mixer using Discrete Element Method (DEM), Ali Hassanpour, Hongsing Tan, Andrew Bayly, Prasad Gopalkrishnan, Boonho Ng, Mojtaba Ghadiri, 206, 1–2, 189–194. Copyright (2011) Elsevier*

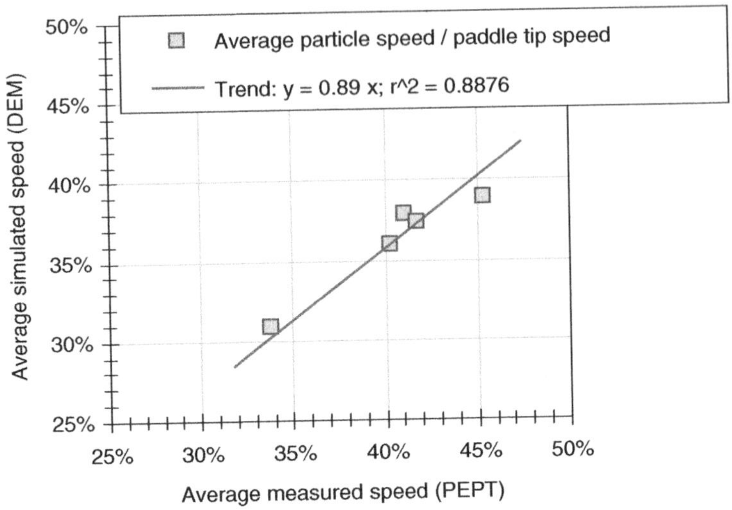

Figure 17.20 *Comparison of DEM simulation vs. PEPT measurement of time-averaged particle speed, normalized to paddle tip speed, for a range of conditions with different mixer speed, particle density and mixer fill level. Reprinted with permission from* Powder Technology, *Analysis of particle motion in a paddle mixer using Discrete Element Method (DEM), Ali Hassanpour, Hongsing Tan, Andrew Bayly, Prasad Gopalkrishnan, Boonho Ng, Mojtaba Ghadiri, 206, 1–2, 189–194. Copyright (2011) Elsevier*

A number of considerations should be taken into account when a comparison of DEM simulation is made with PEPT experimental results. One consideration should be the effect of single tracer particle sampling method used by PEPT, as discussed earlier. For a precise evaluation, the results of PEPT should be compared to those of a single representative particle in DEM, for which longer simulations (more than 15 min in real time) are needed. Particle shape could be another factor that significantly affects the simulations as irregular particles are expected to gain less rotational velocity (compared to spherical particles), hence their kinetic energy could be more in form of linear motion.

17.4 Concluding Remarks

The review of capability of DEM for simulating powder mixing suggests that the technique is useful for the process design and optimization in terms of minimizing tradition trial and error and lowering the cost of process development. Recent advances in the computational capabilities in terms of hardware and software developments have enabled simulation of vessels with complex geometry; however, the technique is still incapable of simulating full population of powders in an industrial scale. Use of larger particles could be an option to reduce the number of elements in the simulation; however, a sensitivity analysis should be carried for the specific application. Furthermore, comparison of simulations and experiments for the validation should be made with cautions; so in order to avoid misleading simulations, the results obtained from the latter should be compared with exactly identical observations in the experiments.

References

Antonyuk, S., Khanal, M., Tomas, J., Heinrich, S., Mörl, L., (2006), Impact breakage of spherical granules: experimental study and DEM simulation, *Chemical Engineering and Processing: Process Intensification*, 45(10), 835–856.

Arratia, P.E, Duong, N.H., Muzzio, F.J., Godbole, P.E., Reynolds, S., (2006), A study of the mixing & segregation mechanisms in the Bohle blender via DEM simulations, *Powder Technology*, 164, 50–57.

Bridgwater, J, (1976), Fundamental powder mixing mechanisms, *Particle Technology*, 15, 215–236.

Bridgwater J., (2012), Mixing of powders and granular materials by mechanical means –A perspective, *Particuology*, 10(4), 397–427.

Calvert, G., Hassanpour, A., Ghadiri, M., (2011), Mechanistic analysis and computer simulation of the aerodynamic dispersion of loose aggregates, *Chemical Engineering Research & Design*, 89, 519–525.

Chandratilleke, G.R., Yu, A.B., Bridgwater, J., (2012), A DEM study of the mixing of particles induced by a flat blade, *Chemical Engineering Science*, 79, 54–74

Chaudhuri, B., Muzzio, F.J., Tomassone, M.S., (2006), Modeling of heat transfer in granular flow in rotating vessels, *Chemical Engineering Science*, 61, 6348–6360.

Chu, K.W., Yu, A.B., (2008), Numerical simulation of complex particle-fluid flows, *Powder Technology*, 179, 104–114.

Cundall, P.A., (1971), A computer model for simulating progressive large scale movements in blocky rock systems, *ISRM Symp., Nancy, France, Proc. 2*, pp. 129–136.

Cundall, P.A., Strack, O.D.L., (1979), Discrete numerical model for granular assemblies, *Geotechnique*, 29(Compendex), 47–65.

Datta, A., Mishra, B.K., Das, S.P., Sahu, A., (2008), A DEM analysis of flow characteristics of noncohesive particles in hopper, *Materials and Manufacturing Processes*, 23, 196–203.

Delaney G.W., Cleary P.W., (2009), Fundamental relations between particle shape and the properties of granular packings, *Powders and Grains*, 1145, 837–840.

Di Maio, F.P., Di Renzo, A., (2005), Modelling particle contacts in distinct element simulations – Linear and non-linear approach, *Chemical Engineering Research and Design*, 83, 1287–1297.

Di Renzo A., Di Maio, A., Girimonte F.P., Formisani R. B., (2008), DEM simulation of the mixing equilibrium in fluidized beds of two solids differing in density, *Powder Technology*, 184, 214–223.

Favier, J.F., Abbaspour-Fard, M.H., Kremmer, M., Raji, A.O., (1999), Shape representation of axi-symmetrical, non-spherical particles in Discrete Element Simulation using multi-element model particles, *Engineering Computations*, 16, 467–480.

Golchert, D., Moreno, R., Ghadiri, M., Litster, J., (2004), Effect of granule morphology on breakage behaviour during compression, *Powder Technology*, 143, 84–96.

Hassanpour A., Kwan C. C., Ng B. H., Rahmanian , N., Ding, Y.L., Antony S.J., Jia X.D., Ghadiri M., (2009), Effect of granulation scale-up on the strength of granules, *Powder Technology*, 189, 304–312.

Hassanpour A., Pasha M., Susana L., Rahmanian R., Santomaso A. C., Ghadiri, M., (2013), Analysis of seeded granulation in high shear granulators by discrete element method, *Powder Technology*, 238, 50–55.

Hassanpour, A., Tan, H.S., Bayly, A., Gopalkrishnan, P., Ng, B., Ghadiri, M. (2011), Analysis of particle motion in a paddle mixer using Discrete Element Method (DEM), *Powder Technology*, 206, 189–194.

Higashitani, K., Iimura, K., Sanda, H., (2001), Simulation of deformation and breakup of large aggregates in flows of viscous fluids, *Chemical Engineering Science*, 56, 2927–2938.

Hogue, C., (1998), Shape representation and contact detection for discrete element simulations of arbitrary geometries, *Engineering Computation*, 15, 374–390.

Jia X., Gan M., Williams R.A., Rhodes D., (2007), Validation of a digital packing algorithm in predicting powder packing densities, *Powder Technology*, 174, 10–13.

Johnson, K.L., Kendall, K., Roberts, A.D., (1971), *Surface Energy and the Contact of Elastic Solids, Proceeding of the Royal Society A*, 324, 301–313.

Kalman, H, Rodnianski, V., Haim M, (2009), A new method to implement comminution functions into DEM simulation of a size reduction system due to particle-wall collisions, *Granular Matter*, 11(4), 253–266.

Kaneko, Y., Shiojima, T., Horio, M., (2000), Numerical analysis of particle mixing characteristics in a single helical ribbon agitator using DEM simulation, *Powder Technology* 108, 55–64.

Kuang, S.B., Chu, K.W., Yu, A.B., Zou, Z.S., Feng, Y.Q., (2008), Computational investigation of horizontal slug flow in pneumatic conveying, *Industrial & Engineering Chemistry Research*, 47, 470–480.

Kuo, H.P., Knight, P.C., Parket, D.J., Seville, J.P.K. (2005). Solids circulation and axial dispersion of cohesion-less particles in a V-mixer, *Powder Technology*, 152, 133–140.

Laurent, B.F.C., Bridgwater, J., (2000), Motion in a particle bed agitated by a single blade, *AIChE Journal*, 46, 1723–1734.

Lemieux, M., Léonard, G., Doucet, J., Leclaire, L.-A., Viens, F., Chaouki, J., Bertrand, F., (2008), Large-scale numerical investigation of solids mixing in a V-blender using the discrete element method, *Particulate Processes in the Pharmaceutical Industry*, 181(2), 205–216.

Li, J., Wassgren C., Litster J.D., (2013), Multi-scale modeling of a spray coating process in a paddle mixer/coater: the effect of particle size distribution on particle segregation and coating uniformity, *Chemical Engineering Science*, 95, 203–210.

Luding, S., (2008), Cohesive, frictional powders: contact models for tension, *Granular Matter*, 10, 235–246.

Marigo, M., Cairns, D.L., Davies, M., Ingram, A., Stitt, E.H., (2011), Developing mechanistic understanding of granular behaviour in complex moving geometry using the discrete element method. Part B: Investigation of flow and mixing in the Turbula® mixer, *Powder Technology*, 212, 17–24.

Marigo, M., Davies, M., Leadbeater, T., Cairns D. L., Ingram A., Stitt, E.H., (2013), Application of positron emission particle tracking (PEPT) to validate a Discrete Element Method (DEM) model of granular flow and mixing in the Turbula mixer, *International Journal of Pharmaceutics*, 446(1–2), 46–58.

Moakher, M., Shinbrot, T., Muzzio, F.J., (2000), Experimentally validated computations of flow, mixing and segregation of non-cohesive grains in 3D tumbling blenders, *Powder Technology*, 109, 58–71.

Moreno, R., Ghadiri, M., (2006), Mechanistic analysis and computer simulation of impact breakage of agglomerates: Effect of surface energy, *Chemical Engineering Science*, 61(8), 2476–2481.

Muguruma, Y., Tanaka, T., Kawatake, S., Tsuji, Y., (1997), Discrete particle simulation of a rotary vessel mixer with baffles, *Powder Technology*, 93, 261–266.

Ng, B.H., Kwan, C.C., Ding, Y.L., Ghadiri, M., Fan, Z.F., (2007), Solids motion in a conical frustum-shaped high shear mixer graulator, *Chemical Engineering Science*, 62(3), 756–765.

Pasha, M., Dogbe, S., Hare, C., Hassanpour, A., Ghadiri, M., (2014), A linear model of elasto-plastic and adhesive contact deformation, *Granular Matter*, 16, 151–162.

Portillo, P.M, Ierapetritou, M.G., Muzzio, F.J., (2007), Characterization of continuous convective powder mixing processes, *Powder Technology*, 182, 368–378.

Potapov, A.V., Campbell, C.S., 1997, Computer simulation of shear-induced particle attrition, *Powder Technology*, 94, 109–122.

Sarkar, A., Wassgren, C.R., (2012), Comparison of flow microdynamics for a continuous granular mixer with predictions from periodic slice DEM simulations, *Powder Technology*, 221, 325–336.

Sato, Y., Nakamura H., Watano S., (2008), Numerical analysis of agitation torque and particle motion in a high shear mixer, *Powder Technology*, 186, 130–136.

Savkoor, A.R., Briggs, G.A.D., (1977), The effect of the tangential force on the contact of elastic solids in adhesion, *Proceeding of the Royal Society of London A.*, 356, 103–114.

Schutyser, M.A.I., Briels, W.J., Rinzema, A., Boom, R.M., (2003), Numerical simulation and PEPT measurements of a 3D conical helical-blade mixer: A high potential solids mixer for solid-state fermentation, *Biotechnology and Bioengineering*, 84(1), 29–39.

Stewart, R.L., Bridgwater, J., Zhou, Y.C., Yu, A.B., (2001), Simulated and measured flow of granules in a bladed mixer – a detailed comparison, *Chemical Engineering Science*, 56, 5457–5471.

Tahvildarian, P., Ein-Mozaffari, F., Upreti, S.R., (2013), Circulation intensity and axial dispersion of non-cohesive solid particles in a V-blender via DEM simulation, *Particuology*, 11, 619–626.

Thakur, S.C., Morrissey, J.P., Sun, J., Chen, J.-F., Ooi, J.Y., (2014), Micromechanical analysis of cohesive granular materials using the discrete element method with an adhesive elasto-plastic contact model, *Granular Matter*, 16, 383–400.

Thornton, C., Ning, Z., (1998), A theoretical model for the stick/bounce behaviour of adhesive elastic-plastic spheres, *Powder Technology*, 99, 154–162.

Thornton, C., Cummins, S.J., Cleary, P.W., (2013), An investigation of the comparative behaviour of alternative contact force models during inelastic collisions, *Powder Technology*, 233, 30–46.

Tomas, J. (2007), Adhesion of ultrafine particles-A micromechanical approach, *Chemical Engineering Science*, 62, 1997–2010.

Tsuji, Y., Kawaguchi, T., Tanaka, T., (1993), Discrete particle simulation of two-dimensional fluidized bed, *Powder Technology*, 77, 79–87.

Wassgren, C.R., Hunt, M.L., Freese, P.J., Palamara, J., Brennen, C.E., (2002), Effects of vertical vibration on hopper flows of granular material, *Physics of Fluids*, 14, 3439–3448.

Xu, Y., Xu, C., Zhou, Z., Du, J., Hu, D., (2010), 2D DEM simulation of particle mixing in rotating drum: a parametric study, *Particuology*, 8, 141–149.

Yang, R.Y., Zou, R.P., Yu, A.B. (2003), Microdynamic analysis of particle flow in a horizontal rotating drum, *Powder Technology*, 130, 138–146.

Yang, R.Y., Yu, A.B., McElroy, L., Bao, J., (2008), Numerical simulation of particle dynamics in different flow regimes in a rotating drum, *Powder Technology*, 188, 170–177.

Walton, O.R., Braun, R.L., (1986), Viscosity, granular-temperature, and stress calculations for shearing assemblies of inelastic, frictional disks, *Journal of Rheology*, 30, 949–980.

Zhou, Q., Liu, X., (2004), Analysis on errors of derived slope and aspect related to DEM data properties, *Computer and Geosciences*, 30(4), 369–378.

Zhu, H., Zhou, Z., Yang, R., Yu, A., (2008), Discrete particle simulation of particulate systems: A review of major applications and findings, *Chemical Engineering Science*, 5728–5770.

Index

Note: Page numbers in *italics* refer to Figures; those in **bold** to Tables.

Pharmaceutical Blending and Mixing, First Edition. Edited by P.J. Cullen, Rodolfo J. Romañach, Nicolas Abatzoglou and Chris D. Rielly.

Printed and bound by CPI Group (UK) Ltd, Croydon, CR0 4YY
16/09/2026
14963385-0002